NUTRITION

Principles and Clinical Practice

NUTRITION

Principles
and Clinical
Practice

SARA M. HUNT, PH.D., R.D.
Professor and Chairman
Department of Community
Health Nutrition
Georgia State University

JAMES L. GROFF, PH.D.
Associate Professor
Department of Medical Technology
Georgia State University

JOHN M. HOLBROOK, PH.D.
Associate Professor
Department of Biomedical Sciences
Mercer University
School of Pharmacy

JOHN WILEY & SONS
New York   Chichester   Brisbane   Toronto

Library of Congress Cataloging in Publication Data:

Hunt, Sara M   1921–
  Nutrition.

  Includes index.
  1. Nutrition. 2. Metabolism. 3. Diet therapy.
4. Nutrition disorders. I. Groff, James L., joint
author. II. Holbrook, John M., joint author.
III. Title.

QP141.H83   613.2   79-25899
ISBN 0-471-03149-6

Printed in the United States of America

10 9 8 7 6 5 4 3 2 1

PREFACE

No book can adequately cover all the information needed by the student of clinical dietetics, but certain subject areas are more vital than others to the emerging practitioner. Remembering past difficulties as a student and practitioner in integrating information from various sources into a body of working knowledge and being acutely aware as an instructor of the problems in preparing lesson plans that have real meaning for students, I have attempted with the help of clinical chemist and a pharmacologist to organize into one text the information that the three of us believe can provide a firm foundation for an understanding of total health care. Past and present experiences have convinced me a textbook is needed that not only integrates normal and therapeutic nutrition, but also acquaints the student of clinical dietetics with the various types of information in patients' medical records that can provide insight into overall health status. I must explain at the onset, however, that this book, when used as a text for dietetics students, should be accompanied by a good diet manual, because we have intentionally included only the rationale for the various therapeutic dietary managements with no attempt to provide diet patterns.

The health team approach is a popular concept, but for this concept to become a reality, all the health team members must understand the language of the various disciplines represented on the team. The clinical dietitian can no longer be concerned only with following physicians' orders in the feeding of the patient during hospitalization; he or she must also share the responsibility for the total nutritional management of the patient, including the provision of continuity of excellent nutritional care and/or rehabilitation.

The dietitian will not be diagnosing disease states, but if he/she aspires to providing total nutritional care of patients and to functioning as a true member of the health team, he/she must be able to make rapid nutritional assessments of patients. Because nutritional assessments are based on objective as well as subjective data, dietitians must be able to interpret all those objective data found in medical records that could influence nutritional status. A dietitian who has knowledge of biochemistry, physiology, and pharmacology as well as foods is in an unusual position to be of real service to patients and to other members of the health team. He/she will be the *one* person who can appropriately educate patients and colleagues about their diets; furthermore, such a dietitian can answer questions about "why" certain dietary modifications are valuable to the prevention or treatment of disease.

This book is written primarily for students in clinical dietetics, but can be utilized equally well as a desk reference by dietitians and nutritionists. It may have appeal, also, for other health professionals, particularly medical, pharmacy, and nursing students who are interested in nutrition as an applied science and who are concerned over the interrelationships among various nutrients and drugs as they may affect health and treatment of disease. The integrated approach used in the text can be particularly helpful to the medical student, resident, and practicing physician because it bridges the gap between scientific theory and the actual application of biochemistry and physiology in the provision of nutritional care. In addition, the delineation and description of activities that should be performed by dietitians/nutritionists can provide physicians with information about services they may expect from well-educated nutrition personnel.

Although the emphasis of the book is primarily on clinical nutrition, review chapters are included on the cell and the major nutrients. These chapters are followed by a section on fluid and electrolyte balance, in which problems associated with surgery and burns are considered. Throughout the rest of the text, discussion of clinical nutrition is divided according to systems or organs, with each system or organ being introduced by a brief review of its anatomical makeup and its physiological function.

Following this introduction to the system or organ, we examine normal metabolism of specific nutrients and the interrelationship between nutrient metabolism and the functioning of the various systems or organs. Coordinated with this consideration of normal metabolism is a discussion of consequences incurred by body systems and organs when aberrations in nutrient digestion, absorption and/or metabolism occur. The appropriate dietary and drug therapy for various pathological conditions is outlined with special emphasis placed upon the synergistic or adverse effects that may result from simultaneously occurring dietary modifications and drug dosage. An attempt is made throughout to integrate the interpretation of various important biochemical measurements of health status, the most commonly prescribed drugs for different disease conditions, and the science of nutrition as related to maintenance of human health and prevention or management of disease states.

With this approach nutrition students can begin to think and function realistically as health professionals. They will not only be able to augment the care begun by the physicians, but will also have the capability to initiate special aspects of care beneficial to the patient's recovery and/or maintenance of health.

Sara M. Hunt
James L. Groff
John M. Holbrook

ACKNOWLEDGMENTS

The senior author wishes to express her appreciation to Judy Bonner, Ph.D., who contributed the section on cystic fibrosis and offered many helpful suggestions for the organization of the material. Many thanks go to Corinne Cataldo, M.S., Ruth Kocher, M.S., and Barry Rosenbaum, M.D., who spent much time in reviewing the contents for readability, relevance, and accuracy. Mrs. Cataldo, a former student of the senior author, not only worked very hard in helping with completion of the text but also offered the viewpoint of nutrition students. Words are not sufficient to express the authors' thanks to her.

The authors are particularly grateful to Phyllis Acosta, Dr. P.H., for the chapter on nutrition in inherited disease. Inclusion of such a comprehensive treatment of inborn errors of metabolism would have been impossible without the contribution of this chapter.

S.M.H.
J.L.G.
J.M.H.

CONTENTS

CHAPTER 1

Introduction to Life — An Overview of Cell Structure and Function

INTRODUCTION

The term "cell" was commonly used in the seventeenth century to describe the small, bare sleeping quarters found in monasteries. In 1665, Robert Hooke, the noted biologist, applied the term "cell" to the tiny, empty chambers he observed while examining the structure of dried cork under the light microscope. Since the time of Hooke's first observation, knowledge of the cell has increased dramatically and has led to the present concept of the cell as a vastly complicated structure containing numerous subcellular components capable of performing complex tasks. This brief introductory chapter concerning the cell is designed only as an overview of cellular structure and function to prepare the reader for the understanding of materials presented in this text.

The cell is the smallest structural unit of living matter able to survive independently by utilizing nonliving materials. In the multicellular organism, cells are differentiated and specialized in order to perform certain tasks required for the survival of the organism. All cells, however, share certain characteristic physiological properties that distinguish them from nonliving materials. These properties include the following:

1. *Irritability, conductivity, and contractility.* Irritability refers to the ability of the cell to respond to a specific stimulus. Cells vary in their ability to respond to stimuli, but all possess this ability to some degree. Two types of response to stimuli are conductivity and contractility. Conductivity is the ability of the cell to transmit a wave of electrical excitability from the point of the stimulation to all areas of the cell surface. Contractility is a response manifested by shortening of some portion of the cell. Irritability and conductivity are developed to a high degree in nerve cells while contractility is an important characteristic of muscle cells.
2. *Absorption.* All cells have the ability to absorb nutrients and, at times, other substances through their surfaces which are termed cell or unit membranes.
3. *Assimilation.* Assimilation or anabolism is the process by which nutrients are converted into living matter.
4. *Secretion.* Certain specialized cells of the multicellular organism have

1

the capability of synthesizing specific substances, which can be released (secreted) into the blood stream or elaborated externally to the body surface or through a body orifice. Examples of secreted compounds include lacrimal fluids, sweat, hormones, and plasma proteins.

5. *Excretion.* All cells have the ability to discharge waste products from nutrient metabolism.

6. *Respiration.* Cellular respiration is the process by which nutrients are oxidized within the cell to provide energy. This highly specialized function occurs in the mitochondrion, a subcellular organelle.

7. *Growth and Reproduction.* In multicellular organisms, cells usually remain at an optimal size. Therefore, cellular growth occurs by increases in the number of cells rather than by increases in cellular size. An exception to this general characteristic occurs with the adipocyte, a cell whose size apparently can increase indefinitely.

CELLULAR COMPONENTS

When a cell is viewed under the light microscope, its apparent essential characteristics are a cell edge which surrounds the cellular substance and a dense mass or nucleus usually situated near the center of the cell. However, techniques utilizing the electron microscope, which greatly magnifies the cell, have revealed that the cell is a much more complicated structure than the one viewed through the light microscope. In actuality, the cell contains, in addition to a cellular (unit) membrane and nucleus, a number of subcellular structures termed organelles (Fig. 1.1). These organelles are found within the cellular substance, termed the cytoplasm, and are responsible for performing those specific functions that allow the cell to exist as a unit as well as to carry out specialized functions required by the organism.

The cell membrane (plasma or unit membrane) surrounds the cytoplasm and nucleus and makes the cell a unit unto itself. This membrane possesses characteristics that allow for the occurrence of processes such as absorption, assimilation, secretion, and excretion. The cell membrane can be permeated to varying degrees by certain substances, being more permeable to lipid-soluble compounds and small molecules and less permeable to water-soluble compounds and large molecules. This characteristic of selective permeablility allows for the transport of substances into and out of the cell in an ordered fashion and, in addition, maintains an electrical gradient between the cell's interior and the external environment by selectively allowing or preventing the movement of charged particles through the unit membrane. These charged particles (ions or electrolytes) are ionization products of compounds that are taken into the body and can form positively charged particles (cations) and negatively

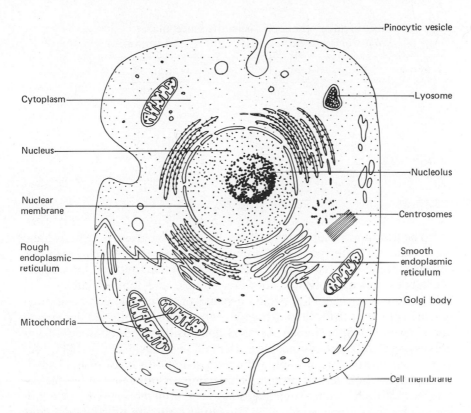

Figure 1.1 Diagram of a typical cell.

charged particles (anions) when they are solubilized in the body fluids. The electrical gradient that exists at the cell membrane makes possible the transfer of electrical impulses across the surface of certain specialized cells such as those found in cardiac tissue, nerve tissue, skeletal muscle, and smooth muscle. The movement of the electrical impulse across the cardiac, skeletal, and smooth muscle cells acts as the stimulus that produces muscle contraction, while movement of electrical impulses along nerve tissue provides communication between the central nervous system and the body. Table 1.1 lists the electrolytes and their concentrations in the intracellular and extracellular fluid compartments. While the distribution of cations and anions is quite different between the two compartments, within each compartment the total number of milliequivalents of cations and anions is balanced. This balance of positive and negative charges is called electrical neutrality and is essential for the maintenance of cellular integrity. See Chapter 4 for further information concerning electrolyte and fluid balance.

Table 1.1 Electrolytes in Intracellular and Extracellular
Fluid Compartments

Electrolyte	Extracellular (mEq/liter)	Intracellular (mEq/liter)
Na^+	142	10
K^+	5	141
Ca^{++}	5	<1
Mg^{++}	3	58
Cl^-	103	4
HCO_3^-	28	10
Phosphates	4	75
SO_4^{--}	1	2

The transport of substances across the cell membrane is selective and may occur due to one of several processes. As previously mentioned, the cell membrane is selectively permeable to lipid-soluble (or fat-soluble) substances and impermeable to water-soluble and ionized substances. This selective permeablility occurs because of the unique composition of the membrane, a trilamelar (three-layer) structure with the inner and outer layers having a similar chemical composition and the middle layer possessing a different composition. Danielli and Davidson, in 1935, proposed that this trilamelar composition consisted of a layer of lipid sandwiched between layers of protein. This composition would allow for the transport of lipid-soluble substances across the membrane while excluding more water-soluble substances. However, this membrane model does not explain all of the properties displayed by the cell membrane, and newer theories have, therefore, been postulated. One such theory views the membrane as consisting of lipid micelles, coated with protein and separated by protein septae. Another theory proposes that the membrane consists of a fluid lipid bilayer in which globular proteins are partially or completely imbedded (1). Figure 1.2 depicts the globular protein concept of the cellular membrane.

The selective permeability of the cellular membrane to very small molecules has been explained by the presence of pores or very small channels that pass across the cell membrane and allow for the movement of small molecules into and out of the cell. This process is termed simple diffusion. Simple diffusion does not require the expenditure of energy and involves the movement of molecules from an area of high concentration to an area of lower concentration.

The transport of large molecules, water-soluble molecules, and certain anions and cations across the cell membrane against concentration and/or electrical gradients occurs through the process of active transport. This process requires the expenditure of energy and usually involves a carrier that is protein in nature. This carrier attaches to the molecule to be transported on one side of the membrane and carries it to the other side.

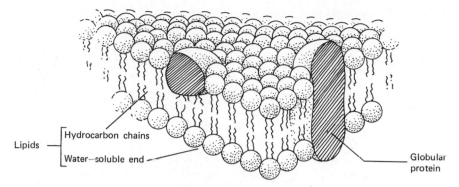

Figure 1.2 Globular protein concept of the cell membrane.

Some substances of high molecular weight such as proteins may be transported across the cell membrane by the process of pinocytosis ("cell drinking"). Pinocytosis is an energy-requiring process which involves the surrounding of the substance by the cell membrane, forming a vacuole that enters the cytoplasm as a free-floating structure.

The cytoplasm of the cell consists of two primary types of components, the matrix (ground substance) and the organelles. The cell matrix is a colloidal solution of enzymatic and nonenzymatic proteins which contains absorbed nutrients, waste products awaiting excretion, and certain inclusion materials such as glycogen, fat, and pigments. The organelles are the specialized structures of the cell that carry out many of the functions essential to the life of the organism.

Nutrients such as glucose, fatty acids, and amino acids after entering the cell through the cellular membrane are metabolized within various compartments of the cell. Glucose is converted in the cytoplasm to pyruvic acid by the process of glycolysis and fatty acids are converted by beta-oxidation to acetyl coenzyme A in the mitochondrion. Pyruvate, formed from glucose in the cytoplasm, can enter the mitochondrion where it too can be converted to acetyl coenzyme A. Acetyl coenzyme A serves as the starting product for the production of most of the energy utilized by the cell. Amino acids, as well as being used in protein synthesis, can be converted into pyruvate or other metabolites and used for energy.

Within the cytoplasm, materials are transported between organelles in an orderly process. Each organelle performs its specific functions in the preparation, synthesis, and secretion of products needed by the cell as well as those which may be elaborated by the cell. Each organelle has its own individual function within the framework of overall cellular function, and the activity of each complements that of the others.

The mitochondria are scattered throughout the cell as granules or filaments numbering from 300 to 300,000 depending upon the type of cell. These organelles are composed of three membranes: an outer limiting membrane, a middle transverse membrane (cristae), and an inner limiting membrane. The transverse membranes or cristae are actually folds of the inner limiting membrane and it is on these cristae that a group of enzymes catalyze reactions that provide the cell with energy in the form of the compound adenosine triphosphate (ATP). This process of energy production is termed cellular respiration and will be discussed further in Chapter 3. Also contained within the mitochondria are the enzymes of the citric acid cycle and those necessary for the catabolism of fatty acids. The acetyl coenzyme A mentioned earlier is utilized in the mitochondria as a starting substrate for the enzymes of the citric acid cycle.

The ribosomes are cytoplasmic organelles that are found in one of two forms. They may be scattered throughout the cytoplasm as free entities not attached to any membrane surface, or they may be found attached to walls of another organelle, the endoplasmic reticulum. The ribosomes consist of protein and ribonucleic acid (ribosomal ribonucleic acid or rRNA) and are involved with the synthesis of proteins. The ribosomes attached to the endoplasmic reticulum are associated with the synthesis of proteins needed to maintain the normal functioning of the cell.

The endoplasmic reticulum of the cell also occurs in one of two forms. One type is called the rough endoplasmic reticulum to which the previously mentioned ribosomes were attached. This rough endoplasmic reticulum is found in most cells but is seen in largest quantities in cells that are actively secreting protein, such as the acinar cells of the pancreas. The endoplasmic reticulum of this type serves as the channels and storage areas or cisterns in which the synthesized proteins can be sequestered from other cellular components until they are secreted by the cell. The second form of endoplasmic reticulum is called the smooth endoplasmic reticulum. This organelle is also found in most cells and appears to be involved in lipid synthesis and, in some cells, with steroid biosynthesis. In skeletal muscle, the smooth endoplasmic reticulum is called the sarcoplasmic reticulum and is associated with the uptake of calcium ions into the cell.

The Golgi apparatus is a cellular organelle about which little was known until recent years although this structure was identified as early as 1890. The Golgi apparatus is actually part of the endoplasmic reticulum and is now known to perform many complex tasks in the cell. Its primary function appears to be the packaging of substances for secretion from the cell, for example, plasma proteins, enzymes, and hormones.

Lysosomes are membranous organelles that contain various types of hydrolytic enzymes, for example, the hydrolases, which are used by the cell to produce amino acids from protein molecules. Lysosomes function in the digestion of substances that are brought into the cell or that may be formed within the cell. The lysosomal membrane serves to contain these powerful digestive enzymes, thus preventing the autodigestion of the cell.

However, under certain conditions such as anoxia or viral infections, the cell is damaged, and the released enzymes may result in the destruction of the cell.

The last primary structure of the cell to be included in this brief discussion is the cell nucleus, considered the brain of the cell. The various organelles and structures previously discussed exist and function under the influence of the cell nucleus. All cells, with the exception of the mature erythrocyte, have a nucleus surrounded by a membrane that contains one or two nucleoli. The genetic material deoxyribonucleic acid (DNA), which is responsible for heredity and for directing the synthesis of cellular proteins, is found in the nucleus. The reproductive function of the nucleus assures that when a cell divides, all of the information of the cell is transferred to two daughter cells. The nucleus controls the function of the cell by directing the synthesis of all of the enzymes and organelles that are required for the specialized function of the cell.

GENETIC CODE AND
BIOSYNTHESIS OF PROTEIN

Of all the specialized functions of the cell, the one that has been the target of most investigative research in recent years is the mechanism by which the cell's genetic structure dictates the synthesis of enzymes and other specialized proteins. From the knowledge acquired, there have emerged remarkably sophisticated manipulative procedures for artificially altering a cell's genetic character. It has now become possible to induce a cell to synthesize totally different proteins from those to which it was committed naturally. This is accomplished by destroying the cell's natural genetic structure and implanting it with a structure of different biosynthetic specificity, a manipulation commonly referred to as genetic engineering. A sensational example of such a manipulation is the science of cloning, by which exact duplicates of living organisms can be produced. The successful cloning of lower forms of life is established. Whether it can be applied to phylogenetically advanced living things is a matter of scientific conjecture at this time. The implication of such experimentation is awesome, and cloning research is obviously a topic of considerable controversy.

The nuclear nucleic acid, deoxyribonucleic acid (DNA), serves both to replicate itself and to direct the synthesis of proteins through ribonucleic acid (RNA) intermediates. That the information for protein biosynthesis flows from DNA to RNA to protein rests with a concept proposed by Crick in 1958, called the central dogma of molecular genetics. Except for a minor revision in 1970 necessitated by the discovery that DNA polymerization may, in some instances, be directed by RNA, this unidirectional flow of information is accepted in full by the scientific community. The central dogma further defined three major processes in the preservation and transmission of genetic information:

a. Replication, the copying of DNA to form identical daughter molecules.
b. Transcription, the means by which the genetic information coded into the DNA molecule is transcribed into the form of RNA (messenger RNA) to be carried to the ribosomes of the cell.
c. Translation, the decoding of the genetic message on the RNA, which leads to the synthesis of proteins on the ribosomes.

To these could be added elongation, which refers to the incorporation of incoming amino acids into the growing polypeptide (protein) chain in a highly ordered sequence, under the direction of the genetic code of the messenger (mRNA).

The salient features of DNA-directed protein biosynthesis will be reviewed. The reader is referred to Chapter 2 for the chemical structure of nucleotides, nucleic acids, amino acids, and proteins. The literature dealing with the subject of protein biosynthesis is extensive, and for a more detailed account of the processes involved, the reader is referred to Ref. 2 listed at end of chapter.

In each of the three divisions of the central dogma: replication, transcription, and translation, the specificity of the molecular interactions is accomplished through the base-pairing of nucleotides. The pairing occurs between purine- and pyrimidine-type nucleotides, that is, in a given pairing, one member will be a purine and the other will be a pyrimidine base nucleotide. The binding force is due to hydrogen bonding between the amino and carbonyl functions on the heterocyclic rings of the purine and pyrimidine nuclei. It is steric hindrance that obviates the pairing of two purine or two pyrimidine nucleotides. For the purpose of simplicity, the five nucleotides that comprise the DNA and RNA structure are abbreviated, using the first letter of the name of the nitrogenous base, as indicated:

Purine Bases	*Pyrimidine Bases*
Adenine (A)	Cytosine (C)
Guanine (G)	Uracil (U)
	Thymine (T)

Thymine-base nucleotides are found in DNA but not RNA; uracil nucleotides are in RNA but not DNA, and adenine, guanine and cytosine appear in both nucleic acids.

Replication

DNA, located in the nucleus of the cell, exists as two, large strands of nucleic acids intertwined to form the double helical conformation. Each strand has a terminal 5'-phosphate group at one end and a terminal 3'-

phosphate at the other. The two strands are said to be antiparallel, meaning that the terminal 3′ nucleotide of one strand is base-paired with the terminal 5′ nucleotide of the second strand. In the process of cell division, the two strands unravel at one end. At the same time, new strands are synthesized on the parent strands simultaneously through the complementary base-pairing already described. Incoming nucleotides are introduced as their 5′-triphosphate derivatives and pyrophosphate (shown below) is split from the molecules as the phosphate diesters are formed

$$
(HO{-}\overset{\overset{\displaystyle O}{\|}}{\underset{\underset{\displaystyle O{-}}{|}}{P}}{-}O{-}\overset{\overset{\displaystyle O}{\|}}{\underset{\underset{\displaystyle O{-}}{|}}{P}}{-}OH)
$$

(see nucleic acid structures, Chapter 2). As mentioned above, the sequence of nucleotides in the new strands is dictated by the complementary base-pairing, while the actual synthesis of the strands is accomplished by the concerted action of the enzymes DNA polymerase, DNA ligase, and endonuclease. The end result is the synthesis of two new DNA chains "read" from the two unraveled parent chains, thereby producing two double helical molecules from the single parent molecule. The essential concept of base-pairing in the replication process is represented in Figure 1.3. The scheme is simplified, however, and the reader is again alerted to the second reference for a more detailed treatment of the process.

Transcription

While nuclear DNA is ultimately responsible for directing protein biosynthesis through its genetic code, the cellular site of protein synthesis is not in the nucleus, but on the ribosomes. It is evident that some form of messenger must convey the genetic information from nucleus to ribosome. The messenger was found to be ribonucleic acid and is called messenger RNA or mRNA.

Most proteins, in order to exhibit full biological activity, must have the amino acids of which they are comprised arranged in a specific sequence. Even minor deviations from an established sequence can lead to serious if not fatal consequences and inborn errors of metabolism discussed in Chapter 9 are primarily due to sequencing errors in certain enzymes. Enzymes are proteins that have the function of catalyzing the metabolic reactions within the body. Because DNA directs the sequence of amino acids in a protein, the question arises as to how a molecule with only four different repeating units (the A, G, C, and T nucleotides) can dictate the synthesis of another molecule (protein) that has 20 different repeating units (the naturally occurring amino acids). The question has been answered through a masterpiece of biological research—sequences

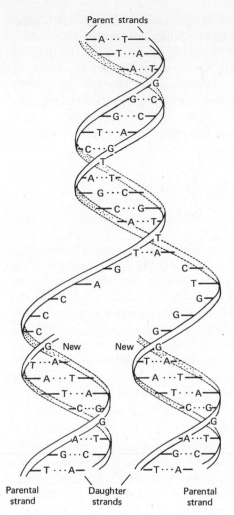

Parent strands

Parental strand

Daughter strands

Parental strand

Figure 1.3 Proposed replication of DNA.

of three adjacent nucleotides in DNA specify the order of amino acids. The "genetic code" therefore consists of the known sequences of triplet nucleotides specific for each amino acid. DNA molecules consist of many segments called genes or cistrons. Each gene can direct the synthesis of one protein or one RNA molecule.

In transcription, mRNA is synthesized on DNA template strands in much the same manner as the replication of DNA. The nucleotide sequences of mRNA, tRNA and ribosomal RNA (rRNA) are determined by complementary base-pairing between the polymerizing nucleotides and the nucleotides of the DNA. The sequence is read from a single strand of the DNA duplex called the sense strand and the mRNA so formed is said to have been transcribed from DNA. As in replication, nucleotides enter as triphosphate derivatives and pyrophosphate is eliminated as the phosphate diester bonds are formed. The reaction is catalyzed by RNA polymerase.

As a result of transcription, the genetic code is now contained in the mRNA molecule. Each segment of three adjacent mRNA nucleotides is coded for a particular amino acid. These triplet nucleotides are called codons and nucleotide sequences within the codons specific for all 20 amino acids are now known. Messenger RNA, with its genetic information, leaves the nucleus after transcription and enters the cytoplasm.

Translation

The division of protein biosynthesis referred to as translation encompasses the reactions by which the code on the mRNA is read so as to incorporate the amino acids specified by the mRNA codons into protein. The reactions require, in addition to mRNA, a smaller ribonucleic acid called transfer RNA (tRNA), ribosomes, and enzymes for catalyzing the various reactions.

Each of the 20 amino acids has its own specific tRNA. Prior to incorporation into protein, the amino acids must be activated in an energy-consuming reaction and then attached to their specific tRNA. The enzymes that catalyze these reactions are called aminoacyl-tRNA synthetases. They are highly specific for both the amino acid and its corresponding tRNA. The uniqueness of each tRNA molecule has been revealed by nucleotide sequence studies. Each tRNA has a specific nucleotide triplet within its chain that distinguishes it from other tRNAs. This triplet is now known to be an anticodon that binds to the mRNA codon by complementary base-pairing. The tRNAs are known to exist in a configuration resembling a cloverleaf with several appendages. The sites for the attachment of the amino acid and the anticodon triplet are located on the distal portion of two of the arms and are spatially well separated. This arrangement provides for sterically favorable base-pairing between anticodon and codon. Figure 1.4 illustrates the characteristic features of a tRNA: its cloverleaf configuration, the location of anticodon and site for amino acid attachment, and the fact that its terminal nucleotide sequence at the free 3'-OH end is always -C-C-A. A guanidine nucleotide usually occupies the other end.

Aminoacyl tRNAs are condensed into protein on ribosomes. Functional ribosomes consist of two major subunits, one of which brings amino-acid tRNAs to the messenger RNA strand, initiating the codon–anticodon base-pairing interaction. The second subunit facilitates the closure of the first subunit's tRNA onto the mRNA at the first codon site at the end of the mRNA strand. As shown in Figure 1.5, the ribosome then

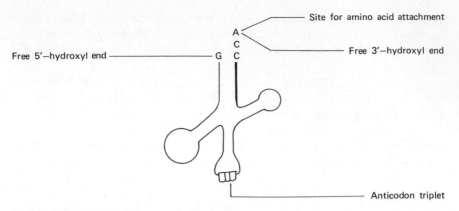

Figure 1.4 General structure of tRNA.

moves along the mRNA to the second codon where the complementary tRNA with its specific amino acid is base-paired. The two amino acids, juxtaposed in this manner, are covalently joined through a peptide bond, and the first tRNA, now freed of its amino acid, is released from the mRNA. The ribosome then moves to the third codon where still another tRNA base-pairs and its amino acid is bonded to the second, thereby forming a tripeptide whose sequence was directed by the specific codon–anticodon base-pairing. The cycle is repeated as the ribosome scans the segment of mRNA capable of coding an entire protein, and the chain elongates by one amino acid for each reading of a new codon.

From this overview of protein systhesis, it becomes clear how mutations within the DNA molecule, such as deleted, added, or substituted nucleotides would be manifested as sequencing errors in the protein synthesized through the affected genes. The clinical consequences of such errors will be described later under inborn errors of metabolism. (Chapter 9)

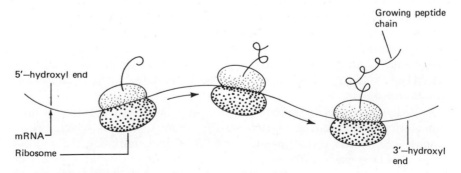

Figure 1.5 Illustration of the movement of a ribosome along a segment of mRNA and the elongation of a protein chain coincident with the "reading" of the mRNA code.

ENZYMES—THE CATALYSTS OF THE CELL

Enzymes are proteins endowed with the capability for catalyzing in a highly specific manner each of the thousands of chemical reactions in the cell. Some enzymes are purely protein; however, in most cases, the functional activity of an enzyme derives not only from the protein portion of the molecule, but also from nonprotein entities called coenzymes. Coenzymes are relativley small (compared with the protein portion) organic compounds that work in partnership with the protein portion (called the apoenzyme) in bringing about the functional activity. In some instances the enzyme may require, instead of a coenzyme, a specific metal ion referred to as an activator. Many of the coenzymes are derived directly from the B-complex vitamins through structural modifications, which are themselves catalyzed by enzymes. Examples of activators are magnesium, zinc, copper, manganese, and iron ions. The dietary requirements for the B-complex vitamins and for the metals mentioned are therefore evident.

The terminology for describing enzyme-catalyzed reactions, simply stated, is that the enzyme (E) catalyzes the conversion of a compound, the substrate (S), into a structurally different compound, the product (P). In the process, the enzyme binds fleetingly with the substrate to form an enzyme-substrate complex (ES) and then releases the product. The enzyme, in compliance with the definition of a true catalyst, is neither altered nor consumed in the reaction. The overall reaction may be represented as:

$$E + S \underset{①}{\rightleftharpoons} ES \underset{②}{\rightleftharpoons} E + P$$

Many enzymes catalyze their specific reactions reversibly as indicated by the double arrows, in which case it could be said that in an isolated system the enzyme hastens the rate at which an equilibrium is attained between the concentration of substrate and product. In reading the reverse reaction, the product, designated as P, obviously becomes the substrate and the substrate of the forward (or left to right) reaction becomes the product. Other enzymes catalyze unidirectionally (in one direction) meaning that reaction ② above proceeds only from left to right. Whether or not the enzyme catalyzes reversibly or unidirectionally, reaction 1 is always reversible, and the tendency of the ES complex to dissociate is, of course, inversely related to the affinity of the enzyme for its substrate.

Enzyme Specificity

Many enzymes display a nearly absolute specificity for their particular substrate, which means that they will react with that compound only and will not convert even closely related substances. On the other hand, there are those enzymes that exhibit a relatively broad specificity, reacting with a number of compounds that share a common structural feature. In general, however, the enzymes involved in cellular metabolism do exhibit a high degree of specificity. This is necessary to prevent an assortment of undesired side reactions, which would disrupt the regimentation of cellular events.

The specificity of the reaction is vested in what is known as the active site of the enzyme, a relatively small region or pocket within the folds of the polypeptide chain which is structurally complementary to the structure of the substrate. There is still a great deal to be learned about the enzyme–substrate interaction, but from the extensive research in enzymology there has emerged the observation that for some enzymes, at least, the active site is composed of two distinct features, a positioning site and a catalytic site. It is proposed that the specificity resides in the alignment of the substrate within the positioning site. This site, in turn, serves the additional function of positioning the substrate so that the susceptible bond (or bonds) is properly located within the catalytic site. It is the catalytic site that causes the chemical transformation of substrate into product. The positioning and catalytic sites must, therefore, lie in proximity to each other, and if a coenzyme or activator is required for enzymatic activity these must form an integral part of the enzyme and occupy a position favorable for facilitating the substrate–product conversion. Certain coenzymes are bound loosely to their enzymes and readily dissociate from and reassociate with the apoenzyme reversibly. Other coenzymes are tightly bound to the apoenzyme through nondissociable covalent or coordinate covalent bonds. More will be said about coenzymes in Chapter 2.

Allosteric Enzymes and the Regulation of Metabolism

Metabolism in a living cell consists of a multitude of simultaneous, enzyme-catalyzed reactions. The enzymes are compartmentalized within the cell and they function in sequential chains called multienzyme systems or pathways. This means that the product of one enzymatic reaction becomes the substrate for the next, etc., until the final product (end product) is formed. A symbolic representation of such a pathway is shown below:

$$A \xrightarrow{E_1} B \rightleftharpoons^{E_2} C \rightleftharpoons^{E_3} D \xrightarrow{E_4} E \rightleftharpoons^{E_5} F \xrightarrow{E_6} G$$

In this particular multienzyme system, compound A is ultimately converted to compound G via the intermediate compounds B, C, D, E, and F. Each "step" or reaction in this sequence is catalyzed by a different enzyme, $E_1, E_2, \ldots$ and so on. As indicated, some reactions in such pathways are reversible while others are unidirectional. However, it is important to understand that despite the reversibility of a reaction, the continuous removal of one of the products drives the reaction toward the formation of more of that product. This driving force, therefore, never permits a true equilibrium to be established as it would be in an isolated system, and encourages the sequential reactions to proceed primarily in the desired direction.

The complexity of the integrated pathways of metabolism necessitates a regulation or control of the rate of reaction systems. In most multienzyme systems, one or more of the enzymes involved serves to regulate the rate of the overall sequence. These are called regulatory or allosteric enzymes, and the first enzyme in a metabolic sequence usually functions in this manner. These enzymes are called allosteric because they possess an "allosteric site," a specific "other" site from that of the catalytic site. It is to this allosteric site that certain substances, called modulators, can be bound. Modulators exert a profound influence on the enzyme's activity, presumably by altering the binding of the substrate with the active site through changes in the conformation of the polypeptide chain or chains of the enzyme. In other words, the interaction of the modulator substance with the allosteric site changes the manner of folding of the enzyme (its conformation) which in turn affects the affinity of the enzyme's active site for its substrate. Modulators may enhance the binding of substrate, in which case they are called positive modulators. Negative modulators are those that diminish the binding of the substrate and, therefore, decrease the activity of the enzyme. Modulators, also called effectors, are very often the end product of a sequence of reactions. As the end product accumulates above a certain critical concentration, it inhibits, through negative modulation, the allosteric enzyme of the sequence. In referring to the symbolic pathway shown above, product G may be a negative modulator for allosteric enzyme E_1, thus slowing the reactivity of the entire sequence.

Enzyme Classification

There exists an international classification of enzymes based on the type of reaction catalyzed. The multitude of known enzymatic reactions are encompassed within six general classifications:

1. *Oxido-reductases* catalyze a wide variety of oxidation–reduction reactions. Included in this group are the so-called dehydrogenases, oxidases, and peroxidases. Enzymes in this class frequently require coenzymes such as nicotinamide adenine dinucleotide (NAD), nicotinamide adenine dinucleotide phosphate (NADP), flavin adenine dinucleotide (FAD), coenzyme Q and others. These coenzymes will be described in Chapter 2.

2. *Transferases* catalyze the transfer of various kinds of functional groups from one compound to another.
3. *Hydrolases* catalyze the breaking of bonds between carbon atoms and other kinds of atoms by the addition of water.
4. *Lyases* catalyze the breaking of carbon–carbon, carbon–sulfur, and carbon–nitrogen (other than peptide) bonds.
5. *Isomerases* catalyze the interconversion of optical or geometric isomers.
6. *Ligases* catalyze the formation of bonds between carbon and oxygen, sulfur, nitrogen, and other atoms. Ligases generally require energy released from the hydrolysis of adenosine triphosphate (ATP) for bond formation.

There is considerable information available to the interested reader on the subject of enzyme reactions. Discussion of topics such as enzyme kinetics, inhibition, mechanisms of catalysis and the effect of substrate concentration, pH and temperature on the reaction rates will not be discussed here, but can be found in standard biochemistry texts.

REFERENCES

1. Ross, L. M. *The Cell*. Ciba Clinical Symposia, R. K. Shapter, ed. **25**(4):10 –13, Summit, N. J.: Ciba Pharmaceutical Co., 1973.
2. Orten, J. M. and O. W. Neuhaus. *Human Biochemistry*. 9th ed. St. Louis: C. W. Mosby, 1975; pp. 29–123.

Questions

1. If the concentration of a nutrient inside a cell is greater than outside, why wouldn't additional nutrient enter the cell by simple diffusion? Is there a mechanism, and if so what, by which nutrients can enter a cell against such a concentration gradient?
2. Within which of the cellular organelles discussed is most of the cell's energy, in the form of ATP, generated? Which organelle serves as the site for protein biosynthesis?
3. The biosynthesis of protein is an energy-requiring process. What does this fact, together with the answers to question #2, suggest about the freedom of ATP movement within the cytoplasm?
4. Many metabolic diseases, caused by the individual's inability to synthesize certain enzymes, are inherited disorders. How is this explained on the basis of the central dogma of molecular genetics?
5. Enzymes can catalyze reactions either reversibly or unidirectionally. Allosteric enzymes would predictably be which type? Why?

CHAPTER 2

Major Nutrients — Structural Characteristics

The term *nutrients,* as used in this and subsequent chapters, refers to dietary substances that either furnish energy through their metabolic oxidation or are otherwise required to maintain normal metabolism. The major nutrients are categorized according to chemical structure into the major divisions—carbohydrates, fats (lipids), proteins, vitamins, and minerals. Water also is a nutrient, but its discussion is beyond the scope of this chapter.

CARBOHYDRATES

Carbohydrates are polyalcohols of carbonyl (aldehyde or ketone) compounds. In their simplest or nonderivatized form, they are constructed from the atoms of carbon, oxygen, and hydrogen which occur in proportion approximating that of a "hydrate of carbon", or $C(H_2O)$. The carbohydrates have classically been subdivided into three major classes according to molecular size: monosaccharides, oligosaccharides, and polysaccharides. The latter two are simply polymeric forms of monosaccharides and, therefore, retain the monosaccharides' empirical composition of carbon, oxygen, and hydrogen.

Monosaccharides

Monosaccharides are the simplest form of carbohydrate. Referred to as "simple sugars," they cannot be broken down into smaller units by acid hydrolysis. Naturally occurring monosaccharides contain from three to seven carbon atoms, and on this basis are classified as trioses, tetroses, pentoses, hexoses, and heptoses. Among these, only the hexoses glucose, fructose, and galactose occur in foods, and therefore deserve the most attention from the nutritional standpoint. Nevertheless, heptoses, pentoses, tetroses, and trioses appear as products of intermediary metabolism and in combination with other biomolecules. They are also, therefore, of much importance to the living organism.

It has already been mentioned that carbonyl functions occur in the simple sugars. These may be aldehydes or ketones, necessitating a more specific classification based, in addition to the number of carbon atoms,

Table 2.1 Examples of Monosaccharide Classification

Name	Classification	Formula	Structure
glyceraldehyde	aldotriose	$C_3H_6O_3$	CH=O | CH—OH | CH_2—OH
dihydroxyacetone	ketotriose	$C_3H_6O_3$	CH_2—OH | C=O | CH_2—OH
ribose	aldopentose	$C_5H_{10}O_5$	CH=O | (CH—OH)$_3$ | CH_2—OH
glucose	aldohexose	$C_6H_{12}O_6$	CH=O | (CH—OH)$_4$ | CH_2OH
fructose	ketohexose	$C_6H_{12}O_6$	CH_2—OH | C=O | (CH—OH)$_3$ | CH_2—OH

on the type of carbonyl function. Accordingly, a five-carbon monosaccharide possessing a ketone function is called a ketopentose; a six-carbon aldehyde-containing sugar, an aldohexose, and so on. Examples of this classification for several monosaccharides are indicated in Table 2.1.

Stereoisomerism and Optical Activity. Many naturally occurring organic compounds, including the carbohydrates, will rotate the plane of polarized light when such light is passed through a solution of the compound. This property is attributed to the presence in the molecules of one or more asymmetric centers, which are carbon atoms having each of their four covalent bonds attached to different atoms or groups of atoms. Such substances are therefore said to be "optically active" because of their ability to turn the plane of a beam of polarized light.

The angles of the four bonds of a carbon atom are such that if the carbon atom is pictured as being at the geometric center of a tetrahedron, the bonds will point toward the corners of that tetrahedron:

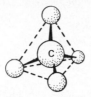

An optically active substance may rotate polarized light either to the right or to the left, and the substance is said to be either *dextrorotatory* or *levorotatory*, respectively. Furthermore, every optically active compound has a counterpart, identical to itself from the standpoint of structural formula, but which rotates polarized light the same number of degrees in the opposite direction. It is known that this is due to the different orientation of the groups bonded to the asymmetric carbon. For example, consider the tetrahedral model in the two forms shown:

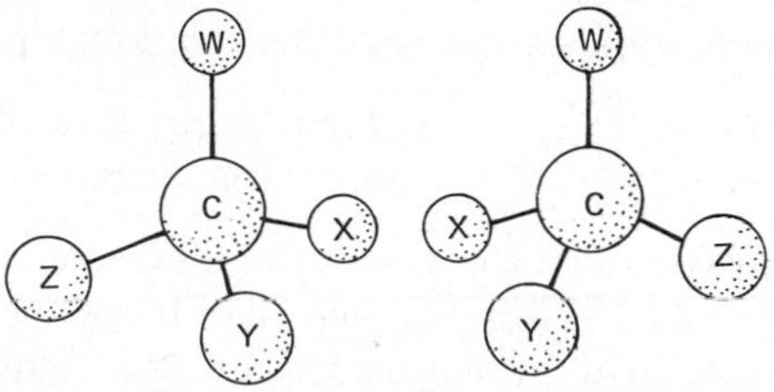

Mental manipulation of the forms will show that the two are not superimposable. The two forms are, in fact, mirror images of each other; they are said to be *enantiomers*.

The monosaccharides exist in either the stereoisomeric D or L form, which does not indicate the direction of rotation of plane-polarized light, that is, if the form is dextro- or levorotatory. It simply indicates structural analogy to the reference compound, glyceraldehyde, whose D- and L-forms are, by convention, drawn as shown:

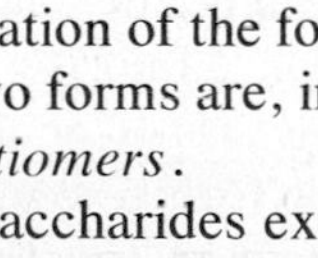

$$
\begin{array}{cc}
\mathrm{CH{=}O} & \mathrm{CH{=}O} \\
| & | \\
\mathrm{H{-}C{-}OH} & \mathrm{HO{-}C{-}H} \\
| & | \\
\mathrm{CH_2OH} & \mathrm{CH_2OH} \\
\text{D-glyceraldehyde} & \text{L-glyceraldehyde}
\end{array}
$$

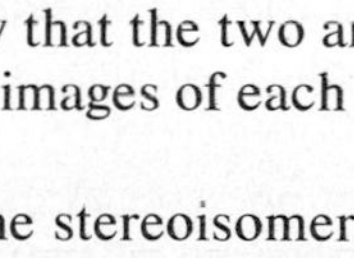

The distinction therefore rests with the direction of the —OH bond on the single asymmetric carbon of this molecule. Monosaccharides having more than three carbon atoms possess more than one asymmetric center, only one of which is the structural indicator as to whether the sugar is of the D- or L- configuration. The highest numbered asymmetric center serves as the indicator, the —OH positioned to the right in the D-form and to the left in the L- form. The examples shown are represented in so-called *Fischer projection structures* to clarify the concept of D-L stereoisomerism.

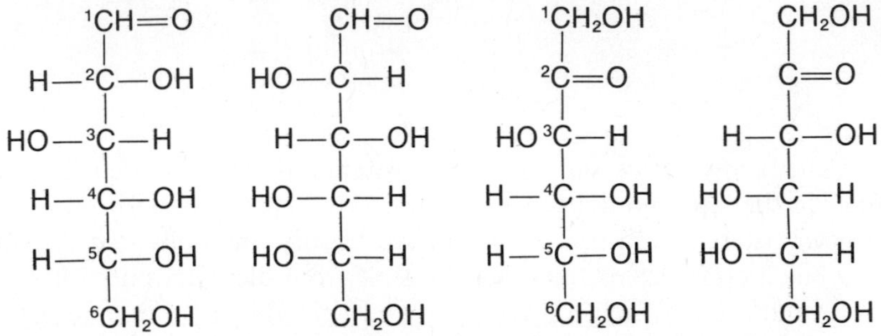

$$
\begin{array}{cccc}
\text{D-glucose} & \text{L-glucose} & \text{D-fructose} & \text{L-fructose}
\end{array}
$$

${}^1CH{=}O$	$CH{=}O$	${}^1CH_2OH$	CH_2OH
$H{-}{}^2C{-}OH$	$HO{-}C{-}H$	${}^2C{=}O$	$C{=}O$
$HO{-}{}^3C{-}H$	$H{-}C{-}OH$	$HO\,{}^3C{-}H$	$H{-}C{-}OH$
$H{-}{}^4C{-}OH$	$HO{-}C{-}H$	$H{-}{}^4C{-}OH$	$HO{-}C{-}H$
$H{-}{}^5C{-}OH$	$HO{-}C{-}H$	$H{-}{}^5C{-}OH$	$HO{-}C{-}H$
${}^6CH_2OH$	CH_2OH	${}^6CH_2OH$	CH_2OH
D-glucose	L-glucose	D-fructose	L-fructose

The number of stereoisomeric structures that can be drawn for an optically active compound is predictable from the number of asymmetric carbons in the compound according to the relationship:

$$\text{Maximum number of optical isomers} = 2^n$$

where n is equal to the number of asymmetric carbons

Therefore, for a hexose, which contains four asymmetric centers, 16 optical isomers are possible. Of these, eight will be of the D- series, that is with the hydroxyl at position five directed to the right, in a two-dimensional representation. The remaining eight will be the enantiomers or mirror images of each of the D- forms and will comprise the L- series of stereoisomers.

The projection structures, or open-chain forms, shown do not represent the true structure of these sugars. Indications for this stemmed from the fact that the aldoses and ketoses do not undergo reactions characteristic of true aldehydes and ketones, and it is now known that the carbonyl carbon (called the anomeric carbon atom in carbohydrate terminology) forms a bond with its most distant asymmetric carbon to generate a cyclic structure. The bond is called a *hemiacetal,* formed as the product of the reaction between an aldehyde and an alcohol, or a *hemiketal,* produced from a ketone and an alcohol.

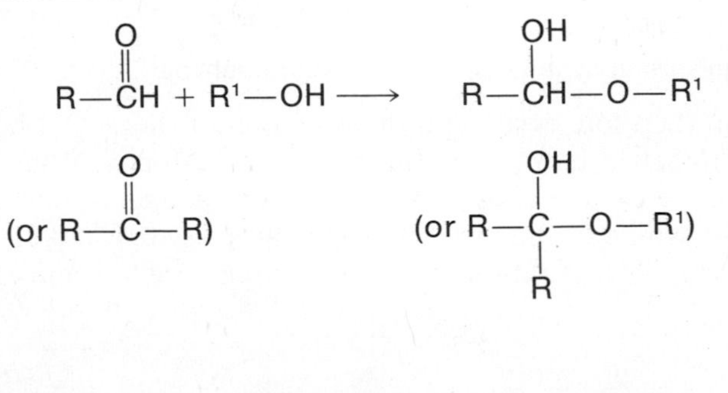

$$R{-}\overset{O}{\overset{\|}{C}}H + R^1{-}OH \longrightarrow R{-}\overset{OH}{\underset{|}{C}}H{-}O{-}R^1 \quad \text{(Hemiacetal)}$$

$$(\text{or } R{-}\overset{O}{\overset{\|}{C}}{-}R) \qquad (\text{or } R{-}\overset{OH}{\underset{\underset{R}{|}}{\underset{|}{C}}}{-}O{-}R^1) \quad \text{(Hemiketal)}$$

Because, in the case of the aldoses and ketoses, both functional groups are present in the same molecule, the hemiacetal is "internal", resulting in a cyclic structure. The cycle will be comprised of either four or five carbons and a single oxygen atom. For D-glucose:

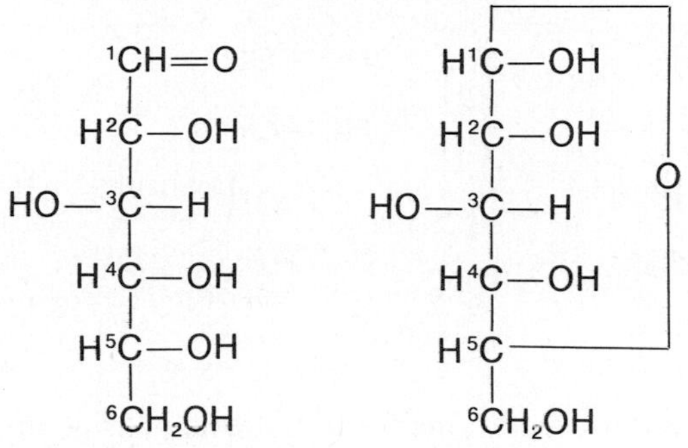

$$
\begin{array}{c}
^1CH{=}O \\
H{^2}C{-}OH \\
HO{-}{^3}C{-}H \\
H{^4}C{-}OH \\
H{^5}C{-}OH \\
{^6}CH_2OH
\end{array}
\qquad
\begin{array}{c}
H{^1}C{-}OH \\
H{^2}C{-}OH \\
HO{-}{^3}C{-}H \quad O \\
H{^4}C{-}OH \\
H{^5}C \\
{^6}CH_2OH
\end{array}
$$

and for D-fructose:

$$
\begin{array}{c}
^1CH_2OH \\
^2C{=}O \\
HO{-}{^3}CH \\
C{^4}H{-}OH \\
C{^5}H{-}OH \\
{^6}CH_2OH
\end{array}
\qquad
\begin{array}{c}
^1CH_2OH \\
\quad OH \\
^2C \\
HO{-}{^3}CH \quad O \\
^4CH{-}OH \\
^5CH \\
{^6}CH_2OH
\end{array}
$$

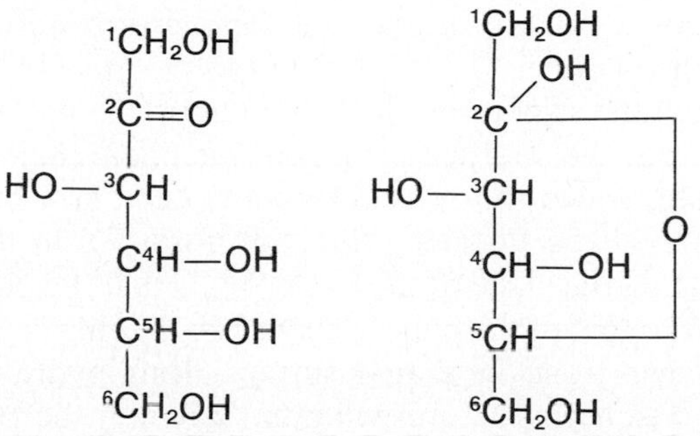

The formation of the hemiacetal produces a new asymmetric center at the anomeric carbon atom and, therefore, the bond direction of the newly formed hydroxyl group becomes significant. In the reactions above, the hydroxyls at position 1 for D-glucose, and position 2 for D-fructose, are arbitrarily directed to the right, resulting in an alpha (α) configuration. Should the hydroxyl at the anomeric carbon be directed to the left, the beta (β) configuration results. α and β forms of the same sugar are called *anomers* because the configurational difference resides at the anomeric carbon atom. In aqueous solution, an equilibrium mixture of α and β anomers exists, with the concentration of the β form being roughly twice that of the α. If a pure solution of either of the two anomers is formed, the optical rotation will change as the equilibrium concentrations are approached. This change in optical rotation is referred to as mutarotation. It results from the interconversion of α and β isomers through the open chain (no hemiacetal) forms as shown below for glucose:

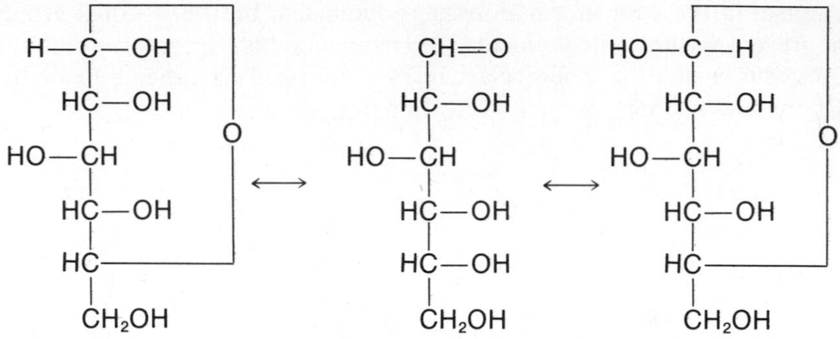

$$
\begin{array}{ccc}
\underset{\alpha\text{-D-glucose}}{
\begin{array}{l}
\text{H}-\text{C}-\text{OH} \\
\text{HC}-\text{OH} \\
\text{HO}-\text{CH} \\
\text{HC}-\text{OH} \\
\text{HC} \\
\text{CH}_2\text{OH}
\end{array}} \quad O
&
\longleftrightarrow
\underset{\substack{\text{Open chain}\\ \text{(Fischer projection)}}}{
\begin{array}{l}
\text{CH}{=}\text{O} \\
\text{HC}-\text{OH} \\
\text{HO}-\text{CH} \\
\text{HC}-\text{OH} \\
\text{HC}-\text{OH} \\
\text{CH}_2\text{OH}
\end{array}}
\longleftrightarrow
\underset{\beta\text{-D-glucose}}{
\begin{array}{l}
\text{HO}-\text{C}-\text{H} \\
\text{HC}-\text{OH} \\
\text{HO}-\text{CH} \\
\text{HC}-\text{OH} \\
\text{HC} \\
\text{CH}_2\text{OH}
\end{array}} \quad O
\end{array}
$$

Such cyclic representations for a monosaccharide are technically inappropriate. For the sake of convenience as well as structural accuracy, the *Haworth* perspective formulae were developed. These representations will be used throughout the remainder of the text. Table 2.2 illustrates the structural relationship among simple projection formulae and Haworth models.

Inspection of the structures shows that a few simple rules are applied in converting from the Fischer projection or open chain models to the more appropriate, Haworth forms. The conversion may be accomplished by rotating the cyclized Fischer projection form 90° in the plane of the paper, then rotating the plane of the cycle 90° so that the plane of the cycle is perpendicular to that of the paper. Therefore the ring is viewed from the "edge" rather than from the planar surface. Ring hydroxyls pointing to the right in the Fischer structure will point down in the Haworth model, and those to the left will point up in the Haworth form. It will be recalled that in a monosaccharide having an α configuration, the anomeric hydroxyl would therefore point to the right in a Fischer structure, and down in a Haworth, while a β configuration would have the anomeric hydroxyl directed to the left in the Fischer and up in the Haworth form. Notice that in the simplified Haworth representation, hydroxyls are indicated by vertical lines, hydroxy methyl groups by right angle straight lines, and hydrogens are ignored. Writing this type of structural representation is obviously of great advantage in the interest of time and space.

Disaccharides

These substances are composed of two monosaccharide units joined together through an acetal bond, referred to as glycosidic bond in carbohydrate chemistry terminology. Acetal bonds are formed through the reac-

Table 2.2 Various Structural Representations Among the Hexoses—
Glucose, Fructose, and Galactose

Hexose	Fischer projection	Cyclized Fischer projection	Haworth	Simplified Haworth
α-D-glucose	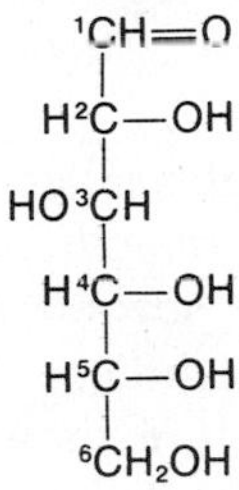	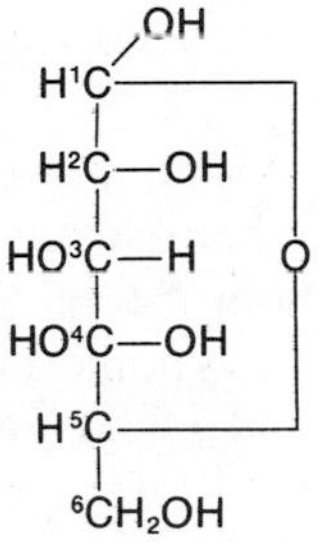	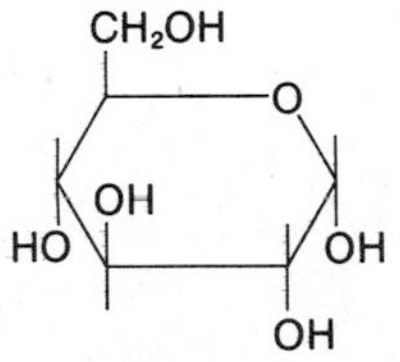	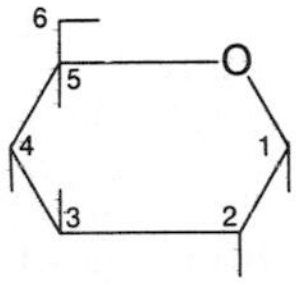
β-D-galactose	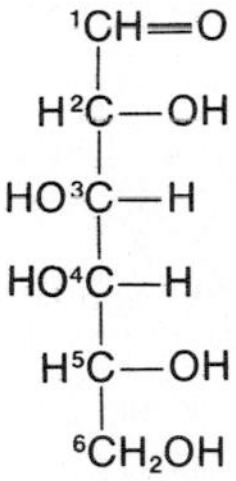	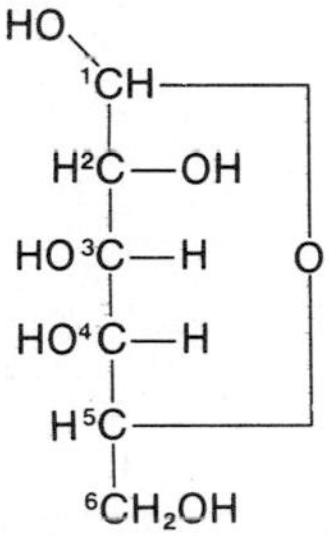	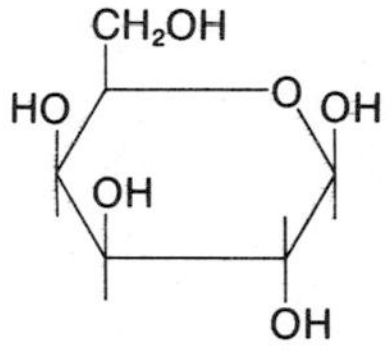	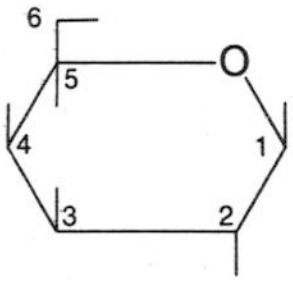
β-D-fructose	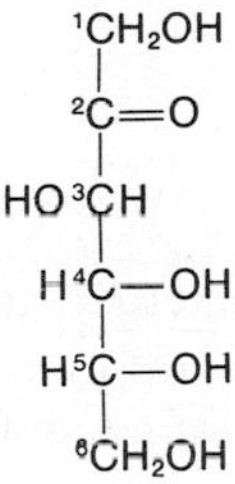	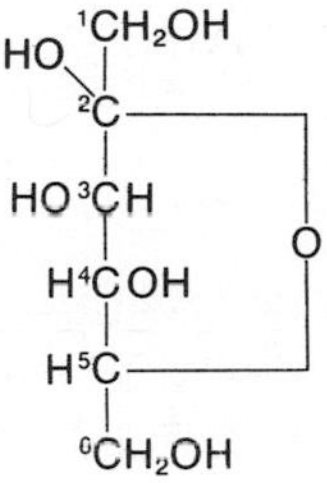	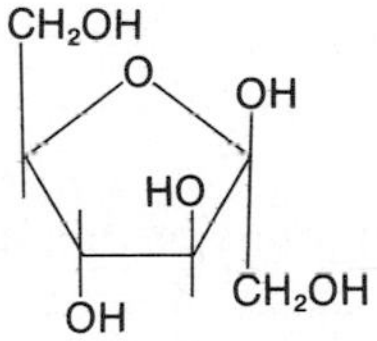	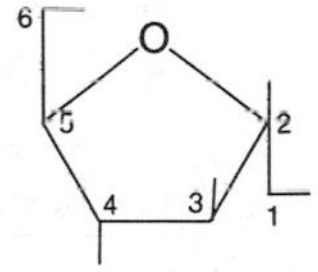

tion of a hemiacetal with an alcohol function, and in the special case of the glycosidic bond, the alcohol is contributed by the second monosaccharide of the pair making up the disaccharide. Disaccharides can be hydrolyzed by acids or, in the body, by enzymes into two monosaccharide units.

Among the oligosaccharides (carbohydrates containing from two to 10 monosaccharide units) found in nature, the disaccharides are the most abundant. The most common disaccharides are maltose, derived mainly from the partial hydrolysis of the polysaccharide, starch; lactose, the sugar found in milk; and sucrose, or cane sugar, used extensively for the sweetening of foods and beverages.

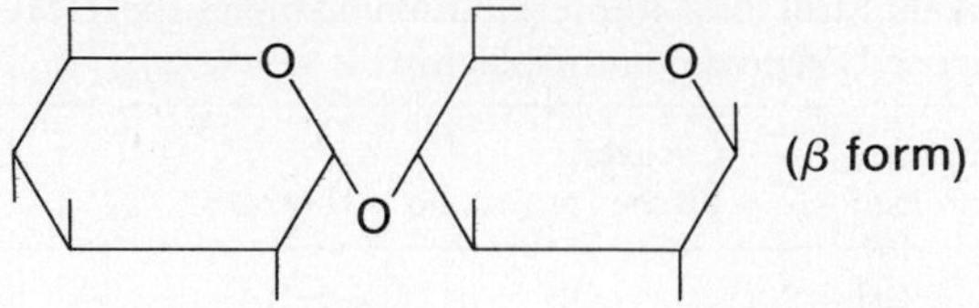

(β form)

maltose

Maltose consists of two glucose units linked through a glycosidic bond involving the hydroxyl function of the hemiacetal of the glucose residue on the left and the hydroxyl at carbon #4 of the second glucose. The direction of the glycosidic bond at the anomeric carbon is alpha, and the bond is therefore symbolized $\alpha(1 \rightarrow 4)$. The structure shown is the beta form, indicating the orientation of the —OH group at the anomeric carbon not involved in the glycosidic bond. Maltose can also exist in an alpha form.

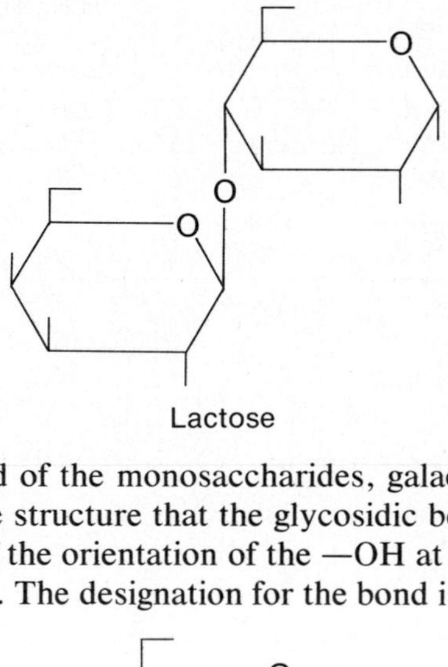

Lactose

Lactose is composed of the monosaccharides, galactose and glucose. It can be seen from the structure that the glycosidic bond joining them is a beta type because of the orientation of the —OH at the anomeric carbon involved in the bond. The designation for the bond is therefore $\beta(1 \rightarrow 4)$.

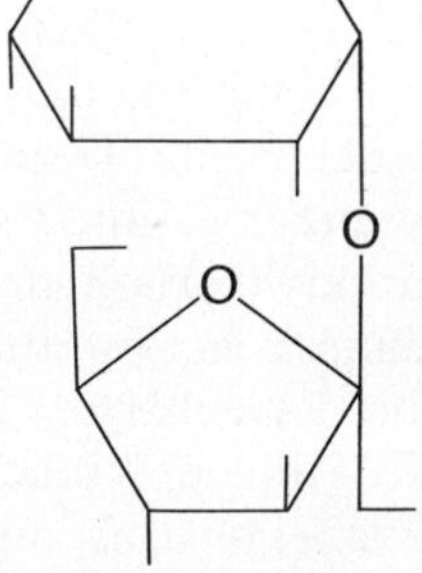

Sucrose

The glycosidic bond of sucrose is somewhat unique in that it involves the anomeric hydroxyl of *both* monosaccharide units, which are glucose and fructose. The linkage is alpha with respect to glucose, and beta, with respect to fructose.

Any mono- or disaccharide that possesses a hemiacetal or hemiketal, and that therefore can equilibrate with an open chain aldehyde or ketone, is capable of chemically reducing certain substances such as the copper ion (Cu^{++}). An inspection of the structures of the sugars discussed in this chapter shows that such hemiacetals do exist in all but sucrose. On this basis, sugars may be classified as reducing or, in the case of sucrose, nonreducing. Certain qualitative and quantitative tests for glucose in the clinical laboratory are based on the reducing properties of this sugar.

Polysaccharides

Just as two monosaccharides may be joined through a glycosidic bond to form a disaccharide, this union may be repeated hundreds of times producing a high molecular weight substance called a polysaccharide. If it consists of a single type of monomeric unit it is called a *homopolysaccharide*, and if two or more different types of monosaccharides comprise its structure, it is called a *heteropolysaccharide*. Either type of polymer may exist in a strictly linear arrangement of its monosaccharide units or it may be branched to various degrees. Polysaccharides are of great importance in nutrition because of the abundance of the substance in many natural foods. They are the chief storage form of carbohydrate in both the plant and animal kingdom.

Starch. Starch is the major form in which carbohydrate is stored in plants, and it can exist in two forms, *amylose* and *amylopectin*. Amylose is a linear (unbranched) polymer of D-glucose in which the units are connected through $\alpha(1 \rightarrow 4)$ glycosidic bonds as they are in maltose. These polymers range in molecular weight from a few thousand to 500,000. Like amylose, amylopectin is made up solely of polymeric D-glucose, but it has, in addition to $\alpha(1 \rightarrow 4)$ glycosidic bonds, $\alpha(1 \rightarrow 6)$ bonds, which create branch points. Figure 2.1 illustrates the formation of such a branch point.

Glycogen. The major form of stored carbohydrate in animal tissues is glycogen. It is localized primarily in liver and skeletal muscle. Structurally, it resembles amylopectin in that it is highly branched through numerous $\alpha(1 \rightarrow 6)$ bonding (see Fig. 2.1). In mammals, glycogen is enzymatically hydrolyzed to glucose which is a major source of energy. This hydrolysis is hormonally influenced according to the body's energy requirements at a given time. Such mechanisms will be discussed in Chapter 3.

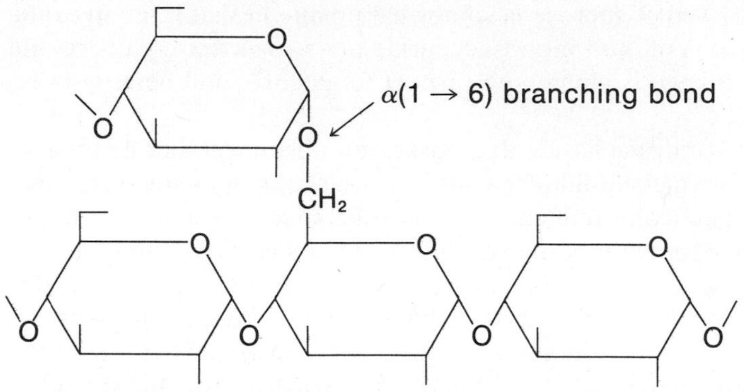

Figure 2.1 The chemistry of polysaccharide branch points.

Cellulose. Cellulose is considered a structural polysaccharide because it is a major component of cell walls in plants, and the wood portion of a vegetation is approximately 50 percent cellulose. Chemically, cellulose is a homopolysaccharide, but differ from the other polysaccharides discussed in that the D-glucose units are connected by $\beta(1 \rightarrow 4)$ glycoside bonds rather than $\alpha(1 \rightarrow 4)$. Humans lack the enzymes that are able to hydrolyze $\beta(1 \rightarrow 4)$ bonds. Ruminants such as cattle, sheep, and goats do derive nutritional benefit from cellulose because the bacterial population in the rumen of these animals has the necessary hydrolytic enzymes. Such bacteria in the stomach of the termite account for this insect's appetite for wood and its ability to "get fat" on the cellulose therein. Although humans cannot derive energy from cellulose, it is a source of fiber or "roughage" in their diets and assumes importance as a bulking agent.

There are numerous heteropolysaccharides of widely diverse composition that are found throughout nature but are particularly important in bacterial cell wall structure. They will not be discussed in this text because they have less importance in human nutrition and energy metabolism.

LIPIDS

The second major class of nutrients that will be considered is the lipids, a structurally heterogeneous group of substances that share the common characteristic of being soluble in organic solvents rather than aqueous solvents. This property requires that, for transport throughout the aqueous milieu of the body, the lipids must be in chemical combination with the relatively large, hydrophilic plasma proteins.

As a family of compounds, lipids may be said to serve two important functions:

1. Storage form of metabolic fuel for energy.
2. Structural components of membranes.

If, however, the definition of lipids is broad enough to include all biological substances exhibiting solubility in organic rather than in aqueous solvents, the list of functions would need to be expanded. Steroid hormones and fat-soluble vitamins, for example, are lipids according to this definition.

Fatty Acids

Fatty acids vary in chain length and are aliphatic carboxylic acids. They do not represent a class of lipid in themselves because they do not normally occur in the free state, but their importance lies in the fact that they form a part of the structure of most of the major lipids. When they do occur in the free state it is because they are released by hydrolysis from the compounds of which they are a part.

The chain of the fatty acid generally contains between 12 and 24 carbon atoms, but the most abundant are those containing 16 or 18 carbon atoms. Table 2.3 lists some naturally occurring fatty acids.

Fatty acid chains may be saturated or they may possess one or more double bonds. The chain length and degree of unsaturation have a signifi-

Table 2.3 Some Naturally Occurring Fatty Acids

Carbon atoms	Structure	Systematic name	Common name
Saturated fatty acids			
12	$CH_3(CH_2)_{10}COOH$	n-Dodecanoic	Lauric acid
14	$CH_3(CH_2)_{12}COOH$	n-Tetradecanoic	Myristic
16	$CH_3(CH_2)_{14}COOH$	n-Hexadecanoic	Palmitic
18	$CH_3(CH_2)_{16}COOH$	n-Octadecanoic	Stearic
20	$CH_3(CH_2)_{18}COOH$	n-Eicosanoic	Arachidic
24	$CH_3(CH_2)_{22}COOH$	n-Tetracosanoic	Lignoceric
Unsaturated fatty acids			
16:1*	$CH_3(CH_2)_5CH{=}CH(CH_2)_7COOH$		Palmitoleic
18:1	$CH_3(CH_2)_7CH{=}CH(CH_2)_7COOH$		Oleic
18:2	$CH_3(CH_2)_4CH{=}CHCH_2CH{=}CH(CH_2)_7COOH$		Linoleic
18:3	$CH_3CH_2CH{=}CHCH_2CH{=}CHCH_2CH{=}CH(CH_2)_7COOH$		Linolenic
20:4	$CH_3(CH_2)_4CH{=}CHCH_2CH{=}CHCH_2CH{=}CHCH_2CH{=}$ $CH(CH_2)_3COOH$		Arachidonic

*16 refers to number of carbon atoms; 1 refers to number of double bonds.

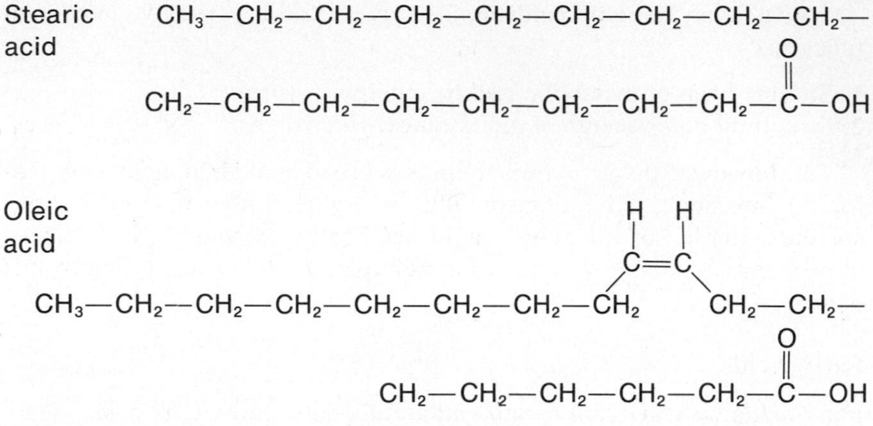

Stearic acid

$$CH_3—CH_2—CH_2—CH_2—CH_2—CH_2—CH_2—CH_2—CH_2—$$

$$CH_2—CH_2—CH_2—CH_2—CH_2—CH_2—CH_2—CH_2—\overset{\overset{\displaystyle O}{\|}}{C}—OH$$

Oleic acid

$$CH_3—CH_2—CH_2—CH_2—CH_2—CH_2—CH_2—CH_2 \quad \overset{\overset{\displaystyle H \quad H}{|\quad\;|}}{C=C} \quad CH_2—CH_2—$$

$$CH_2—CH_2—CH_2—CH_2—CH_2—\overset{\overset{\displaystyle O}{\|}}{C}—OH$$

Figure 2.2 A comparison of chain configuration in an 18-carbon saturated and unsaturated fatty acid.

cant effect on the chemical and physical properties of the fatty acid. For example, saturated fatty acids, in the C_{12} to C_{24} chain length range, are solids at room temperature; they are flexible and elongated in their configuration. On the other hand, unsaturated fatty acids of comparable chain length have more rigid and kinked conformation, and they have lower melting points, existing as liquids at room temperature. Unsaturated organic molecules exhibit either *cis* or *trans* isomerism. Among the unsaturated fatty acids, however, the orientation is nearly always *cis*, resulting in the kinking of the chain, and accounting for reduced molecular interaction which in turn accounts for a lower melting point. An example of an 18-carbon saturated and unsaturated fatty acid is shown in Figure 2.2.

Fats of animal origin contain fatty acids which are primarily of the saturated variety. Due to their higher melting points they are referred to as "hard" fats. Fats derived from vegetables and cold-blooded animals are constructed chiefly from unsaturated, or "soft" fats. Double bonds are loci for certain chemical reactions, and the unsaturated fats accordingly display chemical reactivities not shared by saturated fats. An example of such a reaction, which is of interest in dietetics, is *rancidity,* the development of unpleasant odor and taste in fats. This is due to oxidation of the double bonds to hydroperoxides which in turn are hydrolyzed to shorter chain, keto acids. In addition to oxygen, light, heat, moisture, and bacterial action all contribute to rancidity. This oxidation can be inhibited by substances called *antioxidants,* and many of these occur naturally within the fat itself. Phenols, naphthols, and quinones exhibit this property, but the most common natural antioxidant is vitamin E which is frequently added to foods to minimize rancidity.

Triglycerides (Neutral Fats)

Among the classes of lipids, the triglycerides are the most abundant. The major form of stored fat in the body, called adipose tissue, is triglyceride, and, therefore, most of our dietary fat of animal origin consists of these substances.

Chemically, triglycerides are esters formed from the reaction of the trihydric alcohol, glycerol, with three molecules of fatty acids. The carbon atoms of glycerol, shown below, are commonly designated α, β, and α' so that the position of certain fatty acids with which it is esterified can be indicated.

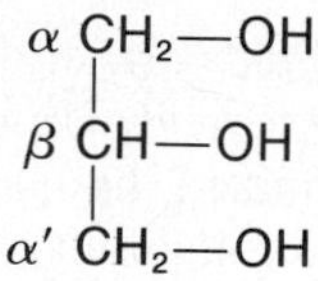

$$\alpha \ CH_2—OH$$
$$\beta \ CH—OH$$
$$\alpha' \ CH_2—OH$$

The general structure of a triglyceride can be represented as:

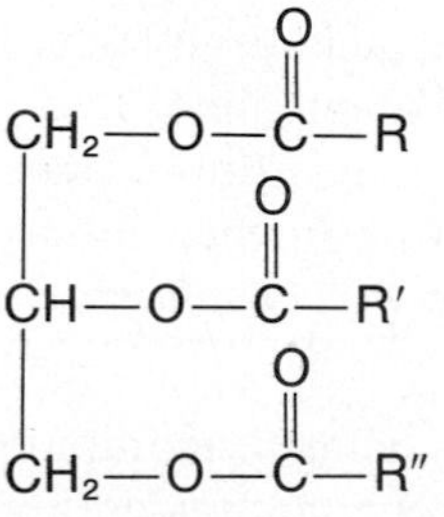

$$
\begin{array}{c}
\quad\quad\quad O \\
\quad\quad\quad \| \\
CH_2—O—C—R \\
\quad\quad\quad O \\
\quad\quad\quad \| \\
CH—O—C—R' \\
\quad\quad\quad O \\
\quad\quad\quad \| \\
CH_2—O—C—R''
\end{array}
$$

in which R refers to the aliphatic chain of the fatty acid. In a single triglyceride molecule, the fatty acids may be saturated or unsaturated or both. If the fatty acids within a single triglyceride molecule are all the same, the lipid is called a *simple triglyceride,* and is named according to the fatty acid involved and the prefix *tri;* for example, tripalmitin, triolein, and so on. When different fatty acids are incorporated into the same molecule, the triglyceride is called a *mixed triglyceride,* and the nomenclature should indicate the position of the fatty acids. Examples would be α-stearo-β, α' diolein, or β-palmito-α, α' distearin. The complete structure of the latter is shown as a typical mixed triglyceride.

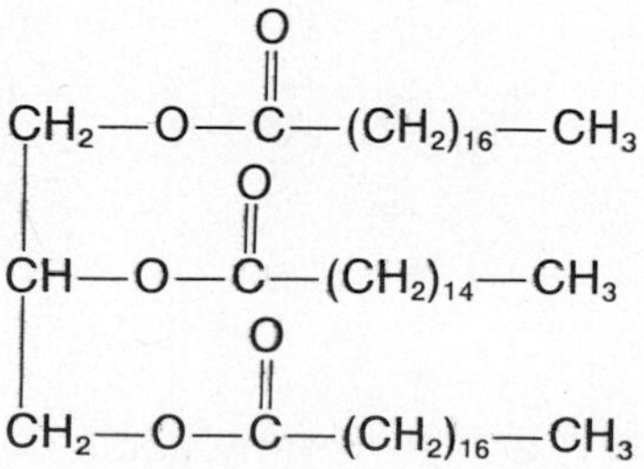

$$
\begin{array}{c}
\quad\quad\quad O \\
\quad\quad\quad \| \\
CH_2—O—C—(CH_2)_{16}—CH_3 \\
\quad\quad\quad O \\
\quad\quad\quad \| \\
CH—O—C—(CH_2)_{14}—CH_3 \\
\quad\quad\quad O \\
\quad\quad\quad \| \\
CH_2—O—C—(CH_2)_{16}—CH_3
\end{array}
$$

Esters are hydrolyzable bonds, and in the laboratory, triglycerides can be converted to free glycerol and three moles of fatty acids by hydrolysis of the three ester bonds. Hydrolysis can be accomplished by acids or alkalies, and in the special case of alkaline hydrolysis, the reaction is called *saponification*. The products of triglyceride saponification are slightly different from the products of acid hydrolysis in that the alkali used produces soluble salts of the fatty acids (e.g., sodium palmitate) which are soaps. In the body, dietary triglyceride is hydrolyzed in the small intestine by enzymes called lipases which are of pancreatic origin.

Phospholipids

As the name implies, phospholipids are substances that are lipids and that contain phosphate as phosphoric acid. Unlike the neutral fats, the acidic phosphate group bestows an ionized, hydrophilic center on the molecule. Because of their increased water solubility, these molecules function differently from the neutral fats in that they are found almost exclusively in cell membranes where their polarity regulates the transport of materials through the membrane. Among naturally occurring lipids, they are second only to the triglycerides in abundance, and yet, they are not stored in large amounts. Depot fat contains only traces of stored phospholipid.

This class of lipids can be further subdivided, on the basis of their structural components, into *glycerophosphatides* and *sphingophosphatides*.

Glycerophosphatides. This subclass encompasses the major portion of cellular phospholipids. Glycerophosphatides are assembled from glycerol, two fatty acids, phosphoric acid, and another component having an alcohol function. This alcohol component is principally choline, although serine, ethanolamine, and inositol may also serve in this function. The α and β hydroxyls of glycerol are esterified with fatty acids, just as in the triglyceride structure. The third hydroxyl, however, is esterfied with phosphoric acid, and the resulting structure is called *phosphatidic acid,* a general term because it does not identify the particular fatty acids involved.

$$
\begin{array}{c}
\quad\quad\quad\quad\quad \overset{\displaystyle O}{\overset{\displaystyle \|}{}} \\
CH_2\!-\!O\!-\!C\!-\!R \\
\quad\quad\quad\quad\quad \overset{\displaystyle O}{\overset{\displaystyle \|}{}} \\
CH_2\!-\!O\!-\!C\!-\!R' \\
\quad\quad\quad\quad\quad \overset{\displaystyle O}{\overset{\displaystyle \|}{}} \\
CH_2\!-\!O\!-\!P\!-\!OH \\
\quad\quad\quad\quad\quad | \\
\quad\quad\quad\quad\quad O_-
\end{array}
$$

R and R′ = fatty acids

Phosphatidic acid

The phosphoric acid ester is exceedingly important in the biochemical events that underlie nutrition, and the formation of these esters will be reviewed briefly here.

Esters are formed between alcohols and acids through a condensation reaction, which means that the elements of water are removed from the reactants, allowing the reactants to combine. One molecule of water is released in the reaction. The reaction of a carboxylic acid with an alcohol is generally represented as follows:

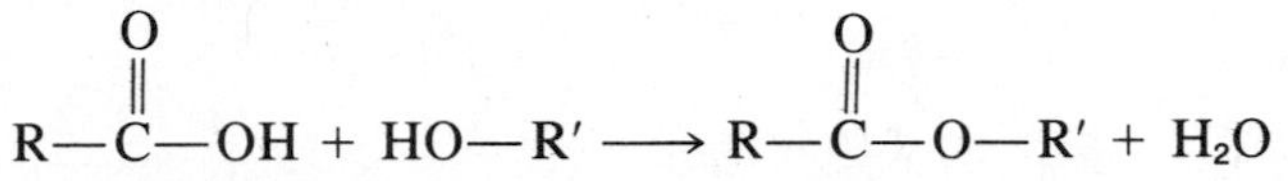

$$\underset{\substack{\|\\O}}{R-C}-OH + HO-R' \longrightarrow \underset{\substack{\|\\O}}{R-C}-O-R' + H_2O$$

Phosphoric acid reacts with alcohols in the same manner to form phosphoric acid esters:

$$HO-\underset{\substack{|\\OH}}{\overset{\overset{O}{\|}}{P}}-OH + HO-R \longrightarrow HO-\underset{\substack{|\\OH}}{\overset{\overset{O}{\|}}{P}}-O-R + H_2O$$

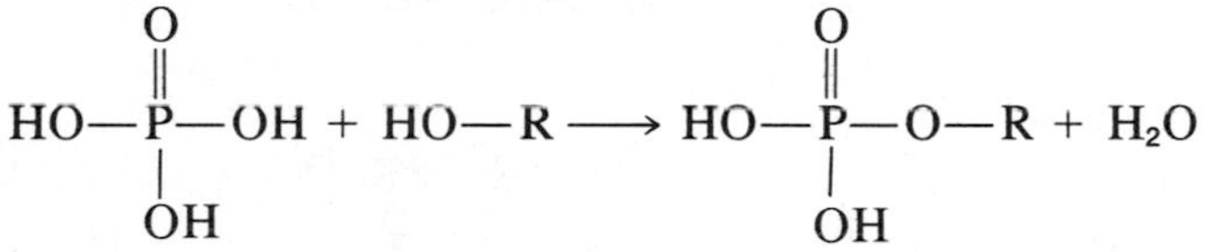

It is important to recognize that the phosphoric acid esterified to an alcohol still has unreacted —OH sites which are also capable of ester formation and which, therefore, can combine with a second molecule of alcohol. For example:

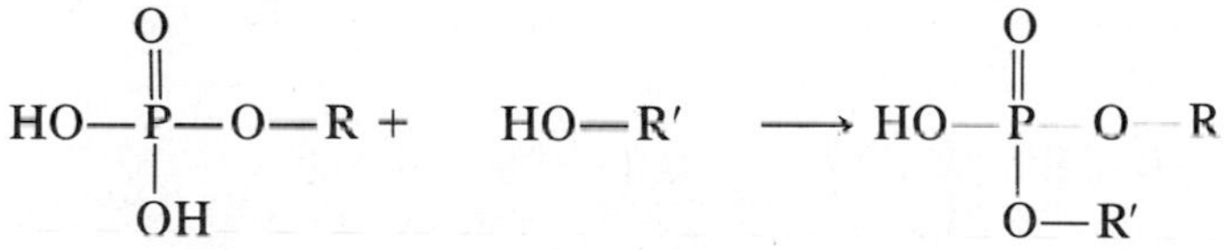

$$HO-\underset{\substack{|\\OH}}{\overset{\overset{O}{\|}}{P}}-O-R + \quad HO-R' \longrightarrow HO-\underset{\substack{|\\O-R'}}{\overset{\overset{O}{\|}}{P}}\quad O\quad R$$

| Phosphoric acid ester | Second molecule of alcohol | Phosphoric acid diester |

The remaining —OH of the diester does not undergo esterification. The hydrogen is acidic, and at the pH of the body fluids, it would be partly dissociated. Therefore the diester could be represented:

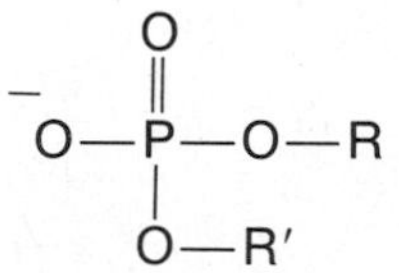

$$^-O-\underset{\substack{|\\O-R'}}{\overset{\overset{O}{\|}}{P}}-O-R$$

Diesters of phosphoric acid are found in the glycerophosphatides. It has already been shown that phosphoric acid is esterified to a hydroxyl of glycerol in phosphatidic acid. The acid undergoes a second esterification with alcohols such as choline, serine, ethanolamine, or inositol, forming the phosphatidyl derivatives of these alcohols as shown:

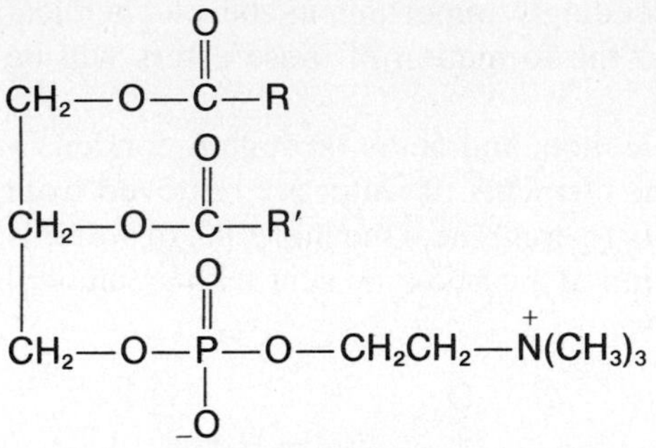

$$CH_2-O-\overset{\overset{\displaystyle O}{\|}}{C}-R$$

$$CH_2-O-\overset{\overset{\displaystyle O}{\|}}{C}-R'$$

$$CH_2-O-\overset{\overset{\displaystyle O}{\|}}{\underset{\underset{\displaystyle O}{|}}{P}}-O-CH_2CH_2-\overset{+}{N}(CH_3)_3$$

R and R' = fatty acid residues

Phosphatidyl choline
(lecithin)

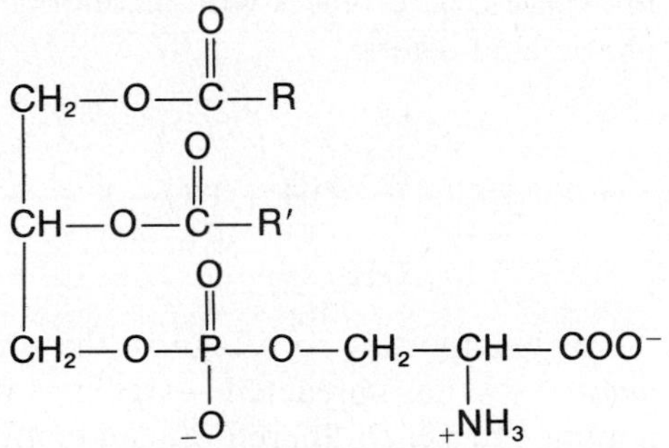

$$CH_2-O-\overset{\overset{\displaystyle O}{\|}}{C}-R$$

$$CH-O-\overset{\overset{\displaystyle O}{\|}}{C}-R'$$

$$CH_2-O-\overset{\overset{\displaystyle O}{\|}}{\underset{\underset{\displaystyle O}{|}}{P}}-O-CH_2-CH-COO^-$$
$$\underset{+NH_3}{|}$$

Phosphatidyl serine

$$CH_2-O-\overset{\overset{\displaystyle O}{\|}}{C}-R$$

$$CH-O-\overset{\overset{\displaystyle O}{\|}}{C}-R'$$

$$CH_2-O-\overset{\overset{\displaystyle O}{\|}}{\underset{\underset{\displaystyle O}{|}}{P}}-O-CH_2-CH_2-\overset{+}{N}H_3$$

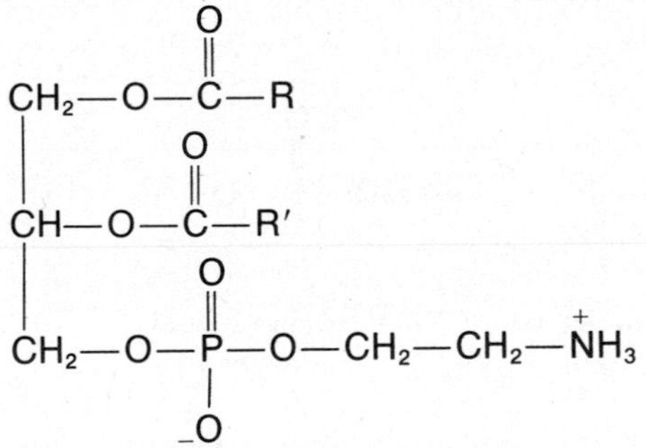

Phosphatidyl ethanolamine

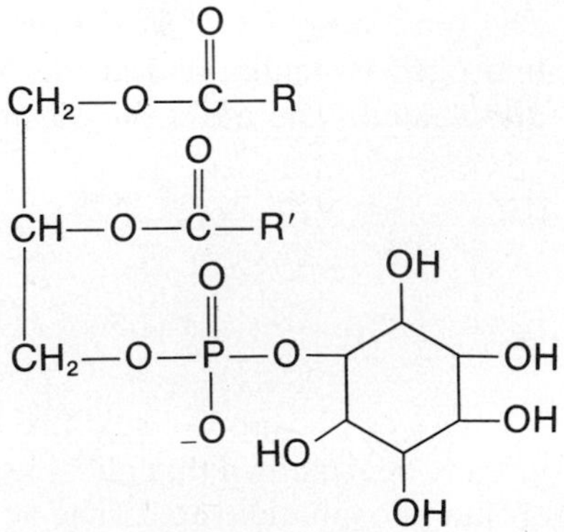

$$CH_2-O-\overset{\overset{\displaystyle O}{\|}}{C}-R$$

$$CH-O-\overset{\overset{\displaystyle O}{\|}}{C}-R'$$

$$CH_2-O-\overset{\overset{\displaystyle O}{\|}}{\underset{\underset{\displaystyle O}{|}}{P}}-O-$$

Phosphatidyl inositol

Phosphatidyl choline is commonly referred to as *lecithin* and the other three glycerophosphatides, *cephalins*.

Digestion of glycerophosphatides requires the action of a family of enzymes called the *phospholipases,* each of which hydrolyzes a specific ester bond in the molecule. The enzymes are designated phospholipase A, B, C, and D, and their specificity (the ester bonds specifically hydrolyzed) is shown below, using lecithin as a model substrate:

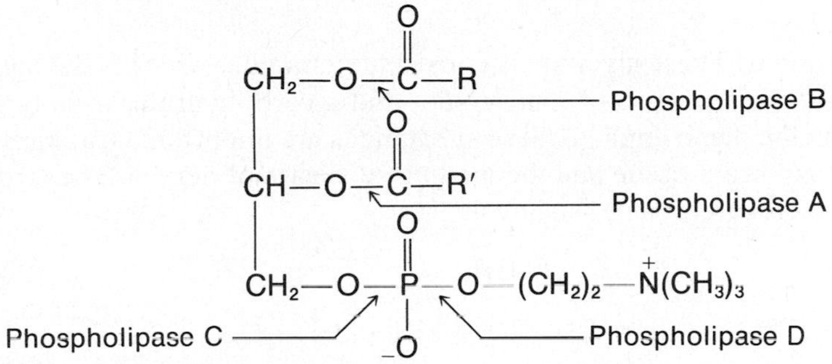

It is clear, therefore, that the concerted action of the phospholipases can hydrolyze a glycerophosphatide into its five components: glycerol, two fatty acids, free phosphoric acid, and alcohol component.

Sphingophosphatides. These lipids are concentrated largely in the brain and other nervous tissue. The simplest and most abundant sphingophosphatide is *sphingomyelin,* which, on hydrolysis yields the components sphingosine, a fatty acid, phosphoric acid, and choline. Sphingosine is an 18-carbon, unsaturated amino alcohol, having the structure shown below:

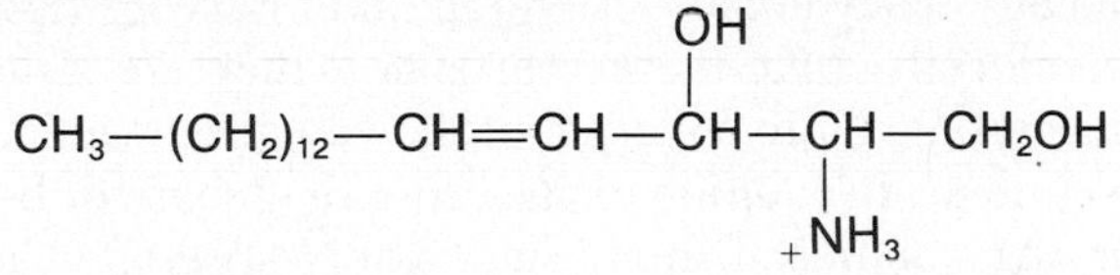

It is also known to exist as its saturated counterpart, dihydrosphingosine. The assemblage of the components to form the sphingomyelin molecule is as shown:

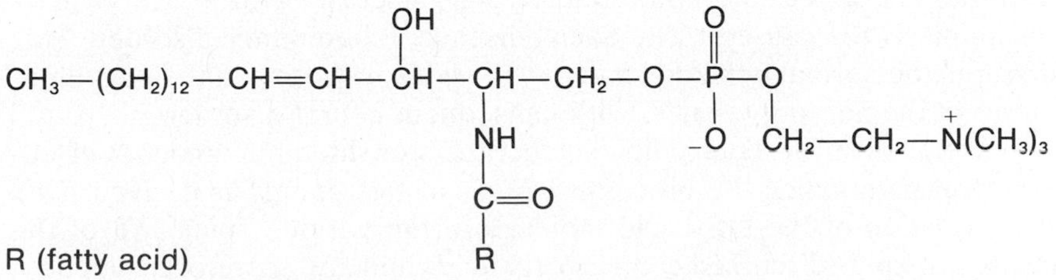

Glycolipids

The prefix *glyco-* implies the presence of carbohydrate. The main structural characteristics of this family of lipids are the presence of one or more monosaccharide residues or derivatives of them, and the absence of phosphate. In addition, they are comprised of sphingosine and a fatty acid. They may be subdivided, on the basis of the nature of the carbohydrate moiety of the structure, into *cerebrosides* and *gangliosides*.

Cerebrosides. These glycolipids consist of ceramide, which is the sphingosine-fatty acid portion of a molecule, and a carbohydrate, usually galactose. As the name implies, these substances are important structural components of brain tissue and the medullary sheath of nerves. The structure of a galactocerebroside is shown:

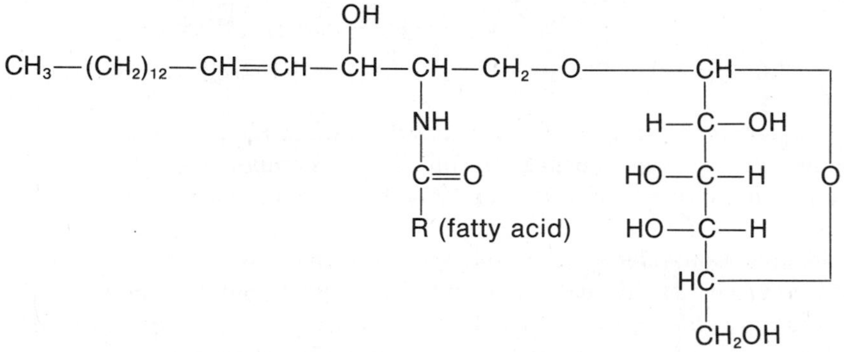

$$CH_3—(CH_2)_{12}—CH{=}CH—\overset{\overset{\displaystyle OH}{|}}{CH}—CH—CH_2—O———CH—$$

$$NH \qquad H—C—OH$$

$$C{=}O \qquad HO—C—H \qquad O$$

$$R \text{ (fatty acid)} \qquad HO—C—H$$

$$HC———$$

$$CH_2OH$$

Gangliosides. Gangliosides are so named because of their being isolated from ganglion cells. They are also found in other nervous tissue, erythrocytes, and spleen cells. Like the cerebrosides, they are structured from ceramide and a carbohydrate moiety, but they do differ significantly in the carbohydrate content. In addition to galactose or glucose or both, gangliosides have varying amounts of amino sugars or N-acetylated amino sugars linked to each other through glycosidic bonds. Examples of these derivatized monosaccharides are N-acetylgalactosamine and N-acetylneuraminic acid.

A deficiency of the enzyme hexosaminidase A, which normally hydrolyzes the glycosidic bond connecting galactose with N-acetylgalactosamine, is the cause of Tay-Sachs disease, a hereditary disorder. This disrupts the normal breakdown of gangliosides, resulting in their accumulation in the nervous tissues, with subsequent neural disorders.

Metabolism of dietary lipids generates considerable amounts of energy for maintaining life processes. Most of this energy is derived from the oxidation of the fatty acid moieties in the various lipids. All of the classes of lipids discussed contain fatty acids and are, therefore, suppliers of energy. There are two additional classes of compounds that are not energy-producing nutrients. However, they are considered lipids according to the solubility criterion mentioned earlier. Furthermore, they serve important biochemical functions, and therefore warrant mention at this time.

Steroids

Steroids are derivatives of the *cyclopentanoperhydrophenanthrene* nucleus. Its structure is given here, along with the numbering system for its carbon atoms and the lettering of its rings.

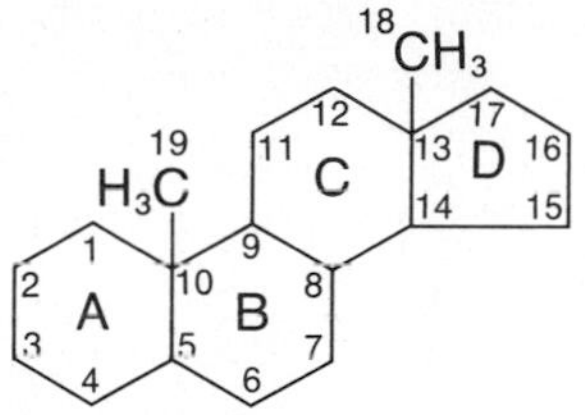

Most of the active steroids have functions or side chains at certain positions on the nucleus. These originate most commonly at carbons 17, 3, and 11. Included among the steroids are sterols, such as cholesterol, bile acids, sex hormones, adrenocortical hormones, cardiac aglycones, and D vitamins. In the body, cholesterol serves as the precursor from which most of the other steroids are formed. Cholesterol can be gotten through the diet or it can be synthesized by nearly all the tissues in the body, but particularly the liver and intestinal mucosa. The structure of this important steroid is shown. Terminating straight lines indicate methyl (CH_3—) groups.

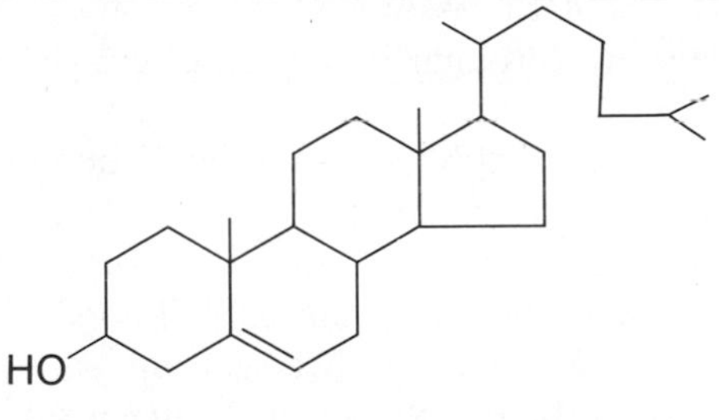

Terpenes

These naturally occurring hydrocarbons or substituted hydrocarbons are constructed from multiples of the five-carbon unit *isoprene* (2-methyl-1,3-butadiene):

$$-CH_2{=}C{-}CH{=}CH_2$$

with CH_3 on the central carbon.

Several of the fat-soluble vitamins, such as vitamins A, K, and E have *isoprenoid* side chains and are therefore classified as terpenes. The structure of vitamin E (α-tocopherol) is given here as an example. The segments of the side chain contributed by isoprene units are indicated parenthetically.

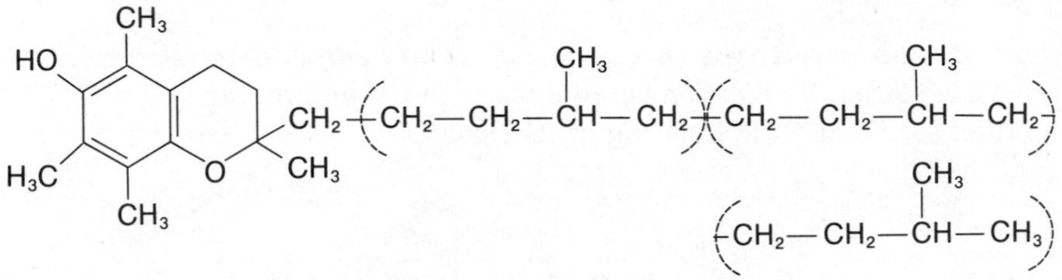

Vitamin E (α-tocopherol)

AMINO ACIDS AND PROTEINS

Proteins occupy a position of primary importance in the maintenance of the living body through a multitude of diverse functions. Among their general biological functions are:

1. Structural integrity, such as connective tissue, musculature, and cell membranes.
2. Transportation of substances such as lipids, certain catabolic products, oxygen, and electrons (e.g., the cytochromes in biological oxidations).
3. Maintenance of osmotic pressure by the plasma proteins.
4. Metabolic regulation, through the action of enzymes and protein hormones.
5. Defense mechanism, through the antibodies found in the gamma globulin fraction of the plasma proteins.

Proteins are biopolymers in which the building block units are amino acids. They are synthesized in the body from amino acids which are derived from the enzymatic hydrolysis of dietary protein. As discussed in Chapter 1, the proper sequencing of amino acids, that is the linear order of the various amino acids within a protein, is under genetic influence, dictated by deoxyribonucleic acid (DNA) and ribonucleic acid (RNA) in cells. The inborn errors of metabolism, discussed in Chapter 9, are attributed to improper sequencing of amino acids in certain enzymes, resulting in diminished or abolished activity of those enzymes.

Amino Acids

All the amino acids have the basic structure of an amino group and a carboxylic acid group connected through an alpha carbon atom as shown:

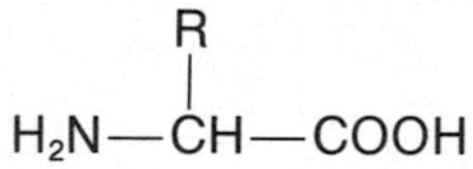

$$\begin{array}{c} R \\ | \\ H_2N-CH-COOH \end{array}$$

It is the side chain group, designated as R in the structure, which differs from one amino acid to the next. The side group may range from simply a hydrogen atom (the amino acid glycine) to bicyclic aromatic groups. Twenty different amino acids occur in proteins. With the exception of glycine, the alpha carbon atom in the amino acids is asymmetric, therefore bestowing optical activity on the molecules. The asymmetry of the alpha carbon means the amino acid can exist in a D or L configuration (see pages 19 and 20). Nearly all amino acids occurring in proteins are of the L configuration, and they are called alpha amino acids because the amino group is joined to the alpha carbon, that is, the one adjacent to the carboxyl group.

In vivo, the pH of the body fluids will cause the amino and carboxyl functions to ionize. Therefore, the amino acid general structure is more correctly written in the *Zwitterion* form shown:

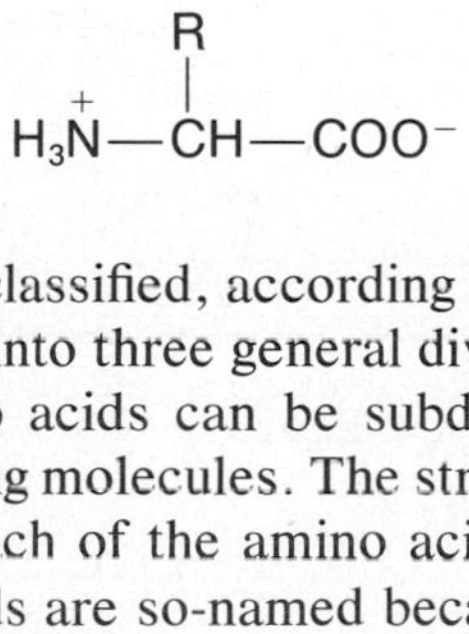

$$\begin{array}{c} R \\ | \\ \overset{+}{H_3N}-CH-COO^- \end{array}$$

Amino acids may be classified, according to the net electrical charge they carry at a pH of 5.5, into three general divisions: neutral, basic, and acidic. The neutral amino acids can be subdivided into aliphatic, aromatic, and sulfur-containing molecules. The structures, names, and three-letter abbreviations for each of the amino acids are given in Table 2.4.

The acidic amino acids are so-named because they contain, in addition to the α carboxyl, a carboxylic acid function in their side chain. As shown in the structures in Table 2.4, this group carries a negative charge (is ionized) at physiological pH. The basic amino acids have basic amino groups in their side chains. These are capable of accepting protons and becoming positively ionized.

The Peptide Bond

A peptide bond is formed when two amino acids are joined by the union of the α-carboxyl of one amino acid with the α-amino group of the second.

Table 2.4 The Amino Acids Common to Proteins

Monoamino Monocarboxylic

Glycine (Gly)

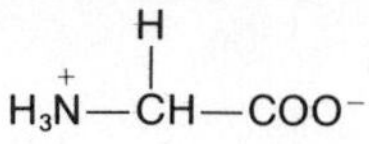

$$\overset{\overset{\displaystyle H}{|}}{\underset{+}{H_3N}}-CH-COO^-$$

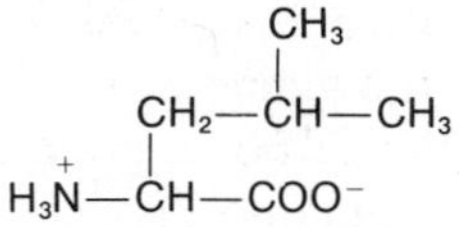

Isoleucine (Ile)

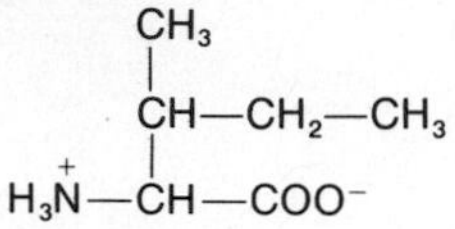

$$\overset{\overset{\displaystyle CH_3}{|}}{\underset{\displaystyle H_3N-CH-COO^-}{CH-CH_2-CH_3}}$$

Alanine (Ala)

$$\overset{\overset{\displaystyle CH_3}{|}}{H_3N}-CH-COO^-$$

Serine (Ser)

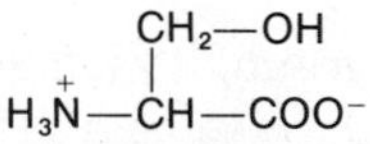

$$\overset{\overset{\displaystyle CH_2-OH}{|}}{H_3N}-CH-COO^-$$

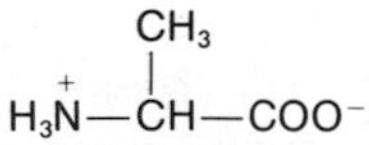

Valine (Val)

$$\overset{\overset{\displaystyle CH_3}{|}}{\underset{\displaystyle H_3N-CH-COO^-}{CH-CH_3}}$$

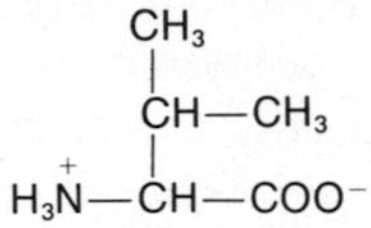

Threonine (Thr)

$$\overset{\overset{\displaystyle CH_3}{|}}{\underset{\displaystyle H_3N-CH-COO^-}{CH-OH}}$$

Leucine (Leu)

$$\overset{\overset{\displaystyle CH_3}{|}}{\underset{\displaystyle H_3N-CH-COO^-}{CH_2-CH-CH_3}}$$

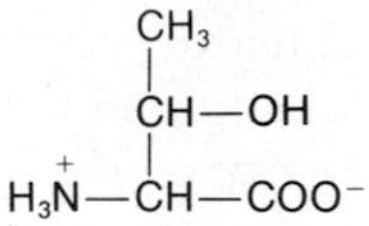

Heterocyclic

Proline (Pro)

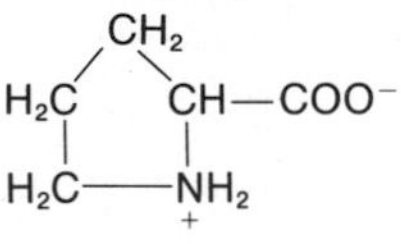

$$\begin{array}{c} CH_2 \\ H_2C \quad CH-COO^- \\ H_2C-NH_2 \end{array}$$

Hydroxyproline (Hyp)

$$\begin{array}{c} CH_2 \\ HO-CH \quad CH-COO^- \\ H_2C-NH_2 \end{array}$$

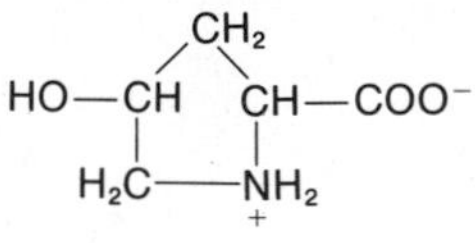

Aromatic

Phenylalanine (Phe)

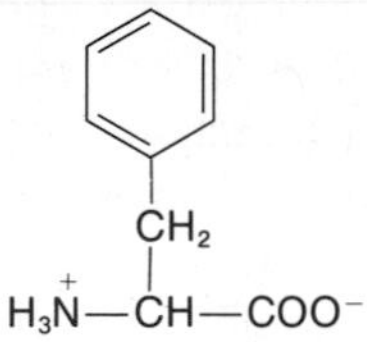

$$\overset{\overset{\displaystyle CH_2}{|}}{H_3N}-CH-COO^-$$

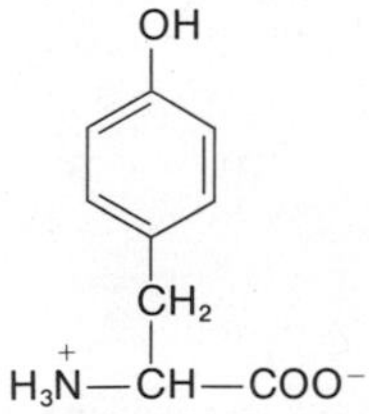

Tryptophan (Trp)

$$\overset{\overset{\displaystyle CH_2}{|}}{H_3N}-CH-COO^-$$

Tyrosine (Tyr)

$$\begin{array}{c} OH \\ CH_2 \\ H_3N-CH-COO^- \end{array}$$

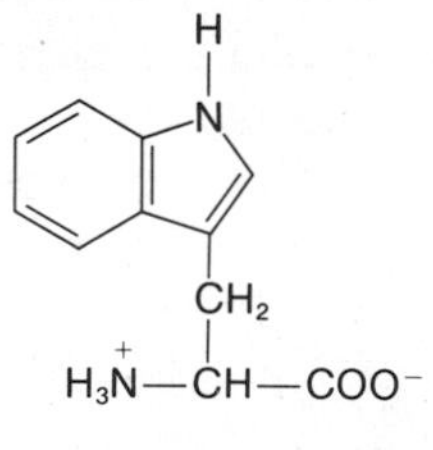

Table 2.4 (*continued*)

Sulfur-containing

Cysteine (Cys)

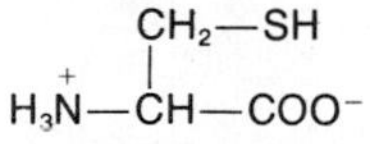

$$CH_2\text{—}SH$$
$$H_3\overset{+}{N}\text{—}CH\text{—}COO^-$$

Methionine (Met)

$$CH_2\text{—}S\text{—}CH_3$$
$$CH_2$$
$$H_3\overset{+}{N}\text{—}CH\text{—}COO^-$$

Cystine (Cysteine dimer)

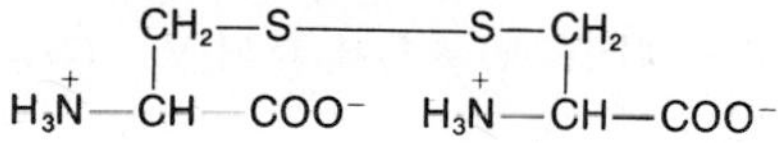

$$CH_2\text{—}S\text{———}S\text{—}CH_2$$
$$H_3\overset{+}{N}\text{—}CH \quad COO^- \quad H_3\overset{+}{N}\text{—}CH\text{—}COO^-$$

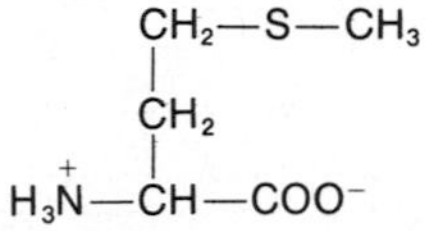

Basic

Lysine (Lys)

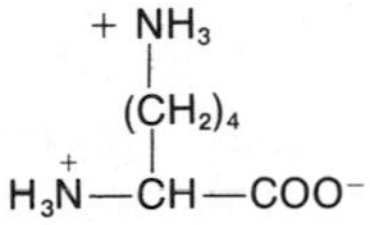

$$+ NH_3$$
$$(CH_2)_4$$
$$H_3\overset{+}{N}\text{—}CH\text{—}COO^-$$

Histidine (His)

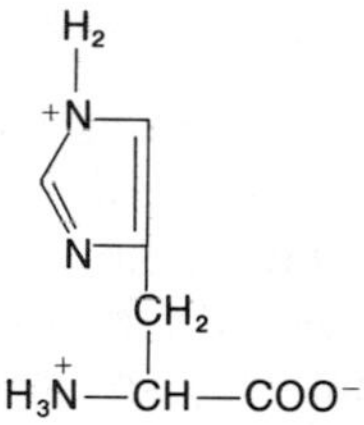

$$H_2$$
$$\overset{+}{N}$$
$$N$$
$$CH_2$$
$$H_3\overset{+}{N}\text{—}CH\text{—}COO^-$$

Arginine (Arg)

$$+ NH_2$$
$$NH\text{—}C\text{—}NH_2$$
$$+ (CH_2)_3$$
$$H_3\overset{+}{N}\text{—}CH\text{—}COO^-$$

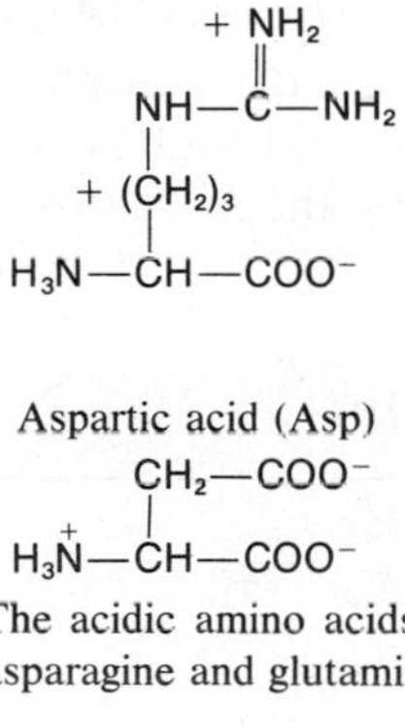

Acidic

Aspartic acid (Asp)

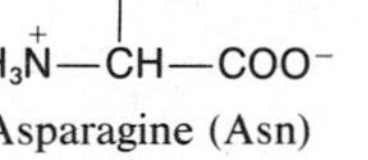

$$CH_2\text{—}COO^-$$
$$H_3\overset{+}{N}\text{—}CH\text{—}COO^-$$

Glutamic acid (Glu)

$$CH_2\text{—}CH_2\text{—}COO^-$$
$$H_3\overset{+}{N}\text{—}CH\text{—}COO^-$$

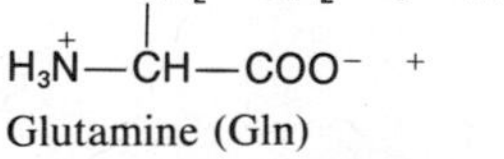

The acidic amino acids frequently occur in proteins as their corresponding acid amides, asparagine and glutamine.

$$O$$
$$\parallel$$
$$CH_2\text{—}C\text{—}NH_2$$
$$H_3\overset{+}{N}\text{—}CH\text{—}COO^-$$

Asparagine (Asn)

$$O$$
$$\parallel$$
$$CH_2\text{—}CH_2\text{—}C\text{—}NH_2$$
$$H_3\overset{+}{N}\text{—}CH\text{—}COO^- \quad +$$

Glutamine (Gln)

The bond is actually an amide bond and is formed through the elimination of the elements of water within the reacting groups.

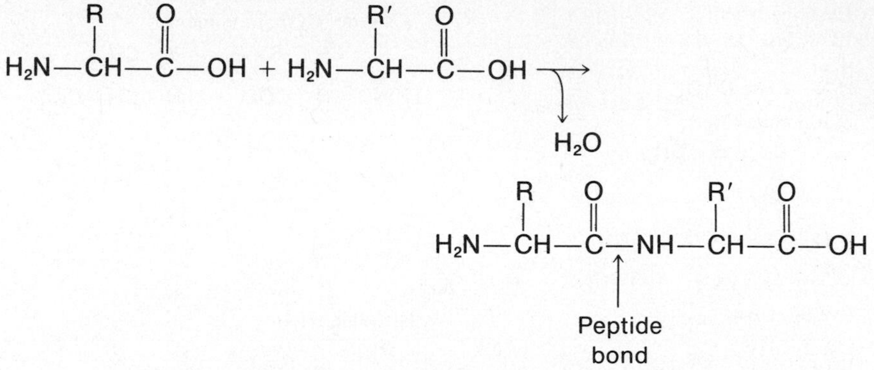

$$
\begin{array}{cc}
R & O \\
| & \| \\
H_2N-CH-C-OH \end{array} + \begin{array}{cc} R' & O \\ | & \| \\ H_2N-CH-C-OH \end{array} \longrightarrow
$$

$$H_2O$$

$$
\begin{array}{cccc}
R & O & R' & O \\
| & \| & | & \| \\
H_2N-CH-C-NH-CH-C-OH \end{array}
$$

Peptide
bond

The resulting structure is called a *dipeptide*. The reaction can be repetitive with a third amino acid, which attaches to the dipeptide through an additional peptide bond forming a tripeptide. In the same fashion, *tetra-*, *penta-*, *hexa-*, peptides can be formed, and in fact the chain of amino acids may elongate into large polypeptides called proteins which may contain from about 50 to several thousand amino acids. The structure of a hypothetical pentapeptide is shown below, along with the name of the structure to illustrate the convention used in naming peptides and polypeptides. The dotted lines indicate the position of the peptide bonds and therefore the division of the five amino acids comprising the structure.

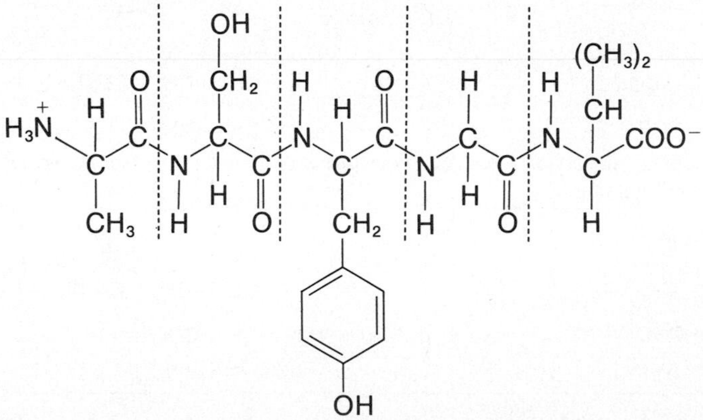

Alanyl-seryl-tyrosyl-glycyl-valine

Proteins

Proteins may be considered as large polypeptides ranging in size from a molecular weight of around 6000 to greater than 1,000,000. The linking together of several hundred amino acids, the number found in an average-sized protein, does not produce a strictly linear biopolymer. Due to chemical interactions among the side chains of the composite amino acids, resulting in forces that may be attractive to repulsive, the chain, in its most stable orientation may be twisted like a coil and folded in a complex, three-dimensional configuration. To describe fully a protein's structure, four aspects must be considered:

Primary structure

Secondary structure

Tertiary structure

Quaternary structure

Briefly, the *primary structure* refers to the sequence of amino acids in the protein. Therefore, if it can be said that the primary structure of a certain protein is known, or established, this means that the precise order or sequence of each of the amino acid residues in the protein has been determined. Until recent years, such a determination was an immense task; however, modern technology and instrumentation have greatly facilitated "sequencing" studies. It should be pointed out that a protein, composed of a single polypeptide chain, has at its one end an amino acid having a free α-amino group. This amino acid is called the *N-terminal amino acid*. At the other end of the chain is the *C-terminal amino acid,* the one possessing the free or unreacted α-carboxyl function.

The *secondary structure* of a protein refers to the orientation of amino acids as viewed along the cross section of a segment of the protein. Although there are certain structural constraints in a protein due to a lack of free rotation around the peptide bonds, portions of a protein chain commonly assume a twisted or helical configuration called an *α-helix*. In some proteins such as keratin (hair protein) and silk fibroin, studies have shown that the planes in which the amide (peptide) bonds lie form alternating angles with each other, resulting in a pattern of "pleats." For this reason, this type of secondary structure is called the *pleated sheet structure* or a *β-configuration*. The forces that stabilize the secondary structure are primarily hydrogen bonds between the amide nitrogen of one peptide bond and the carbonyl oxygen of another. Those proteins or portions of proteins that are not in a helical or a pleated pattern are said to have a *random* configuration.

The *tertiary structure* refers to the folding of the peptide chain in space, that is, its three-dimensional conformation. All proteins exhibit this folding which occurs so that the ionic and polar amino acids project from the outer surface of the structure, while the hydrophobic or nonpolar residues are turned inward toward the core of the molecule. This arrangement enhances the water solubility of the protein. The tertiary structure is stabilized by such forces as hydrogen bonds, ionic interactions, hydrophobic attractions among nonpolar amino acid residues, and van der

Waals interactions. Individually, these bonds or interactions are not strong, but there are a great number of them, and collectively they are able to maintain a specific conformation of the protein. The forces that stabilize the tertiary structure can be disrupted, however, by such factors as heat, pH extremes of the protein solution, perturbation by organic solvents, or even mechanical agitation such as vigorous shaking of the solution. As the interactions weaken, the protein tends to unfold, usually with a partial or a total loss of biological activity. When this occurs, the protein is said to be *denatured,* and in many cases of extensive denaturation, the protein actually aggregates and precipitates from solution. The congealing of egg white in a hot skillet is a classic example of heat denaturation of a protein, in this case, albumin. A *native* protein, on the other hand, is one whose structural integrity and biological activity are unaltered. In addition to these noncovalent bonds, the tertiary structure may also be stabilized by covalent, disulfide bonds made possible by the amino acid cystine. The structure of cystine is such that it contains two sets of α-amino and α-carboxyl functions, meaning that it can form peptide bonds at two different sites along a single polypeptide chain or at sites on different chains. In either case the sites are united through the disulfide bond of the amino acid. If the disulfide bond involves different polypeptide chains, it is called an *interchain disulfide bond*. If the connection is between "half cystines" within the same chain, it is called an *intrachain disulfide bond*. It is shown below how cystine, enclosed within the dotted frame, can be involved in intra- and interchain attachments:

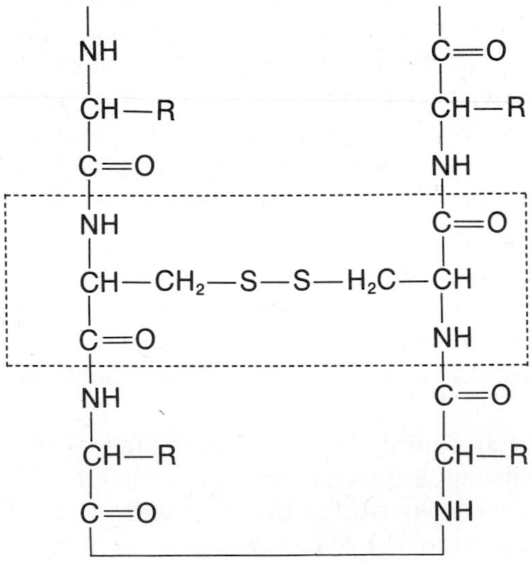

Single
polypeptide
chain

Intrachain disulfide bond

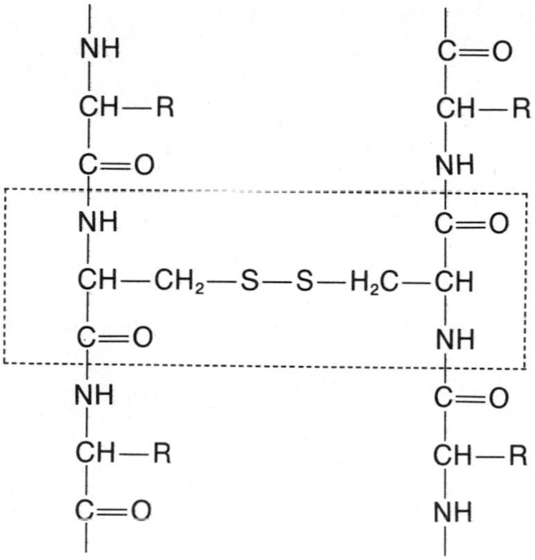

$$
\begin{array}{ll}
\text{NH} & \text{C=O} \\
\text{CH—R} & \text{CH—R} \\
\text{C=O} & \text{NH} \\
\text{NH} & \text{C=O} \\
\text{CH—CH}_2\text{—S—S—H}_2\text{C—CH} \\
\text{C=O} & \text{NH} \\
\text{NH} & \text{C=O} \\
\text{CH—R} & \text{CH—R} \\
\text{C=O} & \text{NH}
\end{array}
$$

Different
polypeptide
chains

Interchain disulfide bond

The *quaternary structure* describes the grouping or aggregation of subunit polypeptide chains in forming a "total" protein. An example of a protein having a quaternary structure is hemoglobin, the oxygen-transporting protein in red blood cells. It consists of four subunit polypeptides (two alpha chains and two beta chains) each having a molecular weight of 16,500. The subunit chains in a protein having a quaternary structure are not covalently attached, and they are freely dissociable by changes in pH and/or ionic strength. When chains are linked through disulfide bonds, the total structure is a single molecule and therefore does not possess a quaternary structure.

To students of nutrition, the most interesting aspect of protein structure is the *amino acid composition* of the proteins. Among the amino acids listed in Table 2.4, some are *essential*, meaning that they must be acquired through the diet. Others are *nonessential* which indicates that they can be synthesized biochemically from other amino acids or precursors other than amino acids. The source of essential amino acids is dietary protein, and the nutritional value of a protein is measured by the number of different essential amino acids and the amount of each incorporated into its structure. The amino acid composition describes the number of each type of amino acid residue found in the protein.

Conjugated Proteins

As they occur in nature, proteins are commonly associated with nonprotein moieties. Such proteins are called *conjugated proteins* to distinguish

Table 2.5 Examples of Conjugated Proteins

Proteins	Prosthetic group	Examples
Nucleoproteins	Nucleic acids	Nuclei in cells Viruses
Glycoproteins	Carbohydrates	Connective tissue Vitreous humor Mucus
Lipoproteins	Lipids	Serum lipoproteins Egg yolk proteins
Phosphoproteins	Phosphate ester	Casein of milk Vitellin of eggs
Chromoproteins	Iron, porphyrin	Hemoglobin Cytochromes
Metalloproteins	Copper, zinc, iron	Plasma proteins: transferrin, ceruloplasmin, carbonic anhydrase

them from *simple proteins* which are comprised entirely of amino acids. The nonprotein portion of the conjugated proteins are called prosthetic groups. Table 2.5 lists some common conjugated proteins along with their prosthetic groups.

NUCLEOTIDES AND NUCLEIC ACIDS

The nucleic acids, ribonucleic acid (RNA) and deoxyribonucleic acid (DNA), are of extreme interest because of their involvement in cell replication, transfer of genetic information, and protein biosynthesis. They are of considerably less importance in the diet because the body's need for them is satisfied by the biosysthesis from simple precursors. Nucleic acids, however, do occur in many of the foods in the average diet, and are particularly abundant in organ meats.

Nucleotides

Nucleotides consist of three parts, a heterocyclic nitrogenous "base," ribose or deoxyribose, and one or more phosphate groups. The nucleotides that will be discussed in this section are restricted to those comprising the nucleic acids, RNA and DNA. The nitrogenous base is an analog of either purine or pyrimidine:

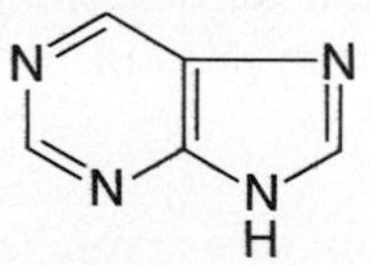

Purine 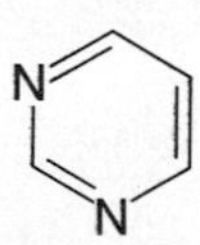   Pyrimidine

A given nucleotide may be formed from either of two purine-type bases or any of three pyrimidine bases:

Purine

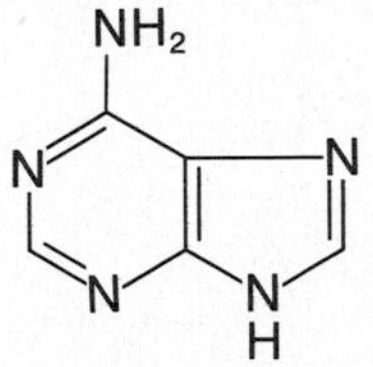

Adenine

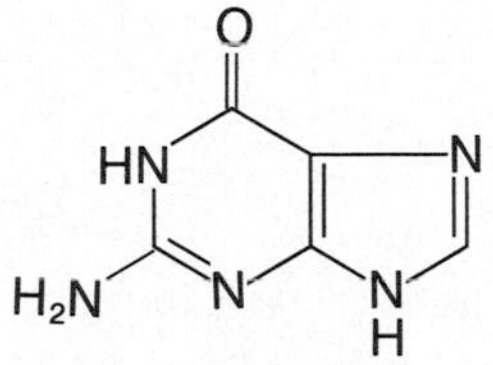

Guanine

Pyrimidine

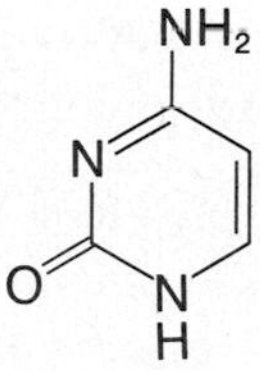

Cytosine 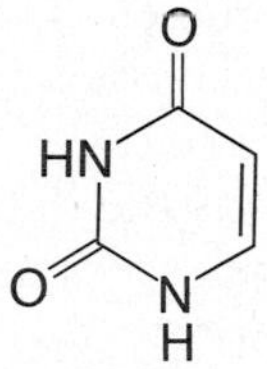   Uracil 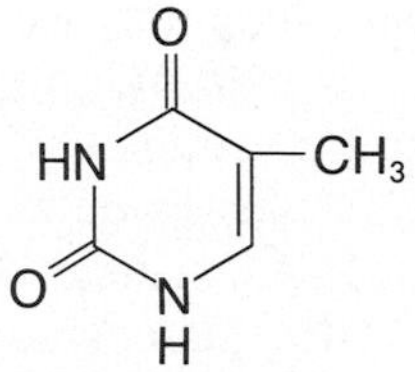   Thymine

A pentose sugar (ribose or deoxyribose) is connected to the nitrogenous base through an N-glycosidic bond between carbon-1 of the sugar and the heterocyclic nitrogen of the base as shown. The phosphate is attached as an ester of phosphoric acid to the 5′ carbon of the pentose (the carbons of the pentose are assigned prime numbers to distinguish them from the carbons of the nitrogenous base).

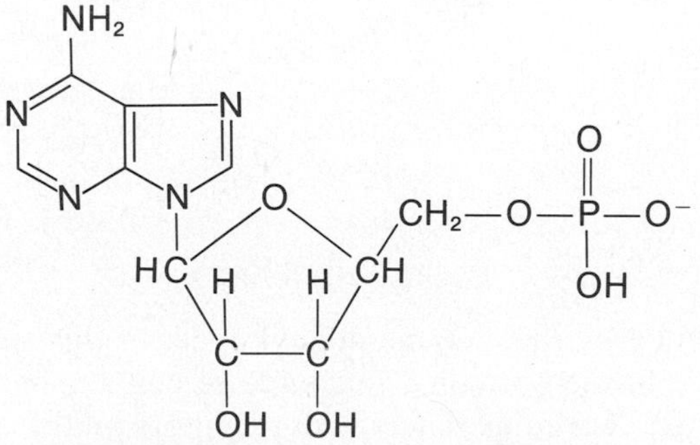

Adenosine 5′ monophosphate
(an example of a purine nucleotide)

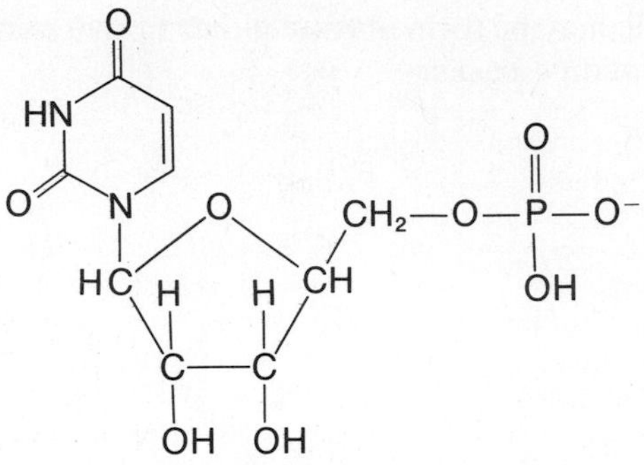

Cytidine 5' monophosphate
(an example of a pyrimidine nucleotide)

A nucleotide without the phosphate is termed a nucleoside. Nucleosides and their corresponding nucleotides having a single phosphate group at carbon 5' have specific names, derived from the particular nitrogenous base from which they were constructed. Table 2.6 presents a listing of the nitrogenous bases along with the names of their corresponding nucleosides and nucleotides.

The nucleotides listed also exist as the di- and triphosphate derivatives, and nucleotides such as adenosine triphosphate (ATP), adenosine diphosphate (ADP), guanosine triphosphate (GTP), and uridine triphosphate (UTP) and diphosphate (UDP) are extremely important mediators in both the conversion of nutrients into energy and in many biosynthetic pathways in metabolism. A particularly exciting adenine nucleotide is adenosine-3',5'-monophosphate, or cyclic AMP (cAMP).

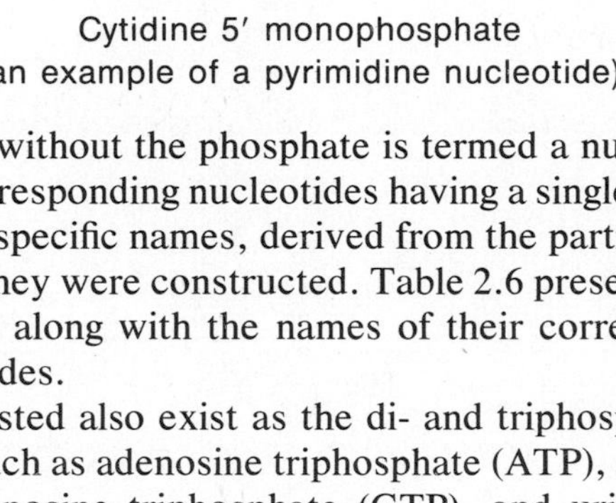

Cyclic AMP (cAMP)

Formed from ATP by the enzyme adenyl cyclase, this substance acts as an intermediary in the hormonal influence of cellular metabolism. More specifically, after a hormone reacts with receptors on the cells of its target tissue, adenyl cyclase is stimulated to generate more intracellular cAMP

Table 2.6 Nomenclature for the Nucleosides and 5′ Phosphate Nucleotides of Purines and Pyrimidines

Nitrogenous base	Nucleoside	Nucleotide
Purines		
Adenine	Adenosine	Adenosine monophosphate (AMP) or adenylic acid
Guanine	Guanosine	Guanosine monophosphate (GMP) or guanylic acid
Pyrimidines		
Cytosine	Cytidine	Cytidine monophosphate (CMP) or cytidylic acid
Uracil	Uridine	Uridine monophosphate (UMP) or uridylic acid
Thymine	Thymidine	Thymidine monophosphate (TMP) or thymidylic acid

which in turn creates the metabolic change dictated by the hormone. For this reason, cAMP has been described as a *second messenger*. Some of the hormones that act through this mechanism include the catecholamines (epinephrine and norepinephrine), glucagon, vasopressin, luteinizing hormone, prostaglandins, and parathyroid hormone.

Nucleic Acids

These molecules are extremely large with molecular weights in the many millions. They are polymers of purine and pyrimidine nucleotides which are connected through phosphate diesters between the 5′ carbon of one nucleotide and the 3′ carbon of the next, as illustrated in Figure 2.3. The nucleotides in the illustration are named according to the purine or pyrimidine from which they were derived rather than the specific nucleotide.

Nucleic acids may exist as two types, DNA (deoxyribonucleic acid) and RNA (ribonucleic acid), and there are two important chemical distinctions between the two. The pentose sugar portion of DNA nucleotides is always deoxyribose, in which the —OH group at position 2′ has been replaced by a hydrogen atom. Also, DNA contains thymine nucleotides but not uracil nucleotides.

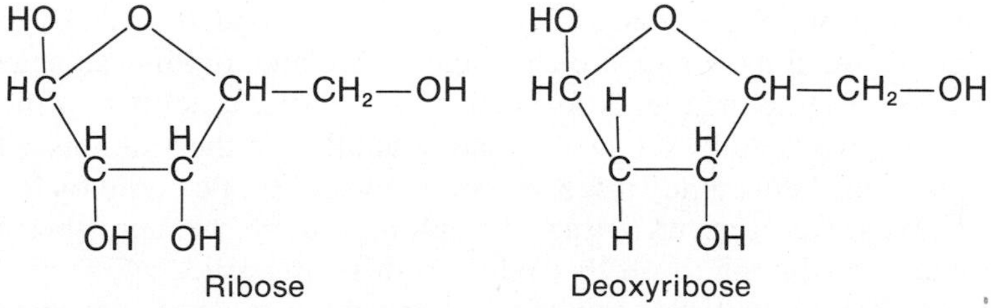

Ribose   Deoxyribose

The nucleotides of RNA, on the other hand, have ribose in their structure rather than deoxyribose, and RNA has uracil nucleotides but not thymine nucleotides.

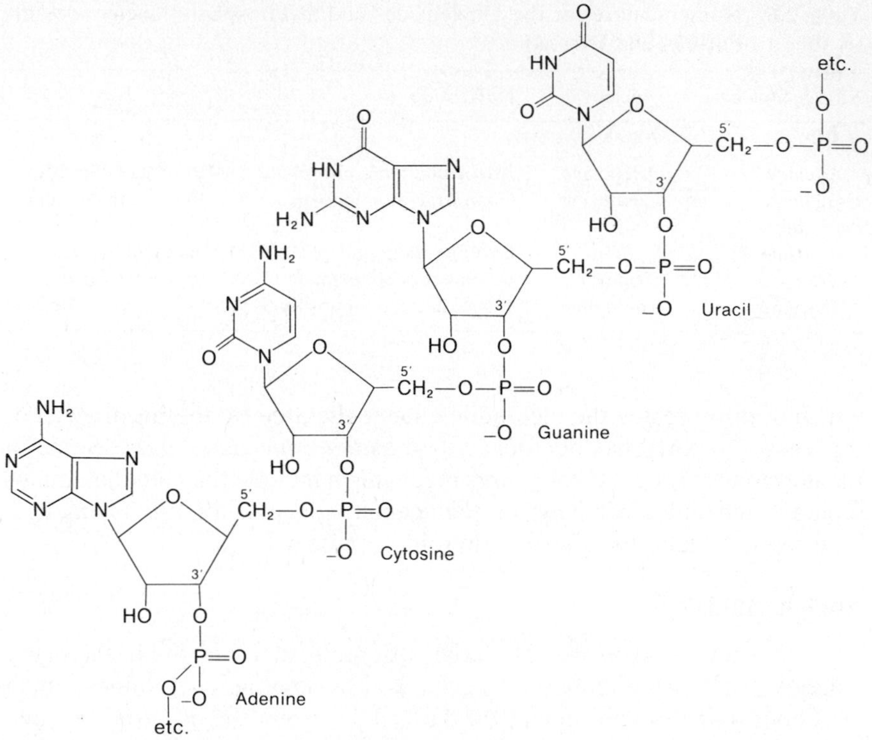

Figure 2.3 A small, four-nucleotide segment of RNA.

VITAMINS

The nutrients discussed up to this point, the carbohydrates, fats, and proteins, serve as sources of energy. Vitamins are not sources of energy, per se, but some of the vitamins (e.g., thiamine, riboflavin, niacin, pantothenic acid) are necessary for the release of energy from carbohydrate, fat, and/or protein (see discussion on glycolysis and the Krebs cycle, Chapter 3). Vitamins, which are chemically unrelated organic substances, are required in trace amounts for specific metabolic reactions in the cell and must be provided by the diet. If one or another of the vitamins is lacking, a nutritional deficiency disease results, which can be cured by feeding the missing trace nutrient. Diseases such as scurvy, pellagra, beri-beri, and rickets are among those that fall into this category.

Coincident with the recognition of the vitamin deficiency diseases was the discovery that certain vitamins were required for the biosynthesis of certain coenzymes of which they are a component. Today it is known that most of the vitamins, in particular the water-soluble ones, function in this manner.

Vitamins are divided into two classes, *water-soluble* and *fat-soluble*. A discussion of the structure, function, and corresponding coenzyme (if known) of the major vitamins follows.

The Water-soluble Vitamins

Thiamine (Vitamin B₁)

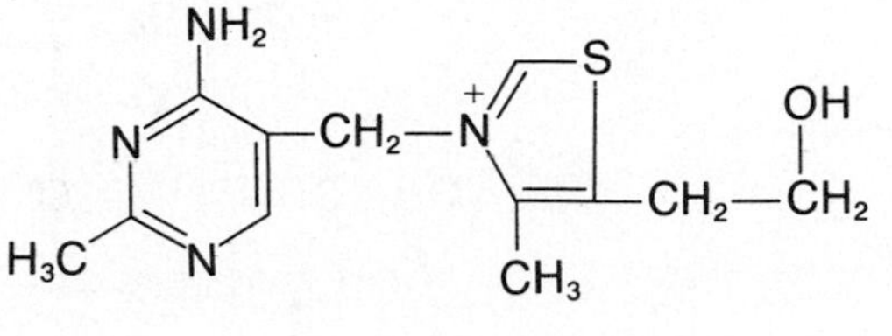

Thiamine Pyrophosphate

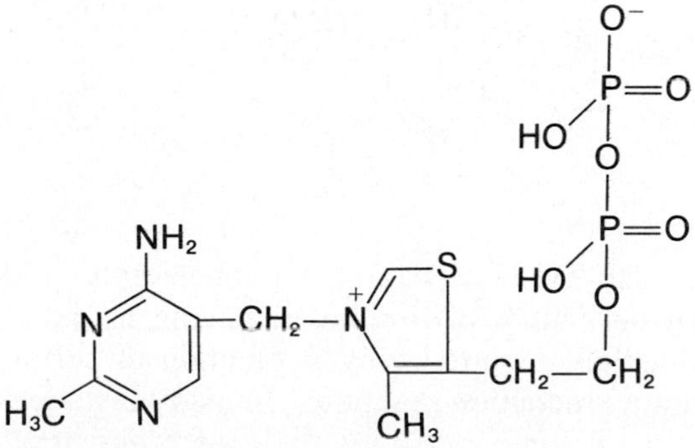

A deficiency of thiamine in the diet of man is the cause of the disease beri-beri. Dietary thiamine is phosphorylated in the body to form its active coenzyme derivative, *thiamine pyrophosphate* (abbreviated TPP), also called *cocarboxylase*.

The primary function of thiamine pyrophosphate and its enzymes in metabolism is the oxidative decarboxylation of substrates. This involves removal of carboxyl groups as carbon dioxide coupled with oxidation of the decarboxylated substrate (see decarboxylation of pyruvate to acetyl-CoA in Krebs cycle, chapter 3).

Riboflavin (Vitamin B₂)

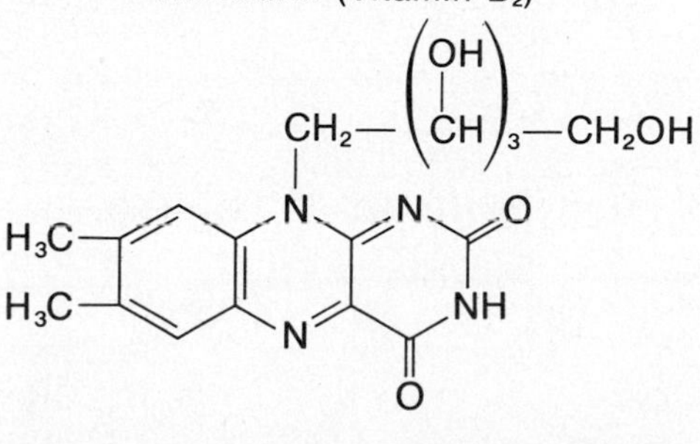

Flavin Adenine Dinucleotide (FAD)

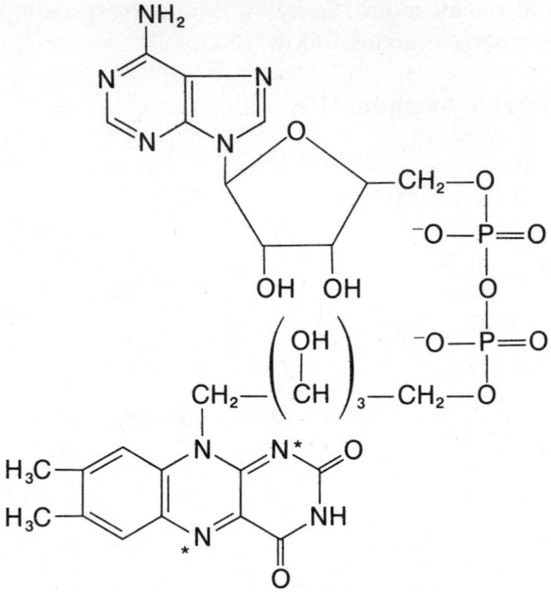

The coenzyme also exists as flavin mononucleotide (FMN), the mono-phosphorylated derivative of riboflavin, having no adenine nucleotide. These coenzymes are required for the function of certain enzymes that catalyze oxidation–reduction reactions. In many instances, the oxidation of a substrate by a flavin enzyme involves the removal of two hydrogens from the substrate. The hydrogens are transferred enzymatically to FAD or FMN, reducing the coenzymes to the hydrogenated forms: $FADH_2$ and $FMNH_2$. The sites at which the hydrogens bind on the coenzymes are at the nitrogen atoms marked by an asterisk in the structure above.

Nicotinic Acid

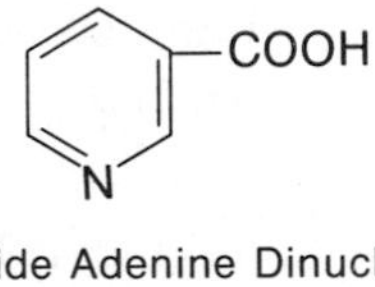

Nicotinamide Adenine Dinucleotide (NAD)

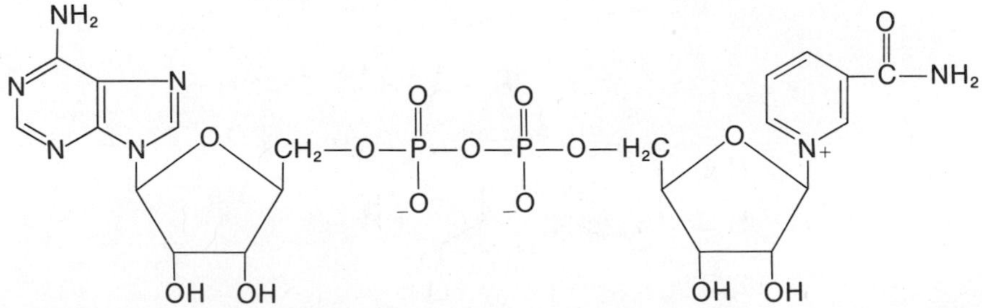

Both nicotinic acid and its amide, nicotinamide, are active in preventing the disease pellagra and a condition known as black tongue in dogs. Nicotinic acid is commonly referred to as *niacin*. Niacin can be formed from the amino acid tryptophan. In fact, it has been known for over 50 years that the symptoms of pellagra could be successfully treated with tryptophan. Although the amino acid does have a sparing effect on the vitamin, the rate of niacin synthesis from tryptophan in a normal diet is inadequate to supply the amount of the vitamin needed.

Like the flavin coenzymes, NAD and its phosphorylated derivative, nicotinamide adenine dinucleotide phosphate (NADP), are active in dehydrogenation reactions. These coenzymes also receive hydrogens transferred from a substrate undergoing oxidation. One of the two hydrogens removed from the substrate is added to the nicotinamide ring while the other is released as a proton. A substrate oxidation (dehydrogenation) by NAD is represented below. Only the nicotinamide portion of the coenzyme is shown:

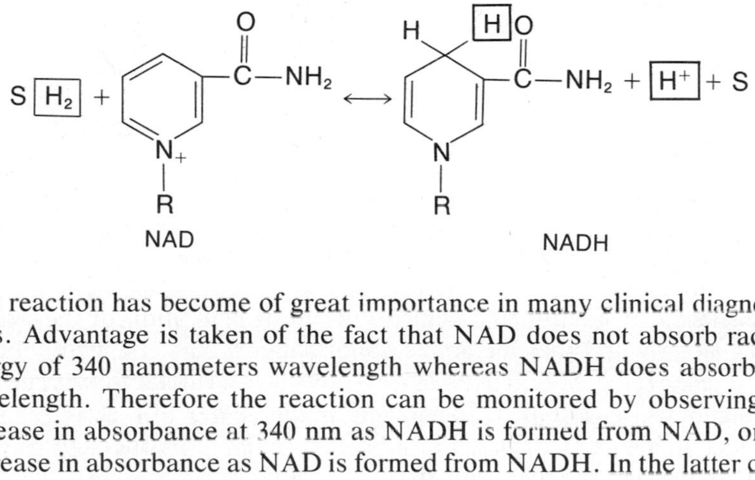

This reaction has become of great importance in many clinical diagnostic tests. Advantage is taken of the fact that NAD does not absorb radiant energy of 340 nanometers wavelength whereas NADH does absorb this wavelength. Therefore the reaction can be monitored by observing the increase in absorbance at 340 nm as NADH is formed from NAD, or the decrease in absorbance as NAD is formed from NADH. In the latter case, a substrate is being reduced:

$$S + NADH + H^+ \rightarrow SH_2 + NAD$$

The clinical application of the reaction will be discussed further in Chapter 14. Examples of oxidation–reduction reactions involving both NAD and FAD can be found in Chapter 3.

Pantothenic Acid

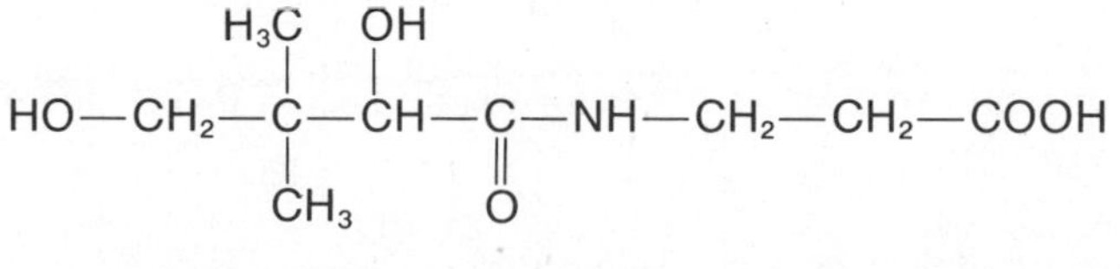

Coenzyme A

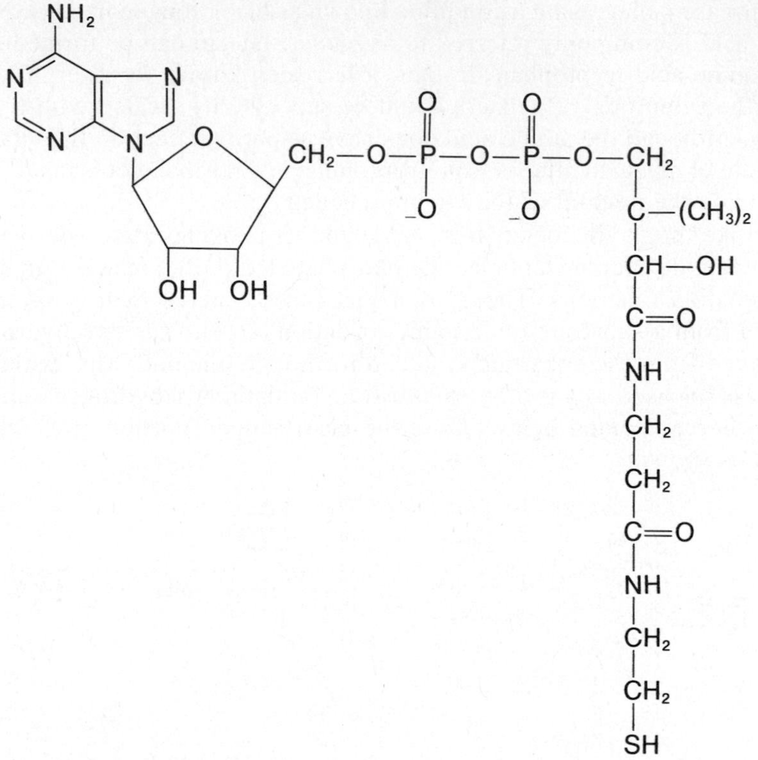

A deficiency of pantothenic acid results in degeneration of the adrenal cortex along with other metabolic abnormalities. The coenzyme formed from it, coenzyme A, functions in metabolism as a carrier for acyl groups. The sulfhydryl group of the coenzyme is the center of reactivity in this function. It becomes acylated and later deacylated as the acyl group is transferred from donor to acceptor molecule.

Pyridoxal (Vitamin B$_6$)

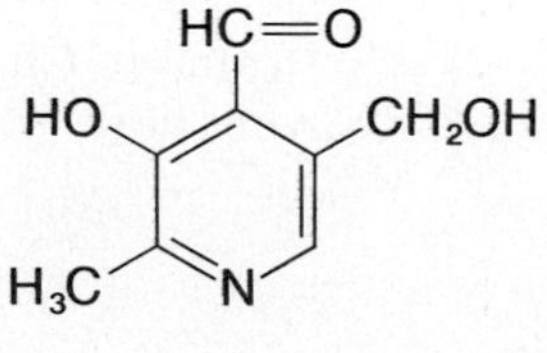

Pyridoxal Phosphate

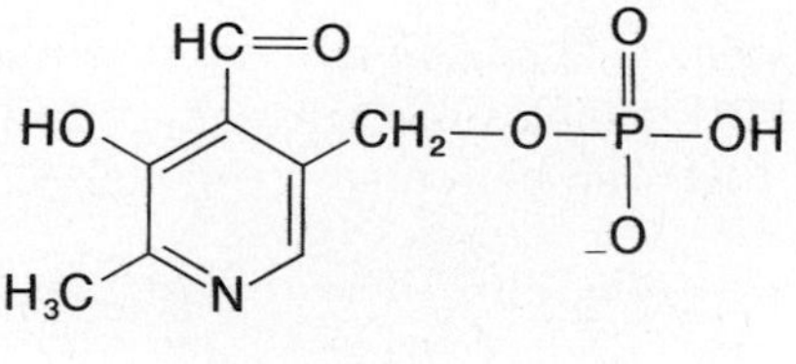

In addition to pyridoxal, other forms of vitamin B$_6$ include *pyridoxine* and *pyridoxamine*.

Pyridoxine

CH$_2$OH

HO

CH$_2$OH

H$_3$C   N

Pyridoxamine

CH$_2$—NH$_2$

HO

CH$_2$OH

H$_3$C   N

The corresponding coenzymes, pyridoxal, pyridoxine, and pyridoxamine phosphates are active in different types of reactions. Primarily, however, they participate in reactions catalyzed by enzymes called *transaminases* or *aminotransferases,* in which an amino group is transferred between molecules. The coenzyme serves as the carrier of the group in this transfer process.

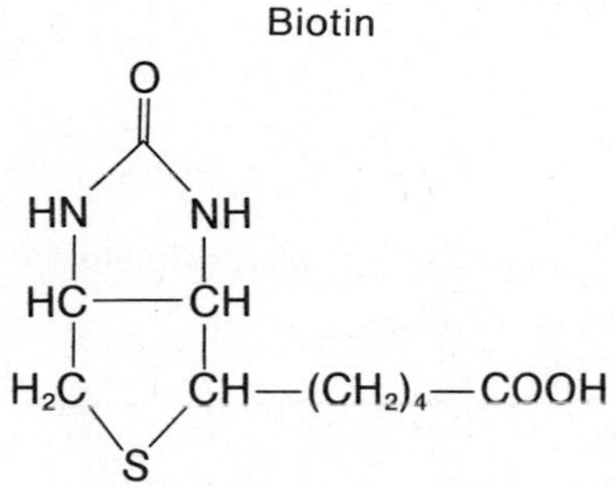

Biotin

O

HN   NH

HC——CH

H$_2$C   CH—(CH$_2$)$_4$—COOH

S

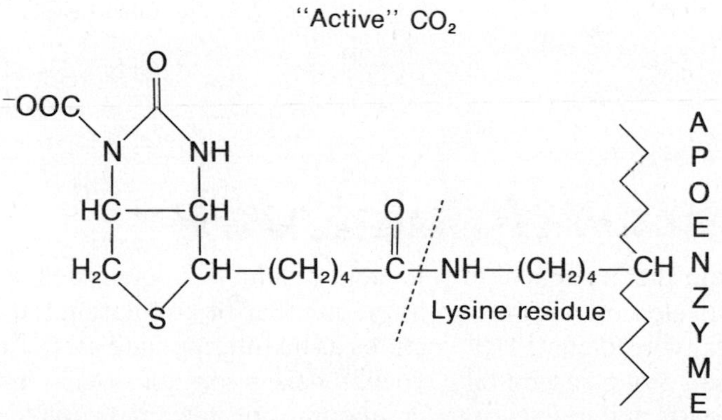

"Active" CO$_2$

$^-$OOC

O

N   NH

HC——CH

H$_2$C   CH—(CH$_2$)$_4$—C—NH—(CH$_2$)$_4$—CH

S

Lysine residue

A
P
O
E
N
Z
Y
M
E

A biotin deficiency can be induced by the feeding of large amounts of raw egg white. This is due to the presence in egg white of *avidin,* a substance that can bind biotin tightly and prevent its utilization. The biochemically active form of biotin is the N-carboxy derivative which becomes linked to a specific enzyme through a lysine residue in the enzyme as shown. The major function of the coenzyme is to serve as a carboxyl group donor in so-called carboxylation reactions.

Folic Acid

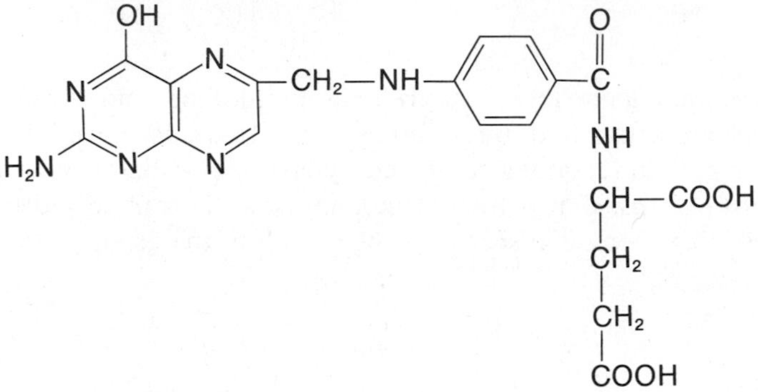

Methylenetetrahydrofolate

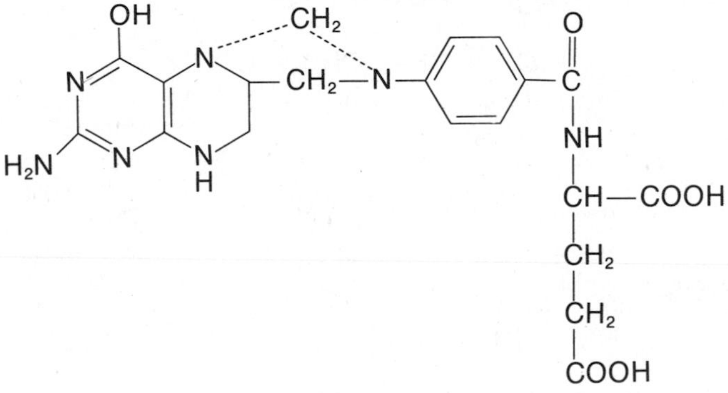

Insufficient dietary intake of folic acid results in a folate-deficiency anemia manifested by a reduction in the number of circulating red cells.

Tetrahydrofolate (FH_4) functions as an intermediate carrier of certain one-carbon groups used in the biosynthesis of various compounds. There are three related one-carbon compounds of tetrahydrofolate—formyl FH_4, methenyl FH_4, and methylene FH_4, each of which can donate its single carbon atom. The active carbon of methylenetetrahydrofolate is bonded to two nitrogen atoms as shown in the structure. Among the important synthetic functions of methylene FH_4 is the synthesis of purines, components of the nucleic acids, DNA and RNA.

Cyanocobalamin (Vitamin B$_{12}$)   Deoxyadenosylcobalamin

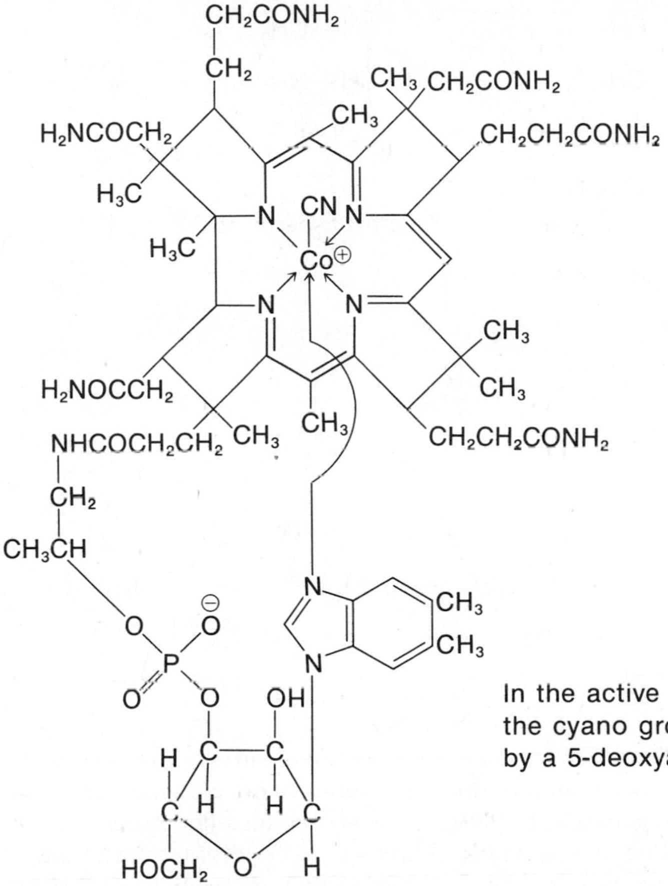

In the active B$_{12}$ coenzyme, the cyano group is replaced by a 5-deoxyadenosine moiety.

Vitamin B$_{12}$ is found in foods of animal origin, but little, if any, is found in plants. Therefore, in a strictly vegetarian diet, it becomes important to supplement the intake of this vitamin. Deficiency of vitamin B$_{12}$ results in anemic symptoms similar to that of folate deficiency. *Pernicious anemia* is a vitamin B$_{12}$ deficiency disease caused by the lack of a protein called *intrinsic factor* that is normally synthesized in the gastric mucosa. Intrinsic factor complexes with vitamin B$_{12}$, a reaction that is necessary for the intestinal absorption of the vitamin.

The coenzyme form is involved in fascinating reactions that cause rearrangements within a substrate molecule. Such rearrangements result from the transfer of a group from one carbon atom to another within a single molecule. An example of such a reaction is the methylaspartate mutase reaction:

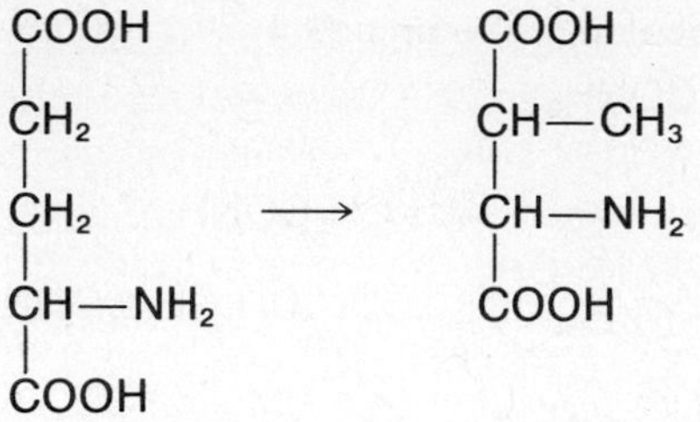

$$
\begin{array}{ccc}
\text{COOH} & & \text{COOH} \\
| & & | \\
\text{CH}_2 & & \text{CH—CH}_3 \\
| & & | \\
\text{CH}_2 & \longrightarrow & \text{CH—NH}_2 \\
| & & | \\
\text{CH—NH}_2 & & \text{COOH} \\
| & & \\
\text{COOH} & &
\end{array}
$$

Glutamic acid $\qquad$ β-methyl aspartic acid

Lipoic Acid

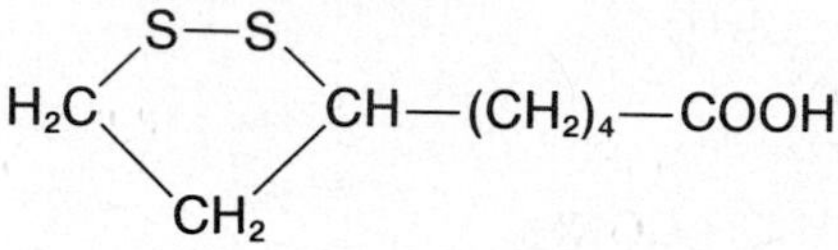

$$
\text{H}_2\text{C} \overset{\displaystyle \text{S—S}}{\underset{\displaystyle \text{CH}_2}{\diagdown \diagup}} \text{CH—(CH}_2)_4\text{—COOH}
$$

Lipoamide

$$
\text{H}_2\text{C} \overset{\displaystyle \text{S—S}}{\underset{\displaystyle \text{CH}_2}{\diagdown \diagup}} \text{CH—(CH}_2)_4\text{—}\overset{\displaystyle \text{O}}{\overset{\displaystyle \|}{\text{C}}}\text{—NH—(CH}_2)_4\text{—CH}
$$

Lysine residue

A P O E N Z Y M E

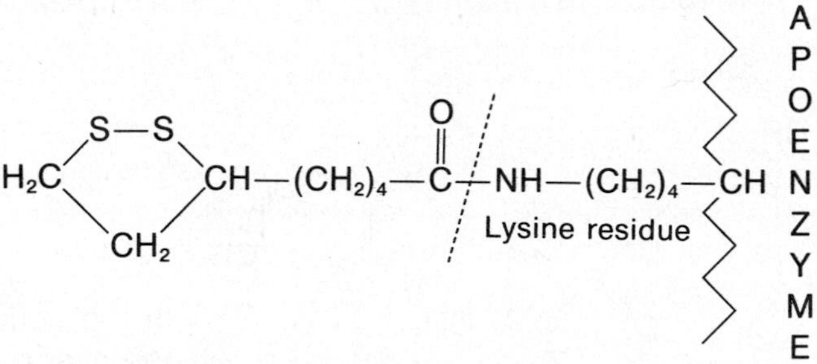

In its coenzyme form, lipoic acid is attached covalently to a specific lysine residue in the apoenzyme. It functions along with enzymes called α-keto acid dehydrogenases. In these reactions the disulfide bond acquires hydrogen atoms becoming reduced to two sulfhydryl groups, one of which in turn serves as carrier of acyl groups that are being transferred to coenzyme A.

Ascorbic Acid (Vitamin C)

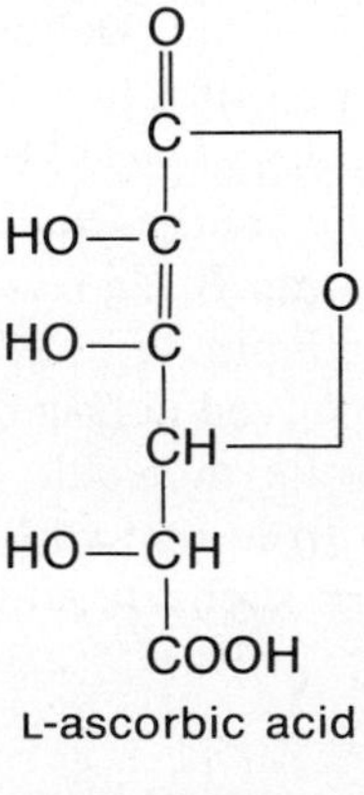

$$
\begin{array}{c}
\text{O} \\
\| \\
\text{C} \!-\!\!\!\!\!\!\!\!\!\!\!\!\rceil \\
\text{HO—C} | \\
\| \text{O} \\
\text{HO—C} | \\
\text{CH}\!-\!\!\!\!\!\!\!\!\!\rfloor \\
| \\
\text{HO—CH} \\
| \\
\text{COOH}
\end{array}
$$

L-ascorbic acid

A deficiency of vitamin C is associated with the disease *scurvy*. It has not yet been established if a coenzyme form of vitamin C exists. However, the vitamin is known to participate in various biochemical systems, such as the biosynthesis of collagen, the structural protein of connective tissue. It also appears that the vitamin is necessary for certain hydroxylation reactions such as the formation of hydroxyproline from proline and the formation of 5-hydroxytryptophan from the amino acid tryptophan. Ascorbic acid is known to be a reducing agent, although it is not clear if this property has any physiological significance. Iron metabolism and transport, however, requires reversible oxidation and reduction of the mineral, and ascorbic acid has been shown to be specific in this reducing function.

Fat-soluble Vitamins

This group of vitamins, which are classified as lipids because of their insolubility in water and solubility in organic solvents, include vitamins A, D, E, and K. They share the common denominator of having been ultimately constructed from isoprenoid building blocks.

The function of the fat-soluble vitamins in animal tissues is fairly well understood. Unlike the water-soluble vitamins, there is no evidence that they function as coenzymes. Their structure and physiological roles will be presented.

Vitamin A (Retinol)

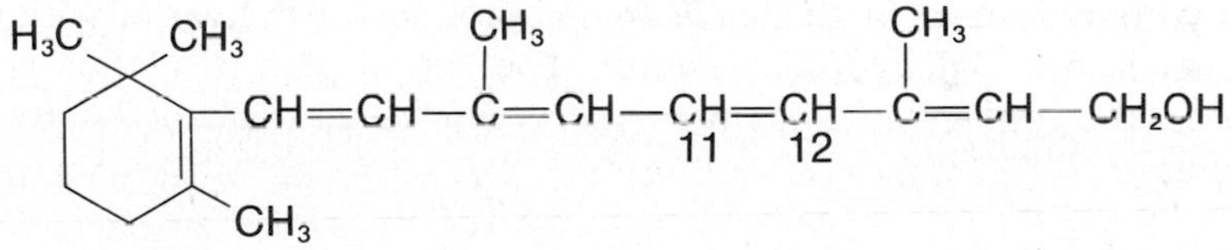

The unsaturated isoprenoid side chain can exist in all *trans* form or as the 11-cis isomer. The vitamin occurs as such in liver, with fish liver oils being particularly rich in vitamin A. Precursors of vitamin A are found in plants in the form of *carotenes*. The substance β-carotene gives rise to vitamin A because it is oxidatively cleaved at a centrally located double bond to yield two molecules of retinal, an aldehyde, which is subsequently reduced to the alcohol (retinol).

Deficiency of vitamin A is most commonly associated with night blindness in humans, although skin lesions, disturbances in bone formation, and abnormal adrenal cortex function are additional consequences. In general, the vitamin is required for the maintenance of normal epithelial tissue, but its precise mode of action is not well understood. Unlike water-soluble vitamins, of which excesses are readily excreted in the urine, vitamin A can accumulate to toxic levels in the wake of excessive intake. The condition of *hypervitaminosis* can produce lethargy, headache, abdominal pain, and other symptoms.

Vitamin D

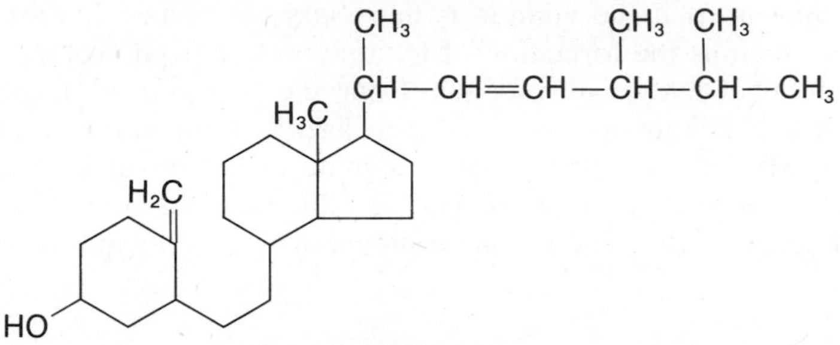

Calciferol

Vitamin D actually consists of a group of closely related steroids, the most important being *calciferol,* shown above, and *cholecalciferol.* Vitamin D deficiency in childhood results in a disease known as *rickets* in which the growing portion of the bones is affected.

Although calciferol and cholecalciferol are the active forms of the vitamin, they are derived from the precursor substances, *ergosterol* and *7-dehydrocholesterol,* respectively, through photooxidation by ultraviolet light. The beneficial effects of sunlight in the prevention of rickets is, therefore, explainable biochemically. Ergosterol is a plant steroid while 7-dehydrocholesterol originates in animal products; fish liver oils are particularly rich in 7-dehydrocholesterol. The site of photooxidation is the same for the conversion of the precursors. For the example of 7-dehydrocholesterol:

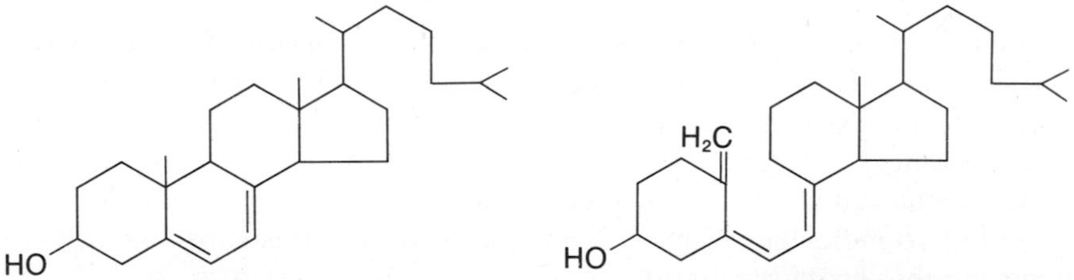

7-dehydrocholesterol   cholecalciferol

The effect of the light is to cleave a carbon–carbon bond in the second ring of the nucleus resulting in the opening of the ring. Vitamin D enhances the absorption of dietary calcium into the intestinal mucosal cells, therefore accounting for its importance in normal bone growth. The proposed mechanism of this action is that a metabolite of cholecalciferol, possibly 1,25-dihydroxycholecalciferol, induces the synthesis of the transport protein for calcium ions in the mucosal cells.

Vitamin E

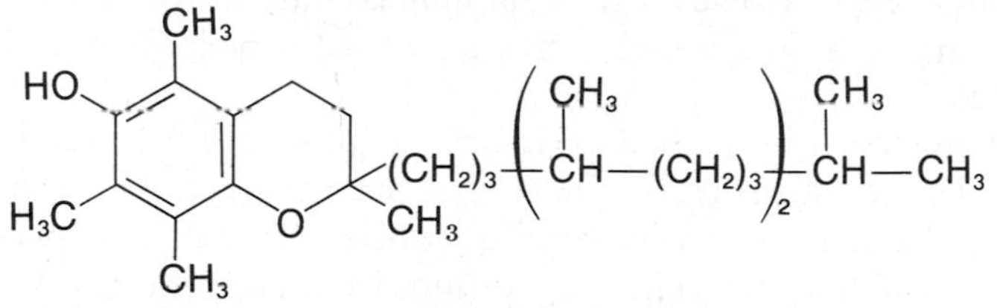

α-tocopherol

The most active form of vitamin E is α-tocopherol, although there also exist β- and γ-tocopherols, which differ from the α-form in the nature of the substituents on the aromatic ring. The biological function of vitamin E is uncertain, although like vitamin C, it has been identified with a list of alleged beneficial effects. Most of these have not been scientifically substantiated. For example, there is no evidence that it displays antisterility properties in humans or that it improves sexual performance. The vitamin does have antioxidant properties, and it is believed to function in part as an inhibitor of the peroxidation of unsaturated lipids in cell membranes.

Vitamin K

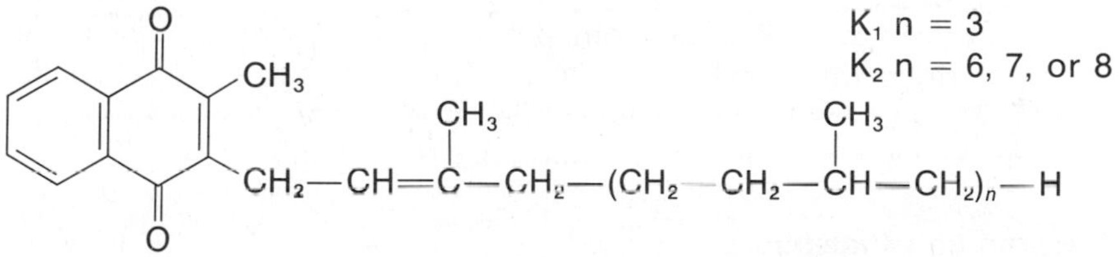

K_1 n = 3
K_2 n = 6, 7, or 8

As the above structure indicates, there are several active forms of vitamin K, the structures of which vary with respect to the number of isoprenoid units in the side chain. Notice the values for n in the K_1 and K_2 forms of the vitamin. Vitamin K is a derivative of *menadione* which is the dicyclic naphthoquinone portion, in which a hydrogen replaces the isoprenoid side chain.

Vitamin K is required for the blood-clotting process and, therefore, its deficiency results in hemorrhagic episodes. One of the major sources for this vitamin is the bacterial flora in the intestine. Extensive antibiotic therapy destroys these bacteria and may result in vitamin K deficiency.

It is important to realize that being fat-soluble, the vitamins so classified are dependent on the presence of bile for their emulsification and eventual absorption. Any liver or biliary tract disease that obstructs the normal flow of bile into the small intestine may in turn produce a fat-soluble vitamin deficiency.

MINERALS

Minerals, like vitamins, are not bulk nutrients in that they are not dietary sources of energy. However, certain minerals are absolutely essential in metabolism and a brief account of some of the principal minerals is warranted here.

Minerals exist in the body primarily as inorganic ions sometimes referred to as the electrolytes. Those that are known to be essential, and that are present in relatively large quantities are calcium, phosphorus, potassium, sodium, chloride, magnesium, iron, and sulfur.

Sodium, Potassium, and Chloride

Collectively, these ions form the bulk of the electrolyte concentration in biological fluids, and therefore are important in maintaining the osmotic pressure of the fluids and the fluid volumes (see Chapter 4). Sodium and chloride are concentrated mainly in the extracellular fluids whereas potassium is largely within the cells. Potassium is essential for certain enzymatic processes and chloride is a necessary activator for the enzyme amylase which converts starch to glucose and maltose. Sodium and potassium ions function cooperatively in the transmission of nerve impulses.

The suppressive action of potassium on muscle contractibility is striking. The heart, for example, will show weakened contractions and may even cease to contract as serum potassium levels rise. This is the single most critical threat to life in a patient in renal failure—the accumulation of potassium with consequent cardiac suppression. Low levels of potassium exert the opposite effect, muscular excitability.

Calcium and Phosphorus

The bulk of the body's calcium and phosphorus is found in the hard structures of bone and teeth. The principal component of these structures is calcium phosphate in the form of hydroxyapatite (Ca_{10} $(PO_4)_6$ $(OH)_2$). There is an ongoing exchange of these minerals between the bone structure and circulating fluids, an exchange that is under hormonal influence, principally parathyroid hormone and thyrocalcitonin.

Calcium, like potassium, has a profound effect on neuromuscular excitability, suppressing contractility as its concentration increases. The hypercontractility associated with low levels of calcium results in an uncontrolled, spasmodic muscular contraction called *tetany*. Calcium also is obligatory in the process of blood coagulation, and is required for the activity of some enzymes.

Phosphate is an essential part of the active form of many intermediary metabolites, existing mainly as phosphoric acid esters within the compounds. The importance of phosphate esters in intermediary metabolism cannot be overemphasized. This will be discussed in greater depth in Chapter 3.

Magnesium

Magnesium is extremely important in metabolism because of its requirement in reactions involving the hydrolysis of ATP, the major energy-producing reaction. Its effect on neuromuscular excitability is similar to that of calcium. High concentration of magnesium reduces the heart rate and can ultimately cause cardiac arrest. As would be expected, low levels produce a hypercontractility of muscle, producing symptoms that mimic a calcium deficiency tetany. Clinical tests for serum magnesium and calcium are necessary to ascertain the cause of tetany in a patient. There is evidence that an antagonism exists between calcium and magnesium. High levels of Ca^{++} tend to aggravate low levels of Mg^{++}, presumably because of interference with Mg^{++} requiring enzymes.

Iron

Iron is required for the synthesis of the heme moiety of *hemoglobin* and *myoglobin*. It is attached to the four pyrrole nitrogen atoms of the porphyrin nucleus within these proteins and it also serves as the site to which molecular oxygen is bound in its transport from lungs to tissue. Porphyrin-bound iron is also a component of a family of compounds called the *cytochromes*. Concentrated in the cell mitochondria, the cytochromes serve as electron carriers in the oxidation of metabolites by molecular oxygen.

Iron is stored in the body in the form of *ferritin* located chiefly in the liver, spleen, and bone marrow. In this form, the iron exists as ferric hydroxide–ferric phosphate complexes bound to the protein, apoferritin. Iron is transported in the plasma, from the stores to the sites of synthesis of physiologically active forms, by the protein *transferrin*.

Iron is conserved efficiently by the body, but deficiencies can occur as a result of blood loss. Iron insufficiency, whether through hemorrhage or low dietary intake gives rise to iron-deficiency anemia.

Sulfur

This element is a component of the amino acids cysteine and methionine, coenzyme A, the vitamins thiamine and biotin, and other indispensable substances. Dietary protein is the major source of sulfur.

There are other minerals required for normal metabolism in addition to those discussed above. Included among these are copper, zinc, manganese, cobalt, molybdenum, chromium, selenium, and iodine. Because of the low concentrations at which they occur in the body, they are referred to as essential *trace* elements. The precise physiological function of some is known while for others it is not. For a discussion of the minerals, consult Orten, J. M. and Neuhaus, O. W., *Human Biochemistry*, 9th ed. C. V. Mosby, St. Louis, 1975, pp. 529–553.

Questions

1. What is the biochemical basis for the lack of caloric value of cellulose? Of what dietary value is cellulose?
2. What structural characteristics of phospholipids account for their importance in stabilizing circulating lipids? Would it be expected that phospholipids would comprise surface or "core" lipids of chylomicrons? Why?
3. Considering the structures of the B-complex vitamins and their corresponding coenzyme forms, account for the importance of ATP in the "activation" of the vitamins.
4. Methotrexate is a drug that prevents the normal utilization of methylene THFA. What important effect would this drug have, therefore, on cell structure and function?
5. A patient suffering from gallstones had, in addition to the expected gastrointestinal symptoms, visual disturbances and a prolonged clotting time. What accounts for these symptoms?
6. In the clinical laboratory, the finding of a high potassium level in a patient is required to be reported to the attending physician immediately. Why is there greater urgency associated with results of this test compared with most other assays?

CHAPTER 3

Metabolic Interrelationship Among the Nutrients: Energy Transformation

AN OVERVIEW OF INTERMEDIARY METABOLISM

The term *intermediary,* as it applies to metabolism, originates from the fact that metabolism occurs through sequential enzyme-catalyzed reactions that produce intermediate compounds. These compounds are commonly referred to as *metabolites.*

Metabolism can be broadly divided into *catabolism,* referring to the degradative phase of metabolism, and *anabolism,* the biosynthetic aspect of metabolism. Catabolic processes generally refer to the degradation, usually oxidative, of the bulk nutrients into simpler end products. End products, such as urea, uric acid, and creatinine are excreted as waste products, whereas complete oxidation of foodstuffs yields carbon dioxide, eliminated by exhalation, and water, which, depending on fluid balance, may also be excreted. Catabolism is accompanied by the release of energy, as the bonds within the highly structured nutrient molecules are broken. Anabolic reactions, on the other hand, generate through biosynthetic pathways functional cellular molecules from simpler precursor substances. Obviously, new bonds must be formed as biosynthesis proceeds, requiring the input of energy. Therefore, an energy balance exists within the cell. The energy required for anabolism or biosynthesis is furnished by the catabolic events that are occurring simultaneously. No understanding of life, let alone appreciation for nutrition, is possible without a grasp of energy metabolism.

Reaction Energetics and Coupled Systems

All material possesses a certain amount of intrinsic energy which is contained in the bonds that hold the atoms together in highly structured molecules. The processes of life are founded on energy, which is available to the living organism in the form of nutrients. The energy contained within the nutrient molecules can be symbolized by the letter G, and is referred to as the free energy. The catabolic products of the nutrients are also vested with a certain free energy level. However, because the overall catabolic process causes a release of energy, as discussed above, this energy must have originated within the molecules themselves, and therefore it would be expected that the free energy of the products must be less than that of the reactants (nutrients). The *difference* between the free energy of reactants and products can therefore be represented as:

$$G_{\text{REACTANTS}} - G_{\text{PRODUCTS}} = \Delta G$$

where the symbol Δ refers to a "change of," in this case, the change of free energy between reactant and product. For any chemical reaction that proceeds *spontaneously,* that is, without the continuous input of energy, the G of the products will always be less than G of the reactants, and ΔG will therefore be less than zero (will carry a negative value). Such reactions are called *exergonic,* or energy releasing. Sometimes they are described as "downhill" reactions, which implies that there is a decrease in G in going from reactant to product. Conversely there are those reactions that do not occur spontaneously. They require an extrinsic source of energy to maintain them, their ΔG is greater than zero (positive), and they are referred to as *endergonic,* energy consuming, or "uphill" reactions. Merging these definitions with the concepts of catabolism and anabolism, it can be said that catabolism has a net decrease in free energy $(-\Delta G)$, while anabolic reactions collectively consume energy, and therefore have a net increase in free energy $(+\Delta G)$.

It is important to understand that *all* the reactions in a catabolic pathway may not be exergonic or downhill even though the net free energy change for the overall sequence is negative. Individual reactions that are not spontaneous can proceed in the desired direction through *coupled reaction systems*. The concept can be explained by considering the following sequence of hypothetical reactions which could represent a metabolic pathway or portion thereof.

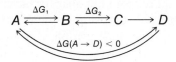

The fact that the ΔG for the overall sequence $A \rightarrow D$ is less than zero (negative) suggests that the *sequence* is exergonic. Suppose that ΔG_2 is positive, meaning that the $B \rightarrow C$ reaction is uphill, and suppose additionally that ΔG_1 has a negative value of greater magnitude than the positive value of ΔG_2. This would mean that reaction 2 actually favors the formation of B from C, because if its ΔG is positive for the $B \rightarrow C$ direction, it must be negative, and of the same value, for the opposite direction $(C \rightarrow B)$. However, since ΔG_1 is less than zero and its negative value is of greater magnitude than the positive value of ΔG_2, reaction 1 significantly increases the concentration of B which upsets the equilibrium of reaction

2, "pushing" the conversion of B into C. The law of mass action accounts for the driving force, in that the elevated concentration of B increases the chance that the enzyme catalyzing reaction 2 will react with it rather than with metabolite C. Simply stated, it can be said that exergonic reaction 1 can be coupled to drive the endergonic reaction 2.

Energy Production in Cells

Organic molecules such as glucose contain considerable potential or free energy. When it is oxidized completely to CO_2 and H_2O it releases free energy because the energy level of the products is lower than that of the glucose. The most familiar example of oxidation is *combustion,* or burning, which very rapidly oxidizes organic material to CO_2 and H_2O, while releasing the intrinsic energy as heat. The process, like all oxidations, requires oxygen which is consumed.

Biological oxidation is not rapid like combustion, and it is a flameless, low-temperature process. Nevertheless it is true oxidation in that molecular oxygen is the ultimate oxidizing agent, and CO_2 and H_2O are the products. Like combustion, it generates energy, not in the form of heat but in the formation of new high-energy compounds, the free energy of which can be utilized to drive the many energy-requiring processes of the body. This reservoir of chemical energy is harnessed and stored primarily in the form of high-energy phosphate bonds within compounds, the most important being adenosine triphosphate, or ATP. A schematic comparison of combustion and biological oxidation is shown below.

$$C_6H_{12}O_6 + 6O_2 \rightarrow 6CO_2 + 6H_2O \left\{ \begin{array}{l} + \text{ Heat (Combustion)} \\ + \text{ 36 ATP (Biological oxidation)} \end{array} \right.$$

Glucose

The generation of 36 moles of ATP for each mole of glucose oxidized is a "debit" on the energy balance sheet of intermediary metabolism. How it is precisely accomplished will be discussed later under metabolism.

Adenosine Triphosphate (ATP)
As Energy Source

As discussed previously in this chapter, all chemical reactions exhibit a certain free energy change (ΔG) which relates to the equilibrium constant of the reaction. For the simplest example of compound A being converted to compound B ($A \rightarrow B$), the equilibrium constant (K_{eq}) can be expressed in terms of the ratio of the concentrations of each *at equilibrium:*

$$K_{eq} = \frac{[B]}{[A]}$$

and the free energy change of the reaction is calculated as:

$$\Delta G = -2.303 \; RT\log_{10}K_{eq}$$

where R is the gas constant (1.987 cal/degree-mole) and T the absolute temperature. It can be seen from the relationship that ΔG will be negative if the ratio $[B]/[A]$ is greater than one, that is, if the equilibrium favors the formation of B from A rather than vice versa. It follows that ΔG will be positive (endergonic) for the reaction if the ratio $[B]/[A]$ is less than one, meaning that the formation of A is favored. Suppose that for the reaction $A \rightarrow B$, $\Delta G = -1000$ cal/mole; it would consequently hold true that for $B \rightarrow A$, $\Delta G = +1000$ cal/mole.

The three phosphate groups of ATP are linked to the ribose component of the nucleotide by an ester bond, and they are connected to each other by anhydride bonds as shown:

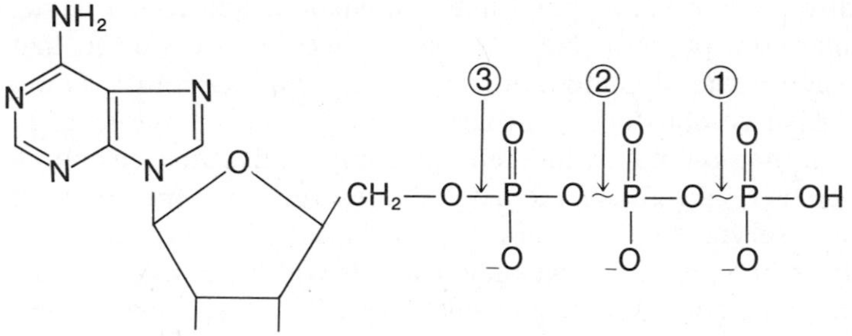

Figure 3.1 Adenosine triphosphate. High energy bonds are indicated by wavy lines.

The hydrolysis (splitting with water) of high-energy phosphate bond ① produces free phosphate and adenosine diphosphate (ADP). There is a drastic reduction in free energy in going from ATP to ADP, and therefore the reaction is strongly exergonic with a high negative value for ΔG.

ATP + $H_2O \rightleftarrows$ ADP + P_i (inorganic phosphate) $\Delta G = -7300$ cal/mole

Similarly, the hydrolysis of bond ② liberates an equivalent amount of energy. The products are *adenosine monophosphate* (AMP) and *pyrophosphate* (PP$_i$):

ATP + $H_2O \rightleftarrows$ AMP + PP$_i$ $\Delta G = -7300$ cal/mole

Phosphate bond ③ is not a high energy bond and its hydrolysis is not used to furnish energy.

In metabolism, the hydrolysis of ATP is performed enzymatically, and the released energy is utilized to "activate" or "energize" other compounds so that they can be properly metabolized. The phosphorylation of glucose is a fitting example of this concept.

Glucose must be phosphorylated before it can be oxidized in the cell. This is accomplished through a transfer of the third (terminal) phosphate of ATP to the hydroxyl group at carbon number 6 of glucose forming a phosphate ester bond at that position. The product is called glucose 6 phosphate. The energetics of the transfer can be illustrated by the following reactions:

1. glucose + P_i ⇄ glucose 6-P $\qquad\qquad$ $\Delta G = +3300$ cal/mole
2. ATP + H_2O ⇄ ADP + P_i $\qquad\qquad$ $\Delta G = -7300$ cal/mole
3. ATP + glucose ⇄ glucose 6-P + ADP $\Delta G = -4000$ cal/mole

Reaction 1 indicates that the phosphorylation of glucose is endergonic (positive ΔG). It requires the *input* of 3300 cal/mole, and therefore is an uphill reaction, the direction of which would *not* favor the formation of glucose 6-P. However, the energy derived from the hydrolytic removal of the phosphate from ATP is more than enough to "drive" reaction 1 to the right. Therefore, as indicated by the coupled reaction (3), the transfer of phosphate from ATP to glucose is exergonic and energetically favorable, with the net ΔG for the overall reaction being -4000 cal/mole.

The role of ATP in metabolism can be broadly summarized by Figure 3.2 which depicts what could be thought of as the ATP–ADP cycle. Energy-producing reactions are able to generate ATP from ADP and phosphate, and the intrinsic energy of the ATP so formed is utilized for a variety of endergonic or energy-requiring events.

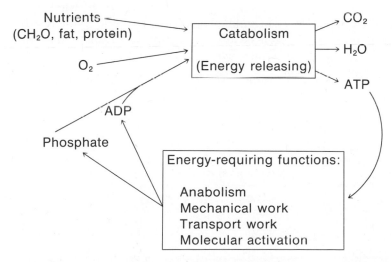

Figure 3.2 An illustration of the generation and utilization of ATP in metabolism.

Formation of ATP

It may be puzzling to the reader at this point as to how a compound with such a high intrinsic energy as ATP can be formed. Because the hydrolysis of the terminal phosphate group of ATP liberates approximately 7300 cal/mole, it follows that this amount of energy must be *consumed* in forming ATP from ADP and phosphate. Therefore, outside sources of considerable energy are necessary to effect the phosphorylation of ADP. The two major mechanisms by which this is accomplished are *substrate level phosphorylation* and *oxidative,* or *respiratory chain phosphorylation,* which will be discussed. In this context, *phosphorylation* implies the phosphorylation of ADP, producing ATP.

Substrate Level Phosphorylation. The fact that different phosphorylated compounds have different free energies of hydrolysis of their phosphate groups has already been discussed. Some phosphate compounds release more energy than ATP upon hydrolysis, while others release less energy. These compounds can therefore be characterized according to their *phosphate group transfer potential* which is a measure of their tendency to donate phosphate groups to other substances. The more negative the value for the ΔG of hydrolysis, the greater is the phosphate group transfer potential. Several representative compounds are given in Table 3.1.

In theory, a compound that releases more energy on hydrolysis can transfer its phosphate, by a specific enzymatic reaction, to an acceptor molecule lower on the scale. Therefore, just as ATP can phosphorylate glucose to glucose 6-phosphate, the scale also shows that ADP can be phosphorylated by any of the three, high-energy compounds listed above ATP. This does in fact occur in metabolism. The phosphorylation of ADP by creatine phosphate represents a major route for ATP formation in muscle, and it exemplifies a substrate level phosphorylation.

$$\text{creatine-P} + \text{ADP} \rightleftarrows \text{creatine} + \text{ATP} \qquad \Delta G = -3000 \text{ cal/mole}$$

Table 3.1 Free Energy of Hydrolysis of Some Phosphorylated Compounds

	ΔG (calories)
Phosphoenolpyruvate	$-14{,}800$
1,3 diphosphoglycerate	$-11{,}800$
Creatine phosphate	$-10{,}300$
ATP	$-7{,}300$
Glucose 1-phosphate	$-5{,}000$
Glucose 6-phosphate	$-3{,}300$

Oxidative Phosphorylation. This mechanism provides the principal means by which ATP is formed in the cell. The energy for "forcing" the phosphorylation of ADP is tapped from a reservoir of energy generated from the flow of electrons from a substrate undergoing oxidation to molecular oxygen which consequently is reduced to H_2O. When a metabolite becomes oxidized by a specific dehydrogenase enzyme, hydrogens and electrons are stripped from the metabolite and conveyed through a series of intermediate, carrier compounds to oxygen. These compounds constitute what is called the *respiratory chain,* which operates within the cell mitochondria. Because the respiratory chain, through oxidative phosphorylation, is the major source of energy in the form of generated ATP, the mitochondria are referred to as the power plants of the cell (Chapter 1).

The components of the respiratory chain are listed below. Each is reversibly reduced and oxidized as it accepts hydrogens or electrons or both from a reduced component and in turn transfers them on to an oxidized component which thus becomes reduced, and the transfer continues.

	Reduced	*Oxidized*
Nicotinamide system:	$NADH + H^+$	NAD
Flavoprotein system:	$FADH_2$	FAD
Coenzyme Q system:	CoQ (reduced)	CoQ (oxidized)
Cytochrome system:	cyt b (Fe^{+2})	cyt b (Fe^{+3})
	cyt c_1 (Fe^{+2})	cyt c_1 (Fe^{+3})
	cyt c (Fe^{+2})	cyt c (Fe^{+3})
	cyt a $-$ a$_3$ (Fe^{+2})	cyt a $-$ a$_3$ (Fe^{+3})

The oxidized and reduced structures of NAD and FAD have been discussed and are illustrated in Chapter 2. Coenzyme Q is a quinone with an isoprenoid side chain. When it accepts hydrogens from a donor component, in this case $FADH_2$, they attach at the quinone oxygens, converting the structure to a hydroquinone.

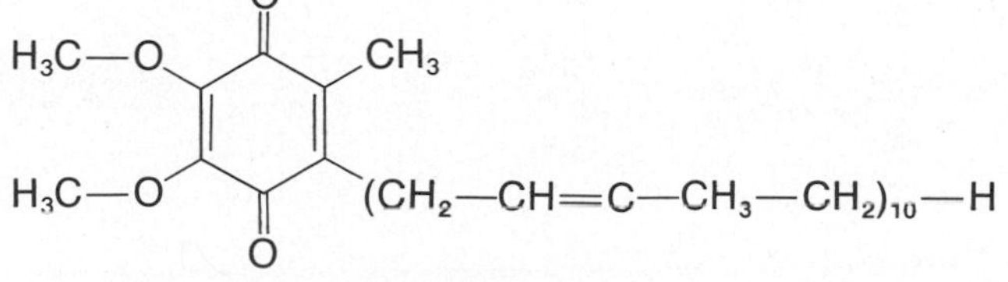

Oxidized coenzyme Q

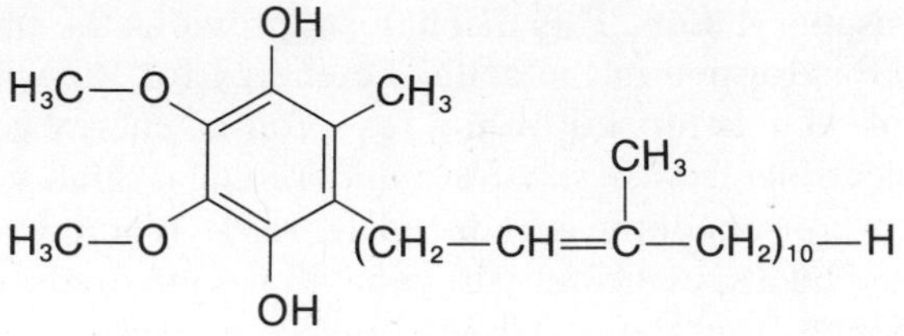

Reduced coenzyme Q

The cytochromes consist of heme groups (iron + porphyrin) attached to protein. As these components become reversibly reduced and oxidized the iron atom acquires, and in turn, donates electrons. Therefore the iron, as it accepts electrons, becomes reduced to Fe^{+2} and then is oxidized to Fe^{+3} as the electrons are transferred on. There is no transfer of hydrogens along the cytochrome segment of the respiratory chain.

The complete respiratory chain is summarized in Figure 3.4. The symbol M represents any metabolite that is oxidized by NAD-requiring dehydrogenase enzymes. Notice that hydrogen and electron transfer occurs only through the CoQ component. Thereafter, only electron transfer is effected, and for that reason, the cytochrome segment is regarded as the *electron transport chain.*

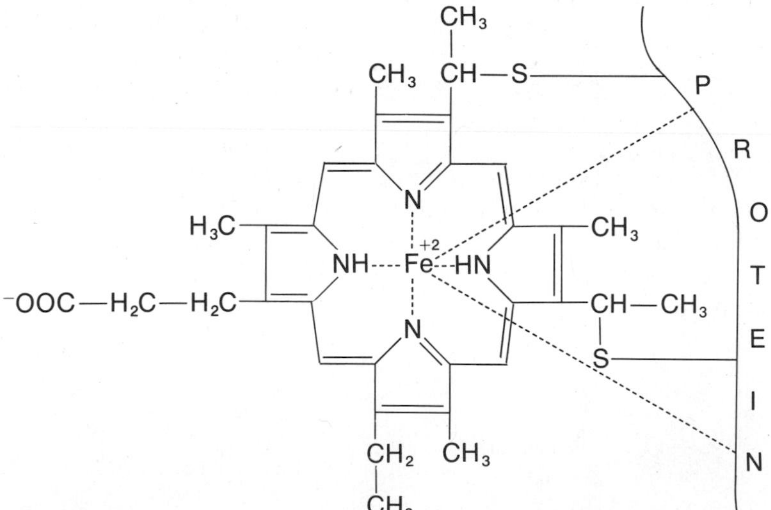

Figure 3.3 Reduced cytochrome c. In the oxidized form of cytochrome c, the iron is in the form of Fe^{+3}.

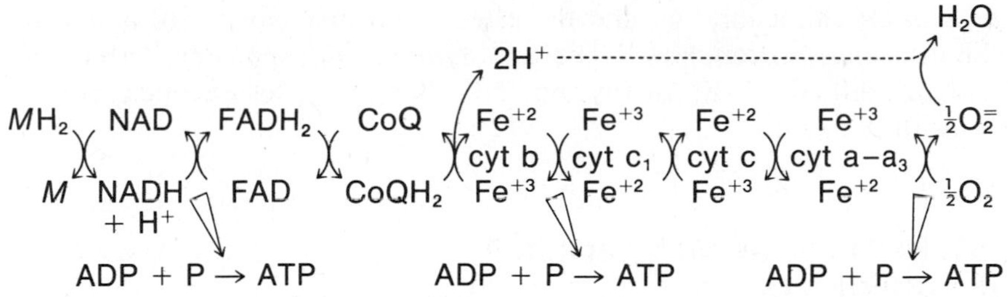

Figure 3.4 The respiratory chain. The scheme shows how a reduced metabolite (MH_2) can be oxidized (M) ultimately by molecular oxygen through a series of electron and/or hydrogen-transferring carriers. Also shown are the stages at which energy is drawn off for the synthesis of ATP.

Each component in the respiratory chain has a particular reducing potential. The magnitude of this reduction potential relative to that of the component it is reducing is directly proportional to the free energy change of that particular transfer. Each step in the respiratory chain, therefore, has a certain ΔG. These are shown in Table 3.2.

Because about 7300 cal are required to phosphorylate ADP, there are clearly three sites at which sufficient energy is produced. These are indicated in Figure 3.4. Therefore, for each mole of metabolite oxidized, one gram atom of oxygen is consumed, one mole of H_2O is formed, and *three* moles of ATP are generated at the expense of ADP and P. Phosphorylation by this mechanism is called *oxidative phosphorylation*.

It is of interest to calculate the energy efficiency of the respiratory chain. As seen in Table 3.2, a single *oxidation step* of a metabolite in a metabolic pathway liberates 52,580 cal of energy. However, the energy *conserved* as ATP is only about 22,000 cal (3 × 7300 cal). Therefore the efficiency is (22,000/52,580) × 100 = 40%, and the additional energy, not salvaged as ATP, is given off as heat in helping to maintain normal body temperature.

Much has been written about oxidative phosphorylation, particularly on the theories of the mechanism itself, the localization of the compo-

Table 3.2 Free Energy Changes at the Different Steps of Respiratory Chain

Reaction	ΔG (calories)
1 NAD → FAD	−12,450
2 FAD → cyt b	− 4,150
3 cyt b → cyt c_1	−10,150
4 cyt c → cyt a–a_3	− 1,380
5 cyt a–a_3 → $\frac{1}{2}O_2$	−24,450
Total:	−52,580

nents in the mitochondria, and the effects and mechanisms of action of inhibitors and "uncouplers." The text, *Human Biochemistry* (Orten and Neuhaus, 9th ed, C. V. Mosby, pp. 210–219), provides excellent coverage of the subject.

DIGESTION AND METABOLISM OF NUTRIENTS

Carbohydrates

Digestion. The major source of carbohydrate in the average diet is the polysaccharide, starch, and the disaccharides, sucrose and lactose. The structures of these compounds are shown in Chapter 2, under chemistry of the carbohydrates. In the process of digestion, these dietary carbohydrates are hydrolyzed to their component monosaccharides which are subsequently absorbed into the circulation via the mucosal cells of the small intestine.

The digestive enzyme that hydrolyzes starch in man is called α-amylase, the action of which is to cleave the α-$(1 \rightarrow 4)$ glycosidic bonds randomly, thereby liberating free glucose and maltose. Amylase activity is found in both saliva and in exocrine secretions of the pancreas. Therefore, some hydrolysis occurs in the mouth before the food is swallowed, but most of the hydrolysis takes place in the small intestine. It is also in the small intestine that hydrolysis of the disaccharides takes place. In addition to ingested sucrose and lactose, the maltose that is derived from the incomplete digestion of starch by amylase must be broken down before absorption can occur.

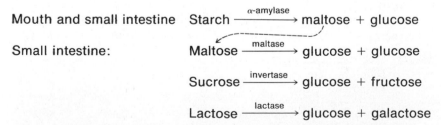

Mouth and small intestine   Starch $\xrightarrow{\alpha\text{-amylase}}$ maltose + glucose

Small intestine: Maltose $\xrightarrow{\text{maltase}}$ glucose + glucose

Sucrose $\xrightarrow{\text{invertase}}$ glucose + fructose

Lactose $\xrightarrow{\text{lactase}}$ glucose + galactose

Figure 3.5 Digestion of carbohydrates, indicating specific enzymes involved.

The monosaccharides can be oxidized for energy or converted into liver or muscle glycogen by pathways that will be discussed. In the liver, the monosaccharides are phosphorylated by specific enzymes called kinases which transfer a phosphate from ATP to the particular hexose:

$$\text{glucose} + \text{ATP} \xrightarrow{\text{glucokinase}} \text{glucose 1-P} + \text{ADP}$$

$$\text{fructose} + \text{ATP} \xrightarrow{\text{fructokinase}} \text{fructose 1-P} + \text{ADP}$$

$$\text{galactose} + \text{ATP} \xrightarrow{\text{galactokinase}} \text{galactose 1-P} + \text{ADP}$$

In addition to the specific enzymes shown above, a family of enzymes called *hexokinases* which exist in various tissues catalyze the phosphorylation of all the monosaccharides at the 6 position. The entry of fructose and galactose into the pathway of metabolism is shown in Figure 3.7.

Glycogenesis. Glycogenesis refers to the pathway by which glucose is converted into glycogen. This pathway is depicted in Figure 3.6.

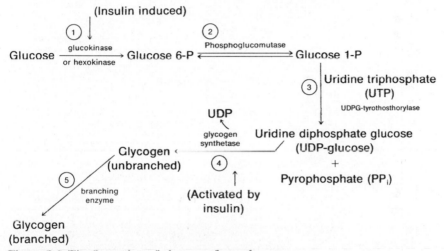

Figure 3.6 The formation of glycogen from glucose.

Comments on Selected Reactions

② A complex reaction by which 6-phosphate and 1-phosphate derivatives of glucose are interconverted.

③ Glucose must be activated by being coupled with the nucleotide UTP, as UDP glucose, before it can be incorporated into glycogen.

④ Glycogen synthetase requires some preformed glycogen (glycogen primer), to which it adds the incoming glucose units.

⑤ Glycogen synthetase cannot make the $\alpha(1 \rightarrow 6)$ bonds found in the branch points of glycogen. The branching enzyme catalyzes the transfer of a terminal oligosaccharide, containing six or seven glucose residues from the end of the main chain, consisting only of $\alpha(1 \rightarrow 4)$ linkages, to the 6-hydroxyl group within the chain to form an $\alpha(1 \rightarrow 6)$ branch point.

Glycogenesis is an energy-consuming sequence because reaction ① consumes one mole of ATP per mole of glucose.

Glycolysis. Glycolysis is the pathway by which glucose is converted anaerobically (in the absence of molecular oxygen) into lactic acid. Glycolysis also provides the initial sequence of reactions necessary for glucose to be

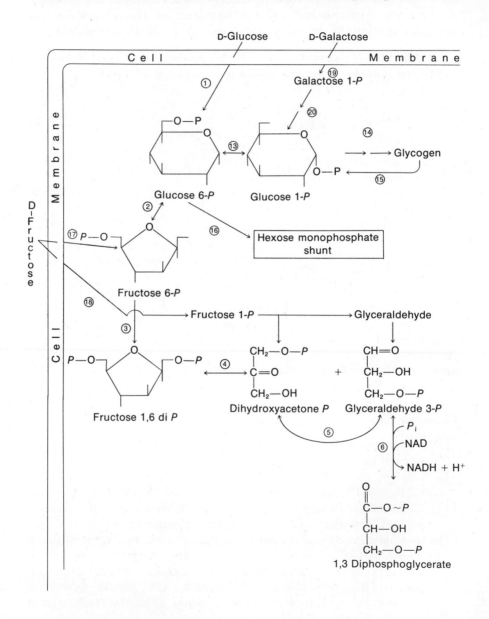

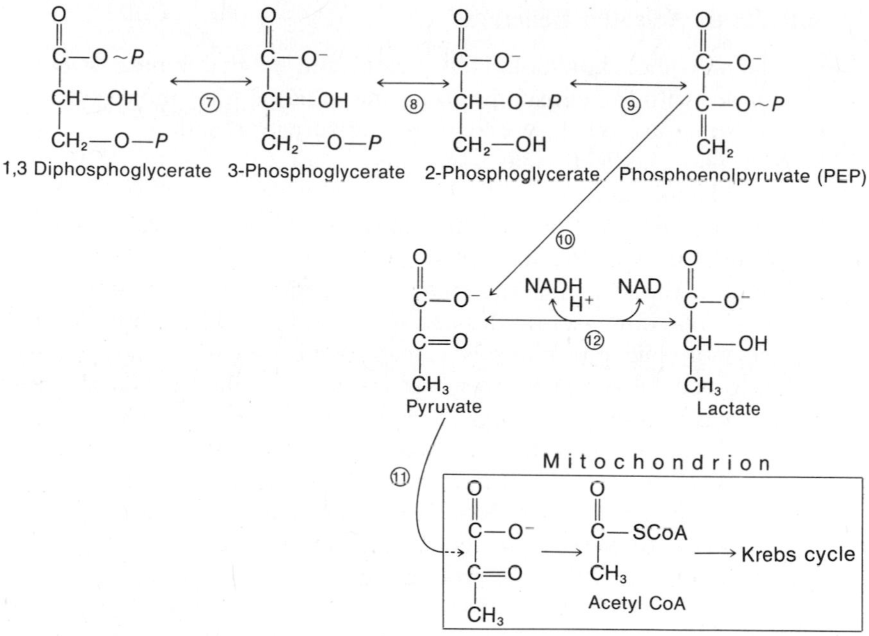

Figure 3.7 Glycolysis, showing the entry of dietary glucose, fructose, and galactose into the pathway.

oxidized completely to CO_2 and H_2O via the Krebs cycle; through which a large amount of chemical energy (ATP) is generated.

The pathway of glycolysis is summarized in Figure 3.7. All of the reactions leading to the formation of pyruvate and lactate are catalyzed by enzymes present in the cytoplasm of the cell. Many cell types are involved in glycolysis, but most of the body's carbohydrate-derived energy originates in the cells of liver, muscle, and adipose tissue.

In the illustration of metabolic pathways, the letter P represents a phosphate group joined to a parent compound through the elimination of water resulting in phosphate esters or anhydrides and occasionally amino phosphates. This is for the purpose of simplification, and it is important to understand that the structure of a phosphate ester is more accurately depicted as:

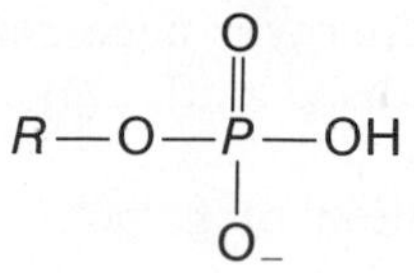

$$R-O-\overset{\overset{\displaystyle O}{\|}}{\underset{\underset{\displaystyle O_-}{|}}{P}}-OH \qquad \text{where } R \text{ is the parent compound}$$

Comments on Selected Reactions

1. The phosphorylation of glucose catalyzed by glucokinase or hexo-kinase, with the consumption of one mole of ATP/mole glucose.
2. An isomerase (glucose phosphate isomerase) reaction.
3. The phosphofructokinase reaction. Another mole of ATP consumed/mole glucose.
4. The aldolase reaction, resulting in the splitting of a hexose diphosphate into two triose phosphates.
5. The triose phosphate isomerase catalyzed interconversions.
6. In this reaction, glyceraldehyde 3-P is oxidized to a carboxylic acid and inorganic phosphate is incorporated as a high-energy anhydride phosphate. The enzyme is glyceraldehyde 3-P dehydrogenase, which utilizes NAD as the hydrogen acceptor. Under anaerobic conditions, with the reaction sequence proceeding to lactate, the NAD consumed is returned to the system by reaction 12. In aerobic metabolism any NADH formed in an oxidation reaction is reoxidized to NAD by molecular oxygen via the respiratory chain (see Fig. 3.4) with the production of energy as ATP. In glycolysis, however, the lactate dehydrogenase reaction (12) assures the continuous repetition of reaction 6 by restoring the NAD used. It is for this reason that glycolysis is an anaerobic pathway.
7. An example of substrate level phosphorylation of ADP. The energy derived from the hydrolysis of the high-energy anhydride phosphate of diphosphoglycerate is more than sufficient to force the phosphorylation of ADP to form 2 moles ATP/mole glucose.
10. Another substrate level phosphorylation made possible by the splitting of the high-energy phosphate bond of phosphoenol pyruvate (PEP). The reaction, catalyzed by pyruvate kinase, generates two more ATP/mole glucose.
11. This step is not a chemical conversion. Is shows how the two moles of pyruvate formed from one glucose are able to enter the mitochondria. It is in the mitochondria that the Krebs cycle enzymes ultimately oxidize the pyruvate to CO_2 and H_2O with the production of a large amount of energy.
17.
18. These two reactions are the means by which dietary fructose can be metabolized for energy. Of the two, reaction 18, catalyzed by fructokinase, is carried out in the liver and is the most important route for fructose utilization. Notice that energy is necessarily expended in phosphorylating fructose and subsequently, glyceraldehyde.
19. Galactokinase catalyzes the phosphorylation of galactose, consuming one mole of ATP.

⑳ In a reaction utilizing UTP, the UDP derivative of galactose is epimerized by a specific enzyme to form UDP glucose. This derivative is subsequently split in such a way as to liberate the glucose 1-*P*. In the metabolic disease, *galactosemia,* the enzyme that couples galactose 1-*P* with UTP is deficient. The enzyme is called galactose 1-phosphate uridyl transferase. Galactosemia patients are unable to metabolize galactose, the major source of which would be the disaccharide lactose, and consequently the galactose blood level rises to toxic amounts.

⑮ The phosphorylase reaction. This will be discussed in detail under glycogenolysis.

⑯ Shows the entry of glucose 6-*P* into the hexose monophosphate shunt, or pentose phosphate pathway. In this pathway, two oxidations occur, catalyzed by dehydrogenases which require NADP as coenzyme. Consequently, significant amounts of NADPH are formed, and this reduced coenzyme is utilized for other important metabolic functions such as the biosynthesis of fatty acids and the maintenance of reducing substances in red blood cells necessary to assure the integrity of the cells. Another important function of the hexose monophosphate shunt is to provide pentose sugars necessary for the synthesis of the purine and pyrimidine nucleotides of RNA and DNA. Within the pathway, 6-phosphogluconic acid, formed from the oxidation of glucose 6-phosphate, is oxidatively decarboxylated (loss of one carbon atom as CO_2) to produce the pentose, ribulose 5-phosphate. Three, four, and seven carbon phosphate sugars are also formed in the pathway, and through molecular rearrangements catalyzed by the fragment-transferring enzymes *transketolase* and *transaldolase,* fructose 6-phosphate is ultimately formed as a "return" to the glycolytic sequence of reactions, thus completing the shunt.

Glycogenolysis. A large amount of stored energy exists in the glucose residues stored as liver and muscle glycogen. When the body's energy demands require it, these residues can be systematically cleaved from the glycogen reservoir as glucose 1-phosphate (reaction 15 in Fig. 3.7) and utilized for energy via the glycolytic and Krebs cycle pathways. The process is called *glycogenolysis* (Fig. 3.8) Glycogen metabolism is regulated by the hormones *epinephrine* and *glucagon* which stimulate glycogen breakdown and by the hormone *insulin* which promotes glycogen formation. Epinephrine and glucagon cause activation of the phosphorylase reaction via cAMP while insulin inhibits the phosphorylase reaction and activates glycogen synthetase. (Refer to Fig. 3.6 for mechanisms involved in glycogenesis.)

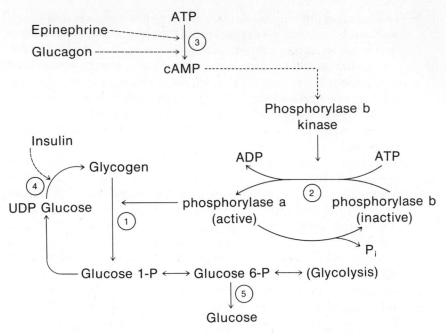

Figure 3.8 Glycogenolysis. The scheme indicates the hormonal influence in glycogen metabolism. Dashed lines represent stimulation of the particular reaction.

Comments on Selected Reactions

(1) The enzyme *phosphorylase a* catalyzes the phosphorolysis of glycogen (splitting of glycosidic bonds by inorganic phosphate) to form glucose 1-phosphate. The phosphorolysis sequentially removes glucose residues from the nonreducing ends of the glycogen branches. The reaction is specific for α-1,4 glycosidic bonds. A second enzyme, the *debranching enzyme,* is required to hydrolyze the α-1,6 linkages at the branch points.

(2) *Phosphorylase a is a phosphorylated form of the enzyme.* Removal of these phosphate groups by *phosphorylase a phosphatase* results in enzymatically inactive *phosphorylase b.* The phosphorylation of phosphorylase b to the active form is stimulated by cyclic AMP (cAMP), which in turn is formed from ATP by the enzyme adenyl cyclase (reaction 3). The stimulatory effect of epinephrine and glucagon on glycogenolysis is attributed to the enhancement of adenyl cyclase activity by these hormones. The structure of cyclic AMP along with a brief account of its important role as "second messenger" in the hormonal control of cellular metabolism is found in Chapter 2. Therefore, the statement of "getting the adrenaline (epi-

nephrine) flowing'' in times of stress is biochemically valid. The energy demands on the body in times of stress are answered by the accelerated breakdown of the glycogen stores.

(5) The cells of the liver contain the enzyme *glucose 6-phosphatase* which forms free glucose from its phosphate derivative. The glucose is free to enter the general circulation (blood glucose) and to be transported to various other tissues for oxidation. Muscle cells, on the other hand, are devoid of glucose 6-phosphatase activity, and therefore the oxidation of the glucose residues of muscle glycogen is confined to muscle tissue only. However, lactate formed in muscle by glycolysis can be returned to the liver for reconversion to glucose by gluconeogenesis. The utilization of muscle lactate by the liver, and the circulatory transport of glucose from liver to muscle is referred to as the *Cori cycle*.

The Krebs Cycle. The Krebs cycle, also referred to as the tricarboxylic acid cycle or the citric acid cycle, is the focal point of energy production in the body. It can be thought of as the *common* or *final metabolic pathway* because products of carbohydrate, fat, and protein metabolism feed into this pathway where their complete oxidation to CO_2 and H_2O generates large amounts of ATP. The cycle is an aerobic pathway and it is compartmentalized within the mitochondria. Therefore, the reduced coenzymes, NADH and $FADH_2$, resulting from the oxidation reactions occurring within the cycle, are oxidized via the respiratory chain, the components of which are neighbors to the enzymes of the cycle in the mitochondria. Therefore, nearly all the energy generated in the Krebs cycle is by oxidative phosphorylation of ADP.

In addition to its energy output, the Krebs cycle produces most of the carbon dioxide which is ultimately exhaled through the lungs. It also provides important precursors needed in the synthesis of various molecules such as hemoglobin and the amino acids. It is through the cycle that the various nutrients interrelate. For example, material coming to it from carbohydrate sources might leave it to form fat or protein, and products of protein metabolism may be converted to carbohydrate. The only block in these interconversions is that which would lead from fatty acids to carbohydrate. There is no *net* synthesis of carbohydrate from fatty acids. Only the glycerol portion of dietary fats can be converted into carbohydrate resulting in net synthesis of the latter.

The reactions of the Krebs cycle are summarized in Figure 3.9. Included in the scheme are the reactions by which fatty acids enter the cycle, as well as the major auxiliary reactions that assure an adequate level of the cycle intermediate, oxaloacetate. Emphasized are the oxidation reactions, catalyzed by dehydrogenase enzymes, which generate re-

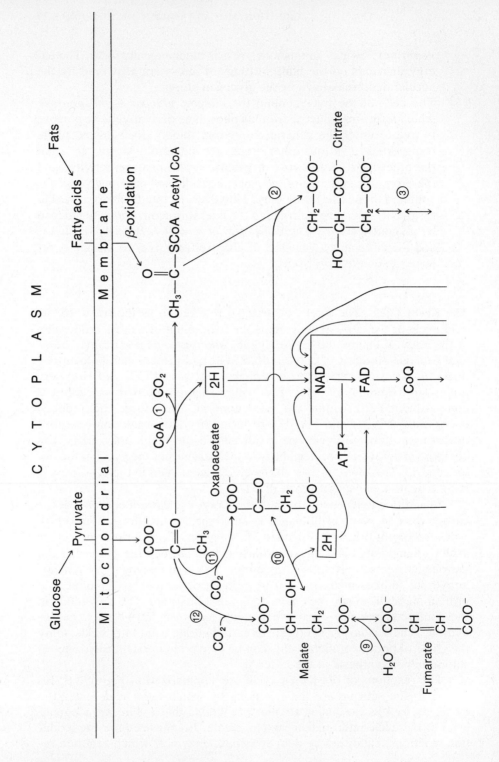

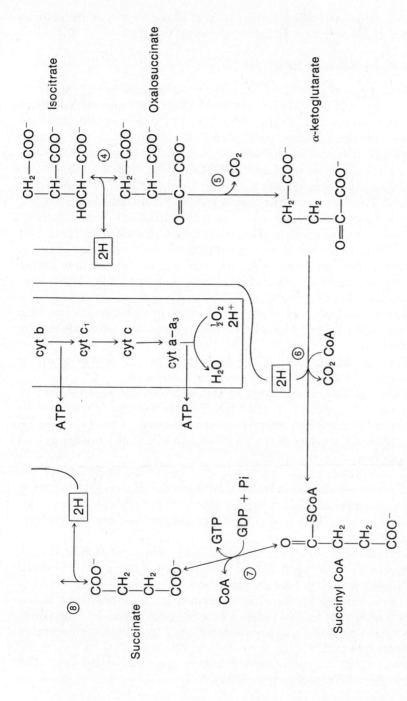

Figure 3.9 The Kreb's cycle, emphasizing energy production through respiratory chain phosphorylation.

duced coenzymes and which in turn are reoxidized by way of the respiratory chain producing large amounts of energy as ATP.

Comments on Selected Reactions

① This reaction is referred to as the pyruvate dehydrogenase reaction, but is in actuality a very complex reaction requiring a multienzyme system and several cofactors. The enzymes and cofactors are contained within a unit called the *pyruvate dehydrogenase complex* which is stable enough to be isolated from many cells as a unit. The functional cofactors of the complex include coenzyme A, thiamine pyrophosphate, magnesium ion, NAD, FAD, and lipoic acid. The enzymes of the complex are pyruvate dehydrogenase, dihydrolipoyl dehydrogenase, and dihydrolipoyl transacetylase. Within the complex, NAD is the ultimate hydrogen acceptor, and the NADH formed is reoxidized through the respiratory chain.

② Sometimes called the *condensing reaction,* the formation of citrate from oxaloacetate and acetyl CoA is catalyzed by the highly specific enzyme *citrate synthetase.*

③ The isomerization of citrate to isocitrate involves an intermediate metabolite called *cis*aconitate and the reaction is catalyzed by *aconitase.*

④ NAD is the acceptor of the hydrogens in this dehydrogenation reaction catalyzed by *isocitrate dehydrogenase.*

⑥ This reaction is analogous to the decarboxylation–oxidation of pyruvate (reaction ①) and it operates through the complex mechanism described in that reaction. Reactions ①, ⑤, and ⑥ account for the loss of the 3-carbon equivalent of pyruvate as carbon dioxide.

⑦ A substrate-level phosphorylation of guanosine diphosphate, one of the few instances in which GDP is preferred over ADP as phosphate acceptor. The energy for this "uphill" phosphorylation derives from the hydrolysis of the high-energy thioester bond of succinyl CoA.

⑧ The *succinate dehydrogenase* reaction utilizes FAD as hydrogen acceptor rather than NAD. The $FADH_2$ formed is reoxidized through the components of the respiratory chain; however, less energy is generated in the process because the ATP-producing oxidation of NADH by FAD in the chain has been bypassed. Therefore, for each mole of succinate oxidized, only two ATPs are generated instead of three.

⑩ The *malate dehydrogenase* reaction completes the cycle. The transfer of hydrogens is to NAD.

⑪
⑫ These reactions are called the *anaplerotic ("filling up") reactions*

because they assure an adequate supply of oxaloacetate required to combine with acetyl CoA in the citrate synthetase reaction. An excessive influx of acetyl CoA, as for example in the case of accelerated oxidation of fatty acids, can deplete the levels of oxaloacetate. This is the situation in diabetes mellitus or in starvation. In these conditions, carbohydrate is not available as an energy source, resulting in insufficient oxaloacetate (formed from pyruvate) to react with the acetyl CoA produced from the unrestrained oxidation of fats. The consequent accumulation of acetyl CoA causes the "venting" of the compound through a series of reactions that produce organic acids and acetone (ketone bodies). High serum and urine concentrations of the ketone bodies are a biochemical manifestation of diabetes or a low carbohydrate diet. Of the two anaplerotic reactions, reaction ⑪, catalyzed by *pyruvate carboxylase* is the more important.

The energy yield for the complete oxidation of one mole of glucose can be summarized as follows: 1 Glucose → 2 Pyruvate. There is a net synthesis of six ATPs within this pathway. Two of these are from substrate level phosphorylation, and the remaining four from oxidative phosphorylation made possible by the respiratory chain oxidation of the two NADHs formed in the glyceraldehyde 3-P dehydrogenase reaction (Fig. 3.7). Since the NADH is extramitochondrial, only two ATPs are generated per mole NADH instead of three.

Pyruvate → Oxaloacetate (Krebs cycle): Reactions ①, ④, ⑥, ⑧, and ⑩ generate a total of *28 ATPs** by oxidative phosphorylation, and *two more* are formed in reaction ⑦ as *GTP*.

For both pathways, therefore, a total of 36 ATPs are formed, meaning that approximately 36 × 7300 cal/mole or 262.8 kcal of energy are salvaged as useful energy. Actually, this is only about 40 percent of the *total* energy produced, because only this percentage of the respiratory chain energy is harnessed as ATP (see page 71). The remainder of the energy released serves to maintain body temperature.

Gluconeogenesis. D-glucose is essential for the proper function of most cells, particularly those of the brain and other tissues of the central nervous system. When adequate amounts of glucose are not provided in the diet, the serum glucose level falls, triggering the accelerated synthesis of glucose from noncarbohydrate sources. The process is called *gluconeogenesis*.

* Reaction 8 is responsible for the formation of 4 ATP rather than 6 because the hydrogen ions and electrons are introduced into the respiratory chain via FAD rather than via NAD.

The carbon source for gluconeogenesis is several of the Krebs cycle metabolites that are derived from L-amino acids (Fig. 6.4). The reactions by which certain amino acids can be converted to the Krebs cycle intermediates are called *transamination* and *oxidative deamination* and will be discussed under protein metabolism. The metabolites formed from amino acids are principally α-ketoglutarate, succinate, pyruvate, and oxaloacetate. Except for pyruvate, which is able to shuttle from cytoplasm to mitochondrion, the metabolites are primarily localized within the mitochondrion. The reactions of gluconeogenesis are cytoplasmic, and therefore there must exist a mechanism for garnering within the cytoplasm substrates originating in the mitochondrion. This is accomplished by malate into which the other metabolites are converted (see Fig. 3.9), and which can be translocated from the mitochondrion into the cytoplasm.

Gluconeogenesis is essentially a reversal of the glucose → pyruvate pathway. It will be recalled that all but three of the reactions in that pathway are reversible (Fig. 3.7) and therefore most of the enzymes catalyzing the glycolytic breakdown of glucose also catalyze the reactions of gluconeogenesis. The reactions shown in Figure 3.7 that are not reversible are the hexokinase and phosphofructokinase reactions, numbered ① and ③, and reaction ⑩, the pyruvate kinase reaction. In the direction of gluconeogenesis, specific phosphatases catalyze the "reversal" of reactions ① and ③, glucose 6-phosphatase and fructose 1,6 diphosphatase respectively. Reaction ⑩ is essentially unidirectional because of the very large positive ΔG for the phosphorylation of pyruvate. The reaction is, therefore, bypassed as illustrated in Figure 3.10. Mitochondrial malate is translocated into the cytoplasm where it is oxidized to oxaloacetate by the enzyme malate dehydrogenase. The oxaloacetate is subsequently decarboxylated and phosphorylated (GTP serving as phosphate donor) by the action of the enzyme phosphoenolpyruvate carboxykinase. From PEP, glucose can be produced through the action of the glycolytic enzymes as described.

Lipids

Digestion. Approximately 40 to 45 percent of the dietary caloric intake is lipid. Most of this dietary lipid is in the form of triglycerides, but also ingested are small amounts of glycerophosphatides, cholesterol esters, and cholesterol. The digestion of these lipids proceeds through the hydrolysis of ester bonds by specific esterases secreted into the duodenum by the pancreas. There is virtually no digestion of lipids in the stomach because the high acidity of the gastric secretion is not conducive to the activity of the lipid-hydrolyzing enzymes which function optimally at a pH between 7 and 8.

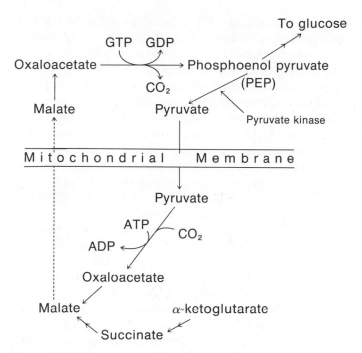

Figure 3.10 The pyruvate kinase bypass in gluconeogenesis.

Because lipids are not water soluble, and yet the enzymes that act upon them must function in an aqueous environment, it is necessary that the fat be emulsified into tiny droplets or *micelles* so as to maximize the surface area of the fat in the aqueous chyme. This emulsification is brought about by the bile, which is produced in the liver, stored in the gall bladder, and released into the lumen of the duodenum in response to fat ingestion. In the absence of the gall bladder, only small amounts of bile can be released at any one time.

Three lipid hydrolyzing enzymes are produced by the exocrine pancreas and secreted into the duodenum. These are pancreatic lipase, cholesterol esterase, and phospholipase. These enzymes remove fatty acids from parent molecules as shown:

$$\text{Triglyceride} + 2H_2O \xrightarrow{\text{Lipase}} \text{Monoglyceride} + 2 \text{ Fatty Acids}$$

$$\text{Cholesterol ester} + H_2O \xrightarrow{\text{Cholesterol esterase}} \text{Cholesterol} + \text{Fatty Acid}$$

$$\text{Thosthatidyl choline} + 2H_2O \xrightarrow{\text{Phospholipase}} \text{Glycerophosphphoryl choline} + 2 \text{ Fatty Acids}$$

The products of the enzymatic hydrolysis are absorbed passively into the intestinal mucosal cells where resynthesis of the fat molecules occurs. The breakdown is necessary because intact fats are not absorbable into the mucosa. Much of the resynthesized fat takes the form of macroscopic lipid droplets made up largely of triglycerides with a small amount of protein and phospholipid on the surface. The polar proteins and phospholipids tend to stabilize the hydrophobic droplets which would otherwise coalesce in an aqueous environment. These lipoprotein droplets are called *chylomicrons*, and they are released from the intestinal mucosa into the lymph and finally the venous blood. It is the chylomicrons that cause the serum to be turbid or opalescent soon after the ingestion of fat. Two or three hours postprandially, however, the serum normally once again becomes clear. This "clearing" of the serum is brought about by a plasma enzyme called *lipoprotein lipase* which once again hydrolyzes the triglycerides within the chylomicrons. The released fatty acids are taken up by tissues, principally the adipose tissue and the liver, where resynthesis into triglyceride and phospholipid is initiated once again. In the adipose tissue the accumulated triglyceride (storage fat) serves as a reservoir for energy which can be summoned when dietary carbohydrate can no longer meet the energy needs of the body.

In the liver, the resynthesized fat is combined with proteins, the purpose of which is to solubilize the lipids by taking advantage of the high degree of solubility of the hydrophilic proteins. These lipid–protein conjugates are called *lipoproteins* and represent the chief transport form of lipids from tissue to tissue via the circulation. Such mobilization of fat is constantly occurring among the intestine, liver, adipose tissue, and other tissues that may be utilizing the fats for energy. Depending on the relative concentration of lipids present and the ratio of lipids to protein within a conjugate, the lipoproteins exhibit different densities. This has led to an important classification of the lipoproteins, from a clinical standpoint, based on their centrifugal properties. The major classes are the chylomicrons (lowest density), the very low density (VLDL), the low density (LDL), and the high density (HDL) lipoproteins. There is considerable clinical interest in the relative concentrations of these fractions because of the possible relationship between elevated levels of certain lipoproteins and development of atherosclerosis (see Chapter 7). A currently popular estimation of risk of cardiovascular disease is based on the determination of the *cholesterol* in LDL versus that found in HDL fractions. Studies have suggested that risk is reduced as the HDL cholesterol is increased and/or the LDL cholesterol decreased relative to a normal or statistically average value. The risk factor is usually estimated from the ratio of the fractions (LDLC/HDLC), the risk increasing as the ratio value increases.

Fatty Acid Oxidation. Fatty acids are a major source of energy in the body because carbohydrate is available in only a limited supply. In response to energy demands, the fatty acids are released from the triglycerides in adipose tissue by hormone-sensitive tissue lipase, and transported to various other tissues for oxidation. In the process of oxidation, two-carbon fragments are successively removed from the carboxyl end of the molecule as acetyl CoA. This process of oxidation, called beta-oxidation, occurs in the mitochondria. The acetyl CoA formed gives rise to energy and in the process is metabolized to CO_2 and H_2O by enzymes in the Krebs cycle. The beta-oxidation sequence is summarized in Figure 3.11 for the fatty acid, palmitate.

For each turn of the oxidation cycle, one acetyl CoA is released. Therefore, the sequence of reactions shown would need to be repeated

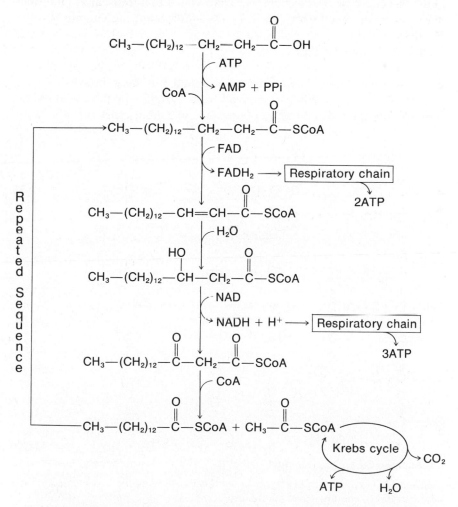

Figure 3.11 Beta oxidation of palmitate.

seven times to oxidize completely 16-carbon palmitate. The high-energy yield of fatty acids is evident from Figure 3.11. Energy is derived not only from the Krebs cycle oxidation of acetyl CoA, but the FAD and NAD reactions leading to the splitting off of the two-carbon unit generate ATP via respiratory chain phosphorylation. The oxidation of fat generates more energy as ATP than does an equal weight of carbohydrate, thus accounting for the higher caloric value of fat.

Unsaturated fatty acids are oxidized in the same manner as the saturated ones. Because these substances are already at a higher level of oxidation, the total energy yield is somewhat less than that for saturated fatty acids. Fatty acids containing an odd number of carbons are also degraded by β-oxidation. The three-carbon propionyl CoA, which would be formed in the last cleavage of the chain, is carboxylated to a four-carbon intermediate, methylmalonyl CoA. Then, in a reaction requiring vitamin B_{12}, the methylmalonyl CoA is isomerized to succinyl CoA which is oxidized as a Krebs Cycle intermediate.

Fatty Acid Synthesis. The starting compound for the synthesis of fatty acids is acetyl CoA. Whether derived from pyruvate or fatty acid oxidation, this compound is intramitochondrial and cannot cross the mitochon-

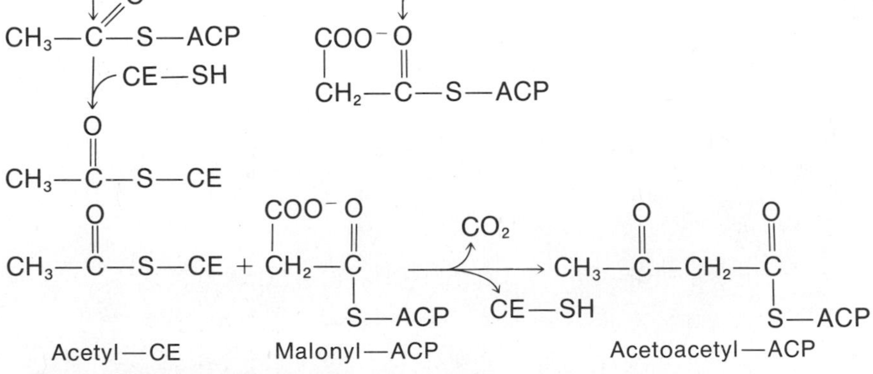

Figure 3.12 The initiation of fatty acid synthesis, showing the involvement of the acyl carriers of the fatty acid synthetase complex.

drial membrane. Fatty acid synthesis occurs in the cytoplasm, however, and a mechanism must, therefore, be in effect for transporting the acetyl CoA from the mitochondria for the synthetic process. It is now known that acetyl CoA leaves the mitochondria as *citrate* which, once in the cytoplasm, is cleaved to acetyl CoA and oxaloacetate in an ATP-requiring reaction catalyzed by citrate lyase. This enzyme and all the others involved in de novo fatty acid synthesis are increased in the liver following the feeding of carbohydrate but are depressed during fasting.

Fatty acids are synthesized by a conglomerate of enzymes and carrier molecules collectively referred to as the *fatty acid synthetase complex*. The components *acyl carrier protein* (ACP-SH) and the *condensing enzyme* (CE-SH) are sulfhydryl compounds that function as carriers of acyl groups. They combine with the acyl groups through a thioester bond in the same manner as CoA activation of acyl substances. The carbons of the fatty acid are derived from acetyl CoA and from malonyl CoA, formed from acetyl CoA by carboxylation. The acyl portions of each are transferred to ACP-SH, or CE-SH as shown in Fig. 3.12.

The acetoacetyl CoA formed by the sequence of reactions shown in Figure 3.12 is reduced to butyryl-S-ACP by the remaining enzymes of the complex. NADPH serves as the hydrogen source in the reduction as shown below:

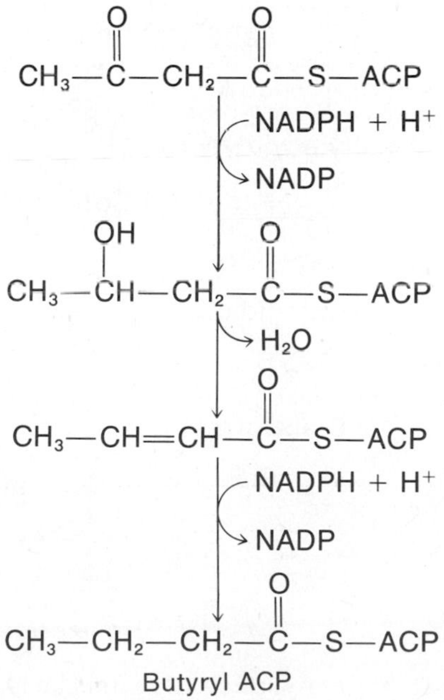

$$CH_3-\overset{\overset{\textstyle O}{\|}}{C}-CH_2-\overset{\overset{\textstyle O}{\|}}{C}-S-ACP$$

NADPH + H$^+$

NADP

$$CH_3-\overset{\overset{\textstyle OH}{|}}{CH}-CH_2-\overset{\overset{\textstyle O}{\|}}{C}-S-ACP$$

H$_2$O

$$CH_3-CH=CH-\overset{\overset{\textstyle O}{\|}}{C}-S-ACP$$

NADPH + H$^+$

NADP

$$CH_3-CH_2-CH_2-\overset{\overset{\textstyle O}{\|}}{C}-S-ACP$$

Butyryl ACP

After this series of events, the sequence is repeated. The butyryl group is transferred to condensing enzyme just as was the original acetyl group, and the butyryl-S-CE reacts with more malonyl-S-ACP, concomitant with decarboxylation, just as in the reaction shown in Figure 3.12. The product is now the six-carbon unit:

$$CH_3—CH_2—CH_2—\overset{\overset{\displaystyle O}{\|}}{C}—CH_2—\overset{\overset{\displaystyle O}{\|}}{C}—S—ACP$$

which is reduced as shown above for butyryl-S-ACP formation.

In summary, only the two carbons at the methyl end of the fatty acid chain are contributed by acetyl CoA per se. All the remaining carbons are incorporated as two-carbon units derived from malonyl groups. The incorporation is accompanied by simultaneous decarboxylation.

The synthesis of an unsaturated fatty acid proceeds by the same pathway. The desaturation (double-bond formation) is catalyzed by a desaturase enzyme *after* the elongation of the fatty acid chain. Dietary linoleic acid, which has two double bonds, can be converted by chain elongation

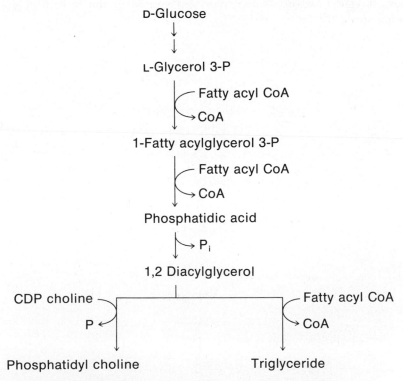

Figure 3.13 Pathways for the biosynthesis of lecithin and triglyceride.

and desaturation to arachidonic acid which has four double bonds. Although linoleic acid is the only unsaturated fatty acid that must be supplied by the diet, the three polyenoic acids, (linoleic (18:2), linolenic (18:3) and arachidonic acids (20:4)) are sometimes referred to as essential fatty acids in humans.

Triglyceride and Glycerophosphatide Synthesis. There are several pathways by which phosphatidyl choline (lecithin) can be synthesized. Two of these pathways will be considered here, one of which also serves as the pathway for triglyceride formation. The glyceryl moiety is furnished through intermediates in the glycolytic breakdown of glucose. The pathway in Figure 3.13 occurs primarily in liver and adipose tissue.

An alternative major pathway accounts for the formation of other glycerophosphatides as well as lecithin. This pathway is shown in Figure 3.14.

Because of the greater polarity of phospholipids compared with other lipid fractions, they tend to stabilize the plasma lipids in the aqueous environment of plasma. For this reason phospholipids are required for the normal transport of lipids. Severe protein deficiency as well as hepatic cell damage, due to excessive alcohol intake or to poisoning by certain chlorinated hydrocarbons such as chloroform or carbon tetrachloride, can result in the condition known as *fatty liver*. This condition is attributed to

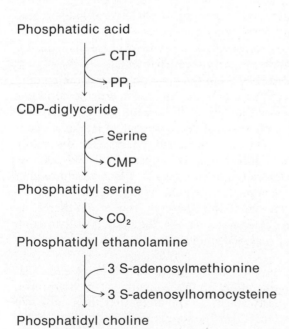

Phosphatidic acid

CTP

PP$_i$

CDP-diglyceride

Serine

CMP

Phosphatidyl serine

CO$_2$

Phosphatidyl ethanolamine

3 S-adenosylmethionine

3 S-adenosylhomocysteine

Phosphatidyl choline

Figure 3.14 Pathway for the biosynthesis of glycerophosphatides.

inadequate phospholipid synthesis in the liver and/or lack of protein which leads to reduced mobility of the triglycerides as lipoproteins. The accumulating triglycerides give rise to the clinical findings.

Cholesterol Synthesis and Metabolism. Cholesterol, like the fatty acids, is produced from acetyl CoA which can be derived from carbohydrate, protein, and/or fat (Figs. 3.9 and 3.17). Because of its complexity, however, the synthetic pathway of cholesterol will not be described in its entirety. Of perhaps greater interest is the effect dietary cholesterol has on the body's production of this sterol.

The synthesis of cholesterol occurs primarily in the liver where dietary cholesterol can exert an inhibitory feedback on production of the sterol, but another important site of synthesis is the intestine where no such feedback mechanism is apparent. Smaller amounts of cholesterol are produced in the endocrine glands from which steroid hormones are secreted, for example, adrenal cortex, testes, and ovaries.

Cholesterol is an essential compound for the proper functioning of the body because it provides the basis for the production of bile acids and all the steroid hormones. All too often, however, this importance is overlooked because of concern for its possible overabundance in the body. Because man does not possess the enzymes necessary for breaking the sterol nucleus, cholesterol cannot be catabolized to CO_2 and H_2O for excretion. The most important catabolic pathway for cholesterol is bile acid production, but because these bile acids are conserved through the *enterohepatic circulation,* only a small amount of cholesterol is excreated through this route. As a result of the body's conservation of cholesterol, an overabundance of serum cholesterol can occur whenever mechanisms for its regulation are not operating properly (see Chapter 7).

Although cholesterol absorbed from the diet can depress the amount produced endogenously, even large amounts of ingested cholesterol can reduce biosynthesis by no more than about 40 percent. This is partly due to the fact that absorption of cholesterol decreases when intake exceeds approximately 500 mg. daily. On the other hand, cholesterol absorption becomes more efficient when intake ranges between 400 and 500 mg. daily. Even a diet severely restricted in cholesterol, which would require that all circulating cholesterol come from endogenous production, can reduce serum cholesterol only about 10 to 15 percent. It appears, therefore, that although a feedback mechanism does exist, the body is able to compensate better for a lack of ingested cholesterol than for an overabundance of it.

Figure 3.15 illustrates the site where dietary cholesterol exerts its more or less imperfect inhibiting effect on the biosynthesis of cholesterol. The inhibition occurs at an early stage, immediately after three moles of acetyl CoA have been condensed into a six-carbon intermediate, 3-hy-

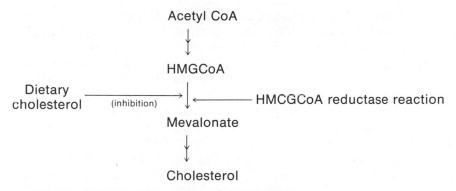

Acetyl CoA

HMGCoA

Dietary cholesterol ⟶ (inhibition) ⟵ HMCGCoA reductase reaction

Mevalonate

Cholesterol

Figure 3.15 Regulation of hepatic cholesterol synthesis.

droxy-3-methylglutaryl CoA (HMGCoA). Dietary cholesterol apparently inhibits cholesterol production by decreasing the synthesis of HMGCoA reductase, the rate-limiting enzyme in the synthetic pathway. HMGCoA is dependent upon its reductase to be transformed into mevalonate, the parent compound of cholesterol. In addition to its negative effect on synthesis of the enzyme, dietary cholesterol possibly may have a negative allosteric effect on its action (see discussion of allosteric enzymes in Chapter 1).

Proteins and Amino Acids

Digestion of Protein. It is through the action of proteolytic enzymes in the gastrointestinal tract that dietary proteins are hydrolyzed to their constituent amino acids. Proteolytic enzymes are specialized hydrolases that hydrolyze the peptide bonds that unite amino acids in the protein. Some of the enzymes are highly specific in their action, hydrolyzing only those peptide bonds contributed by certain amino acids. Others are nonspecific, hydrolyzing randomly the peptide bonds within the protein. Some are called *endopeptidases* which means they cleave peptide bonds within the inner reaches of the protein chain. The *exopeptidases* hydrolyze only the bond connecting the terminal amino acid residue with the penultimate (second from the end) residue. Some exopeptidases react at the carboxyl terminal end of the protein while others remove residues at the amino terminal end.

Digestion begins in the stomach where the endopeptidase *pepsin* hydrolyzes proteins into many smaller peptides. Pepsin is unique in that it is optimally active at the very low pH of the gastric secretions. In patients suffering from *achlorhydria* (absence of gastric hydrochloric acid), sometimes associated with pernicious anemia or gastric carcinoma, protein digestion may be incomplete. Consequently a distaste for high protein foods is sometimes reported by these patients. In the duodenum, the peptides are acted upon by a variety of pancreatic proteases, the most important of which are the endopeptidases *trypsin* and *chymotrypsin,* and the exopeptidase, *carboxypeptidase.* The elevated pH in the duodenum due to the influx of bile and pancreatic bicarbonate allows these enzymes to function optimally. There are also enzymes within the intestinal mucosal cells called *aminopeptidase* and *dipeptidases* which act on the very small peptides and dipeptides that enter the cells. Therefore, in passage through the mucosal cells enroute to the circulation, further hydrolysis occurs so that the final hydrolytic products that enter the bloodstream are free amino acids. The circulating amino acids comprise what is known as the *amino acid pool,* and from this point they may enter any of several metabolic routes depending on the body's requirements. The metabolic fate of the circulating amino acids is summarized in Figure 3.16.

As Figure 3.16 indicates, the composition of the amino acids within the pool is in a state of dynamic equilibrium. The hydrolysis of dietary pro-

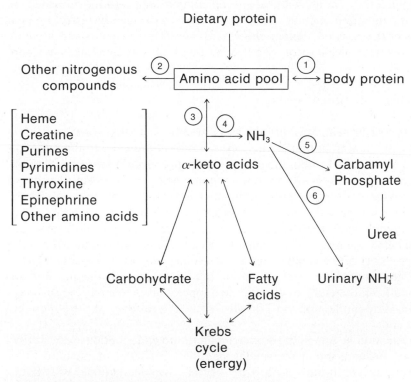

Figure 3.16 A summary of amino acid metabolism.

teins and body proteins supplies the pool with amino acids while the reactions by which they are utilized continuously remove them from the pool. For the sake of convenience in discussing the major reactions, the reactions shown in Figure 3.16 have been numbered.

Reaction ① indicates the interconversion of body protein amino acids and the amino acids of the pool. If the amino acid pool should become depleted through starvation, the breakdown of body protein is the major restorative source of amino acids. During starvation, amino acids are derived first from the plasma proteins, particularly albumin. Other rapidly metabolizing tissues such as liver, pancreas, and intestinal mucosa also tend to lose protein rapidly. Muscle protein is catabolized much more slowly. However, because of the large total mass of body muscle, this tissue represents the largest potential source of amino acids. When fat supplies are exhausted, the body may lose as much as 6 percent of its protein mass per day for energy.

Reaction ② illustrates how amino acids can be converted into a variety of other substances. The amino acids can furnish both carbon and nitrogen atoms for the synthesis of the compounds, a partial listing of which is shown in the illustration. The fact that *certain* amino acids can be synthesized from different amino acids or indirectly from carbohydrate sources (reaction ③) introduces the concept of nonessentiality in amino acids. Amino acids that are designated as *essential* or indispensable must be obtained from the diet in order for normal growth and development to proceed while nonessential amino acids can be synthesized from other sources within the organism at a rate sufficient to meet the body's needs. A third category, called *semiessential,* is composed of those amino acids that can be synthesized by the body but not at an optimal rate, so that a dietary source is also necessary. Some amino acids in this category are semiessential from another standpoint. They are nonessential only if the amino acids from which they are derived are provided in the diet in quantities sufficient to supply the necessary requirements of both. Examples are tyrosine and cystine which are derived from phenylalanine and methionine, respectively.

Reactions ③ and ④ represent the means by which amino acids become α-keto acids which are or can be converted to Krebs cycle intermediates. Therefore, these interconversions are a means by which amino acids can be oxidized for energy. The general reactions by which this is accomplished are called *transamination* and *oxidative deamination.*

Transamination. Reactions in transamination involve the transfer of the amino group from an amino acid to the carbonyl carbon of an α-keto acid, usually α-ketoglutarate. The α-ketoglutarate becomes aminated in the process, becoming glutamate, and the amino acid donating the amino

Table 3.3 Nutritive Classification of the Amino Acids

Essential	Semiessential	Nonessential
Lysine	Arginine	Glutamic acid
Tryptophan	Tyrosine	Aspartic acid
Phenylalanine	Cystine	Alanine
Methionine	Glycine	Proline
Threonine	Serine	Hydroxyproline
Leucine		
Isoleucine		
Valine		
Histidine		

group becomes the corresponding α-keto acid analog of the amino acid. An example of a transamination reaction is shown below.

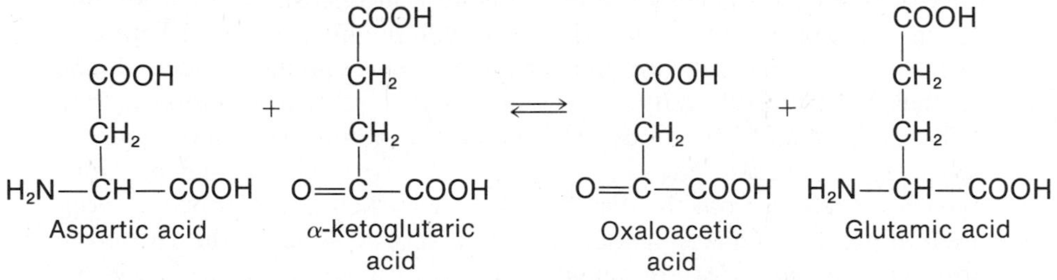

$$
\begin{array}{c}
\text{COOH} \\
|\\
\text{CH}_2 \\
|\\
\text{H}_2\text{N}-\text{CH}-\text{COOH} \\
\text{Aspartic acid}
\end{array}
\;+\;
\begin{array}{c}
\text{COOH} \\
|\\
\text{CH}_2 \\
|\\
\text{CH}_2 \\
|\\
\text{O}=\text{C}-\text{COOH} \\
\alpha\text{-ketoglutaric acid}
\end{array}
\;\rightleftharpoons\;
\begin{array}{c}
\text{COOH} \\
|\\
\text{CH}_2 \\
|\\
\text{O}=\text{C}-\text{COOH} \\
\text{Oxaloacetic acid}
\end{array}
\;+\;
\begin{array}{c}
\text{COOH} \\
|\\
\text{CH}_2 \\
|\\
\text{CH}_2 \\
|\\
\text{H}_2\text{N}-\text{CH}-\text{COOH} \\
\text{Glutamic acid}
\end{array}
$$

This reaction is catalyzed by the enzyme, *aspartate amino transferase* (also called glutamic oxaloacetic transaminase). All transaminases require pyridoxal phosphate as a cofactor, and the reactions are freely reversible. The aspartate amino transferase reaction allows the conversion of two amino acids, aspartate and glutamate, into their respective α-keto acids, oxaloacetate and α-ketoglutarate. In a similar fashion alanine can serve as amino group donor with α-ketoglutarate as the recipient. Alanine would thus become pyruvate and α-ketoglutarate, in aquiring the amino group, would become glutamate. As mentioned previously, the α-keto acids are metabolized via the Krebs cycle for energy. In addition to those already discussed, there are many other amino acids that undergo transamination reactions with α-ketoglutarate. These reactions, therefore, generate large amounts of glutamate which serves as a source of ammonia for the urea cycle which will be discussed later. Most amino acids after undergoing transamination obviously do not become Krebs cycle keto acids directly. However, the carbon skeleton of nearly all the amino acids is ultimately converted to other cycle intermediates. Although these pathways will not be discussed here, the entry of amino acids into the Krebs cycle is summarized in Figure 3.17.

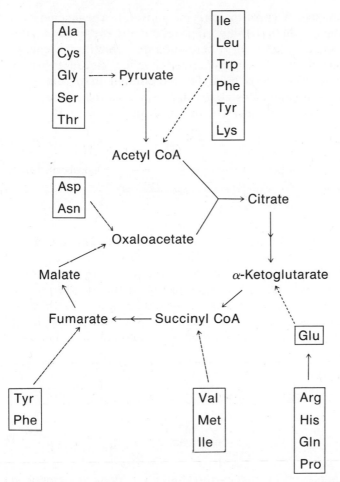

Figure 3.17 Pathways of entry of the carbon skeletons of amino acids into the Krebs cycle.

Oxidative Deamination. A common feature of both oxidative deamination and transamination is that both reactions involve the removal of an amino group from an amino acid, leaving behind an α-keto group. But whereas the amino group is transferred to a keto recipient in transamination, oxidative deamination produces free ammonium ions which eventually are excreted in the urine as such or in the form of urea. These reactions are catalyzed by L-*amino acid oxidase*, an FAD-linked enzyme with a broad specificity. The general reaction can be represented as:

$$\text{L-amino acids} \xrightarrow[\text{FAD} \quad \text{FADH}_2]{} \alpha\text{-keto acids} + NH_4^+$$

Although the broad specificity of the enzyme allows for the deamination of several amino acids, the most important reaction is the oxidative deamination of glutamate, producing α-ketoglutarate, which is an energy source as a Krebs cycle metabolite, and ammonium ion. Because there is such a large amount of glutamate being formed continuously from α-ketoglutarate by transamination, this compound serves as the major intermediary donor of urinary nitrogen. The deamination is catalyzed

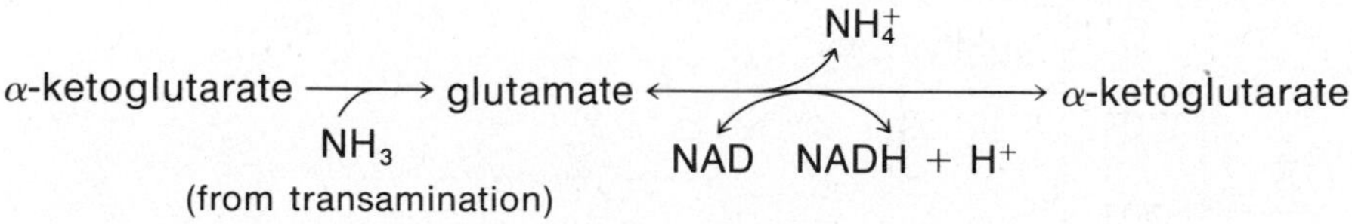

$$\alpha\text{-ketoglutarate} \xrightarrow[\substack{NH_3 \\ \text{(from transamination)}}]{} glutamate \xleftrightarrow[NAD \quad NADH + H^+]{NH_4^+} \alpha\text{-ketoglutarate}$$

by *glutamate dehydrogenase,* an NAD-requiring enzyme. The fate of the large amount of NH_4^+ so formed will be discussed next.

Reaction ⑤, (Fig. 3.16), showing formation of urea from ammonia via carbamyl phosphate, is the major route for the elimination of protein nitrogen. The average adult excretes approximately 30 g of urea per day.

The first step in the formation of urea is the synthesis of *carbamyl phosphate* from carbon dioxide, ammonium ions, and ATP.

$$CO_2 + NH_4^+ + 2ATP \longrightarrow \underbrace{H_2N-\overset{\overset{\displaystyle O}{\|}}{C}-OP}_{\substack{\text{Carbamyl} \\ \text{phosphate}}} + 2ADP + P_i$$

The CO_2 in this reaction, as in most carboxylation reactions, is introduced as a complex with biotin. The complex, referred to as "active CO_2," is shown in Chapter 2 under the topic of biotin structure and function. Most of the NH_4^+ entering the reaction is from oxidative deamination of amino acids, primarily via the glutamate dehydrogenase reaction. Synthesis of carbamyl phosphate is an energy-expending reaction requiring two ATPs per mole of carbamyl phosphate. Urea is formed in the liver through a cycle of reactions called the *urea cycle* (Fig. 3.18).

Free ammonia (as serum NH_4^+) is highly toxic to the central nervous system and must not be allowed to accumulate. It has already been shown in Figures 3.16 (Reaction ⑤) and 3.18 how incorporation of NH_4^+ into carbamyl phosphate and its subsequent excretion as urea prevents accumulation of this toxin. Another means by which ammonium ion is excreted is also represented in Figure 3.16 (Reaction ⑥). In this reaction, NH_4^+ is detoxified by conversion to glutamine which, in turn, is hydrolyzed to free

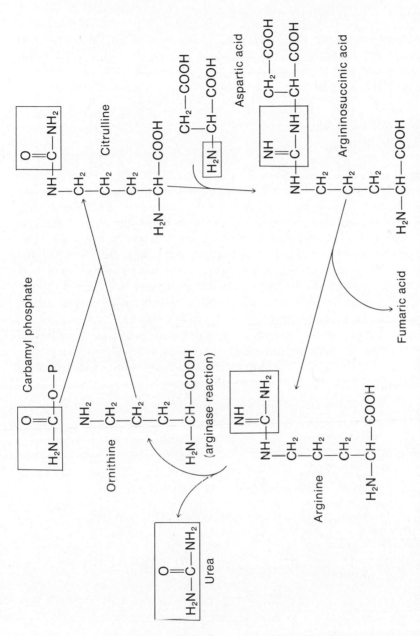

Figure 3.18 The urea cycle. (Portions of the intermediates are enclosed by blocks to trace the atoms comprising the urea molecule).

NH_4^+ in the kidney. Both brain and liver are active in the detoxification reaction, which requires the enzyme *glutamine synthetase*.

$$NH_4^+ + \text{Glutamate} \rightarrow \text{Glutamine}$$

As nontoxic glutamine, the "ammonia" is transported via the general circulation to the kidneys. Within the tubule cells of the kidney, the glutamine is hydrolyzed to glutamate and NH_4^+ by the enzyme, *glutaminase*. The free NH_4^+ is secreted by the tubule cells directly into the urine.

Nucleotide Biosynthesis and Catabolism

Synthesis of Purine Nucleotides. The dependence of life upon RNA and DNA as described in Chapter 1 makes essential an understanding of the metabolism of their purine and pyrimidine components. Both purine and pyrimidine nucleotides can be acquired through the diet. Meat, particularly organ meat such as liver, is a rich source of DNA and RNA. The exopancreas secretes nucleases that hydrolyze the large nucleic acids into their constituent nucleotides, small amounts of which can be absorbed directly and utilized. Most dietary purine, however, is oxidized to uric acid by enzymes in the intestinal mucosa and excreted in this form. Nearly all the purine used for the synthesis of DNA and RNA, is assembled from assorted precursor substances. The detailed biosynthesis pathways will not be covered, although it is of interest to trace the atoms of the purine nucleus to the precursor compounds that furnish them. Adenosine 5'-monophosphate will be discussed in this regard.

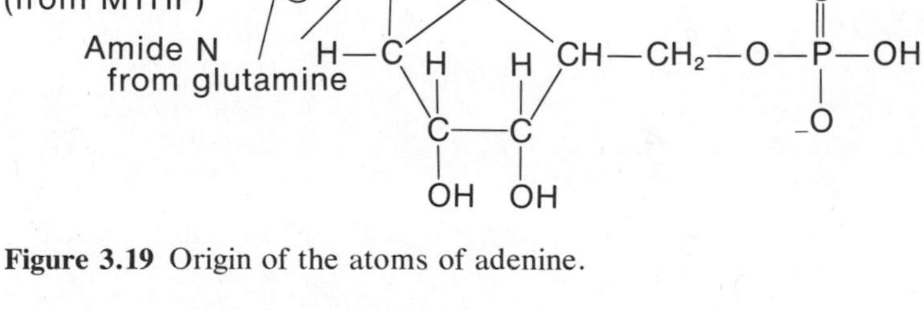

Figure 3.19 Origin of the atoms of adenine.

The biosynthesis is initiated by the reaction between 5-phosphoribo-syl-1-pyrophosphate (PRPP) and glutamine as shown below:

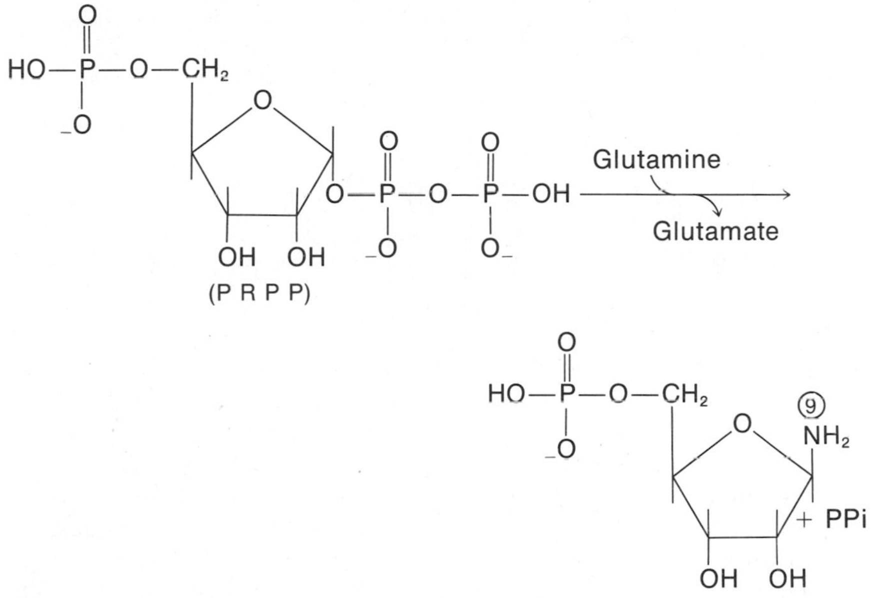

(P R P P)

As indicated, the nitrogen atom numbered nine in the purine nucleus is donated by the amide group of glutamine. Listed below, in the order in which they are introduced, are the remaining atom donors:

1. Glycine; the nitrogen ⑦ and carbons ④ ⑤ are introduced as a single unit.
2. Formate, from methylene tetrahydrofolate ⑧
3. Glutamine amide nitrogen ③
4. CO_2 as "active CO_2" ⑥
5. Aspartic acid nitrogen ①
6. Formate, from methylene tetrahydrofolate ②
7. Aspartic acid nitrogen ⑩

Catabolism of Purine Nucleotides. The ribonucleotides and deoxyribonu-cleotides derived from the hydrolysis of nucleic acids are catabolized to their sugar, phosphate, and purine and pyrimidine bases. The intracellular oxidation of the purine itself culminates in the formation of uric acid which is the excretory product of purines in man. Using adenosine mono-phosphate once again as an example, the oxidation takes place according to the following pathway:

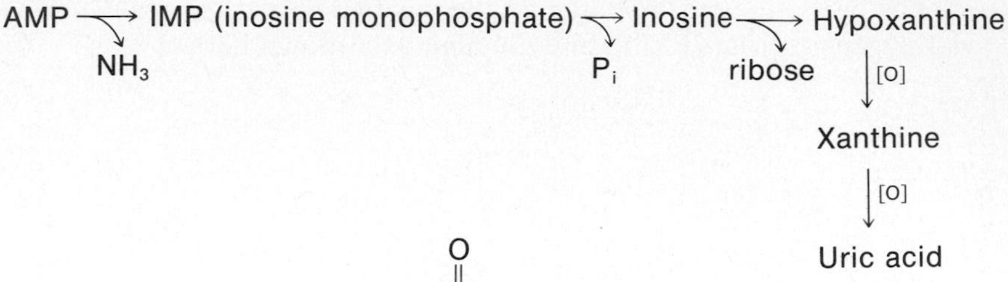

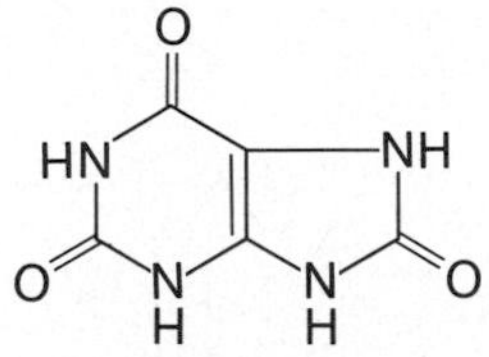

AMP $\longrightarrow$ IMP (inosine monophosphate) $\longrightarrow$ Inosine $\longrightarrow$ Hypoxanthine

$\quad\quad$ NH$_3$ $\quad\quad\quad\quad\quad\quad\quad\quad\quad\quad\quad\quad\quad\quad\quad$ P$_i$ $\quad\quad$ ribose $\quad$ | [O]

$\quad\quad\quad\quad\quad\quad\quad\quad\quad\quad\quad\quad\quad\quad\quad\quad\quad\quad\quad\quad\quad\quad\quad\quad\quad\quad$ Xanthine

$\quad\quad\quad\quad\quad\quad\quad\quad\quad\quad\quad\quad\quad\quad\quad\quad\quad\quad\quad\quad\quad\quad\quad\quad\quad\quad\quad\quad$ | [O]

$\quad\quad\quad\quad\quad\quad\quad\quad\quad\quad\quad\quad\quad\quad\quad\quad\quad\quad\quad\quad\quad\quad\quad\quad\quad\quad$ Uric acid

Uric acid

It can be seen that the reactions of the pathway did not disrupt the core structure of the purine. The oxidation of hypoxanthine to xanthine and the oxidation of xanthine to uric acid are catalyzed by the enzyme *xanthine oxidase,* found in milk, liver, and the intestinal mucosa.

The disease known as *gout* is associated with high levels of serum uric acid and results in the deposition of urate salts in various tissues, primarily cartilage and periarticular structure. Acute inflammation involving the joints, a condition mimicking that of arthritis, is a consequence. The reason for the hyperuricemia is not clearly understood, but the drug allopurinol, which is an inhibitor of xanthine oxidase, sometimes has beneficial effects in the treatment of the disease.

Synthesis of Pyrimidine Nucleotides. Unlike the synthesis of the purine nucleotides, the pyrimidine ring is formed before the ribose phosphate portion is attached. The initial reaction in the sequence is catalyzed by *carbamyl phosphate synthetase,* a cytoplasmic enzyme that forms carbamyl phosphate:

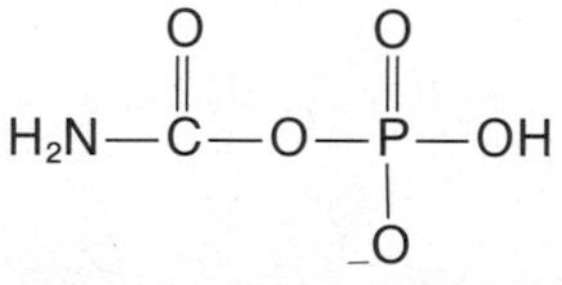

$$H_2N-\overset{\overset{O}{\|}}{C}-O-\overset{\overset{O}{\|}}{\underset{\underset{O}{|}}{P}}-OH$$

from CO_2, ATP, and $\overset{+}{N}H_4$, contributed mainly by glutamate. The ring is formed from the reaction of the carbamyl phosphate with aspartate, with subsequent dehydration to effect ring closure. The origin of the atoms of uridine monophosphate is shown below. In the formation of thymine, the pyrimidine found only in DNA, a methyl group replaces the hydrogen at carbon 5. This methylation is accomplished through the coenzyme 5,10 methylene tetrahydrofolate (5,10 methylene THF). DNA

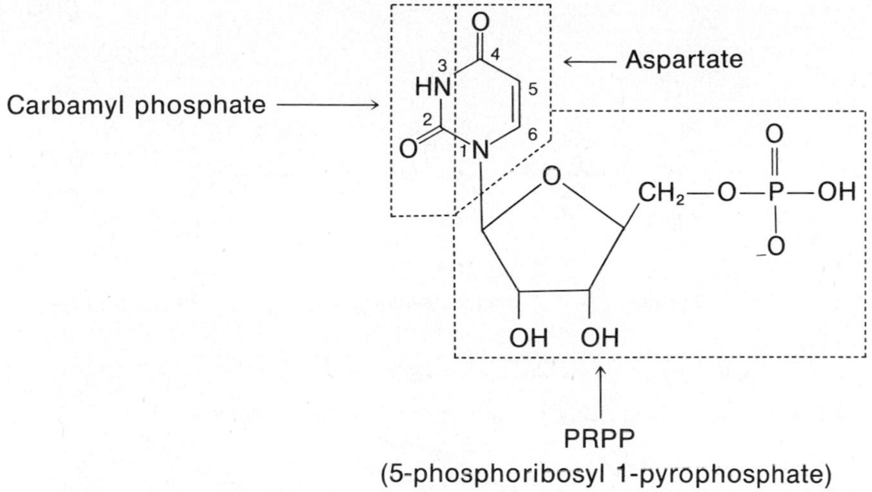

Carbamyl phosphate ⟶

Aspartate ⟵

PRPP
(5-phosphoribosyl 1-pyrophosphate)

synthesis, then, is in fact dependent upon the availability of a vitamin! Here again is an illustration of the interrelationship between nutrients and life.

Catabolism of Pyrimidines. The catabolism of the pyrimidine nucleus is initiated by the reduction of the Δ5 double bond by an NADPH-requiring dehydrogenase. The ring subsequently is opened by a hydrolytic reaction which cleaves the bond between atoms three and four. Ammonia and carbon dioxide are next removed from the carbamyl portion producing β-alanine (H_3^+N—CH_2—CH_2—COO^-), which in turn undergoes transamination to become malonate semi-aldehyde (^-OHC—CH_2—COO^-). The pyrimidine thymine, with its additional methyl group, becomes methyl malonyl through the same sequence of reactions.

Heme Biosynthesis and Catabolism

The synthesis of *heme,* which is the prosthetic group of hemoglobin, myoglobin, and the cytochromes, is an excellent example of how large, complex molecules can be produced from small precursor substances. In this pathway, succinyl CoA, a Krebs cycle metabolite, combines with glycine to initiate the series of reactions. Glycine is, of course, obtainable from dietary protein, but it also can be formed from serine by removal of the —CH_2OH serine side chain by transmethylation, that is, CH_2OH is picked up by tetrahydrofolate to form methylene tetrahydrofolate. The MTHF, in turn, can donate the one-carbon unit for the synthesis of other compounds such as purines (see purine biosynthesis).

The structure of heme, as shown in Figure 3.20, therefore consists of four pyrrole rings connected by methene bridges. In hemoglobin, the fer-

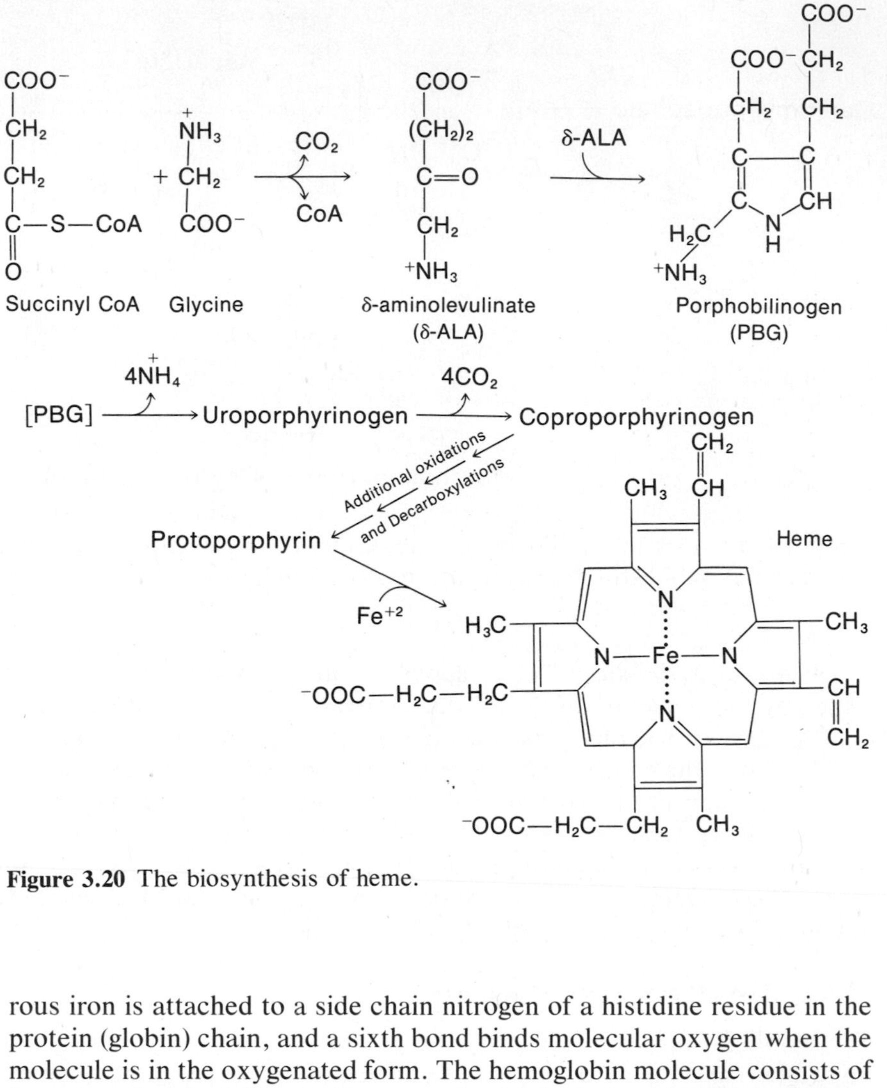

Figure 3.20 The biosynthesis of heme.

rous iron is attached to a side chain nitrogen of a histidine residue in the protein (globin) chain, and a sixth bond binds molecular oxygen when the molecule is in the oxygenated form. The hemoglobin molecule consists of four associated globin chains to each of which is attached one heme group.

The enzymes catalyzing the reactions in heme synthesis are particularly vulnerable to lead toxicity. In fact, the manifestations of lead poisoning are due to blocks in the pathway, leading to the accumulation of intermediates, such as δ-ALA and certain porphyrins. δ-ALA dehydratase, which converts two δ-ALAs to PBG, is especially susceptible to lead toxicity, but other enzymes in the pathway are also affected.

Diseases known as the *porphyrias* are genetic disorders of metabolism attributed to deficiencies of various enzymes in the pathway of heme synthesis. The result is that porphyrins and their precursors accumulate to high levels in various tissues, leading to bizarre manifestations such as intense abdominal pain, seizures, psychoses, and coma.

The *catabolism of heme* follows a brief course leading to the formation of bilirubin, which is excreted by the liver into the bile. Red blood cells have an average life span of 120 days. Damaged or aged cells are removed from the circulation by cells of the reticuloendothelial system, particularly the spleen. In the reticuloendothelial cells, the heme is dissociated from the globin, the iron is removed and enters the iron stores for future utilization, and the porphyrin ring is opened oxidatively. In the latter reaction, the methene opposite the two pyrroles having a propionic acid side chain is oxidatively removed as CO.

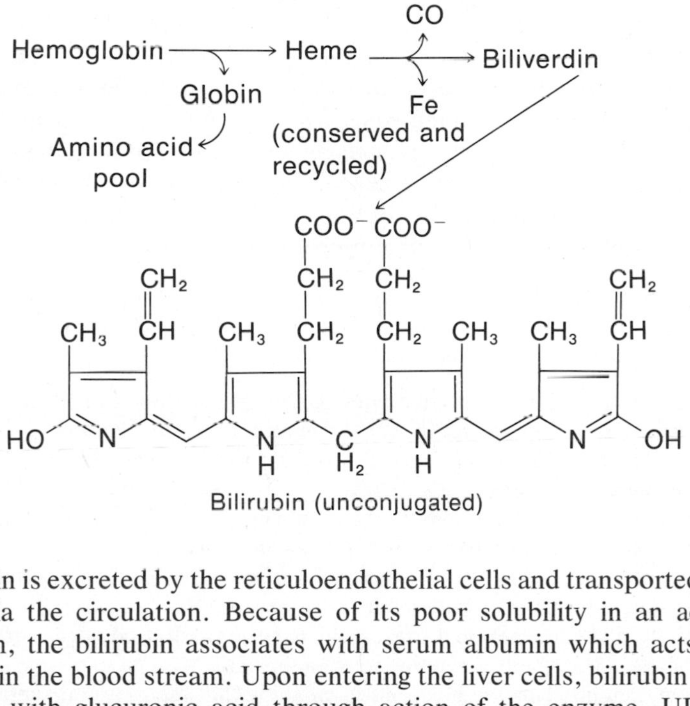

Bilirubin (unconjugated)

Bilirubin is excreted by the reticuloendothelial cells and transported to the liver via the circulation. Because of its poor solubility in an aqueous medium, the bilirubin associates with serum albumin which acts as its carrier in the blood stream. Upon entering the liver cells, bilirubin is conjugated with glucuronic acid through action of the enzyme, UDP-glucuronyl transferase. The conjugation involves the attachment of a glucuronic acid to each of the proprionic acid side chains of the bilirubin. The conjugation, by incorporating hydrophilic centers into the structure, greatly enhances the water solubility of the bilirubin and makes it possible for it to be excreted into the aqueous bile. The product of the conjugation is called conjugated bilirubin.

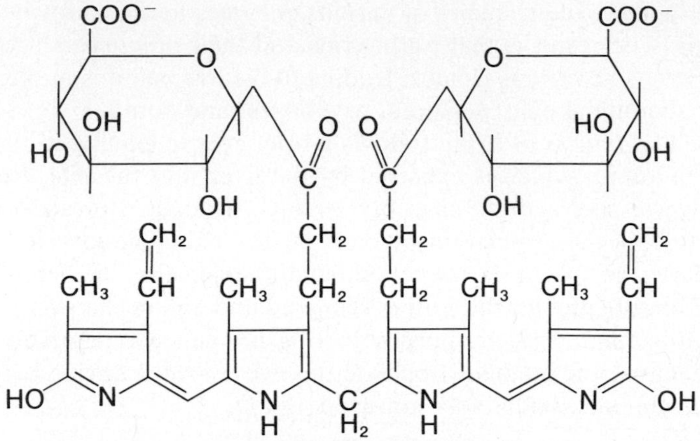

Bilirubin (conjugated)

As discussed in Chapter 8, hepatic dysfunction due to liver disease or bile duct obstruction can result in jaundice, attributable to impaired excretion of the bilirubin with increased concentration in the serum. Still another cause for jaundice, however, is an accelerated breakdown of hemoglobin, such as in hemolytic disease. In such a case, the liver cannot conjugate the excessive amount of bilirubin being delivered to it, resulting in an accumulation of serum unconjugated bilirubin.

Questions

1. Energy production is associated with oxidation reactions in intermediary metabolism. Explain this in terms of the respiratory chain function.
2. Explain the biochemical basis for the ketosis and acidosis observed in starvation or diabetes.
3. Why, under normal conditions, is the serum cholesterol somewhat self-limiting in spite of excessive dietary intake of the compound?
4. Explain the fact that the hexosemonophosphate shunt is very important in adipose tissue while it is of little importance in muscle.
5. What effect would emotional stress (which causes increased release of epinephrine) have on the body's requirement for insulin?
6. a) Some amino acids are glycogenic, meaning that their carbon skeletons can be used for the synthesis of glucose. What is the name for the biosynthesis pathway? List five glycogenic amino acids.
   b) Some amino acids are ketogenic, indicating that their carbon structure is converted into ketonic compounds, such as acetoacetyl CoA and acetyl CoA. Explain the fact that there can consequently be no net synthesis of glucose from ketogenic amino acids.

CHAPTER 4

Fluid and Electrolyte Balance

The human body is an intricate mechanism composed of millions of individual cells which must act collectively as an organism capable of performing numerous functions. While each cellular unit is capable of individual and often highly specialized activity, all of the body's cells must exist together in a uniform and highly constant environment which is conducive to their optimal activity. This constant internal environment in which each cell exists is termed a homeostatic state meaning that while there may be many minor changes occurring at frequent intervals throughout the body, there is almost no discernible change with respect to the total environment, which includes total body fluid volume, fluid pH, and the concentration of electrolytes dissolved in the body fluids. Although acidic and basic compounds are continually taken in or produced by the body, compensatory mechanisms associated with the control of the constancy of fluid volume and the concentration of electrolytes handle these compounds so that they do not affect the homeostatic state adversely.

Virtually every system of the body plays some role in the control of fluids and electrolytes, but the systems that are usually considered to be of major importance are the lungs and the kidneys. The mechanisms by which these systems contribute to the constancy of the internal environment will be discussed at a later point in this chapter, but first, a review of some pertinent information concerning the internal environment of the body is in order.

The total volume of fluid in the body of an average 70 kg adult is 40 liters and is referred to as total body water. Total body water is compartmentalized by numerous membranes into the intracellular fluid, contained within the cells, and the extracellular fluid, which includes all of the remaining fluid not contained within the cells. The primary extracellular fluids are the fluid that surrounds cells (interstitial fluid) and serum, the liquid component of blood, which contains both dissolved and suspended particles. The intracellular and extracellular fluid compartments, while separated by membranes, are in constant contact to allow essential materials and waste products to be interchanged as required by various body components. The interchange of such materials across membranes occurs by one or more of the following processes:

Simple diffusion. This is the process by which substances move from an area of high concentration to an area of lower concentration without the expenditure of energy. Substances that diffuse across biological membranes, if water soluble, must be of low enough molecular weight to pass through the membrane pores. Fat-soluble substances can selectively diffuse through the lipid layers of the membrane. Simple diffusion processes occur as a body mechanism to equalize the concentration of substances on opposite sides of biological membranes. The amount of diffusion that can occur is influenced by the concentration gradient, electrical gradient, and pressure gradient. A concentration gradient is produced by an unequal number of particles on opposite sides of a membrane, while an electrical gradient is produced by an unequal number of charged particles on opposite sides of a membrane. Particles of opposite charge attract each other and diffuse across membranes, thus maintaining electrical neutrality. Even though there are positively charged, nondiffusable ions in biological fluids, this electrical neutrality is maintained by negatively charged particles that can freely diffuse across membranes. Electrical neutrality is further maintained because membrane pores are lined with positively charged calcium ions that prevent the diffusion of other cations and allow the diffusion of anions. The pressure gradient is the difference between the pressure on opposite sides of a membrane. In the body, the higher blood pressure on the arterial side of a capillary will force fluid from the capillary into interstitial fluid spaces, while on the venous side of the capillary the decreased pressure gradient will allow fluid to pass from the interstitium into the venule.

Facilitated diffusion. This is a mechanism by which particles too large for simple diffusion are transported through membranes. With this type of diffusion, the transport of particles from an area of high concentration to an area of lower concentration is facilitated by a carrier protein. This carrier combines with the substance to be transported on one side of the membrane, forming a fat-soluble complex that diffuses to the other side of the membrane where the substance is released. No energy is required for this process.

Active transport. This is the process by which substances are moved across biological membranes against concentration gradients. Active transport resembles facilitated diffusion in that a carrier is required but differs in that energy is required to overcome the concentration gradient. Active transport is responsible for mechanisms such as the movement of glucose across membranes of the gastrointestinal tract and the concentration of sodium outside of nerve cells. Energy for active transport mechanisms is derived from adenosine triphosphate (ATP).

Osmosis. This is the process by which water diffuses across biological membranes. When membranes, which are permeable to water, separate unequal concentrations of particles, water will diffuse through the membrane from an area of high water concentration to an area of low water concentration. This is the same as saying that water moves from an area of low solute concentration to an area of high solute concentration. Osmotic pressure is a measure of the number of particles in a unit volume of liquid and is determined by the total number of particles on either side of a membrane. The distribution of particles in any fluid compartment will determine the water concentration in that compartment.

Diffusion and active transport processes primarily involve the movement of charged particles, gases (oxygen and carbon dioxide) and other small molecules across biological membranes. Various other substances of high molecular weight found in body fluids also add to the total number of particles present and influence osmotic pressure. Such substances are usually nondiffusible and, therefore, cannot cross biological membranes except in the case of the transfer of some high molecular weight substances through membranes by the process of endocytosis. The osmotic pressure produced by nondiffusible particles is termed *colloid osmotic pressure*.

The movement of particles across biological membranes is controlled by the interplay of these mechanisms which allow for the transfer of nutrients and waste products into and out of cells via the interstitial fluids and capillaries. An example of the relationships among capillary pressure, interstitial pressure, interstitial fluid colloid osmotic pressure, and plasma colloid osmotic pressure is illustrated in Figure 4.1. At the arterial end of the capillary, pressure produced by the pumping action of the heart produces a capillary pressure of 25 mm Hg, interstitial fluid pressure is 7.0 mm Hg, interstitial fluid colloid osmotic pressure is 4.5 mm Hg, and plasma colloid osmotic pressure is 28 mm Hg. Therefore, the total force moving fluids from inside the capillary is 36.5 mm Hg and the total inward

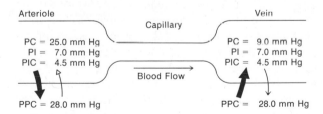

Arteriole   Vein

Capillary

PC = 25.0 mm Hg   PC = 9.0 mm Hg
PI = 7.0 mm Hg   PI = 7.0 mm Hg
PIC = 4.5 mm Hg   PIC = 4.5 mm Hg

Blood Flow

PPC = 28.0 mm Hg   PPC = 28.0 mm Hg

PC = capillary pressure
PI = interstitial fluid pressure
PIC = interstitial fluid colloid osmotic pressure
PPC = plasma colloid osmotic pressure

Figure 4.1 Relationships among capillary pressure, interstitial pressure, interstitial fluid colloid pressure and plasma colloid osmotic pressure.

force is 28 mm Hg. The difference in pressure gradient of 8.5 mm Hg results in the movement of fluids from the capillary into the interstitial spaces. At the venule end of the capillary the capillary pressure is only 9.0 mm Hg and the interstitial fluid pressure and interstitial fluid colloid osmotic pressure remain the same as at the arterial end. The total inward pressure due to plasma colloids also remains at 28.0 mm Hg. Because the outward pressure totals 20.5 mm Hg and the inward pressure is 28 mm Hg, the difference in pressure of 7.5 mm Hg will cause fluids to leave the interstitial spaces and enter the capillary.

As long as the fluid volume in the interstitial spaces remains small, substances will transfer rapidly into and out of the capillaries along electrical or concentration gradients. However, some physical abnormalities such as congestive heart failure, carcinomas, and burns produce alterations in one or more of the factors that control the normal movement of capillary fluids. Such alterations will result in edema, and excessive accumulation of fluid in the interstitial spaces. Edema in turn causes a decrease in the rate of transfer of substances from capillaries into the interstitial spaces and waste products from the interstitial spaces back into the capillaries.

MAINTENANCE OF FLUID BALANCE

Fluid balance in the body is a function of normal compartmentalization of fluids which is governed by osmotic pressure and by the intake and output of fluids by body mechanisms. Water enters the body as a part of beverages, liquids contained in foods, and as water released as a product of chemical reactions. These routes account for daily intake of approximately 2600 ml of fluid. Fluid intake must be adequate because of the importance of water in maintaining blood volume, the transfer of nutrients and waste products, and regulation of metabolic processes. Approximately 2600 ml of water is lost daily from the body via urine (1500 ml), fecal excretion (100 ml), and via the lungs and skin (1000 ml).

The primary organ involved in the control of fluid balance is the kidney, which removes or retains fluids according to the requirements of the body. The anatomy, physiology, and functions of the kidney are discussed in detail in Chapter 10. The basic functional unit of the kidney is the nephron. There are over a million nephrons in each kidney, and each nephron is composed of a glomerulus and a tubule. The glomerulus, a membrane capsule that encloses a group of capillaries, acts as a filter in removing water and other substances including electrolytes, glucose, amino acids, and waste products from plasma. The glomerulus prevents filtration of plasma cells and proteins because of their larger size. The filtered substances are termed the *glomerular filtrate*. The tubule consists of a proximal convoluted portion, descending and ascending limbs of the loop of Henle, distal convoluted portion, and collecting duct. Each of these tubular segments is functionally distinct in its permeability to electrolytes and water. The tubule is surrounded by a network of capillaries, the peritubular capillary plexus, which reabsorbs some substances from the glomerular filtrate and carries them back into the blood stream. The peritubular capillaries may also secrete substances from blood into the renal tubule.

The hormonal substances that affect the kidney are responsible for fluid balance. Antidiuretic hormone (ADH) is produced in the supraoptic nucleus of the hypothalamus but is stored in and secreted by the posterior pituitary gland. The secretion of ADH is stimulated by hypertonicity (increased solute concentration) of plasma. Osmoreceptors, located in the hypothalamus, respond to the hypertonic plasma by stimulating the release of ADH from the pituitary gland. Because hypertonic plasma indicates that the body's water volume is low, ADH is released into the blood stream and transported to the kidney where it causes urine to be excreted in a concentrated form and thus conserves water in the body. If plasma is hypotonic, no ADH will be released from the pituitary and the kidney will excrete a large volume of dilute urine. ADH produces its effects on the distal tubule and collecting ducts, causing them to become more permeable to water. Thus, water leaves the lumen of the tubule and ducts and is reabsorbed into the peritubular capillaries. Solutes remain in the glomerular filtrate and the urine excreted is very concentrated. When a sufficient amount of fluid has been conserved by this mechanism, the plasma passing through the hypothalamus becomes isotonic, due to the return of fluid into the blood stream, and the stimulus for ADH secretion is no longer present.

A second hormone, aldosterone, is produced and secreted by the adrenal cortex. Aldosterone affects fluid volume by causing the reabsorption of sodium from the glomerular filtrate back into the peritubular capillaries and thus into the blood. The increase in sodium reabsorption causes plasma to become hypertonic which, in turn, will stimulate the release of ADH. ADH then stimulates the reabsorption of water which returns the plasma to an isotonic state. The net result of the action of aldosterone and ADH is an increase in extracellular fluid volume.

ELECTROLYTE BALANCE

The kidney is also of primary importance in the regulation of electrolyte balance, that is, the concentration of anions and cations in the body fluid compartments. As the glomerular filtrate moves through the renal tubule, various substances are reabsorbed from the tubule into the peritubular capillaries or secreted from these capillaries into the renal tubule. Most of the reabsorption of solutes from the glomerular filtrate occurs in the proximal convoluted tubule. Glucose and amino acids are almost entirely reabsorbed by an active transport process at this site. In addition, active transport accounts for the reabsorption of 80 percent of sodium, potassium, and other positively charged electrolytes (cations) from the proximal convoluted tubule. Because of the active transport of cations out of the tubule, negatively charged electrolytes (anions) such as chloride and bicarbonate passively diffuse out of the tubule to maintain electrical neutrality. As the solute moves out of the tubule, water also diffuses out to maintain normal osmotic pressure.

The loop of Henle is responsible for dilution of the glomerular filtrate and a further decrease in its volume. Although some water is reabsorbed from the descending limb of the loop of Henle, the ascending limb of the loop of Henle is impermeable to water. Chloride, however, is removed from the filtrate by active transport in the ascending limb. Therefore, the filtrate becomes hypoponic by the time it reaches the end of the loop of Henle.

The distal tubule and collecting ducts are the sites at which final alterations in the concentration of the glomerular filtrate occur. At these sites, aldosterone influences the reabsorption of sodium and ADH increases the reabsorption of water. Also at these sites, hydrogen and potassium ions and ammonia are removed from the fluid of the peritubular capillaries and secreted into the glomerular filtrate. Potassium or hydrogen ions are secreted into the glomerular filtrate as a mechanism of exchange for the sodium ions, which are reabsorbed. This exchange mechanism is necessary in order to maintain electrical neutrality. Whether potassium or hydrogen is exchanged for sodium is probably dependent on the relative concentration of each in body fluids although the exact mechanism for this selection procedure is unknown. This mechanism is of extreme importance to normal body functions because the maintenance of the concentrations of specific cations—sodium, potassium, and calcium—is critical to many body functions. Greatly decreased extracellular potassium (hypokalemia) will produce paralysis, while severely elevated potassium levels (hyperkalemia) will produce cardiac arrhythmias. Excessive extracellular sodium (hypernatremia) will produce fluid retention and decreased plasma calcium (hypocalcemia) will produce tetany by increasing the permeability of nerve cell membranes to sodium. Table 4.1 indicates normal fluid electrolytes and their concentrations.

The exchange of sodium and potassium is also of importance in the generation and propagation of electrical impulses in nerves. In nerve cells, the concentration of sodium is greater on the outside of the membrane and that of potassium is greater on the inside of the membrane. It is thought that the same carrier for this active transport process is responsible for the movement of sodium out of the cell and potassium into the cell. The carrier, an enzyme, undergoes a chemical change that increases its

Table 4.1 Electrolyte Concentrations in Extracellular and Intracellular Fluids*

Electrolyte	Extracellular fluid (mEq/liter)	Intracellular fluid (mEq/liter)
Sodium (Na^+)	142	10
Potassium (K^+)	5	141
Calcium (Ca^{++})	5	<1
Magnesium (Mg^{++})	3	58
Bicarbonate (HCO_3^-)	28	10
Chloride (Cl^-)	103	4
Sulfate (SO_4^{--})	1	2
Phosphates	4	75

*Source: From Guyton, *Textbook of Medical Physiology,* 1976.

affinity for either sodium or potassium. The carrier attaches to potassium ions at the outside of the membrane, transports the potassium through the membrane and releases it on the inside of the cell. The carrier then undergoes a chemical change, attaches to a sodium ion and transports it to the outside of the cellular membrane. The energy for this active transport process is supplied by adenosine triphosphate (ATP). Adenosine triphosphatase acts on ATP in the presence of magnesium to break a high-energy phosphate bond, which creates the energy for this system. Conduction of electrical impulses along nerves occurs due to a change in the cell membrane's permeability to sodium ions which allows sodium to flow to the inside of the cell. This process is termed *depolarization* and its occurrence is regulated by the movement of calcium ions from specific sites on the cell membrane to allow for the inward movement of sodium. As the sodium concentration increases inside the membrane, the outside of the membrane becomes electrically negative to the inside. When sodium concentration reaches a critical level inside the membrane, potassium ions are forced to the outside of the membrane due to the repulsion of like-charged particles. This process is repeated over and over as an impulse travels down a nerve. For the nerve to return to its original condition (repolarization), sodium ions are actively transported to the outside of the membrane and exchanged for potassium ions.

ACID-BASE BALANCE— CONTROL OF HYDROGEN ION CONCENTRATION

Acid-base balance or the control of hydrogen ion concentration in the body fluids is critical to the normal functioning of the body. Hydrogen ion concentration, abbreviated [H^+], is usually expressed with the symbol pH which is defined as the negative logarithm of the hydrogen concentration. This may be represented as

$$pH = -\log[H^+]$$

The hydrogen ion concentration in plasma, expressed exponentially, is 4×10^{-8} equivalents per liter. This may be converted to pH notation as:

$$pH = -\log[H^+]$$

$$pH = -\log[4 \times 10^{-8}]$$

$$pH = \log \frac{1}{4} \times 10^{-8}$$

$$pH = 7.4$$

Utilization of pH notation in the expression of hydrogen ion concentration is much simpler for calculations than the exponential notation form. A low pH value indicates a high hydrogen ion concentration as in acidosis while a high pH value represents a low hydrogen ion concentration as in alkalosis.

The term *equivalent* (as in 4×10^{-8} equivalents per liter) refers to the chemical reactivity or combining power of electrolytes. One equivalent of a substance is the amount of that substance that will combine with one atomic weight of hydrogen. A milliequivalent is $\frac{1}{1000}$ of an equivalent. The term milliequivalent is usually used in describing the concentration of electrolytes (substances that dissociate into ions) in the body fluids because these solutions are dilute and milliequivalent values allow us to work with whole numbers. Substances that do not dissociate in body fluids are usually quantitated in terms of weight such as milligrams per 100 milliliters (mg %) or osmotic pressure exerted, for example, millimeters of mercury (mm Hg).

The equivalent value or chemical reactivity of a compound that dissociates is calculated from its chemical characteristics and is dependent on the ionic charge and concentration in solution.

Equivalents (or usually milliequivalents) are calculated on the basis of the atomic weight of the components of a substance. The atomic weight of an atom is a number that expresses its weight in relation to that of an atom of oxygen whose atomic weight is 16. The molecular weight of a compound is equal to the sum of the atomic weights of all the atoms in one molecule of that compound. For example, the molecular weight of sodium chloride (NaCl) is equal to the sum of the atomic weight of sodium (23) and chloride (35) or 58.

Gram molecular weight is an expression of the molecular weight in grams and is abbreviated mol. One mol of sodium chloride is thus calculated as the sum of the atomic weights of sodium and chloride (23 + 35) and weighs 58 grams. One millimol (mm) or $\frac{1}{1000}$ of a mol of sodium chloride would weigh 58 mg. When one mol of sodium chloride is dissolved in one liter of water, the solution contains one mol per liter (1 mol/L).

When an equivalent is expressed in terms of weight, it is called a gram equivalent weight. The equivalent weight of an ion is determined by dividing the atomic weight expressed in grams by the number of charges associated with the ion (valence). For sodium, the gram equivalent weight is $23/1 = 23$ (atomic weight = 23; valence = 1). The gram equivalent weight of chloride is $35/1$ or 35. One mol of sodium chloride (58 g) would, therefore, contain one equivalent of sodium and one equivalent of chloride.

The distribution of electrolytes in body fluid compartments varies markedly and yet the total chemical reactivity within a compartment is neutral because the total number of milliequivalents of cations is in equilibrium with the total number of milliequivalents of anions. This state is termed electrical neutrality and must be maintained, as previously mentioned, in order for normal physiological activity to occur.

The optimal pH value at which the body operates ranges from 7.35 to 7.45. There are several body mechanisms that work in combination to maintain this normal pH range. Their actions are of extreme importance since a pH below 7.0 or above 7.8 will result in death. The primary mechanisms by which normal pH is maintained involve buffer systems, the lungs, and the kidneys.

The buffer systems are the first line of defense against pH change because of their rapidity of action. A buffer system consists of two or more chemical compounds that combine with strong acid or base to produce a weak acid or base. The buffer systems of the extracellular fluid are plasma proteins and bicarbonate while those of intracellular fluids are proteins, hemoglobin, and phosphate. Urinary pH is buffered by ammonia, bicarbonate and phosphate systems.

Protein buffers are the most potent of the buffer systems. Proteins, composed of amino acids, have free acidic radicals, which dissociate into COO^- and H^+, and free basic radicals, which dissociate into NH_3^+ and OH^-. The hydroxyl radical (OH^-) can combine with hydrogen ions (H^+) to form water and thus remove hydrogen ions from body fluids. Proteins are termed amphoteric because they can act as either an acid or a base.

The bicarbonate buffer of the extracellular fluids is composed of a weak acid, carbonic acid (H_2CO_3), and its salt, sodium bicarbonate ($NaHCO_3$). If a strong acid such as hydrochloric acid (HCl) is added to this system, the following reaction will occur:

$$HCl + NaHCO_3 \rightarrow H_2CO_3 + NaCl$$

Due to this reaction, the strong hydrochloric acid is replaced by the weak carbonic acid. Since carbonic acid is a weak acid, it dissociates to a lesser extent and thus releases fewer hydrogen ions and there is little change in pH.

When a strong base such as sodium hydroxide (NaOH) is added to the bicarbonate buffer system, the following reaction occurs:

$$H_2CO_3 + NaOH \rightarrow NaHCO_3 + H_2O$$

In this reaction the strong base is replaced by a weak base and there is little alteration of pH.

The intracellular fluid phosphate buffer reacts in the same manner as the bicarbonate buffer. The components of the phosphate buffer are disodium phosphate (Na_2HPO_4) and monosodium phosphate (NaH_2PO_4).

Another important mechanism for the regulation of body pH occurs in the lungs and is associated with the rate and depth of respiration which varies the rate of carbon dioxide removal. Carbon dioxide, formed as an end product of many cellular reactions, diffuses from cells into the body fluids and reacts with water to form carbonic acid in the following manner:

$$H_2O + CO_2 \underset{}{\overset{\text{carbonic anhydrase}}{\rightleftharpoons}} H_2CO_3 \rightleftharpoons H^+ + HCO_3^-$$

As plasma levels of carbon dioxide increase, carbonic acid is formed and dissociates to release hydrogen ions, thus decreasing pH. Since this reaction is reversible, the effect of excretion of carbon dioxide by the lungs will force the reaction to the left, resulting in a decrease in free hydrogen ions and an increase in pH. Thus, if respiration is slowed for any reason, carbon dioxide will remain in body fluids and hydrogen ion concentration and acidity will increase.

The third mechanism for the control of body pH is mediated via the kidneys. The kidneys control pH by regulation of the secretion of hydrogen ions, reabsorption of sodium ions, conservation and regeneration of the bicarbonate ion, and the synthesis of ammonia. These processes do not all occur at the same time. Instead, their occurrence is regulated by body concentrations of acids or bases.

Sodium reabsorption from the renal tubule occurs in conjunction with the secretion of hydrogen ions into the renal tubule when hydrogen ions are present in excessive amounts. The sodium ions then combine with bicarbonate ions in extracellular fluid. Figure 4.2 illustrates the mechanisms involved in this reaction. Carbon dioxide, which is formed in cells, diffuses into the plasma and is transported into the renal tubule. From the renal tubule the carbon dioxide diffuses into the cells of the renal tubule and combines with water to form carbonic acid, which dissociates into hydrogen and bicarbonate ions. The hydrogen ion is then actively transported into the renal tubule (secreted) and exchanged for sodium ions which are actively transported out of the renal tubule

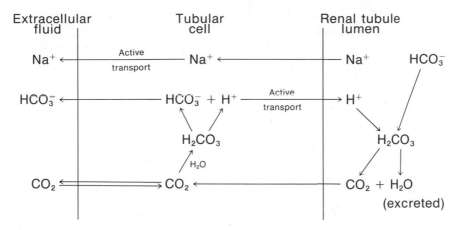

Figure 4.2 Mechanism for the excretion of excessive hydrogen ions into the renal tubule.

(reabsorption). Sodium ions are further actively transported into the extracellular fluid and bicarbonate ions diffuse into extracellular fluid to maintain electrical neutrality. These sodium and bicarbonate ions react to form sodium bicarbonate. In the renal tubule, the secreted hydrogen ions combine with bicarbonate ions to form carbonic acid and/or water. Thus, the presence of excess carbon dioxide or hydrogen ions in the body fluids results in the excretion of hydrogen ions as carbonic acid or water and an increase in total body sodium bicarbonate.

Another mechanism involved in renal regulation of acid–base balance involves the formation of the ammonium ion (NH_4^+). Ammonia (NH_3) is synthesized by cells in the renal tubules and collecting ducts. It diffuses into the tubule and combines with hydrogen to form the ammonium ion (NH_4^+). The ammonium ion can then combine with an anion such as chloride and be excreted via the urine as a salt.

In the control of acid–base balance, the lungs and kidneys play compensatory roles, that is, when kidney function is decreased and excessive hydrogen ions are present in body fluids, respiration rate will increase in an attempt to blow off larger volumes of carbon dioxide. Likewise, when respiratory function is decreased, and respiratory acidosis is present, the kidney responds by increasing hydrogen ion loss through the mechanisms of secretion of hydrogen ions, synthesis of ammonia and retention of bicarbonate. When respiratory alkalosis is present, the kidney responds by decreasing the mechanisms for normal hydrogen ion loss.

Under normal physiological conditions, the mechanisms previously mentioned are sufficient for the regulation of fluid volume, electrolyte and hydrogen ion concentration; however, in certain disease states, the capacity of these mechanisms is not sufficient to prevent serious disturbances of acid–base balance.

Clinically significant acid–base disturbances are categorized as either acidosis (excessive hydrogen ion concentration) or alkalosis (deficient hydrogen ion concentration). Acidosis may occur due to hypoventilation resulting in an accumulation of carbon dioxide and thus excessive hydrogen ions (respiratory acidosis) or may occur due to causes other than hypoventilation (metabolic acidosis). Alkalosis may occur due to hyperventilation which results in an excessive loss of carbon dioxide and thus a deficit of hydrogen ions or it may occur due to causes other than hyperventilation (metabolic alkalosis).

The primary problems associated with abnormalities of acid–base balance involve the central nervous system. Acidosis produces depression of the central nervous system which may lead to coma and death. Alkalosis produces excitation of the central nervous system with possible convulsions followed by postictal depression and death. The physiological parameters used to determine the presence of either acidosis or alkalosis, as well as its etiology, are arterial blood pH and carbon dioxide tension (pCO_2) and total serum carbon dioxide concentration.

Many abnormal physiological conditions or disease states may adversely affect fluid and electrolyte balance. Among hospitalized patients, conditions that require immediate and, at times, heroic treatment are congestive heart failure, emphysema, severe burns, dehydration, renal failure, and postsurgical states. Mechanisms of evaluation and treatment of three of these conditions, severe burns, postsurgical states, and dehydration are presented below.

Fluid and Electrolyte Therapy for Burn Patients

In the case of severe burns, therapy is always multidisciplinary due to the widespread complications associated with this type of trauma. The condition of the patient's fluid volume and electrolyte concentrations changes constantly during periods of recovery, thus requiring constant reevaluation and correctional measures.

Burns are characterized with respect to the amount of body surface involved and the depth of tissue damage. First degree burns affect only the epidermis and, although painful, usually heal spontaneously without medical intervention other than analgesic agents. Second degree burns affect both the dermis and epidermis and may produce damage to capillary beds with resultant fluid leakage. Sterile dressings and antibiotics are needed to prevent infections along with analgesic agents. Third degree burns extend below the dermal layer of the skin and cause severe damage to supportive tissue.

The extent of damage to body surface area must also be considered in assessing the severity of burns. Thus, a third degree burn covering ten percent of the body is considered critical, as are second degree burns over thirty percent of the body.

In any critical burn case, the aim of therapy is to maintain blood volume and electrolyte concentration, prevent renal shutdown and reduce edema.

Fluid and electrolyte shifts are the most prevalent early complications of severe burns because of the loss of fluids through surface areas (exudation) and body mechanisms which reflexly attempt to minimize such losses. During the first 24 to 48 hours after a severe burn, fluids leave damaged blood vessels and enter interstitial spaces as well as leaving the body through burned areas. Because of the decreased fluid volume, aldosterone is secreted to stimulate renal sodium reabsorption and the ensuing hyperosmolar plasma results in ADH secretion, thus promoting water conservation. The decreased fluid volume also decreases renal blood flow and the combination of effects may result in decreased urinary output or total anuria. The sodium-conserving effects of aldosterone are usually offset by sodium loss through exudation and bicarbonate is lost along with the sodium. This loss of bicarbonate will cause a tendency toward metabolic acidosis due to disruption of the bicarbonate buffer system. Therefore, early in therapy both sodium and bicarbonate ions are replaced via intravenous solutions.

Plasma potassium levels also rise during the first 48 hours because tissue damage allows leakage from within the cell into extracellular fluids. Hyperkalemia may be treated by the administration of insulin which forces both glucose and potassium back into cells.

During the second 24 to 48 hours after a severe burn, the fluid and electrolyte shifts begin to reverse themselves. Edema fluids begin to reenter the systemic circulation, increasing fluid volume and decreasing electrolyte concentrations. In the kidney, the increased blood flow will promote diuresis, which may lead to excessive sodium and potassium loss. The concurrent loss of bicarbonate with these cations may continue the tendency toward metabolic acidosis. The level of metabolic acidosis that results will partially be dependent on the kidney's ability to provide compensation in the form of hydrogen ion secretion. Also, during this stage of recovery, potassium is taken back into cells as the cellular membranes again become functional and plasma potassium levels may be deficient. At this stage, intravenous potassium supplements may be necessary.

During the first few days of recovery, tissue destruction and loss of plasma proteins will produce a state of negative nitrogen balance. This condition will be treated with plasma or whole blood administration along with a high protein diet as recovery continues.

Postsurgical Fluid and
Electrolyte Therapy

Prior to planned surgery, a patient will be hydrated and provided with optimal nourishment as a part of the overall preparation for the stress associated with surgery. This presurgical manipulation will include restoration of electrolytes if any are found to be deficient. In addition, just prior to surgery an intravenous infusion of five percent dextrose in water or saline or some similar intravenous fluid will be initiated to promote adequate renal function, provide some nourishment, and serve as a medium for the infusion of drugs or plasma expanders during and after surgery.

Even with optimal presurgical preparation, the stress and trauma associated with most surgical procedures will produce major alterations in fluids and electrolytes which must be readjusted as quickly as possible. Even normal reflex mechanisms, such as fluid retention in response to decreased blood volume following surgery, may need to be mechanically altered to prevent serious damage to renal function.

The trauma of surgery causes the injury and death of cells leading to the release of nitrogenous compounds into extracellular fluids. This excretion of nitrogen leads to a negative nitrogen balance which usually exceeds that which would be expected from the degree of surgical trauma. This excessive response is due to stress-released hormones such as the glucocorticoids (hydrocortisone). To overcome the effects of the stressful situation, the body requires extra glucose for energy. This glucose is supplied from protein whose catabolism is stimulated by the glucocorticoids released due to the action of ACTH from the pituitary gland. When proteins are being hydrolyzed to produce energy, nitrogenous waste products are produced and excreted. When the rate of protein utilization exceeds that of protein synthesis, the body is said to be in a state of negative nitrogen balance which leads to weight loss and possible metabolic acidosis. This process may be at least partially avoided and overcome by the intravenous administration of a glucose solution.

Stress also causes the release of aldosterone, producing sodium retention and, indirectly via ADH, water retention to avoid hypovolemia. Catecholamines are released from the adrenal medulla to stimulate cardiac rate. Force of contraction, also, in response to hypovolemia and vasoconstriction will reflexly occur to maintain an adequate tissue perfusion pressure.

In the postsurgical patient, tissue trauma causes some release of potassium and water into the extracellular fluid. This hyperkalemia is only temporary since the renal mechanisms for conserving sodium will cause potassium to be excreted in its place with hypokalemia as a result. This hypokalemia is reversed within the first 24 hours after surgery by intravenous replacement. Water released due to surgical trauma, in addition to that produced by protein catabolism, results in an increased extracellular volume which is further augmented by the effects of aldosterone and ADH. Thus fluid volume becomes excessive, often resulting in edema, until normal urinary output is resumed and fluids are adequately removed from the body.

As the effects of stress subside, stress hormone secretion decreases and, if protein intake is appropriate, the nitrogen balance will be restored. The return of electrolyte balance to normal is dependent on those compensatory mechanisms associated with the lungs and kidney.

Due to anesthetics used in surgery, respiratory function may be depressed for some time, leading to a state of respiratory acidosis. In this case, renal function must be adequate to remove excessive hydrogen ions. The overhydration previously mentioned is, therefore, beneficial in sustaining urinary output to excrete hydrogen ions as is some degree of sodium retention, which leads to the secretion of hydrogen ions in the exchange mechanism. Postsurgically, hydration will be aimed at keeping urine output at a level of at least 30 ml/hour to assure adequate renal function.

Fluid and Electrolyte Therapy for Dehydration

With regard to fluid and electrolyte balance, one of the more frequently encountered abnormal conditions is dehydration. Dehydration is particularly devastating to the pediatric patient and often may result from severe vomiting and/or diarrhea due to gastroenteritis.

The clinical symptoms of dehydration usually include weakness and lethargy, dry mouth, and a grayish skin. The body temperature may be elevated due to infection or due to the dehydration itself. In severe cases, the extremities may be cold and blue and tachycardia may be present due to impending circulatory collapse. A blood analysis usually reveals an elevated urea level and there may be an increase in hemoglobin and packed cell volume. Electrolyte measurements are used to determine the form of dehydration and thus to indicate the required therapy. A history of the onset of the dehydrated state and the physical condition of the patient will also serve as indicators of the type of therapy necessary. In pediatric patients rapid weight loss is a common feature of dehydration. Decreased urine output is also indicative of dehydration, but this symptom may be difficult to assess, especially in the infant. The source of fluid loss, such as excessive vomiting or diarrhea, should also be noted, because the sudden loss of large volumes of fluid produces a more severe effect than the loss of the same volume over a more extended period of time.

Dehydration may occur as an isotonic, hypotonic, or hypertonic type with reference to serum sodium concentration. In severe cases, the type should be determined before therapy is begun. Even without blood analyses, the type of dehydration may often be adequately determined from physical symptoms and therapy can be rapidly initiated.

Replacement of fluids and electrolytes in the dehydrated patient may be accomplished using either the oral or parenteral route, depending upon the severity of the patient's condition. For milder cases of dehydration, the oral route is usually preferable. If the condition has been produced by diarrhea or vomiting, such as with gastroenteritis, all fluid intake should be withheld for several hours and oral administration should be begun with small volumes of solution such as Pedialyte® (Ross). Severe dehydration should be treated by the parenteral route of administration with the composition and concentration of the solution being dependent on the type of dehydration.

Isotonic dehydration is treated initially with an intravenous solution of normal saline. A volume of 20 to 40 ml per kg body weight should be administered over a two to three hour period followed by a more gradual infusion of normal saline in five percent dextrose at a rate of 200 ml per kg per 24 hours. When it has been determined that renal function is adequate, potassium chloride should be added to the infusion in a concentration of 13 mEq of potassium per 500 ml of solution. In many cases of dehydration, acidosis may be present (especially after prolonged vomiting) and this condition may correct itself with fluid infusion. Should the acidosis not improve spontaneously, the patient should be treated with sodium lactate or sodium bicarbonate.

Hypotonic dehydration occurs in only a small percentage of patients. This type of dehydration is defined clinically as a serum sodium concentration of less than 130 mEq per liter. Sodium is lost due to vomiting and diarrhea and the situation is often worsened by at-home fluid replacement with tap water, which contains few electrolytes. Hypotonic dehydration is treated with a normal saline solution rather than a hypertonic saline solution because too rapid alteration in serum sodium is dangerous.

Hypertonic dehydration also occurs in a small percentage of patients and is seen clinically with a serum sodium concentration of greater than 150 mEq per liter. This condition occurs most frequently in infants with diarrhea who are continued on milk with its high solute concentration. The symptoms of hypertonic dehydration differ from other types of dehydration in that the fluid deficit is related to the intracellular rather than the extracellular fluid volume. The skin takes on a doughy consistency and the patient becomes irritable rather than lethargic. In addition to the elevation of serum sodium, serum chloride levels may be elevated and bicarbonate levels decreased. Even though serum sodium levels are elevated, total body sodium and potassium are usually below normal levels.

Treatment of hypertonic dehydration is accomplished with a slow infusion of electrolytes such as potassium in a normal saline and dextrose solution. A hypotonic saline solution cannot be used under most conditions because water moves into cells more rapidly than electrolytes and the rapid swelling of cells of the brain can cause convulsions.

Intravenous therapy for dehydration should be continued only as long as it is absolutely necessary. Once the patient is able to keep down fluids, oral solutions should be initiated so that the oral fluid intake approaches normal when intravenous therapy is discontinued.

These examples point out clearly the need for proper regulation of fluids and electrolytes in the presence of altered physiological function. When the body's compensatory mechanisms are not adequate to meet the needs of critical situations, immediate rational therapy often makes the difference between the life and death of the patient.

Questions

1. Briefly explain the role of plasma buffer systems in maintaining normal body homeostasis.
2. What clinical characteristics are used to differentiate between hypertonic and hypotonic dehydration?
3. Briefly describe the mechanisms involved in renal excretion of excess hydrogen ions.
4. Describe the function of antidiuretic hormone in maintaining fluid homeostasis.
5. When fluids are lost from the body rapidly, what compensatory mechanisms are activated to maintain some degree of homeostasis?

RECOMMENDED READINGS

Bricker, N. S., ed. *The Sea Within Us: A Clinical Guide to Fluid and Electrolyte Balances*. San Juan, P.R.: Searle and Co., 1977.

A compilation of papers by renowned physicians which deal with derangement and control of fluid balance, acid–base balance, and selected electrolytes.

CHAPTER 5

The Digestive System

ANATOMY AND PHYSIOLOGY

The science of nutrition is primarily the study of nutrient metabolism at the cellular level, but such study is of little impact unless consideration is first given to those mechanisms by which nutrients are made available for use by cells. The alimentary tract, shown in Figure 5.1, serves in a liaison capacity between the external environment which provides potential nutrients in the form of food and the body itself which is maintained through utilization of these nutrients. Within the digestive system are the mechanisms necessary for the ingestion of food, the selective separation of nutrients from the food (digestion), the movement of these nutrients into the body proper (absorption), and finally the passage of food residue back into the external environment (defecation).

Principles of gastrointestinal motility deserve consideration because transit time of food is of critical importance in nourishment of the body. The basic structures of the intestinal wall are identified in Figure 5.2. Of particular importance to the movement of food through the gut are the circular muscle, the longitudinal muscle, and the innervated myenteric plexus which lies between the circular and longitudinal smooth muscular layers.

The circular and longitudinal smooth muscles exhibit tonic and rhythmic contractions which are regulated by the myenteric plexus. Tonic contraction by the muscles is responsible for the amount of steady pressure provided by the gut while the rhythmic contractions make possible the mixing of food and its peristaltic movement through the gut.

The myenteric plexus receives both parasympathetic and sympathetic innervation but is principally under the control of the parasympathetic nerves; consequently, stimulation of the myenteric plexus increases not only the intensity and rate of muscle contractions but also the velocity with which excitatory waves are carried along the intestinal wall. Parasympathetic nerves of particular importance to the upper segments of the digestive tract are the vagus nerves which innervate the esophagus, stomach, and pancreas. To a lesser degree these nerves also stimulate the small intestine, gall bladder, and portions of the colon.

The alimentary canal is a long tube that extends from the mouth to the anus and is composed of the following parts: mouth, pharynx, esopha-

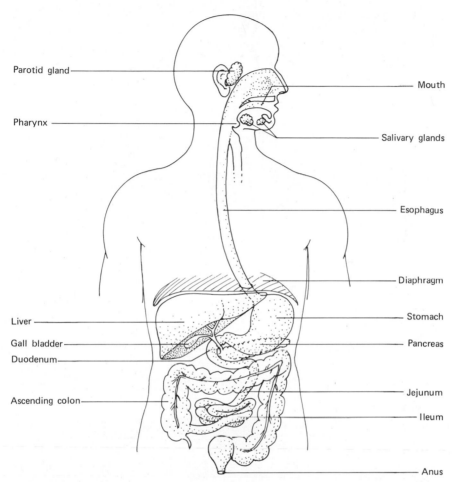

Parotid gland

Pharynx

Mouth

Salivary glands

Esophagus

Diaphragm

Liver

Stomach

Gall bladder

Pancreas

Duodenum

Ascending colon

Jejunum

Ileum

Anus

Figure 5.1 The alimentary tract. (From *Textbook of Medical Physiology*, 5th ed., by Arthur C. Guyton. Copyright 1976 by W.B. Saunders Company. Reprinted by permission of the publisher and author.)

gus, stomach, small intestine, and large intestine or colon. Although the pancreas, liver, and salivary glands are structures separate from the canal itself, they are necessary to the canal and must be included in any discussion of the digestive system because of their specific digestive secretions essential to providing normal nourishment for the body (Table 5.1).

Mouth and Pharynx

The mouth is the site not only for the ingestion of food but also for the beginning of the digestive process. By proper mastication food is divided

Table 5.1 Digestive Enzymes and Their Actions*

Enzymes or Secretory Product	Site of Secretion	Stimuli to Secretion	Action
Salivary amylase (ptyalin)	Mouth Salivary glands (3 pr.)	Psychic: thought, sight, smell, taste of food Mechanical: presence of food in mouth Chemical: contact of sugar, salt, spices on taste buds	Cooked starch ⎤ Glycogen ⎥ → Branched oligosaccharides, some maltose Dextrin ⎦
HCl	Stomach Gastric glands (approx. 35,000,000)	Psychic: as above Mechanical: presence of food in stomach Hormonal: gastrin	Pepsinogen → Pepsin $Fe^{+++} \rightarrow Fe^{++}$ Swelling of proteins Antibacterial effect
Pepsinogen (activated to pepsin by HCl)	Stomach Gastric glands (approx. 35,000,000)		Hydrolyzes peptide bonds between aromatic and dicarboxylic acids ⎤ → Large polypeptides and amino acids ⎦
Rennin (important only in infants)			Casein $\xrightarrow{Ca^{++}}$ Paracaseinate
Tributyrase (negligible importance)			Tributyrin → fatty acids & glycerol
Trypsinogen (activated to *trypsin* by enterokinase and free trypsin)	Pancreas Exocrine secretion	Secretin Cholecystokinin–pancreozymin (CCK–PZ)	Protein & polypeptides → small polypeptides
Chymotrypsinogen (activated to *chymotrypsin* by trypsin)			Protein & polypeptides → small polypeptides
Procarboxypeptidase (activated to carboxypeptidase A and carboxypeptidase B by trypsin)		Secretin CCK–PZ	Polypeptides with free → smaller peptides & carboxyl group aromatic amino acids Polypeptides with free → smaller peptides & carboxyl group dibasic amino acids

Enzyme / Substance	Source	Action
Elastase		Hydrolyzes fibrous proteins
Collagenase		Hydrolyzes collagen
Ribonuclease		Ribonucleic acid → nucleotides
Deoxyribonuclease		Deoxyribonucleic acids → nucleotides
α-amylase		Starch → maltose
Lipase		Fats → monoglycerides, fatty acids, and glycerol
Phospholipase A & B		Removal of fatty acids from lecithin
Cholesterol esterase		Free cholesterol → cholesterol esters (fatty acids)
Retinyl ester hydrolase		Hydrolyzes retinyl esters
Aminopeptidases	Entercrinin	Polypeptides with free → smaller peptides and amino group free amino acids
	Small intestine (Most enzymes located in brush border of villi)	
Dipeptidases		Dipeptides → amino acids
Nucleotidase		Nucleotides → nucleosides + H_3PO_4
Nucleosidase		Nucleosides → purines, pyrimidines, pentose
Alkaline phosphatase		Organic phosphates → free phosphates
Monoglyceride lipase		Monoglycerides → fatty acid and glycerol
Lecithinase		Lecithin → fatty acids, glycerol, phosphoric acid, choline
Disaccharidases		
Sucrase		Sucrose → glucose and fructose
Maltase		Maltose → glucose
Lactase		Lactose → glucose and galactose
Bile	Liver (Gall bladder is storage site from which bile moves into small intestine)	Emulsifies fats
		Stabilizes emulsions
	Cholecystokinin–pancreozymin (CCK–PZ)	Accelerates action of pancreatic lipase

Lipase, Phospholipase A & B, Cholesterol esterase, Retinyl ester hydrolase → require bile salts

*References: Robinson and Lawler, Normal and Therapeutic Nutrition, 15th ed., Macmillan, 1977; Pike and Brown, Nutrition: An Integrated Approach, 2nd ed., Wiley, 1975.

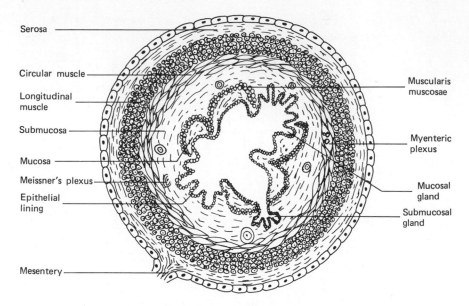

Serosa

Circular muscle

Longitudinal muscle

Submucosa

Mucosa

Meissner's plexus

Epithelial lining

Mesentery

Muscularis muscosae

Myenteric plexus

Mucosal gland

Submucosal gland

Figure 5.2 Basic structure of intestinal wall. (From *Textbook of Medical Physiology,* 5th ed., by Arthur C. Guyton. Copyright 1976 by W.B. Saunders Company. Reprinted by permission of the publisher and author.)

into smaller particles, thereby increasing tremendously the surface area upon which digestive enzymes may act. Of particular importance in mastication is the tremendous force that the jaw muscles working in concert can exert. A pressure of 55 pounds is possible for the cutting incisors with a grinding force potential of 200 pounds for the molars (1). As mastication proceeds, three pairs of salivary glands (sublingual, submaxillary, and parotid) pour secretion over food. This secretion is a slightly acidic fluid called *saliva* (pH 6.8) which serves to moisten ingested foods, hold particles together, lubricate the bolus for swallowing, and initiate digestion of cooked starch. Any hydrolysis of starch into dextrins and possibly maltose that occurs in the mouth is due to salivary amylase (ptyalin), the digestive action of which can continue until activity of the enzyme is destroyed by the acidity of the stomach. Once sufficient mastication has occurred, food can move from the mouth to the esophagus by way of the pharynx or throat. This movement is accomplished through swallowing which begins as a voluntary act but becomes a reflex action as food reaches the pharynx.

Esophagus

The presence of food in the pharynx brings about a stimulation of pharyngeal and esophageal musculature the result of which is a peristaltic wave that moves food very rapidly from the pharynx into the esophagus and on into the stomach. Any food remaining in the esophagus causes peristaltic waves to continue until the tube is swept clean. Just a few centimeters above the juncture of the esophagus with the stomach, the circular muscle of the esophageal tube is slightly hypertrophied to form the *gastro-esophageal sphincter*, the function of which is to prevent reflux of gastric contents into the upper portion of the esophagus. During swallowing the sphincter is relaxed but at other times it remains tonically contracted in contrast to the rest of the esophagus which is always relaxed.

Stomach

The stomach is a J-shaped organ located under the diaphragm and possessing a volume of approximately 50 ml when empty (2). The force of the esophageal peristaltic wave allows food to enter the stomach where first it is stored against the walls of the fundus area and then by the regular muscular contractions of the stomach is mixed with gastric juice and gradually reduced to a paste-like product called chyme. Figure 5.3 shows the gross structure of the stomach with its component parts: fundus, body, antrum, pylorus.

The surface of the stomach is covered with a single layer of epithelium consisting of mucus-producing columnar cells. Pits found in the epithelium are openings leading to gastric glands located primarily in the body area of the stomach. Gastric glands are composed of a central canal

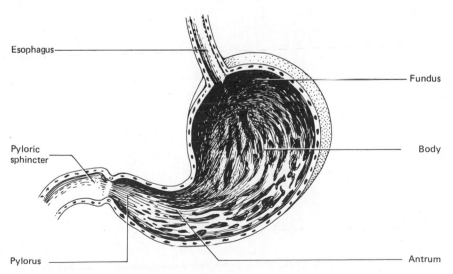

Figure 5.3 Gross anatomy of the stomach. (Adapted from *Human Anatomy and Physiology*, 2nd ed., by J. E. Crouch and J. R. McClintic. Copyright 1976 by John Wiley and Sons, Inc. Reprinted by permission of the publisher.)

surrounded by four different types of cells which pour secretions into the canal: parietal (or oxyntic) cells which secrete hydrochloric acid, chief (or zymogenic) cells which produce the digestive enzymes found in the stomach, mucous neck cells which are the source of mucus and the intrinsic factor, and argentaffin cells, the exact function of which is not known but may be the site of secretion of local hormones (3). The mucus produced by the mucous neck cells and the epithelial cells lining the stomach adheres to the surface of the stomach and protects it against autodigestion. Figure 5.4 illustrates the arrangement of chief, parietal, and mucous cells in the gastric glands.

The sight, smell, thought, or taste of food causes the vagus nerves to stimulate production of gastric juice via gastric glands. Most stimulation of gastric juice production, however, occurs due to the presence of food in the stomach and is mediated not only by the vagus nerves but also by the hormone, gastrin. Gastrin is produced by ductless glands located in the antral mucosa and its production is increased by substances known as secretagogues which include partially digested proteins, most extractives, alcohol, and caffeine, to name a few. Gastrin is carried by the blood stream to parietal cells which are thereby stimulated to produce hydrochloric acid. As soon as gastric juices reach a pH of 2.0 further production of gastrin is inhibited.

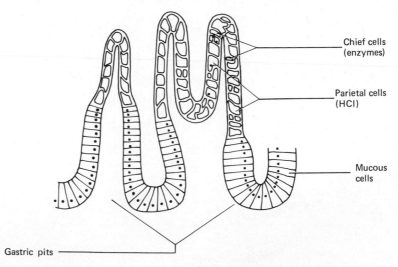

Chief cells (enzymes)

Parietal cells (HCl)

Mucous cells

Gastric pits

Figure 5.4 Cell loci in gastric glands. (From *Human Physiology—The Mechanisms of Body Function* by A. C. Vander, J. H. Sherman, and D. S. Luciano. Copyright 1975 by McGraw-Hill Book Co. Reprinted by permission of the publisher.)

Digestion in the Stomach. The kneading and mixing of food by muscular action in the stomach expose extensive surface areas of substrates upon which digestive enzymes may act. Enzymes produced by the chief cells include:

1. Pepsin which is secreted as pepsinogen but converted to the active enzyme by hydrochloric acid. This enzyme is active only in an acid medium (optimal pH 2.0 to 3.0) and is completely inactivated at a pH higher than 5. Pepsin begins the digestion of all types of protein in the diet, hydrolyzing them into proteoses, peptones, and polypeptides which usually contain from 4 to 12 amino acid residues. Of particular importance is the ability of pepsin to digest collagen which is little affected by other digestive enzymes (1).
2. Renin which is found in more abundance in the stomach of infants than in adults and has an optimum pH of 3.7. This enzyme coagulates milk through its action on the milk protein, casein, and in the presence of calcium ions produces a milk curd, calcium paracaseinate. Decreasing the fluidity of milk slows down its passage through the stomach, thereby increasing the satiety value of an infant's food and allowing its more nearly complete digestion.
3. Tributyrinase which digests butterfat in the infant's stomach but has little or no significance in fat digestion for the adult.

Any absorption in the stomach is quite limited and is confined primarily to water, salts, and some fat soluble materials of low molecular weight, such as alcohol and salicylate compounds (4).

Emptying of stomach contents into the small intestine is promoted by peristaltic waves from the stomach to duodenum and requires approximately 3 to 4 hours for completion. The rate at which food is emptied from stomach into duodenum is controlled (1) by the *enterogastric reflex,* which inhibits antral peristalsis, and (2) by various humoral agents secreted by the intestinal mucosa, which slow down both gastric secretions and motility. Humoral agents having this inhibitory effect are enterogastrone (postulated but never identified with certainty), secretin, cholecystokinin–pancreozymin (CCK–PZ), and gastric inhibitory polypeptide (GIP). The enterogastric reflex increases the emptying time of stomach contents whenever chyme is more or less concentrated than plasma, when chyme is excessively acid, or when too much chyme is already in the small intestine. The presence of fatty foods in chyme slows down the rate of stomach emptying by causing inhibitory humoral agents to be secreted by mucosa of the duodenum. Emotional stress through its effects on the parasympathetic and/or sympathetic nervous system also influences the emptying time of the stomach. When excess stimulation of parasympathetic nerves occurs, motility of the entire gastrointestinal tract is increased, whereas hyperstimulation of the sympathetic system can decrease this movement.

Small Intestine

When chyme reaches the duodenum, much peristaltic activity is already underway in this section of the intestinal tract. This activity occurs because of the *enterogastric reflex* elicited by stomach distention that immediately follows a meal. Chyme, however, is subjected not only to the propulsive movement of peristalsis but also to many contractions and mixing movements by the various muscles in the small intestine:

1. Segmenting contractions which divide the tube into small segments with each contraction occurring at a different place along the intestine. These contractions of the circular muscles occur many times per minute and serve to mix and churn chyme with secretions of the small intestine.
2. Counterclockwise rotations of chyme by the longitudinal muscles which not only mix food with intestinal secretions but also keep it exposed to the mucosa in order that absorption of nutrients can occur.
3. Pendular movements which are actually local contractions of the longitudinal muscle that shorten the length of the gut and by so doing help in the mixing of intestinal contents.
4. Movements elicited by muscularis mucosa which cause folds to appear in the mucosa, thereby increasing the absorptive area of the digestive tract. This muscle also causes periodic elongation and shortening of the villi, and these contractions keep the chyme moving so that new areas of fluid are constantly being presented for absorption.
5. Peristaltic waves occurring primarily through action of the circular muscles and initiated by stimulation of the myenteric plexus. These waves move the chyme along the intestinal mucosa to the ileocecal valve where it must remain until the person eats another meal and the valve opens. A *peristaltic rush* can occur as a result of extreme distention of the intestine or because of an acute irritation to the mucosal surface. Such a rush will cause intestinal contents to move very quickly from the small intestine into the colon.

Digestion in the Small Intestine. The first few centimeters of the duodenum are covered with mucous cells. The secretion from these cells normally protects the duodenal wall from digestion by the gastric juice which is contained in the chyme moving from the stomach into the small intestine. Just distal to these mucous cells is located the duct which allows passage of bile and pancreatic secretions into the small intestine. The presence of chyme in the duodenum elicits mucosal secretion of the hormone, *secre-*

tin, which in turn causes a copious production of pancreatic juice. This secretion is a thin watery fluid containing high levels of bicarbonate. By action of this particular fluid, acid contents from the stomach are neutralized and a pH appropriate for the action of pancreatic enzymes (8.0) is made possible.

A second hormone, cholecystokinin–pancreozymin (CCK–PZ), is also secreted by the duodenal mucosa in response to presence of food in the upper small intestine. This hormone is carried by way of blood to both the pancreas and the gall bladder and produces two responses: (1) secretion of a pancreatic juice very rich in digestive enzymes, and (2) contraction of the gall bladder and release of stored bile. The intestinal mucosa that releases this hormone is particularly sensitive to presence of fat in the duodenum.

Many stimuli contribute to the copious production of intestinal juice by the glands of the small intestine (crypts of Lieberkühn). One stimulus is a hormone, designated as enterocrinin, which is secreted as a result of any tactile contact with the small intestine and elicits secretion of fluid from all glands. Secretion from the small intestine is very similar to extracellular fluid and contains only a small quantity of two enzymes: *amylase* and *enterokinase,* the latter of which is an activator of trypsinogen. The large volume of intestinal juice and the rapidity with which it is absorbed by the villi makes this secretion very valuable to the process of nutrient absorption. The major digestive enzymes produced by the small intestine are found in the microvilli; therefore, the final digestion of food substances may be completed in the process of their absorption. The digestive enzymes are listed and their actions described in Table 5.1. For a discussion of digestion of specific nutrients, see Chapter 3.

The significance of the small intestine in nourishment of the body cannot be overemphasized. Here digestive enzymes are kept in contact with food substances until they are hydrolyzed into those products that can be absorbed by the body. But more importantly, here also is the absorptive surface so constructed that absorption of nutrients proceeds at an optimal rate. Projecting from the entire surface of the small intestine are millions of villi and from each epithelial cell on these villi extend about 600 microvilli to make up the "brushborder." Thus, the absorptive area of the small intestine is increased to such an extent that it equals approximately 550 square meters (1). Figure 5.5 illustrates the functional organization of the villus and shows the optimal arrangement of lacteal and blood vessels for rapid absorption of nutrients.

The villi are particularly profuse in the upper portion of the small intestine and it is here, as can be seen in Figure 5.6 that most of the nutrients are absorbed. Although the small intestine is composed of the duodenum, jejunum, and ileum, it is only through microscopy that the three sections can be distinguished (2).

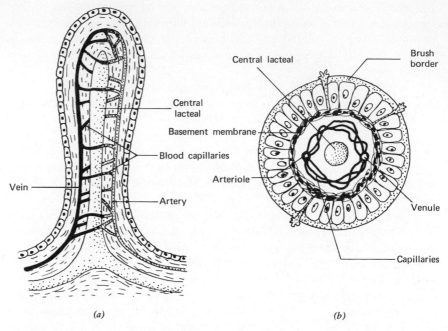

Central lacteal

Brush border

Central lacteal

Basement membrane

Blood capillaries

Arteriole

Vein

Artery

Venule

Capillaries

(a)   (b)

Figure 5.5 The villus: (*a*) Longitudinal section. (*b*) Cross section. (From *Textbook of Medical Physiology,* 5th ed. by Arthur C. Guyton. Copyright 1976 by W.B. Saunders Company. Reprinted by permission of the publisher and author.)

Colon

Movement of chyme from the ileum into the colon is controlled by the ileocecal sphincter, a thickened muscular portion of the ileum just preceding the ileocecal valve. Immediately following each meal, the sphincter relaxes sufficiently to allow a small amount of chyme to pass into the colon. No further digestion of the food substances occurs in the colon, however, since the only secretion of any significance is mucus, the presence of which is necessary to protect the intestinal wall.

The primary functions of the colon are to promote absorption of fluid and electrolytes from the chyme and to act as a storage area for feces until defecation occurs. The chyme is moved through the colon by mixing movements called haustral contractions and by propulsive movements termed "mass movements". Haustral contractions differ from the segmenting contractions that occur in the small intestine in that constrictions of the circular muscle are simultaneously accompanied by contraction of the longitudinal muscle (1). Portions of the colon are forced by these combined contractions to project outward into pouches called haustrations. The haustral contractions move all along the proximal half of the colon thereby allowing absorption of fluid from the fecal matter and serving as a weak propulsion for the feces.

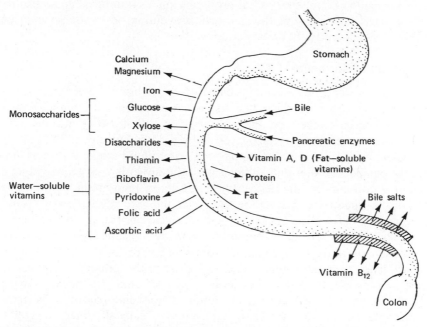

Figure 5.6 Sites of absorption in small intestine. (From "Effect of location along the small intestine on absorption of nutrients" by John Field. *Handbook of Physiology, Alimentary Canal,* Vol. 3. Copyright 1968 by American Physiology Society. Reprinted by permission of the publisher.)

The propulsive movements or "mass movements" occur primarily in the distal portion of the colon and are infrequent in number, occurring only after meals and most commonly following the morning meal. The duodenocolic reflex, which causes an excitation of the colon as a result of the duodenum being filled, is largely responsible for these mass movements. However, any irritation in the colon can also cause mass movements. With these propulsive contractions fecal matter is pushed toward the anus and when the rectum has been reached and distended, the urge for defecation is experienced.

DIAGNOSIS AND THERAPY OF DISEASES OF THE DIGESTIVE TRACT

Discussion of gastrointestinal disorders will be approached in the same manner as description of the normally functioning alimentary tract. Although any gastrointestinal disorder of long duration will be of concern to the dietitian because of the likelihood of associated poor nutritional status, the legion of alimentary tract problems makes it impossible to discuss any disease states except those whose prevention or treatment may be affected significantly by dietary modification.

Mouth and Esophagus

Oral problems of long duration that disturb mastication are of extreme importance in proper nutrition because any interference with mandibular function decreases the type and amount of food that can be ingested. All too often the tremendous force exerted by the jaw muscles in the cutting and grinding of food is underemphasized. When food intake becomes limited to liquids, the dietitian is faced with the difficult task of providing a diet that contains all the necessary nutrients in recommended amounts and at the same time making the food acceptable to the patient (5). Oral problems of particular concern in adults are carcinoma and broken jaw.

When the esophagus is narrowed or made inelastic by some growth or inflammation, dysphagia and odynophagia will result (6). As the esophageal lumen becomes smaller and less elastic, the affected person will find swallowing of any solid food quite difficult. If the narrowing continues, even the swallowing of liquids will become painful or perhaps impossible. Narrowing of the esophageal lumen is usually due to a growth which can be malignant. Cancer of the esophagus in North America is found primarily in persons who smoke and/or drink heavily (4).

Additionally, dysphagia may result from *achalasia,* a condition characterized by an aperistaltic esophagus with a gastroesophageal sphincter that cannot relax, or from *chalasia,* a persistent relaxation of the lower end of the esophagus. The etiology of dysphagia is diagnosed most often by barium swallow.

Chalasia is a problem not uncommon to the pediatric population. When the infant is placed in a horizontal position after feeding, vomiting occurs because of the relaxation of the lower esophageal sphincter. Therapy includes the thickening of foods and keeping the infant in an erect position following feeding.

Achalasia is a common cause for dysphagia is some parts of the world, but in the United States it is a relatively rare disease entity. When the disease does occur in this country, it is found primarily in the 30- to 60-year age groups (7). Since the gastroesophageal sphincter (lower esophageal sphincter or LES as it is commonly called), does not relax and there are no peristaltic waves to push food through the constriction, food and liquid accumulate in the esophagus of the achalasic patient until he/she stands and the hydrostatic pressure gradually forces the esophageal contents into the stomach. In more severe cases of dysphagia and/or achalasia, weight loss and other evidence of poor nutrition status will be apparent. Treatment will be determined by the etiology of the dysphagia. In the case of achalasia, dilation of the LES is essential. In most instances this dilation must be achieved by injury to the muscle through partial instrumental damage or surgical split, because no viable drug therapy exists. Dysphagia due to narrowing of the esophagus by a growth can be relieved only by surgical removal of the mass.

The dietitian indeed faces a challenge in trying to encourage dysphagic patients to consume an adequate diet. Food temperature as well as food consistency can be a real concern (5). Parenteral feedings and/or tube feedings often become very important in the successful treatment of such patients. In cancer patients the side effects of radiotherapy and/or chemotherapy may make oral feeding an impossibility at times.

Paradoxically, a weak and overrelaxed LES is responsible for another condition causing dysphagia, that is, an esophagus narrowed by scarring due to repeated attacks of peptic esophagitis (8). A decrease in the pressure exerted by the LES permits excessive reflux of gastric contents into the esophagus where the mucosa is irritated by the acid gastric juices (heartburn). An inefficient LES has been linked to many factors with a very strong relationship being shown to exist between excessive gastric reflux and the existence of hiatal hernia (6). Other factors causing relaxation of the LES include: (1) secretion of the hormones, secretin and CCK–PZ; (2) intake of coffee, regular and decaffeinated, both of which also increase gastric acid secretion; (3) ingestion of chocolate (defatted as well as regular), alcohol, all foods high in fat, and the carminitives, peppermint and spearmint; (4) cigarette smoking (9,10,11).

Hiatal hernia is a condition in which the junction between the esophagus and the stomach moves upward through the esophageal hiatus and pulls the upper part of the stomach with it. Under normal circumstances despite the upward force of intraabdominal pressure against the diaphragm, the esophagus is held firmly against the diaphragm by the phrenoesophageal ligament and the musculature of the diphragm itself. When, however, this intraabdominal pressure is increased on a recurrent or sustained basis, as may occur with obesity, pregnancy, weight-lifting, ascites, severe coughing or tight corseting, normal resistance of the diaphragm may be overcome and part of the stomach is allowed to slide through the widened hiatus (12). Figure 5.7 illustrates the differences between a normal esophagus and one in which hernia has occurred.

The fact that hiatal hernia is so prevalent in older women has led to the belief that the ligaments and muscles that hold the esophagus in place may weaken with age, thereby fostering herniation. Definitive diagnosis of the problem must rest on radiographic evidence.

Treatment of hiatal hernia short of surgery is directed toward relief of those symptoms characteristic of gastroesophageal reflux and includes the following recommendations:

1. Obese patients should lose weight and avoid use of tight undergarments.

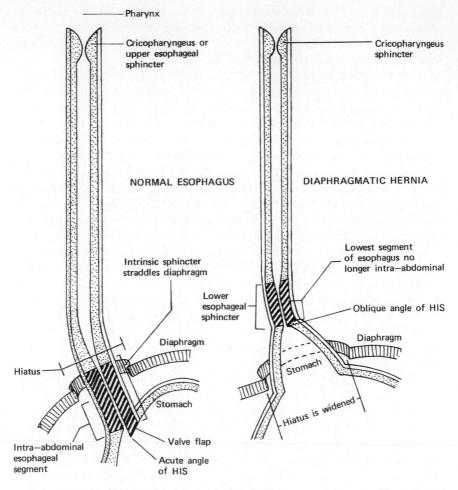

Figure 5.7 Changes in esophogus as result of diaphragmatic hernia. (Reproduced with permission of *Nutrition Today*, January/February 1973.)

2. Only small amounts of food should be eaten at any one time because volume of food in the stomach is correlated with likelihood of gastric reflux. Fat intake also should be restricted because fat increases secretion of CCK–PZ.
3. The last meal of the day should be eaten at least 2 hours prior to retiring; the head of the bed should be positioned on blocks so as to elevate it 4 to 10 inches, thereby lessening the likelihood of nocturnal regurgitation.
4. All practices that cause relaxation of the LES, such as cigarette smoking, ingestion of coffee, chocolate, and so on, should be avoided.

5. Drug therapy directed toward neutralization of stomach acidity and increase in the competency of the lower esophageal sphincter should be utilized. Viscous antacid preparations often are used to decrease the irritant effect of refluxed gastric acid, to increase gastrin secretion, and to increase (possibly) the competency of the esophageal sphincter (13). Antacids are usually administered one hour after meals and at bedtime. One concern associated with chronic administration of antacids is the possibility of inefficient iron absorption. Evaluation of iron status should be routine in these patients.

Because the smooth muscle and sphincters of the gastrointestinal tract are controlled by the parasympathetic portion of the autonomic nervous system, drugs that directly increase the activity of parasympathetic nerve fibers may be used to increase lower esophageal sphincter competency. Two drugs that increase the competency of this sphincter are bethanechol (Urecholine®) and metoclopropamide (Reglan™). Bethanechol, because it is chemically similar to acetylcholine, has the same effect on the esophageal sphincter as does the neurotransmitter itself. However, this drug is more slowly hydrolyzed by the enzyme acetylcholinesterase than is acetylcholine. The pharmacologic properties of bethanechol are similar to those of acetylcholine; therefore, the drug has a number of adverse effects including excessive salivation, sweating, flushing of the skin, urinary urgency, and increased gastrointestinal tone and motility. The usual oral dosage for bethanechol is 10-30 mg three to four times daily (13). Metoclopropamide, a drug presently utilized in Europe and Canada, is still in the clinical trial stage in the United States. Metoclopropamide increases peristalsis in the stomach and small intestine without altering gastric secretions or peristalsis in the colon. The possible side effects of metoclopropamide include headache, drowsiness, insomnia, fatigue, and diarrhea, but these are seen infrequently. The usual dosage is 5 to 20 mg, three or four times daily before meals (14).

Stomach

Common disorders of the stomach include dyspepsia, gastritis and ulcer. Dyspepsia, more commonly called indigestion, is a frequent cause of gastrointestinal distress, but because this disorder is usually functional in nature and caused by emotional tension, little space will be devoted to its discussion. However, one symptom often reported by dyspeptic patients is anorexia. This symptom should always alert the dietitian regardless of its cause because prolonged failure to eat an adequate diet can result in nutritional impairment. A detailed diet history should be taken routinely on any patient complaining of anorexia.

Gastritis, or inflammation of the mucosal lining of the stomach, is a frequently occurring gastrointestinal problem and is classified as acute or chronic in nature. Acute gastritis can occur for no apparent reason but is most often caused by aspirin ingestion, acute alcoholism, or ingestion of certain antiinflammatory drugs. The disorder can be detected by gastroscopy but because the inflammation usually subsides spontaneously, little treatment is necessary except in rare cases of massive bleeders (15).

Chronic gastritis is widespread throughout all age groups but is particularly prevalent among older persons. Development of chronic gastritis is part of normal aging but it is also found in conjunction with many disease states including pernicious anemia, sprue, thyroid disease, chronic iron deficiency, diabetes mellitus, and carcinoma of the stomach. The disorder is characterized by atrophy of gastric cells with a consequent decrease in secretion of gastric juice. However, symptoms that may be experienced by patients with chronic gastritis closely resemble those reported by patients with functional dyspepsia: anorexia, nausea, pain, flatus, and so on.

Diagnosis of chronic gastritis is possible through biopsy directed by gastroscopy, but no specific treatment for the disorder exists. Recommendations to patients generally include use of medications to relieve symptoms and avoidance of foods that appear to elicit any discomfort. Coffee and other caffeine-containing beverages as well as alcohol and salicylates are usually contraindicated.

Peptic ulcer is a term used to identify a gastrointestinal disorder caused by a lesion occurring either in the stomach (gastric ulcer) or in the duodenum (duodenal ulcer). Peptic ulcer is believed to affect at least one person out of 10 during his/her lifetime, being more prevalent in the male than in the premenopausal female and occurring more frequently in the white collar worker than in the laborer (16). Nevertheless, for unknown reasons, the incidence of the disease has been decreasing during the last few years.

Gastric ulcer may appear at any age but is most common in the 45- to 55-year age group, with the ratio of men to women affected being 3.5:1. The lesion occurs most often in the antrum of the stomach or at the juncture of the antrum and the body. Although a usual clinical finding among patients with gastric ulcer is a normal or low acid secretion, there is a strong possibility that regurgitation of bile into the proximal parts of the stomach injures the mucosa, thereby fostering ulceration. Asymptomatic gastric ulcers are not uncommon and lesions may be discovered only by chance or as a result of complications such as perforation or bleeding. Stress ulcers associated with diseases of the central nervous system or occurring in wake of trauma (e.g., severe burns) are found more often in the stomach than in the duodenum.

Duodenal ulcers account for 80 percent of all peptic ulcers and are from three to 10 times more prevalent in men 20 to 50 years old than in premenopausal women. The lesion usually occurs within 3 cm of the pylorus and is of chronic nature, characterized by exacerbation in the spring and/or fall and possible remission during the rest of the year (16). The most common symptom of the disorder is pain in the upper midepigastrium which can be relieved by ingestion of food and/or antacids.

People most susceptible to development of peptic ulcers are those subjected to extreme anxiety for long periods of time, the result of which is excessive stimulation of the vagus nerves. Factors other than neuropsychiatric ones, however, may very well be involved in development of the disorder. Other possible etiologic factors include:

1. Genetic predisposition, because duodenal ulcers are more common in patients with O blood grouping while gastric ulcers may occur more frequently in persons with type A blood;
2. Endocrine factors, because estrogenic hormones appear to protect against appearance of lesions while steroid therapy acts in the opposite manner;
3. Factors related to presence of certain other disease states such as cirrhosis of the liver, chronic pancreatitis or cystic fibrosis, chronic pulmonary emphysema, and rheumatoid arthritis.

An X-ray examination with barium is necessary for a definitive diagnosis of peptic ulcer.

Successful treatment of the patient with peptic ulcer is largely dependent upon the patient and requires of him or her an increased capacity to handle emotions, a willingness to attempt relaxation, securing of sufficient rest and abstinance from cigarette smoking, and a cooperativeness in following a dietary regimen that excludes alcoholic beverages, coffee or caffeine-containing beverages. All members of the health team should offer the ulcer patient much support. The dietitian in particular should help in the careful planning of a dietary regimen with which the patient can live comfortably and in which are incorporated the principles that follow. These principles must be well understood by the dietitian and explained carefully to the patient:

1. Frequent meals so as to avoid hunger and a resultant stimulation of the vagus nerves. Keeping food in the stomach helps neutralize excess acid and dilute gastric juice so that digestive action on mucosa is minimized.
2. Small meals in order to avoid distension of antrum and consequent secretion of gastrin. Duodenal ulcer patients have been shown to secrete much less gastrin when food intake is divided into six small meals rather than three larger ones (17).
3. Adequate protein intake in order to promote healing but not excessive in amount so as to avoid stimulating effect on gastrin secretion.
4. Adequate fat intake for patients not overweight in order to decrease gastric motility through the enterogastrone mechanism.

5. Carefully selected food to assure nutritional adequacy.
6. Avoidance of alcohol, coffee and caffeine-containing beverages, pepper, and meat extractives in order to prevent excessive stimulation of gastric acid secretion.

Reactions of patients to various foods are highly individual; therefore, strict diets with little flexibility are no longer recommended for ulcer patients (18). Initially it is probably wise to place the ulcer patient on a *bland diet* free of those foods found most often to be irritating or to cause flatus (e.g., fried foods, dried legumes, fibrous fruits and vegetables), but as soon as pain has subsided, individualization of the diet should begin. The patient should be made aware of the fact that he/she may be able to include a much wider variety of foods in the diet than is ordinarily considered appropriate for a bland diet. Tolerance to various foods may be established by introducing one food at a time. As soon as one food has been shown to be well tolerated, another food may be tried, and so on. It is always the responsibility of the dietitian to learn about the daily living situation of any patient being placed on a modified diet so that patients can be educated in food choices and patterns of food consumption that will be compatible with their life-style.

Drug therapy for the patient suffering from acute or chronic gastritis or peptic ulcer will usually consist of medications used to relieve pain and decrease stomach motility. To alleviate pain, the most frequently used agents are the antacids, which provide symptomatic relief but probably do not promote healing or prevent recurrence of the problem. The antacids are used to neutralize or decrease stomach acid even though patients with peptic ulcers usually have normal stomach acidity. Antacids are divided into two categories: those that are absorbed and those that are not absorbed from the gastrointestinal tract. The only clinically useful absorbable antacid is sodium bicarbonate. Sodium bicarbonate is the most potent antacid, but because it is absorbed, it may produce systemic alkalosis and resultant kidney damage if administered too frequently.

A number of nonabsorbable antacids are presently available. Table 5.2 indicates some of these preparations which are usually combinations of calcium carbonate, aluminum hydroxide, magnesium oxide, magnesium hydroxide, or magnesium trisilicate. The majority of these antacids also contain some sodium. Aluminum hydroxide is a relatively safe compound but its sustained use may lead to phosphorus depletion due to binding of phosphate by aluminum in the gastrointestinal tract. This binding does not usually pose a clinical problem because the usual ulcer diet provides sufficient amounts of phosphorus for absorption. Aluminum hydroxide also will frequently produce constipation.

Magnesium-containing compounds are also used frequently as antacids and are considered to be almost as effective as sodium bicarbonate.

Table 5.2 Composition of Commonly Used Antacids

Product	Calcium carbonate	Aluminum hydroxide	Magnesium oxide or hydroxide	Magnesium trisilicate	Sodium
Aludrox®		X	X		X
Amphojel®		X			X
Di-Gel®		X	X		X
Gelusil®		X		X	X
Kolantyl®		X	X		
Maalox®		X	X		X
Mylanta®		X	X		X
Phillip's Milk of Magnesia®			X		
Silain-Gel®		X	X		X
Titralac®	X				X
Trisogel®		X	X		X
Tums®	X				X
WinGel®		X	X		X

A disadvantage to the use of magnesium is its cathartic action which on prolonged use will result in diarrhea.

The more frequently used antacids are combinations of aluminum and magnesium. At normal doses and with the daily administration of four or less doses, the combination produces normal gastrointestinal tract activity. In choosing the appropriate antacid, the patient's taste preference is usually the deciding factor.

Drugs that decrease the motility and tone of the gastrointestinal tract are useful in the treatment of gastritis and peptic ulcers because they delay the emptying time of the stomach and thus prolong the retention of antacids and, in some cases, may decrease the secretion of gastric acid. The most frequently used drugs in this category are the anticholinergics. These agents not only antagonize the parasympathetic nervous system control of gastrointestinal motility but also affect other body sites under the control of this system. Thus, they produce frequent side effects such as dry mouth, blurred vision, and urinary retention. The anticholinergic drugs are classified as naturally occurring, semisynthetic, synthetic, and antispasmodic (Table 5.3). All of these agents have the ability to decrease gastrointestinal tract motility, but the semisynthetic and synthetic compounds are more specific in their action on the gastrointestinal tract and produce fewer side effects than the others.

Several newer agents also have been shown to be useful in the treatment of peptic ulcers. Cimetidine (Tagamet™) is classified as an antagonist of histamine at the histamine (H_2) receptors of the parietal cells. Because it inhibits both basal and stimulated secretion of gastric acid,

Table 5.3 Gastrointestinal Anticholinergic Preparations

Naturally Occurring and Semisynthetic

Preparation	Trade Name
Atropine sulfate	Atropine sulfate
Belladonna alkaloids	Bellafoline®
l-hyoscyamine	Levsin®, Anaspaz®
Methscopolamine Br	Pamine®
Scopolamine HBr	Scopolamine HBr

Synthetic Anticholinergics

Preparation	Trade Name
Clindinium Br	Quarzan®
Glycopyrrolate	Robinul®
Isopropamide	Darbid®
Mepenzolate Br	Cantil®
Methantheline Br	Banthine®
Piperidolate HCl	Dactil®
Propantheline	Pro-Banthine®
Tridihexethyl chloride	Pathilon®

Synthetic Antispasmodics

Preparation	Trade Name
Adiphene HCl	Trasentine®
Anisotropine	Valpin®
Dicyclomine HCl	Bentyl®
Triphenamil HCl	Trocinate®

cimetidine is indicated for the short-term therapy of ulcers (up to eight weeks) and for the treatment of pathological hypersecretory conditions.

Carbenoxolone, an experimental drug, increases the rate of healing of peptic ulcers by increasing the secretion of gastric mucoproteins and by increasing the life span of the mucosal cells. Side effects of carbenoxolone may include edema, hypertension and hypokalemia; therefore, it cannot be used in the presence of cardiovascular, pulmonary, or renal disease (13).

Ancillary therapy for the gastritis or ulcer patient may also include sedatives/antianxiety agents such as phenobarbital, chlordiazepoxide (Librium®) or other benzodiazepines, especially if the condition has been brought on by stress.

Only about 10 to 20 percent of patients with peptic ulcer are unable to be handled by medical therapy and must undergo surgery (12). Patients requiring surgery usually are those experiencing gastric retention due to strictures resulting from repeated exacerbations and healing of ulcers located near the pylorus. In such patients the diameter of the pylorodu-

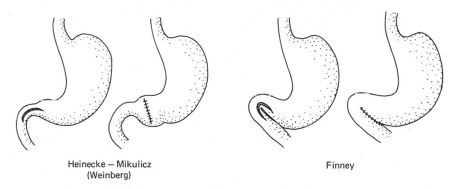

Heinecke — Mikulicz   Finney
(Weinberg)

Figure 5.8 Typical pylorplasty procedures. (From *Textbook of Surgery* by Loyal Davis and Frederick Christopher. Copyright 1972 by W. B. Saunders Co. Reprinted by permission of the publisher and author.)

odenal segment is often narrowed to less than 5 mm, thereby impeding the flow of gastric contents into the jejunum.

Many patients requiring surgery for peptic ulcer are in a poor state nutritionally; therefore, the surgical procedure presenting the least risk is often the one of choice, that is, vagotomy and pyroplasty. Figure 5.8 illustrates two types of pyroplasty in common use. The vagotomy, through disrupting stimulation of the parietal cells, decreases the production of gastric juice but also stops antral peristalsis. In order for the stomach to empty itself the pylorus must be incised and sutured so that the opening to the duodenum is larger. The disadvantage of this surgical procedure is that ulceration may reoccur in 10 to 15 percent of the cases.

More drastic surgical procedures (12,19), two of which are illustrated in Figure 5.9, include:

1. Gastroduodenostomy (or Bilroth I anastomosis) in which approximately 40 to 50 percent of the stomach is removed. The antrum of the stomach is excised and the cut end of the stomach is anastomosed to the transected end of the duodenum.
2. Gastrojejunostomy (or Bilroth II anastomosis) in which a loop of the jejunum is anastomosed to the remnant of the stomach after approximately 75 percent of the organ has been excised.
3. Total gastrectomy in which the entire organ is removed and the jejunum is anastomosed to the esophagus. This drastic procedure is reserved primarily for patients with proximal gastric carcinoma or Zollinger–Ellison syndrome. The latter condition is due to excessive gastrointestinal ulceration resulting from gastrin-producing tumors originating from the pancreas.

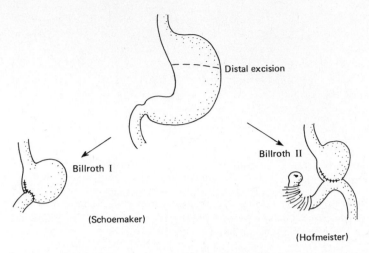

Distal excision

Billroth I

Billroth II

(Schoemaker)

(Hofmeister)

Figure 5.9 Gastrectomy procedures: gastroduodenostomy (Bilroth I Anastomosis) and gastrojejunostomy (Bilroth II Anastomosis). (From *Textbook of Surgery* by Loyal Davis and Frederick Christopher. Copyright 1972 by W.B. Saunders Co. Reprinted by permission of the publisher and author.)

The more extensive the gastric resection the greater the likelihood of postsurgical complications, such as the dumping syndrome.

In 5 to 10 percent of the patients undergoing gastric surgery, excision of the pylorus will cause the stomach to lose its retentive capacity completely and it will literally "dump" its hyperosmolar contents into the small intestine about 20 to 30 minutes following a meal. The larger the opening of the stomach into the intestine, the more likely this dumping becomes. Dilution of the hypertonic solution reaching the small intestine is caused by a rapid influx of fluid from the plasma, the results of which are decreased blood volume and lowered blood pressure. The affected individual experiences a variety of symptoms including weakness, nausea, abdominal cramps, feeling of warmth, palpitation, and diarrhea, many of which can be relieved by recumbent positioning. About two to three hours after eating, the patient may again suffer many of the same symptoms, this time elicited by functional hypoglycemia due to excess insulin secretion or insulin hypersensitivity.

Because carbohydrate foods increase the osmolarity of gastric contents more than proteins and/or fats and because the rapid absorption of carbohydrate results in an exaggerated insulin reaction, treatment of the dumping syndrome is effected through the feeding of small meals low in sugar and starch, high in protein, and moderate in fat. Because fluids taken with food foster production of hyperosmolar solutions, fluids are allowed only between meals, usually about 45 minutes before or after food intake.

The dietitian has a real challenge in the patient with dumping syndrome and it is his/her responsibility not only to see that the diet is modified properly to decrease symptoms and provide adequate nourishment but also to reassure the patient and encourage him/her to eat.

Anemia occurs in 20 to 50 percent of patients undergoing partial gastrectomies, and this condition often represents vitamin B_{12} deficiency as well as iron deficiency. Iron deficiency can be due not only to decreased intake of food but also to blood loss and poor iron absorption as a result of hypochlorhydria and/or bypass of the duodenum where most iron absorption occurs. Vitamin B_{12} deficiency can result from a decrease in intrinsic factor due not only to the reduced number of gastric glands but also to the effect of vagotomy. The dietitian should be alerted to careful nutritional assessment of any patient who has had a partial gastrectomy.

The iron content of preparations utilized in the treatment of an iron deficiency state can range from 90 to 300 mg. Such large quantities of iron are very irritating to the stomach and their administration may result in nausea and either constipation or diarrhea. Therapeutic iron preparations should be administered during or after meals but should not be accompanied by milk or antacids because these substances interfere with the absorption of iron.

Weight loss is common in patients who have had large portions of their stomachs excised, particularly if they suffer from the dumping syndrome. The decreased capacity of the stomach may make it difficult for the individual to ingest sufficient food for maintenance of weight; furthermore, fear of causing the untoward effects of dumping often results in a severely restricted intake.

Malabsorption occurs more commonly in patients who have undergone Bilroth II anastomosis than in those on whom pyroplasty or Bilroth I were performed. The cause of malabsorption is poorly understood but factors implicated include:

1. Poor mixing of chyme with pancreatic juices and bile due to bypassing of the duodenum where stimulus for secretion of secretin and CCK–PZ occurs and into which pass the pancreatic juices and bile.
2. Effects of bacterial overgrowth which may occur in the obstructed afferent loop as a result of stasis of intestinal contents in loop. Organisms produced may cause deconjugation of bile salts which are rapidly reabsorbed and therefore unavailable in the jejunum for normal micelle formation and fat absorption. Excessive growth of microorganisms that use vitamin B_{12} may be responsible for impaired absorption of this vitamin.
3. Decreased intestinal transit time due to loss of storage function of stomach (9,20).

Small Intestine

Figure 5.6, which illustrates the sites of absorption of the various nutrients, makes clear how important healthy mucosal tissue in the small intestine is to the nutritional status of the individual. Failure to thrive in some infants can be traced to Hirschsprung's disease which is a congenital aganglionic megacolon disease. In this disease state, sufficient absorption of nutrients for survival is impossible because food cannot be moved appropriately through the gastrointestinal tract. Abdominal distention and fecal retention are primary symptoms and relief can be accomplished only through surgical removal of the affected portion of the intestinal tract.

Numerous disorders can damage the absorptive mechanisms of the small intestine, thereby making unavailable to the body a large proportion of the ingested nutrients. One such disorder is celiac disease (non tropical sprue or gluten sensitive enteropathy) which presents a classic example of malabsorption syndrome and is caused by the plant protein, gliadin, which together with glutelin makes up gluten. Two theories are suggested for injury to the mucosal tissues which is characteristic of the disease: (1) deficiency of an enzyme necessary for splitting N-glutamyl peptides of gliadin, the accumulation of which exert a toxic effect on mucosal cells of the proximal bowel; (2) immunologic disorder in which mucosa exposed to gluten binds the antigenic peptides of gliadin and locally produces an antibody for reaction with the antigen (21).

Regardless of the cause of celiac disease, the absorptive surface of the small intestine is reduced about 30-fold, as illustrated in Figure 5.10, and the following consequences can result (22):

1. Steatorrhea—the stool may contain 50 percent of ingested fat.
2. Creatorrhea—amino acids and peptides are excreted in larger than normal quantities.
3. Disaccharide intolerance—the disaccharide most commonly not tolerated is lactose.
4. Increase in prothrombin time due to malabsorption of vitamin K.
5. Disturbance in absorption of calcium, magnesium, and vitamin D which if uncorrected can result in tetany and/or osteomalacia.
6. Decreased iron absorption, possibly resulting in microcytic anemia.
7. Decreased absorption of folic acid and vitamin B_{12}, possibly resulting in macrocytic anemia.
8. Disturbed absorption of water, sodium, potassium, and all water-soluble vitamins in severe disease.

Tropical sprue presents a mucosal damage and malabsorption syndrome almost identical to that found in celiac disease but unlike celiac disease, sprue is responsive to treatment with antibiotics and folic acid.

Paradoxically, antibiotics themselves taken in large doses or on a continuous basis may contribute to malabsorption by causing diarrhea.

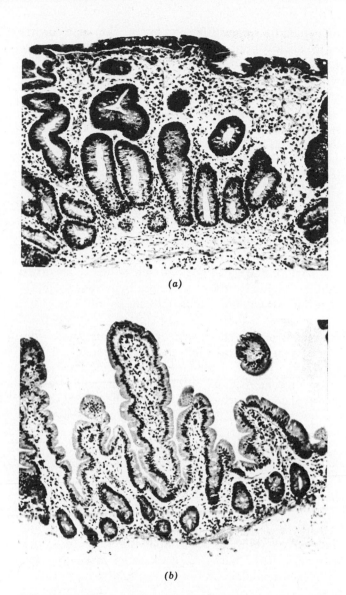

(a)

(b)

Figure 5.10 The small intestine in nontropical sprue. (*a*) Jejunal mucosa in patient with nontropical sprue. (*b*) Mucosa of same patient after nine months on gluten free diet. (From "Disorders of absorption" by George W. Thorn et al. *Harrison's Principles of Internal Medicine,* Copyright 1977 by McGraw-Hill Book Co. Reprinted by permission of the publisher.)

Any condition accompanied by or resulting in malnutrition may further cause diarrhea and consequently contribute to malabsorption. Malabsorption due to malnutrition is related to the decreased synthesis of the epithelial cells lining the villi.

Certain other disease states such as lymphomas, amyloid disease, and Whipple's disease are characterized by total malabsorption similar to that of celiac disease. However, rather than being due to a lack of absorptive surface malabsorption caused by these diseases results from concentration of abnormal cells and/or extracellular material in the lamina propria which prevents normal passage of nutrients into lymph and blood vessels (20). An entirely different type of malabsorption disorder is that seen in lactase deficiency in which only one substance is affected and which causes no damage to the mucosal tissue. This disorder is common among adults, particularly non-Caucasians, and is due to an insufficiency of lactase acitvity in the microvilli of the epithelial cells. Lactose instead of being digested into glucose and galactose and subsequently absorbed remains in the intestinal lumen, thereby producing a hypertonic solution that draws water from the extracellular fluids and causes diarrhea (20).

Diagnostic Tests for Malabsorption. The malabsorption syndromes, from the clinical point of view, can be divided into those associated with generalized malabsorption of fat, protein, and carbohydrate, and those associated with failure to absorb one or more specific substances. Disease of the small intestine, particularly that which would result in a decreased absorptive surface (e.g., celiac disease), would cause a generalized malabsorption because the overall absorptive process would be affected. Tests are available to diagnose impairment of intestinal absorption. A few of these, along with their clinical significance, will be discussed briefly.

Quantitative Determination of Stool Fat. In order to confirm presence of steatorrhea the stool should be collected for 24 to 72 hours and analyzed for total fat. It is necessary to have an accurate record of dietary fat intake in order for fecal fat excretion to be meaningful. Normally 95 percent of ingested fat is absorbed; therefore, if excretion exceeds much more than 5 percent of intake, malabsorption is strongly suspected.

D-Xylose Absorption Test. Xylose, usually found in only small amounts in the blood, is a pentose that is not metabolized but maintains its original molecular form. When given orally, xylose is passively absorbed in the duodenojejunal region of the small intestine, passes unchanged through the liver, and is excreted by the kidneys.

Usually, a 26 g dose is administered orally, and urine voided over the next five hours is collected. The xylose concentration in this specimen and in a blood specimen taken during the collecting period is chemically determined. Normal values for the blood and urine levels are published. The levels will, of course, be significantly reduced if there is impairment of the intestinal absorption. The test has the additional value of being able to distinguish intestinal malabsorption from pancreatic insufficiency. In the latter condition, the absorption of xylose will be essentially normal.

Schilling Test for Vitamin B$_{12}$ Absorption. Vitamin B$_{12}$ can be absorbed only when it has formed a complex with *intrinsic factor,* a mucopolysaccharide secreted by mucous neck cells in gastric glands of the stomach. Absorption of vitamin B$_{12}$, therefore, depends on normal gastric secretion as well as normal intestinal absorption processes. Although the test is designed to diagnose pernicious anemia, a condition caused by the absence of intrinsic factor, the Schilling test is also a useful test for identification of malabsorption syndromes, particularly ileal defects.

A small dose of the vitamin labeled with radioactive cobalt is given, and the amount of radioactivity excreted in the urine is measured. If the malabsorption is due to pernicious anemia, administration of the labeled vitamin together with intrinsic factor results in normal absorption. If it is due to intestinal disease, the malabsorption persists.

Lactose Tolerance Test. Intestinal malabsorption may be due to chemical errors in the mucosal cells as well as to diminished absorptive surface. For example, deficiency of small bowel mucosal lactase (the enzyme responsible for hydrolyzing the disaccharide, lactose, into glucose and galactose) has been found to be a rather common condition in adults. As discussed previously, unabsorbed lactose can cause severe diarrhea due to its hypertonicity.

The test consists of administering 100 g of lactose, followed by a periodic determination of glucose and galactose in the blood during the following several hours. Chemical tests that measure glucose and galactose simultaneously are used. If mucosal lactase is present and active, the blood levels of glucose and galactose should rise rapidly, peak, and then return to fasting levels within a few hours. Lactase deficiency would result in a relatively "flat" tolerance curve (Fig. 5.11). A flat curve may sometimes result from delayed gastric emptying, thereby producing a false positive test. Other useful parameters in evaluating carbohydrate absorption are pH of the stool and presence of reducing sugars. Normally fecal matter is slightly alkaline, but when undigested carbohydrate is present in the stool, the oxidation of aldehydes to acids by intestinal microbes decreases the pH (see Chapter 2). Antibiotic therapy may alter microbial flora and therefore invalidate this test.

The "short bowel syndrome" resulting from extensive excision of the small intestine mimics the "malabsorption syndrome" seen in celiac disease except that carbohydrate intolerance presents no problem in the resected small intestine. Treatment of all malabsorption disorders is

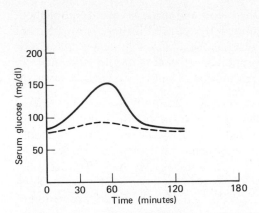

Figure 5.11 Graphical representation of tests to determine lactase deficiency. Following oral administration of lactose, serum glucose is determined periodically as in a glucose tolerance test. The solid line represents a normal curve, while the flattened, dotted line curve illustrates lactase deficiency, resulting in decreased absorption of free glucose.

aimed toward nutritional replacement in order to stabilize weight and to prevent muscle wasting and general malnutrition (23).

Vitamins and minerals can be given parenterally and total parenteral nutrition can be employed in extreme cases of malabsorption; however, long-term practical measures for maintaining or improving the nutritional status of individuals suffering with malabsorption problems must be addressed, and the success of such measures in large degree rests upon the dietitian and/or nutritionist. He/she not only must institute proper dietary treatment in the hospital but also must educate and motivate the affected individuals to continue necessary modifications of diet. This will mean establishing an excellent rapport and spending much time with the patient as he/she gains independence in management of diet.

Scientifically based dietary modifications often necessary in treatment of malabsorption include one or more of the following:

1. Reduction of intake of long chain dietary lipids in patients with steatorrhea in order to (a) place no further burden of fat digestion and absorption on an already inefficiently functioning small intestine and (b) decrease loss of nutrients.
2. Replacement of the long chain dietary lipids with medium chain triglycerides in order to help maintain adequate caloric intake.
3. Avoidance of gluten-containing cereals in gluten-sensitive enteropathy. Exclusion of all products containing wheat, rye, barley as fillers is necessary. Such products often include ice cream, salad dressings, various canned foods, condiments, candy, etc. Beer and ale also must be avoided because of their cereal residues.

4. Omission of specific disaccharides in disaccharidase deficient patients, for example, lactose in lactase insufficiency.
5. Increase of total caloric intake so as to compensate for calories lost through malabsorption of nutrients.

Regional Enteritis (Crohn's disease). Crohn's disease is an inflammatory lesion characterized by granulomas and occurring most commonly in young people, aged 15 to 35 years. In the United States the annual incidence of regional enteritis is two to three per 100,000 but the incidence is on the rise (24). This disorder is a chronic disease of unknown cause that can occur anywhere in the gastrointestinal tract and often spreads to adjoining areas of the intestine. Obstruction is a common complication of the disease. Because malabsorption is a hallmark of the disorder, Crohn's disease is usually identified through differential diagnosis of malabsorption and through radiology. In most instances, treatment involves excision of the diseased bowel but supportive care is very important, particularly in regard to adequate nutrition for those patients whose disease is of long standing.

Other patients, especially those in the early or acute stages of the disease, may benefit from steroid therapy. Large doses of prednisone (40 to 60 mg per day) are administered initially with the dosage being gradually reduced to 10 to 20 mg per day. Use of such a steroid may reduce fever and diarrhea, relieve abdominal pain and tenderness, and improve appetite. Adjunctive therapy such as anticholinergic drugs and narcotic analgesics (tincture of opium or codeine) may be useful in decreasing cramps and diarrhea (13). High caloric chemically defined diets are commonly used to assure adequate nutrition for the patient. Although supplying the nutrients in a form easily assimilated by the small intestine (i.e., nutrients reduced to their simplest forms), elemental preparations are rather unpalatable and their successful use requires much time and effort on the part of the dietitian (see Table 12.4). The dietitian needs to determine which flavors of elemental preparations are most acceptable to the patient and provide support to him/her in the continued ingestion of these dietary supplements. If regular foods are permitted the patient during an acute attack, these should be low in residue in order to prevent danger of obstruction and avoid stimulation of peristalsis (23).

Colon

Diarrhea. This term describes the condition in which there is excessive stimulation of the mucosa and increased motility of the intestinal wall resulting in very frequent passage of stools or passage of quite liquid stools. This condition can accompany numerous disease states characterized by malabsorption but the major causes of diarrhea are: (1) infection of some segment of the gastrointestinal tract, usually the colon, and (2) excessive stimulation of the colon by parasympathetic nerves as a result of nervous tension.

Most acute infectious diarrheas are of brief duration and serve the purpose of ridding the body of the toxic agents. Therefore, treatment usually is aimed at replacement of the fluids and electrolytes orally, if possible, through use of tea, salty broths, and unchilled diluted sweetened fruit juices in sufficient quantities to produce a urinary output of no less than 1500 ml daily (25).

Drug therapy for diarrhea uncomplicated by an infection usually consists of an "antidiarrheal" medication which decreases the motility of the intestinal tract, decreases intestinal inflammation, and favorably modifies the intestinal flora. In these preparations, the following ingredients may be found: opium and anticholinergic agents which decrease gastrointestinal tract motility; attapulgite, kaolin, and pectin which are adsorptive agents; aluminum and bismuth which are used as antacids and adsorptive agents; zinc, which is an intestinal antiseptic and astringent; and bacterial cultures that modify intestinal flora (see Table 5.4). The most commonly used antidiarrheal prescription is a combination of diphenoxylate and atropine (Lomotil®). Diphenoxylate is a derivative of meperidine (a narcotic analgesic) which produces its therapeutic effect by slowing intestinal motility. Atropine is added to the diphenoxylate to discourage deliberate overdosage.

Ulcerative Colitis. This is an inflammatory disease involving the mucosa of the colon, which occurs more often in women than in men and reaches its peak of incidence in the 20- to 25-year age group with a second rise in incidence occurring between the fifth and sixth decades. The disease is characterized by a bloody diarrhea, and irritation to the colon may be so severe that mass movements occur almost continuously rather than occurring only 10 to 20 minutes daily as is normal (1). Although the true etiology is unknown, the disorder has been linked to nervous tension and/or immunologic reactions. Approximately 25,000 to 30,000 new cases of ulcerative colitis are diagnosed each year and the total cases in this country are estimated at between 200,000 and 400,000 (26). The best tool for diagnosing the disorder is sigmoidoscopy.

Because there is no known specific therapy for ulcerative colitis, treatment is primarily supportive and its success depends to a large degree upon the relationship existing between the patient and the health team. Nutritional deficits, especially iron deficiency anemia, are common in patients whose colitis is long-standing, and the dietitian has a critical role in helping to correct these deficits. Getting to know the patient, his/her food preferences and tolerances is essential when attempts are being made to tempt the patient to eat. Visits by the dietitian are probably

Table 5.4 Antidiarrheal Medications

Products	Ingredients				
	Opiates	Adsorbents and/or antacids	Anticholinergics	Astringents	Bacterial cultures
Amogel®	Powdered opium	Bismuth, kaolin, pectin		Zinc	
Bacid®		Carboxymethyl-cellulose			Lactobacillus acidophilus
Donnagel®		Kaolin, pectin	Hyoscine, atropine hyoscyamine		
Donnagel®-PG	Powdered opium	Kaolin, pectin	Hyoscine, atropine hyoscyamine		
Kaopectate®		Kaolin, pectin			
Lactinex®					Lactobacillus acidophilus and L. bulgarius
Paregoric®	Opium tincture				
Pabizol® with Paregoric®	Paregoric	Aluminum, magnesium sulfate, bismuth		Zinc	
Parelixir®	Opium tincture	Pectin			
Parepectolin®	Paregoric	Kaolin, pectin			
Pargel®		Kaolin, pectin			
Pepto-bismol®		Bismuth, calcium carbonate			
Polymagma®		Attapulgite, pectin, alumina gel			

needed before each meal while the patient is in an acute stage of the disease. The nutritional therapy employed depends on the response of individual patients and can range from a low residue diet to minimal residue diet to total parenteral nutrition (TPN). TPN may be indicated for those patients in whom healing of the ulcerated tissue requires complete immobility of the colon. Steroids such as prednisone and sulfasalazine (Azulfidine®) along with various antibiotics are often used in an attempt to control inflammation of the colon.

Constipation. This is slow passage of feces through the colon, usually characterized by hard, dry stools with evacuation occurring irregularly and/or infrequently. The most common cause for constipation not related to organic disease is habitual inhibition of the defecation reflexes which normally occur most often immediately following the breakfast meal. Constipation, however, also may occur due to atony of the colon muscles or may be due to spasm of a small segment of the sigmoid, a condition often referred to as *spastic* or *irritable colon.* Irritable colon accounts for more than 50 percent of all gastrointestinal illnesses and although onset can occur at any age, it usually begins in early adult life (25). The disorder often develops as a result of stress and emotional tension and although symptoms commonly abate during periods of calm life situations, they reoccur when pressures begin to mount again. Symptoms of irritable colon are abdominal pain and passage of small stools at the height of distress. These stools may be hard and dry or soft and pasty, but they are always small and often contain visible mucus. Symptoms and motor disturbances associated with spastic or irritable colon closely resemble those found in diverticular disease. Some investigators believe that irritable colon precedes the development of diverticular disease or that the two disorders coexist.

Before proper treatment for either atonic or spastic constipation can be undertaken, a thorough dietary, medical, and social history must be obtained and analyzed. Information should be obtained about eating and defecatory habits, use of laxatives and drugs, home and work environment with their associated emotional problems. Because therapy is successful only when it is directed toward the patient as a whole rather than just his/her colon, consideration of the patient's attitudes and environmental situation is essential (25).

Although therapy must be individualized, a dietary modification that usually seems appropriate is an increase in those foods providing bulk, that is, fruits, vegetables, whole grain breads, and cereals. Dietary fiber obtained from such foods enlarges the fecal size, thereby stimulating mass movement in the colon, and furthermore it increases the amount of moisture that may be held in the feces. A fecal weight of 140 to 150 grams daily has been suggested as an index for establishment of a recommended intake of dietary fiber (27).

Laxatives are a diverse group of therapeutic agents utilized in drug treatment of constipation. Their function is to promote evacuation of the bowel. The laxatives are divided into the following categories according to their mechanisms of action: saline laxatives which are hyperosmolar compounds that retain water in the lumen of the intestine; irritant (stimulant) laxatives which increase activity in the intestine by a direct action; bulk-producing laxatives which increase the frequency of bowel movements and soften stools by holding water in the stool; lubricant laxatives which lubricate the intestinal mucosa and soften the stool; fecal softeners which are surfactants, thereby promoting water retention in the fecal mass (Table 5.5).

Laxatives are one of the most commonly overused groups of drugs. Their use should be limited to short-term therapy for constipation or specific evacuation of the bowel prior to surgery or examination. Prolonged or excessive use of laxatives, especially the stimulants, may lead to dependence and electrolyte imbalance. Patients who use laxatives should be encouraged to drink sufficient amounts of water, especially with those agents classified as bulk-producing laxatives. A number of the laxatives contain sodium, and these agents should not be used by patients on sodium-restricted diets (28).

Diverticular Disease. Incidence of diverticular disease is difficult to determine because diverticula occur in the colon most often without symptoms. However, it is estimated that 20 percent of all persons over 40 years of age suffer from diverticular disorders (25).

Diverticula are pouches of mucous membrane that protrude from the intestinal lumen and occur most commonly in the sigmoid segment of the colon. These pouches project through and beyond the circular muscles and usually develop at those points in the muscle that are pierced by blood vessels and are, consequently, the weakest sites on the muscle. Diverticula are believed to result from high intraluminal pressures that occur when the circular muscles of the colon contract excessively (extreme haustral contractions). Fecal matter is moved back and forth in the sigmoid for efficient absorption of water and this movement is made possible by these haustral contrictions or segmenting motions. When, however, the segmenting contractions become excessive to the point that the lumen is almost occluded on either side of the haustra, local intrasegmental pressures increase to the point that diverticula are formed. (Figure 5.12 illustrates mechanisms believed responsible for diverticula formation).

N. S. Painter and D. P. Burkitt (29) have postulated that diverticular disease results when colonic muscles have hypertrophied in response to a diet too low in fiber, particularly deficient in wheat bran. Although their hypothesis seems plausible and has some epidemiological support, only about one-third of the population suffering with diverticulosis gives evidence of muscle hypertrophy (30). An alternate hypothesis is that ex-

Table 5.5 Categories of Laxative Preparations According to
Mechanism of Action

Saline Laxatives	
Generic name	*Trade name*
Magnesium sulfate	Epsom Salt
Magnesium hydroxide	Milk of Magnesia
Monosodium phosphate	Sal Hepatica®
Sodium phosphate and sodium biphosphate	Phospho-Soda® and
	Sodium Phosphate and Biphosphate®

Irritant or Stimulant Laxatives	
Generic name	*Trade name*
Cascara sagrada	Cascara Sagrada
	Bileo-Secrin
	Cas-Evac
Danthron	Modane®
	Dorbane®
Calcium salts of sennosides A & B	Glysennid®
Senna	Black Draught®
	Senokot®
	Senolax®
	X-Prep®
	Casafru®
Phenolphathalein	Phenolphthalein
	Prulet Liquitab®
	Alophen®
	Prulet®
	Phenolax®
	Ex-Lax®
	Evac-U-Gen®
	Feen-a-Mint®
Castor oil	Castor oil
	Neoloid®
Bisacodyl	Bisacodyl
	Bisco-Lax
	Bon-O-Lax
	Codylax
	Dulcolax®
	Fleet® Bisacodyl
	Rolax
	SK-Bisacodyl®
	Theralax
	Tulax
	Vactrol
	Laxadan Supules

Bulk-Producing Laxatives	
Generic name	*Trade name*
Methylcellulose	Cologel
	Hydrolose

Table 5.5 Continued

Nondiastatic barley malt extract	Maltsupex®
Psyllium	Mucilose
	Hydrocil®
	L.A. Formula®
	Laxamead, P.H.M.
	Metamucil®
	Modane Bulk®
	Mucillium
	Regacilium
	Syllact TM
	Effersyllium®
	Konsyl®
	Siblin®

Lubricant Laxatives

Mineral oil	Mineral oil
	Neo-Cultol
	Agoral Plain®
	Petrogalar Plain
	Kondremul Plain®

Fecal Softeners

Generic name	*Trade name*
Dioctyl sodium sulfosuccinate (DSS)	Colace®
	D-S-S®
	DioMedicone®
	Disonate®
	Doxinate®
	Afko-Lube®
	Bu-Lax®
	Coloctyl
	Dilax-100
	Diosuccin®
	Diosux
	Duosol
	Laxinate
	Regul-Aids
	Softon
	Doctate 100®
	Molatoc
	Regutol®
	Softeze
	Stulex
	Modane Soft®
	Doss 300®
	Doctate 300®
	Parlax®
Dioctyl calcium sulfosuccinate	Surfax®
Poloxamer 188	Polykol®

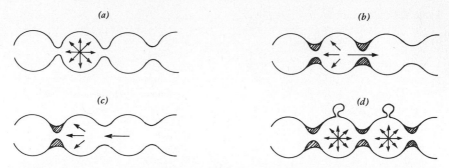

Figure 5.12 Proposed mechanisms for diverticula formation. Role of segmentation in colonic physiology and the pathogenesis of diverticula. Segmentation is concerned in the transportation and halting of feces in the sigmoid colon. Diagram A shows a segmented colon; one segment has produced pressure by contracting. Diagram B shows how relaxation of the contraction ring on one side of this segment allows its contents to move into the next segment which harbors a lower pressure; this is the mechanism by which contents are moved. Diagram C shows how feces are halted; contraction rings act as baffles that slow and finally halt contents and a pressure change results. Segmentation is seen in the sigmoid as feces are shunted back and forth. Diagram D shows a segmented colon acting as a series of "little bladders" whose outflow is obstructed at both ends and which extrude diverticula by generating high localized intrasegmental pressures. Segmentation is essential to the pathogenesis of diverticula. Any factor that causes segmentation to occur more frequently or more efficiently favors the causation of diverticular disease. (From "Diverticular disorders of the colon: a deficiency disease of western civilization" by N. S. Painter and D. P. Burkett. *British Medical Journal.* Copyright May 22, 1971, by British Medical Journal. Reprinted by permission of the publisher and authors.)

cessive intrasegmental pressures are generated due to a diseased longitudinal muscle that prevents the colon from elongating properly (31).

Diverticula become symptomatic only when they become inflamed (diverticulitis). It is estimated that diverticulitis occurs in approximately 25 percent of patients with diverticulosis (12). Fecal matter moving into the diverticula cannot be discharged through the narrow necks of the pouches. With stasis the fecal matter loses its moisture and forms a fecalith which has the potential of eroding the mucosal lining of the diverticulum. Erosion of the mucosa results in inflammation. Stasis also promotes bacterial growth which increases danger of sepsis. Diagnosis is made most frequently by means of radiologic findings after administration of a barium enema.

Dietary management of diverticular disease has traditionally been through the use of the low residue diet. However, during the last ten to fifteen years the trend has been toward the use of a high fiber diet which increases fecal bulk and appears to decrease hypersegmentation of the colon, thereby presumably preventing excessive intrasegmental pressures (31). If, however, diarrhea is associated with diverticular disease, excessive amounts of raw fruits and vegetables are avoided because of their possible increase of bowel irritability. Controversy still abounds concerning the appropriate dietary treatment for diverticular disease because many patients receiving high fiber diets have reported no symptomatic advantage over those being treated with a diet low in fiber (30).

Cancer of the Colon. Carcinoma of the colon and rectum is the second most common malignancy found in the adult population of the United States and is responsible for an annual death rate of approximately 16 to 18 adults per 100,000 population (32).

The disease is usually diagnosed by lower gastrointestinal X-ray series and/or sigmoidscopic examination. During the past several years, however, much interest has centered around a substance known as carcinoembryonic antigen (CEA) which may be a diagnostic indicator of colon and pancreatic carcinoma. CEA is an oncofetal marker of antigen found in fetal and embryonic gut tissue as well as malignant tissue of the gastrointestinal tract. Although oncofetal markers are believed to be normal fetal antigens, they are also produced by malignant tissue as a result of the transformation process.

The determination of serum CEA has been evaluated as a potentially simple and accurate diagnostic test for colonic cancer since it was discovered that over 90 percent of patients with malignancies of the colon or pancreas are CEA positive (33). Hopes were dimmed, however, with the finding of CEA in patients with a wide variety of nonmalignant gastrointestinal disorders. Furthermore, early, curable colon cancers rarely produce sharply elevated levels. The value of CEA determination lies in its relationship to disease progression. Changing CEA levels appear to correlate with progression or remission of the disease, and very high levels are almost invariably associated with metastases (34).

Although the etiology of cancer of the colon is unknown, three factors believed to have influence on the development of the disease are: the environment (of which diet is an important part), heredity, and certain disease states, for example, ulcerative colitis.

Dietary habits that may influence development of colonic cancer include: (1) excess intake of fat which increases the amount of cholesterol and bile acids present in the intestinal lumen, both of which are considered to be potential sources of carcinogens; (2) high consumption of meat which promotes development of bacteria responsible for producing certain carcinogens in the large intestine; and (3) lack of fiber which permits the feces to remain for a longer time in the colon, thereby prolonging the contact of carcinogens with the mucosal tissue (35).

Therapy for an existent colonic cancer can only be immediate surgery, but in the future a change in dietary habits may serve to prevent the disorder. A diet lower in fat content with more of its caloric content being contributed by fiber-containing foods, that is, fruits, vegetables, and whole grain products could be a preventive measure. Much research is being devoted to examination of these theories, and if dietary habits are found to be causal factors in colonic cancer, the role of dietary counseling and nutrition education in preventive medicine will become much better recognized.

Articles reporting various aspects of fiber research have proliferated in the literature but there is a lack of consensus among investigators concerning the value of fiber in preventive medicine. One important fact that has emerged, however, is that this "bulking agent" is made up of many different types of fiber, so different in fact that they cannot be grouped together in regard to function (36). Although present data fail to support many of the claims made in recent years for this long overlooked food constituent, continuing research is aimed at determining just how valuable fiber may be in preventive medicine (37).

Another area of intensive research in the study of fiber is determination of total dietary fiber along with its component parts in a wide variety of food products. Present estimations of fiber content in commonly consumed foods are inaccurate because currently available food composition tables reflect only "crude" fiber, that is, residue after food has been treated in the laboratory with a solvent, hot acid, and hot alkali. The present figures for the fiber in food estimate its lignin content and much of its cellulose, but fail to include the soluble components such as the hemicelluloses, gums, and pectin.

Gastrointestinal Surgery

The dietitian's role in therapy for surgical patients is often overlooked. The patient's course of recovery, however, can be affected significantly by the degree of interest and astuteness exhibited by the dietitian in assessing the individual's nutritional status and in determining what and how much food should be given the patient. The dietitian can be very important to the patient admitted for gastrointestinal surgery, both preoperatively and postoperatively.

Many patients admitted for elective gastrointestinal surgery are already malnourished because their medical problems, (for example, ulcer, Crohn's disease), have prevented them from ingesting or utilizing an adequate diet. These patients are often excellent candidates for nourishment via elemental diets and their diet is so prescribed immediately following admission to the hospital. Should the surgeon, however, elect to order a traditional hospital diet for a patient who could benefit from nutritional therapy, the dietitian has the responsibility of bringing the patient's need to the attention of the surgeon. The dietitian needs to be familiar with all the various types of available supplements and to know not only their nutritional value but also their degree of palatability (see Chapter 12). Many of the elemental preparations, although excellent sources of easily utilizable nutrients, are far from palatable and need to be improved in taste as much as possible by an imaginative dietitian. All people respond to attention and concern for their opinions and well-being; therefore, the really caring dietitian in most instances will be able to encourage patients to consume various nutritious concoctions despite their lack of true taste appeal.

Following gastrointestinal surgery, patients require frequent observation from an astute, assertive dietitian. When a surgeon's busy schedule prevents him/her from progressing the patient's diet as soon as is desirable for the patient's condition, the dietitian should assume the responsibility for seeing that the patient is fed appropriately. The exact nutritional care of the patient may vary from hospital to hospital depending upon the medical and surgical staff, but the principles remain much the same (23,38):

1. Postoperative feeding can begin as soon as flatus is passed or bowel sounds can be detected. Only a small amount of fluid is given initially in order to avoid the swallowing of air which accompanies the drinking of liquids. Some patients find they tolerate dry toast or crackers quite well along with their first liquids. Although most hospitals have standard postoperative dietary routines, individual patients will vary markedly in their rate of progression from clear liquids to a regular diet.
2. Patients recovering from esophageal surgery take about nine to 10 days to progress from the liquid diet through soft solids to a regular diet.
3. Patients who have undergone gastric surgery can begin a standard post-gastrectomy diet as soon as complete function of the gastrointestinal tract has returned. This diet consists of six small meals and should be individualized with the patient being visited before each meal until food tolerances and acceptable meal sizes have been determined. Dietary modifications appropriate for prevention of the "dumping syndrome" are followed for the first two or three days and if there are no symptoms of dumping, foods containing some sugar may be added to the diet.
4. Patients with massive small bowel resection are carefully watched so as to correlate daily weight change with caloric intake of intravenously administered hyperalimentation solution and to determine the number of kilocalories necessary to prevent weight loss. When oral low residue diets can begin, a complete dietary history should be available to serve as a guide to the patient's food preferences. Current research suggests

that oral feedings should begin even while total energy requirements are being met by parenteral nutrition in order that hyperplasia of the small bowel may be stimulated (29,40).

5. Patients with ileostomies and colostomies require special care as their diet progresses. In order to regulate evacuation the diet initially should be low residue and contain only warm foods, because cold ones stimulate peristalsis. Usually in two weeks or less, however, patients should progress to a regular diet. Consequently, ostomy patients need much encouragement and support in order to alleviate their concern over food ingestion. Such support can be provided by the dietitian, particularly when he/she has the excellent counsel of an ostomy technician or nurse.

CASE STUDY: CROHN'S DISEASE

The patient, a white 32-year-old male, was admitted to the hospital with complaint of painful anal drainage. At time of admission his height and weight were recorded at 5' 10" and 135 lbs, respectively. The patient reported a weight loss of approximately 20 lbs during the past three months. An examination by the physician revealed inflamed friable granular rectal mucosa up to 16 cm, with increased amounts of blood and pus in the rectal lumen. A diagnosis of ulcerative colitis had been made approximately 18 months previously and the patient had been treated intermittently with prednisone and Azulfidine. He had been doing reasonably well, being maintained on the Azulfidine tablets daily, until the onset of the painful anal drainage. Over the past six weeks he had been treated for the anal drainage with prednisone, Azulfidine, intermittent antibiotics, and sitz baths which appeared to be controlling the condition until the present admission. A recent examination of the colon by barium enema had shown the colon to be normal with no evidence of shortening or ulceration.

Medical history disclosed that the patient at the time of admission reported having had three to four semiformed bowel movements daily with additional passage of blood and mucus several times daily. There was also intermittent abdominal cramping prior to bowel movements.

The family medical history revealed that both of the patient's parents were living and well. There was no family history of carcinoma, colitis, mental or emotional disorders, diabetes, hematemesis, or liver disease.

Upon admission, the patient at the physician's request was given a hematologic and chemistry screening along with a microscopic examination of the colonic mucosa. Additionally, a low residue diet was ordered for the patient.

Laboratory findings were as follows:

Hemoglobin: 11.6 (norm for males 14.0—18.0 gm/dl)

Hematocrit: 36.3 (norm for males 40.0—54.0 ml/dl)

BUN: 16 (norm 10—20 mg/dl)

Total Protein: 6 (norm 6—8 gm/dl)

Albumin: 3.0 (norm 4.0—5.5 gm/dl)

Alk. Phos: 110 (norm, leucocyte total score 14—100)

SGOT: 24 (norm 15—40 units/ml)

Microscopic examination revealed some colonic glands with areas of acute inflammation and some other areas of ulcerated mucosa. Mucus-producing cells in some glands were markedly diminished and lymphoid tissue was increased in the mucosa. A colonoscopic examination was conducted and disclosed deep longitudinal ulcerations of the rectum. Based on these findings a diagnosis of Crohn's disease was made.

1. Among the laboratory findings, which would have alerted the physician to the possibility of Crohn's disease?
2. Why would the physician have expected the levels of serum alkaline phosphatase and albumin to be abnormal in this disease state?
3. What category of drugs other than steroids and antibiotics might the clinical pharmacist suggest as treatment to relieve the symptoms of the disease?
4. What information about the nutritional status of the patient can the dietitian obtain from the various recorded subjective and objective data?
5. Was a low residue diet the appropriate prescription for the patient?

Discussion

Inflammatory disease of the colon is positively diagnosed through visual inspection of the affected region, made possible by sigmoidoscopy and colonoscopy. The rectal fistulas and regional ulceration are clearly discernible using these techniques. Contrast media (barium) enemas can also be of value in the diagnosis if the lesion is located in regions of the colon not accessible to the colonoscopic probe. Findings from the microscopic examination of the intestinal mucosa would also contribute to the diagnosis. Acute inflammation of the colonic glands and the infiltration of leucocytes would be findings that are compatible with this sort of lesion.

The hematologic and chemical determinations carried out by the laboratory personnel are, in this case, not as important in establishing the diagnosis as the examination methods already described. However, their results are consistent with this type of disease. For example, the somewhat reduced hemoglobin, referred to as a mild hypochromic anemia, is caused by the chronic intestinal bleeding experienced by the patient. Alkaline phosphatase is an enzyme that functions in various tissues, principally that of liver, bone, and intestine. An inflammatory process involving one of these tissues, in this case the intestine, causes an increase in the porosity of the affected cells with the release of cellular enzymes into circulation. The serum alkaline phosphotase is slightly elevated for this reason. This impression could be confirmed through evaluation of the alkaline phosphatase isoenzyme pattern.

Excessive loss of blood can explain the abnormally low (although only marginally) serum albumin. As blood volume is restored following blood loss, the water is replenished more rapidly than the cellular components or dissolved solutes such as serum proteins. The effect is a dilution of the solutes.

Because the presenting symptoms of Crohn's disease are associated with hypermotility of the gastrointestinal tract, anticholinergic drugs such as atropine (as belladonna tincture) or synthetic anticholinergic agents such as propantheline (Banthine®) may be used to decrease gastrointestinal motility. Such agents will decrease diarrhea and smooth muscle cramps, but will also produce unpleasant side effects such as dry mouth and decreased bronchial secretions. The excessive drying of the mouth may be overcome by having the patient hold hard candy (such as peppermint) in the mouth to stimulate salivary secretions.

From the patient's serum albumin level of 3.0 gm/dl and his weight of 135 lbs at a height of 5' 10", the dietitian was able to determine that the patient was at risk nutritionally. Futhermore, the patient's admission of a 20 lb weight loss in the previous three months was also indicative of poor nutritional status.

Because the ideal body weight of this patient was approximately 166 lbs and his serum albumin should have been no less than 4.0 gm/dl, the appropriate dietary prescription should have been high caloric, high protein, low residue rather than just low residue. The need for frequent visits to the patient was indicated in order to determine his food preferences and food tolerances. Supplying the patient with a variety of appropriate supplementary feedings from which he could select an acceptable one would probably have helped to make the progress of his nutrition rehabilitation more rapid. If the malabsorption continued to be severe and the patient was unable to gain weight, the dietitian might have needed to suggest that the physician consider administration of a chemically defined tube feeding for the purpose of augmenting the patient's oral intake or even to propose the use of total parenteral nutrition (TPN) should more complete bowel rest seem indicated clinically.

Any of the above recommendations, however, *always* should be based on careful monitoring of the patient's food intake in order to make an accurate determination of ingested calories and nutrients.

REFERENCES

1. Guyton, A. C. *Textbook of Medical Physiology.* 5th ed. Philadelphia: W. B. Saunders, 1976; pp. 850–901.
2. Crouch, J. E. and J. R. McClintic. *Human Anatomy and Physiology.* 2nd ed. New York: John Wiley & Sons, 1976; pp. 587–628.
3. Bell, G. H., D. Emslie-Smith, and C. R. Paterson. *Textbook of Physiology and Biochemistry.* 9th ed. New York: Churchill Livingstone, 1976; pp. 639–648
4. Inglefinger, F. J. Gastric function. *Nutrition Today* **6:** 2, Sept./Oct. 1971.
5. Fleming, S. M., A. W. Weaver, and J. M. Brown. The patient with cancer affecting head and neck: Problems in nutrition, *J. Am. Diet. Assoc.* **70:** 391, Apr. 1977.
6. Inglefinger, F. J. How to swallow, belch and cope with heartburn. *Nutrition Today* **8:** 4, Jan./Feb. 1973.
7. Almy, T. P. Diaphragmatic hernia, hiatal hernia and reflex esophagitis. In *Textbook of Medicine,* P. Bieson and W. McDermott, eds. Philadelphia: W. B. Saunders, 1975; pp. 1182–1185.
8. Hendrix, T. R. Diseases of the esophagus. In *Harrison's Principles of Internal Medicine,* G. W. Thorn et. al., eds. 8th ed. New York: McGraw-Hill, 1977; pp. 1487–1494.
9. Coffee drinking and peptic ulcer disease, *Nutr. R.* **34:** 167, June 1976.
10. Castell, D. O. Diet and the lower esophageal sphincter. *Am. J. Clin. Nutr.* **28:** 1296, Nov. 1975.
11. Bahka, J. O. and D. O. Castell. On the genesis of heartburn — The effects of specific foods on the lower esophageal sphincter. *Am. J. Clin. Nutr.* **18:** 391, 1973.
12. Dworken, H. J. *The Alimentary Tract.* Philadelphia: W. B. Saunders, 1974.
13. Berkow, R. ed. *The Merck Manual of Diagnosis and Therapy,* 13th ed. Rahway, N.J.: Merck, Sharp and Dohme, 1977; pp. 759–807.
14. Kastrup, E. K. ed. *Facts and Comparisons.* St. Louis: Facts and Comparisons, Inc., 1978; p. 756.
15. MacDonald, W. C. and C. E. Rubin. Cancer, benign tumors, gastritis and other gastric diseases. In *Harrison's Principles of Internal Medicine,* G. W. Thorn et. al., eds. 8th ed. New York: McGraw-Hill, 1977; pp. 1510–1518.
16. Silen, W. Peptic ulcer. In *Harrison's Principles of Internal Medicine,* G. W. Thorn et. al., eds. 8th ed. New York: McGraw-Hill, 1977; pp. 1494–1510.
17. Duodenal ulcer patients secrete much less gastrin on six meals a day. *J. Am. Med. Assoc.* **232:** 695, May 1975.
18. Weinstein, L., R. E. Olson, T. B. Van Itallie, E. Caso, D. Johnson, and F. J. Inglefinger. Diet as related to gastrointestinal function. *J. Am. Med. Assoc.* **176:** 935, Jan. 1961.
19. Behm, V., G. Marchie, and D. R. King. Nutritional care of the patient following gastric surgery. *Ross Timesaver—Dietetic Currents* Mar./Apr. 1974.
20. Greenberger, N. J. and K. J. Isselbacher. Disorders of absorption. In *Harrison's Principles of Internal Medicine,* G. W. Thorn et. al., eds. 8th ed. New York: McGraw-Hill, 1977; pp. 1518–1537.
21. On the pathogenesis of gluten sensitive enteropathy. *Nur. R.* **32:**267, 1974.
22. Inglefinger, F. J.. For want of an enzyme. *Nutrition Today* **3:** 2, Sept. 1968.

23. Richmond, D. and P. W. Curreri. Nutritional management following massive small bowel resection. *Ross Timesaver—Dietetic Currents* July/Aug. 1974.
24. Glickman, R. M. and K. J. Isselbacher. Diseases of the small intestine. In *Harrison's Principles of Internal Medicine,* G. W. Thorn et. al., eds. 8th ed. New York: McGraw-Hill, 1977; pp. 1537–1547.
25. Almy, T. P. Disorders of intestinal mobility. In *Textbook of Medicine,* P. Bieson and W. McDermott, eds. 14th ed. Philadelphia: W. B. Saunders, 1975; pp. 1187–1195.
26. Janowitz, H. D. Chronic inflammatory diseases in the intestine. In *Textbook of Medicine,* P. Bieson and W. McDermott, eds. 14th ed. Philadelphia: W. B. Saunders, 1975; pp. 1256–1274.
27. Briggs, G. M., G. A. Spiller, M. C. Chernoff, E. A. Shipley, and M. A. Beigler. Can fecal weight be used to establish a recommended intake of dietary fiber (plantix)? *Am. J. Clin. Nutr.* **30:** 5, May 1977.
28. Darlington, R. C. Laxative products. In *Handbook of Nonprescription Drugs.* 5th ed. Washington, D.C.: American Pharmaceutical Assoc., 1977; pp. 37–53.
29. Painter, N. S. and D. P. Burkitt. Diverticular disease of the colon—a deficiency disease of civilization. *Brit. Med. J.* **5759:** 450, May 22, 1971.
30. Connell, A. M. Pathogenesis of diverticular disease of the colon. *Advances in Internal Medicine* **22:** 377, 1977.
31. Goldstein, F. Diet and colonic disease. *J. Am. Diet. Assoc.* **60:** 499, 1972.
32. O'Brien, T. F. Neoplasms of the large intestine. In *Textbook of Medicine,* P. Bieson and W. McDermott, eds. 14th ed. Philadelphia: W. B. Saunders, 1975; pp. 1298–1302.
33. Moore, T. L., H. Z. Kupchik, N. Marcon, and N. Zamcheck. Carcioembryonic antigen assay in cancer of colon and pancreas and other digestive tract disorders. *Am. J. Digest. Diseases* **16:** 1, 1971.
34. Booth, S. N. Carcioembryonic antigen in management of colorectal carcinoma. *British Med. J.* **4:** 183, 1974.
35. Hegsted, D. M. Priorities in nutrition in the U.S. *J. Am. Diet. Assoc.* **71:** 9, 1977.
36. Bing, F. C. Dietary fiber in historical perspective. *J. Am. Diet. Assoc.* **69:** 498, 1976.
37. Bradfield, R. B. A review of research on effects of fiber intake on man. *Am. J. Clin. Nutr.* **31:** 142, Jan. 1978.
38. Malt, R. A. Keep it simple. *Nutrition Today* **6:** 30, May/June 1971.
39. Stimulus for hyperplasia of the small bowel. *Nutr. R.* **34:** 345, Nov. 1976.
40. Williamson, R. C. N. and M. Chri. Intestinal adaptation—Structural, functional and cytokinetic changes. *N. Eng. J. Med.* **298:** 1393, June 1978.

RECOMMENDED READINGS

The American Journal of Clinical Nutrition, Supplement vol. 31, Oct. 1978.

This entire issue is devoted to a symposium on Role of Dietary Fiber in Health which was sponsored by the Nutrition Coordinating Committee of the National Institutes of Health.

Bloom, S. R. Gut Hormones. *Proceedings of the Nutrition Society* **37**: 259, Dec. 1978.

This is the introductory paper from a symposium on "Hormones and Food Utilization" and is an excellent, up-to-date, descriptive review of all the hormones secreted throughout the digestive tract.

Ippoliti, A. F., V. Maxwell, and J. I. Isenberg. The effect of various forms of milk on gastric-acid secretion. *Annals of Internal Medicine* **84**: 286, Mar. 1976.

Authors present experimental results on patients with duodenal ulcer during a period of remission and question the advisability of a generous milk intake in the treatment of ulcer.

Mendeloff, A. I., A. M. Connell, and D. Kritchevsky. Fiber. *Nutrition in Disease*, Columbus: Ross Laboratories, Sept. 1978.

This is a concise discussion of the various components of fiber, the fiber content of selected foods, the importance of fiber in gastrointestinal functions and the possible relationship among dietary fiber, lipid metabolism, and cancer.

Sleisenger, M. H. Malabsorption syndrome. *New England Journal of Medicine* **281**: 1111, Nov. 13, 1969.

An excellent review of the malabsorption syndrome is presented, including classification and pathophysiology, basis for clinical picture, laboratory tests used for diagnosis, and specific treatments for the various disease states causing malabsorption.

———. Lactose intolerance. *Dairy Council Digest* **42**: 31, Nov./Dec. 1971.

A concise review of lactose metabolism, causes and diagnosis of lactose intolerance along with its etiology is given. The practical significance of lactose intolerance among various population groups is discussed.

———. Perspective on milk intolerance. *Dairy Council Digest* **49**: 31, Nov./Dec. 1978.

CHAPTER 6

The Pancreas

ANATOMY AND PHYSIOLOGY

In addition to being the site for the production of the most potent digestive enzymes (see Table 5.1), the pancreas secretes insulin and glucagon, the hormones primarily responsible for regulation of blood glucose. Because of the interrelatedness of carbohydrate, fat, and protein metabolism these hormones exert much influence on the body's handling of fat and protein as well as regulating carbohydrate metabolism. Other hormones besides glucagon are involved in the elevation of blood glucose and their influence will be described later in the chapter; however, insulin alone increases the utilization and storage of exogenous glucose, thereby lowering the level of circulating glucose.

The pancreas, a slender, elongated organ ranging in length from about six to nine inches, runs horizontally behind the greater curvature of the stomach and lies between it and the duodenum (Fig. 6.1). The organ is only about one inch wide and is less than one inch thick, weighing approximately 3 oz. Within the pancreas are two distinctive types of active tissue: the acini or ducted exocrine tissue which secretes enzymes, and the ductless endocrine tissue which produces hormones. The exocrine tissue is comprised of cuboidal zymogenic cells arranged into circular glands that are attached to the ducts interposed throughout the tissue. These small collecting ducts carry enzyme secretions into the large main duct of the pancreas, the duct of Wirsung (Fig. 6.2). Scattered among the enzyme-secreting glands and located at capillary bed sites are a million or more clusters of cells called the islets of Langerhans. These islets of Langerhans, comprising only about 2 percent of the pancreatic tissue, are made up of three different types of endocrine cells: the glucagon-producing alpha cells, the insulin-secreting beta cells, and the D cells which secrete somatostatin. The D cells are closely positioned to the alpha cells, and the somatostatin produced by these cells is thought perhaps to be the physiologic regulator of the alpha and beta cell function (Fig. 6.3) (1).

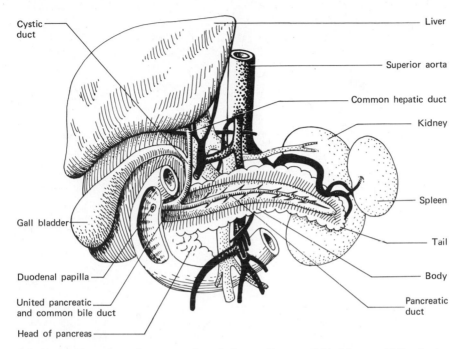

Figure 6.1 Location of pancreas in relation to liver, gall bladder, and bile ducts. (From *Human Anatomy and Physiology,* 2nd ed. by J. E. Crouch and J. R. McClintic. Copyright 1976 by John Wiley and Sons, Inc. Reprinted by permission of the publisher.)

NORMAL CARBOHYDRATE METABOLISM

The absorption of carbohydrate following a meal evokes insulin secretion which continues under the influence of elevated plasma glucose levels. Normal carbohydrate metabolism following a meal is controlled by the body's one "feasting" hormone, insulin. Insulin directs the *storage* of carbohydrate which can be used for energy during the interdigestive periods and promotes efficient *utilization* of that portion of carbohydrate needed to meet immediate energy requirements. However, brain cells (with the exception of the hypothalamus) do not require insulin for utilization of glucose.

Storage of Carbohydrate

Storage of carbohydrate occurs mainly in the liver, muscle tissue, and adipocytes.

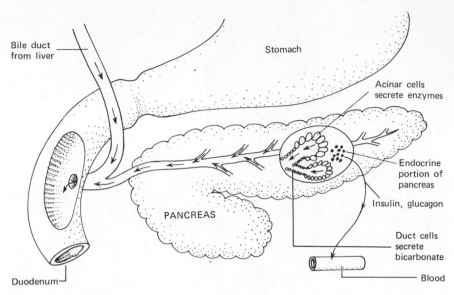

Figure 6.2 Structure of the pancreas. (From *Human Physiology—The Mechanisms of Body Function* by A. C. Vander, J. H. Sherman, and D. S. Luciano. Copyright 1975 by McGraw-Hill Book Co. Reprinted by permission of the publisher.)

Liver. Insulin is not required in order for carbohydrate to enter liver cells, but the hormone does control the level of *glucokinase,* the enzyme that converts glucose to nondiffusible glucose-6-phosphate (pp. 72–73), the first step in *glycogenesis.* Insulin also, through its activation of glycogen synthetase and its inhibition of cAMP and phosphorylase, further promotes glycogen storage (see Fig. 3.6 and 3.8). Consequently, much of the excess blood sugar can be stored as liver glycogen for future utilization.

Most of the carbohydrate absorbed from the digestive tract goes directly to the liver via the portal vein where it is either stored as glycogen or converted to glucose, which is the only form in which carbohydrate can leave the liver. For this reason, only small quantities of fructose may be metabolized as such in the muscles and adipose tissue (2). The entrance of fructose into glycolysis is depicted in Figure 3.7.

Muscle Tissue. Insulin is responsible for the proper transport of glucose through the membrane of muscle cells. Because glucose entering cells is dependent upon a carrier mechanism, it is postulated that insluin exerts its action in the inhibition of an active cellular process that normally blocks the carrier movement (3). Chromium in some way also helps promote the entry of glucose into the cell. It is possible that this trace mineral

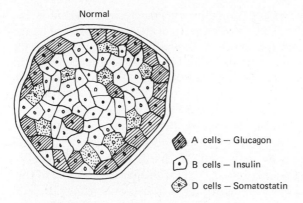

Normal

A cells — Glucagon

B cells — Insulin

D cells — Somatostatin

Figure 6.3 Cellular composition of islets of Langerhans. (From "Somatostatin" by J. E. Gerrich. *Archives of Internal Medicine,* May 1977, Volume 137, pp. 659–666. Copyright 1977, American Medical Association. Reprinted by permission of the publisher and author.)

is necessary for the binding of insulin to cellular hormone receptor sites. Glucose that enters the muscle cell is phosphorylated to glucose-6-P and is trapped there because muscle tissue contains no glucose-6-phosphatase. Accumulated glucose-6-P is converted to glycogen until stores are filled, at which time no more glucose is allowed to enter the cells.

Adipocytes. Insulin is required for entry of carbohydrate into fat cells. Glucose entering the adipocytes not only can furnish acetyl CoA necessary for fatty acid production but also supplies the alpha-glycerophosphate required for triglyceride synthesis. Insulin further promotes the storage of carbohydrate as fat by its inhibitory action on hormone sensitive lipase, thereby preventing lipolysis.

Utilization of Carbohydrate

All glucose transported into cells under the influence of insulin is not stored for future use but may enter the glycolytic pathway, thereby producing two moles of ATP along with two moles of pyruvate or lactate (Fig. 3.7). Pyruvate enters the Krebs cycle via acetyl CoA and is oxidized to produce 15 ATPs per mole. By-products of this oxidation or carbon dioxide and water (Fig. 3.9).

In the liver oxidation of glucose may occur additionally by way of the phosphogluconate pathway (pentose phosphate shunt). About one-third of the glucose oxidized in the liver follows this pathway which is of much importance because of its production of the pentose (ribose) necessary for nucleotide synthesis and its production of NADPH needed in fatty acid and steroid synthesis.

Although most of the effect of insulin on protein metabolism is indirect, that is, increased utilization of carbohydrate spares protein as an energy source, the hormone appears to directly affect protein synthesis as well, particularly in the liver. Part of this influence on protein synthesis can be attributed to the fact that insulin increases transport of amino acids through cell membranes.

During interdigestive periods, an upward regulation of blood glucose levels must occur rather than the downward direction required postprandially. Maintenance of an adequate level of blood glucose is of prime importance because glucose is the only nutrient that can be used in a sufficient quantity to provide the energy required for proper functioning of the brain, retina and germinal epithelia. Normally a constant concentration of 70 to 90 mg glucose per deciliter blood can be maintained by the regulatory action of a variety of hormones, most of which are secreted in response to stimulation from the hypothalamus.

The hypothalamus, which requires insulin for glucose utilization, is very sensitive to decreased blood glucose levels and responds by the following mechanisms: (1) transmission of impulses through sympathetic nervous system which cause release of epinephrine from the adrenal medullae and release of norepinephrine from the adrenals and the sympathetic nerve endings; (2) stimulation of the anterior pituitary to secrete growth hormone, corticotropin, and thyrotropic hormone. Corticotropin and thyrotropic hormone, in turn, stimulate the adrenal cortex and thyroid gland to secrete glucocorticoids and thyroxin, respectively. These hormones along with glucagon (which is secreted by the alpha cells in the islets of Langerhans in response to a lowered blood sugar level), maintain adequate blood glucose during interdigestive periods. Glycogenolysis and/or gluconeogenesis, both of which raise blood sugar (Figs. 3.8 and 3.10), are initiated through the action of those hormones mentioned above.

Liver. Glycogenolysis and gluconeogenesis both occur in the liver in order that this organ can continuously add glucose to the blood in an amount sufficient to equal that being consumed by the extrahepatic tissues. For the adult male approximately 8 to 16 grams of glucose per hour are being released from the liver to the blood stream. Glycogenolysis is initiated by the action of glucagon and/or epinephrine which bind onto liver cell receptor sites provided by the enzyme, adenylate cyclase. The hormonally stimulated cyclase then removes pyrophosphate from ATP and uses the energy thus derived to produce cyclic AMP. Cyclic AMP, in turn, activates cellular protein kinases which, with ATP, phosphorylate the enzymes, glycogen synthetase and glycogen phosphorylase. Phosphorylation depresses the action of the synthetase but converts the phosphorylase into its highly active state. As a result glycogen synthesis is inhibited while degradation of glycogen to glucose-6-P occurs rapidly. Glucose-6-P thus produced can quickly be converted to free glucose by liver glucose-6-phosphatase (Fig. 3.8).

Gluconeogenesis also is begun by hormonal action on adenyl cyclase at the cell membrane. Glucagon activates the cyclase which then causes production of cAMP. This latter product stimulates those enzymatic reactions necessary to convert pyruvate to phosphoenol pyruvate, thereby reversing glycolysis (Fig. 3.7 and 3.10). Glucagon also initiates activation of hepatic lipase which promotes lipolysis and elevation of cellular fatty acids with a resultant decreased utilization of glucose by liver cells. With increased hepatic lipolysis, there is an accumulation of acetyl CoA which inhibits its further formation from pyruvate, thereby enhancing conversion of pyruvate into oxaloacetate through action of the enzyme, pyruvate carboxylase. Oxaloacetate is then decarboxylated by PEP carboxykinase to phosphoenol pyruvate (PEP), the essential compound for glucose synthesis. The glucocorticoids enhance gluconeogenesis through induction of several liver enzymes needed in the gluconeogenic process. Although the glucocorticoids stimulate synthesis of protein in the form of certain liver enzymes needed for gluconeogenesis, they enhance catabolism of other proteins in the liver and muscle tissue, thereby providing free amino acids for glucose synthesis by liver cells.

During the interdigestive period the brain utilizes approximately half of all glucose produced by gluconeogenesis. Figure 6.4 identifies the carbon sources of gluconeogenesis.

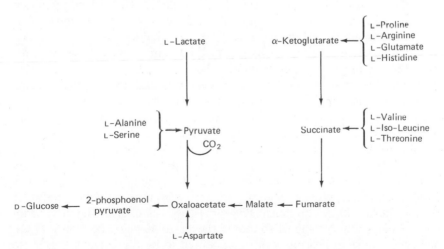

Figure 6.4 Carbon sources for gluconeogenesis. (From Montgomery, Rex, Dryer, R. L., Conway, Thomas W., and Spector, Arthur A.: *Biochemistry: a case oriented approach*, 2nd ed. Copyright 1977 by The C.V. Mosby Co. St. Louis. Reprinted by permission of the publisher and authors.)

Hitting Muscle Tissue. Glycogenolysis is begun in the muscle by the action of epinephrine on adenyl cyclase at the cell membrane. Degradation of glycogen to glucose-6-P proceeds as in the liver but due to the absence of glucose-6-phosphatase in skeletal tissue, free glucose cannot be formed (p. 79). Therefore, glucose-6-phosphate is converted by glycolysis to pyruvate (or lactate) which can be oxidized in the Krebs cycle for production of energy. Lactate not oxidized via pyruvate in the muscles is picked up by the blood and returned to the liver where through gluconeogenesis it is converted into glucose. Lactate returned to the liver from skeletal tissue may account for 10 to 40 percent of the glucose provided by the liver. Figure 6.5 illustrates the relation of blood glucose to carbohydrate metabolism.

Adipocytes. Glucagon, epinephrine, and growth hormone activate hormone sensitive lipase via cAMP; lipolysis occurs and raises the free fatty acid level in the blood. These free fatty acids attached to their albumin carriers are transported to tissues where they are oxidized for energy, thereby depressing carbohydrate utilization and indirectly elevating blood glucose.

Diagnosis and Therapy of Aberrations in Carbohydrate Metabolism

Diabetes Mellitus. Diabetes is a metabolic disease characterized by hyperglycemia resulting from an absolute or relative deficiency of physiologically active insulin. This disorder may be classified according to type: (1) genetic or primary diabetes which may be juvenile- or adult-onset in nature; (2) pancreatic diabetes, in which the islets of Langerhans have been destroyed by some disease state or surgical removal; (3) endocrine diabetes which is associated with various endocrinopathies, for example, hyperpituitarism; (4) iatrogenic diabetes which can result from extensive use of certain drugs, for example, corticosteroids (4).

In the United States diabetes is the fifth leading cause of death by disease and approximately 4.2 million persons suffer from the disorder which in most cases is genetic in nature. According to the U.S. Public Health Service, juvenile diabetes is relatively rare, affecting only 1.3 persons per thousand up to age 17 years. The incidence of the disease increases markedly with aging so that in the 25- to 44-year age group, 17 out of every thousand persons can be expected to be diabetic; in the 65- to 74-year group, the number jumps to approximately 79 per thousand (4,5).

Juvenile- and adult-onset diabetics exhibit the same metabolic abnormalities, that is, inefficient peripheral utilization of glucose and defective control mechanisms for glucose production. These aberrations however are usually more severe and difficult to control in persons with juvenile

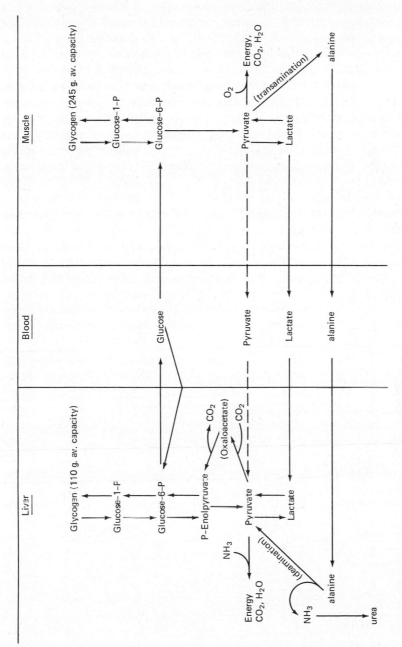

Figure 6.5 Relation of blood glucose to carbohydrate metabolism.

diabetes than in those with the adult-onset type. For example, the juvenile diabetic almost invariably requires exogenous insulin, is ketosis-prone and presents an unstable or brittle condition. On the other hand, the patient with adult-onset diabetes can usually be treated by diet alone, is ketosis-resistant and presents a stable, easily managed condition. The typical adult-onset diabetic is overweight and somewhat insulin resistant. As a result, he/she has insufficient insulin production to maintain a normal glucose level, but unlike the juvenile who secretes little or no insulin, the adult may exhibit normal or above normal amounts of circulating insulin (6). Nevertheless, adult-onset diabetes can occur in lean individuals as well as in the overweight, and when it does, the severity of the disease is variable (7).

Abnormalities in nutrient metabolism are excessively severe in truly uncontrolled diabetes and consequences of insulin lack are depicted in Figures 6.6, 6.7, and 6.8.

It is the view of some investigators (8) that diabetes should be categorized as a bihormonal disorder rather than one due only to a deficiency of insulin. According to this hypothesis, in diabetes not only does a hyposecretion of insulin occur but also a hyposuppressibility of glucagon production. Other investigators (9) dispute this theory and provide evidence to support the belief that underproduction of insulin can account for all

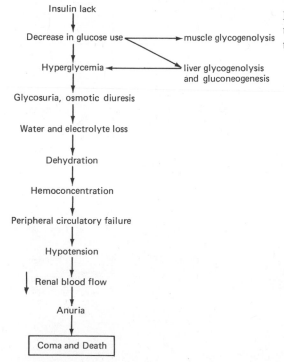

Figure 6.6 Carbohydrate metabolism as affected by uncontrolled diabetes.

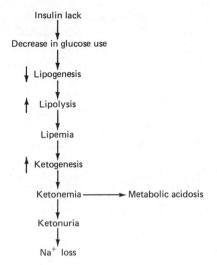

Figure 6.7 Fat metabolism as affected by uncontrolled diabetes.

the symptoms associated with the diabetic state. Glucagon because of its evanescent effect in producing hyperglycemia can cause deterioration of the diabetic state only in cases of absolute insulin deficiency. In their view the primary importance of glucagon in maintaining glucose homeostasis lies in its effect on the prevention of hypoglycemia associated with an increased insulin production in response to elevated plasma amino acids following a protein meal.

Many noteworthy advances in the understanding of diabetes have occurred in recent years. For example, evidence has been presented to

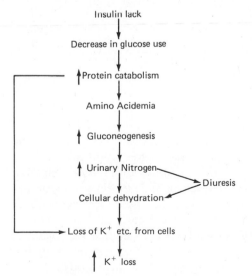

Figure 6.8 Protein metabolism as affected by uncontrolled diabetes.

support the theory that viral infections and aberrant immune mechanisms may be responsible for unmasking in the juvenile a predisposition to diabetes (10,11). It is suggested that viruses attack defective beta cells; then the antibodies attack these dead cells. In ridding the body of dead cells, the antibodies also render ineffective other beta cells. The variability in the manifestations of the disease among affected persons has led to the demonstration that numerous genetic mechanisms and environmental factors are involved in the development of clinical diabetes (12).

Although no startling new treatment for diabetes is available presently, much exciting research aimed toward improved management of the disease is being conducted currently. One area of research centers around the hormone, somatostatin, one function of which is regulation of blood glucose. Although the exact mechanism of this regulation is unclear (1,9,13), and the administration of the hormone presently is not feasible, the possibility exists that in the future somatostatin or its analogues may provide improved treatment for diabetes. Another possibility for improved diabetes therapy in the future is the implantation of an artificial pancreas equipped with sensor device and pump (14). The sensor will monitor blood glucose levels and the pump sequentially deliver insulin in amounts proportional to need.

Perhaps the most promising research in management of diabetes centers around development of an artificial pancreas using living beta cells (15). Beta cells are cultured on outside surfaces of synthetic hollow fibers which are permeable to insulin but impermeable to antibodies and lymphocytes. These beta cell containing devices, when implanted in diabetic experimental animals as arteriovenous shunts, have been able to maintain glucose at relatively normal levels without causing any type of rejection by the body.

The importance of using to best advantage those means presently available for maintaining blood glucose within normal limits, that is, insulin therapy and dietary management, is becoming increasingly apparent. There is mounting evidence that complications of the kidney, eye, and nerves commonly associated with the disease are not necessarily inevitable but can be prevented with proper management of blood glucose levels (10,16,17).

Although primary diabetes is an inherited disease, whether or not the predisposition is unmasked depends to a large degree upon the environment. For the adult-onset diabetic, environmental factors often responsible for overt manifestation of the disease include obesity and/or excessive intake of carbohydrates. Increased intake of carbohydrate causes an increased production of insulin. Initially, if the carbohydrate intake is excessive, circulating insulin may be insufficient to handle the load and blood glucose will be elevated. The islets of Langerhans, however, by hypertrophy adapt to a continued elevation of blood sugar and in a few weeks insulin secretion has increased to a level adequate for handling the glucose (3). As a result of the elevated insulin levels, the excess glucose is transported into fat cells and obesity often results. The engorged adipocytes for some reason become resistant to the action of insulin; therefore, more and more insulin is required to transport the same amount of carbohydrate into cells for storage or immediate utilization. Eventually the beta cells in the person predisposed to diabetes can no longer produce the insulin required for proper utilization of circulating glucose; hyperglycemia occurs and becomes a chronic condition. Prolonged elevation of blood glucose in the predisposed person can cause the beta cells literally to wear themselves out so that insulin production is reduced or may cease entirely in some individuals. Other factors besides excessive food intake that may precipitate development of clinical diabetes include acute stress situations and changes in the secretory patterns of other hormones, that is, glucagon and growth hormone.

Beta cells that are no longer functioning lose their granular appearance and become hyalinized. In most adult-onset diabetics, however, there are sufficient functional beta cells for the handling of normal glucose loads when adipocytes have been reduced in size through adequate weight loss.

Diagnosis of Diabetes Mellitus. The juvenile-type diabetic presents the classic symptoms of the disease: rapid weight loss accompanied by polyphagia, polydipsia, and polyuria. The adult-onset diabetic, on the other hand, may be asymptomatic and suspicion of the disorder arises during a routine physical examination when glycosuria is discovered. Because of the glucose threshold variability among individuals, glycosuria cannot be used to diagnose diabetes but should prompt further tests for hyperglycemia. One diagnostic tool often used is the fasting blood sugar, but this test is not as definitive as a blood sugar determination one or two hours after a breakfast containing approximately 100 grams carbohydrate. A blood sugar of 170 mg percent or higher an hour following such a breakfast is strongly suggestive of diabetes, but an even better diagnostic tool is the oral glucose tolerance test (4). For this test the patient is required to consume 250 to 300 grams carbohydrate daily for three consecutive days; on the morning of the fourth day, following a fasting blood sugar determination, the patient receives 100 grams glucose by mouth. Blood glucose is measured at one-half hour, one hour, two hours, and three hours and urinalysis is performed for determination of sugar. Blood sugar concentrations are plotted against time and the curve obtained is compared with a normal curve. Figure 6.9 shows the blood glucose curves for a normal person and a diabetic following oral doses of glucose. A new method being used for diabetic screening and determination of blood glucose control is measurement of hemoglobin A_{1C}. This is HbA to which has been

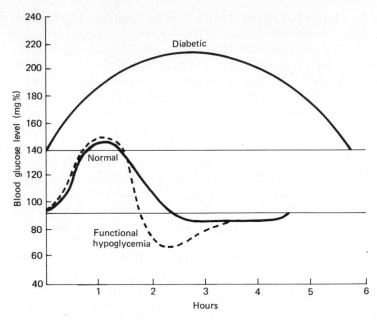

Figure 6.9 Glucose tolerance curve in the normal person, in the diabetic, and in the person with functional hypoglycemia.

attached a glucose molecule (glycosylation of hemoglobin). In patients with diabetes there is two to three times as much circulating HbA_{IC} as is found in the normal population (18).

Complications of Diabetes Mellitus. As was mentioned earlier it is probable that much more importance will be placed on good management of the diabetic patient because the current view is that many complications are resulting from metabolic changes entailed by redirection of excess blood sugar into insulin-insensitive pathways, for example, the polyol pathway, the glycoprotein and mucopolysaccharide precursor pathway (16). Good evidence exists to support the belief that complications of the microvessels and the nerves can be prevented by careful regulation of blood sugar levels (16,17).

The most striking complications of diabetes are the changes that occur in the capillaries of the glomerulus and the retina. The commonest abnormality in diabetic patients is diabetic retinopathy which affects more than 90 percent of the persons who have had the disease for 20 or more years (4,6). This complication is the third leading cause of blindness in the United States, the blindness itself being precipitated by numerous hemorrhages in the retina. Cataracts are also especially common in diabetics and development seems to be influenced by the degree of hyperglycemia (7).

Clinical symptoms of nephropathy are present in about one-fourth of diabetics who have had the disease more than 15 years, but kidneys examined histologically reveal a much higher occurrence of the complication, actually approaching 100 percent (6). The change in the capillaries that is characteristic of diabetes is most striking in the glomerulus. There is a thickening of the basement membrane, the degree of which correlates with the duration of the disease. Analysis of the diabetic glomerular membrane reveals an increased number of the carbohydrate moieties in the collagenlike material. The increased amount of carbohydrate alters the shape of the molecules making up the basement membrane and it is postulated that perhaps the presence of these extra glucose moieties prevent tight packing together of membrane molecules. The thickening of the membrane may be due not only to the presence of above average amounts of protein material but also to increased space between the collagenlike fibers. If this hypothesis is correct, it could explain why a thicker basement membrane in the diabetic is also one that leaks more than normal (5).

Therapy for Diabetes Mellitus. Therapy for the diabetic is directed toward achieving as nearly a perfect balance as possible between food intake and insulin (exogenous and/or endogenous) without interfering unreasonably with the patient's ability to carry on a normal life. Objectives of diet therapy include:

1. Provision of a nutritionally adequate diet.
2. Prevention of excessive postprandial hyperglycemia.
3. Prevention of hypoglycemia in insulin-dependent patients.
4. Attainment and maintenance of ideal body weight.
5. Control of blood lipids.
6. Prevention or hindrance in development of pathologic changes associated with diabetes.

The balance between food intake and insulin is affected by various factors which often necessitate modification of established food intake and/or insulin dosage. One factor of particular importance is exercise because physical activity acts much like insulin in causing glucose to be transported into muscle cells. Increased activity of any duration will necessitate either an increase in the amount of food consumed or a decrease in insulin dosage. Conversely, any infection or illness will increase above normal the requirement for insulin, perhaps because of increased glucagon secretion in response to the protein catabolism usually accompanying any fever-producing illness.

The diet prescription for the diabetic child must provide sufficient calories and nutrients not only for maintenance of health but also for promotion of normal growth. An important point to remember is that the nutrient and caloric needs of the diabetic child are exactly the same as for any other child at his/her stage of development. On the other hand, for the adult-onset diabetic whose growth is completed and who is often overweight, concern centers around provision of adequate nutrients in a calorically restricted diet designed to promote weight loss.

The place of carbohydrate in the diabetic diet has been a subject of much research, and results of recent studies encourage the use of diets much higher in carbohydrate than have been traditional (7). In Table 6.1 comparisons are made among the newer diabetic diets, traditional diabetic diets, and typical American diets. Diabetic patients have been shown to have an improved glucose tolerance as a result of higher intakes of carbohydrate when it is distributed throughout the day. Diets with a higher percentage of calories coming from carbohydrate are naturally lower in fat, and therefore should be helpful in controlling the lipidemias commonly associated with the diabetic state. Diabetics suffering with specific lipidemias, however, should have their diets planned according to the principles recommended for lowering these lipids (see Table 7.2). The usual recommendation for protein intake is approximately 20 percent of the total calories. This level of protein is usually well above the amount needed by the individual, but in order to keep fat intake low and to limit sugar in the diet, protein intake must be increased. For children, pregnant women, and lactating mothers, protein intake should never fall below 1.5 g/kg body weight (7). A suggested division of calories is 50 percent carbohydrate (primarily complex carbohydrates), 20 percent protein, and 30 percent fat.

A diet prescription for a 15-year-old boy weighing 134 lbs or approximately 61 kilograms could be calculated as follows:

Calories: 2745 (61 kg $\times$ 45 kcal/kg)*
Carbohydrate: 345 g (2745 kcal $\times$ 0.50 = 1372.5 $\div$ 4 kcal/g = 343 g)
Protein: 135 g (2745 $\times$ 0.20 = 549 $\div$ 4 kcal/g = 137 g)
Fat: 90 g (2745 $\times$ 0.30 = 823.5 $\div$ 9 kcal/g = 92 g)

The recommendation that fat be reduced to approximately 30 percent of total calories is aimed at control of blood lipids and at retarding development of atherosclerosis, a complication that apparently is eventually inevitable in the diabetic.

The importance of more careful control of fat intake is reflected in the 1976 revision of *Exchange Lists for Meal Planning* (19), a guide designed to promote adequate nutrient intake, to allow easy calculation of caloric content, and to avoid monotony in meal planning. Foods are grouped in

---

* Recommended energy allowances for adolescents are set at 45 kcal/kg for males and 38 kcal/kg for females.

Table 6.1 Distribution of Major Nutrients in Normal and Diabetic Diets (United States)*

Diet	Nutrients (percent of total calories)					
	Starch and other polysaccharides†	Sugars and dextrins‡	Total carbohydrate	Fat	Protein	Alcohol
Typical "normal" diet	25–35	20–30	45–50	35–45 (P:S ratio about 0.3)	12–19	0–10
Traditional diabetic diet	25–30	10–15§	35–40	40–45	16–21	0
Newer diabetic diets	35–45	5–15§	45–55‖	25–35‖ (P:S ratio about 1)	12–24	0–6

*Modified from "Diabetes Mellitus" by Kelly West. *Nutritional Support of Medical Practice*, edited by Schneider et al. Copyright 1977 by Harper and Row, Publishers, Inc. Reprinted by permission of publisher and author.
†A very substantial majority of these calories are starch, but complex carbohydrates also include cellulose, hemicellulose, pentosans, and pectin.
‡These are monosaccharides and disaccharides, mainly sucrose, but also include fructose, glucose, lactose, maltose, and both refined and natural sugars.
§These are almost exclusively natural sugars, mainly in fruit and milk (lactose).
‖Even higher levels of starch and lower levels of fat would be desirable but are seldom possible in Western societies because they differ too much from traditional diets of those cultures.

such a fashion that each list is composed of those food items that provide approximately the same amount of carbohydrate, protein, and fat per serving and contribute similar levels of many other nutrients. These lists were developed by the American Diabetes Association and American Dietetic Association in cooperation with the National Institutes of Arthritis, Metabolism and Digestive Diseases and the National Heart and Lung Institute of the U.S. Department of Health, Education and Welfare. The recent revision of these lists emphasizes the low fat concept by basing milk exchanges on nonfat milk and dividing the meat group into three lists: one for lean meat, one for medium-fat meat, and one for high-fat. In addition, attention is directed toward the type of fat that will be contributing approximately 30 percent of the calories. For those patients who need to maintain a high polyunsaturated to saturated fat ratio, appropriate selections of fats are simplified by a clear identification of all polyunsaturated fats appearing in the List of Fat Exchanges. Table 6.2 lists the carbohydrate, protein, and fat composition of the foods comprising the various exchange groups.

All dietitians should become very familiar with the six groupings of foods that comprise the exchange lists and learn how to use them quickly and accurately in the calculation of diets. Sample work sheets for figuring diabetic diets in exchanges and for converting exchanges into meal plans are given in Figures 6.10 and 6.11.

In addition, dietitians need to make clear to other members of the health team that learning to use exchange lists correctly is no easy task and that much effort and patience are necessary for education of patients in use of this valuable guide. Patients need to understand that foods are grouped together because of their similarity in nutrient and calorie content and, as a consequence, only those foods contained in the same list can be "exchanged" with each other. Teaching this concept will require much interaction between dietitian and patient (and quite frequently, the patient's family, also).

Before any meal plans are devised in terms of exchanges, the dietitian not only should have a good diet history on the patient and know which foods are acceptable, but also should involve the patient in establishing a dietary pattern. Involvement of the patient in decision-making is particularly important in relation to the milk included in meal plans because in most plans at least two milk exchanges are included daily in order to assure an adequate intake of calcium. Advance planning of an acceptable diet as well as one adequate in nutrients eliminates many frustrations for both the patient and the dietitian.

An occasional alcoholic beverage may need to be incorporated into the diabetic diet of those individuals whose habits include consumption of such drinks. West (7) suggests that a convenient method by which this incorporation can be made is to exchange fat calories for alcohol calories

Table 6.2 Composition of Food Exchanges

Exchange groups	Food	Amount	Carbohydrate (grams)	Protein (grams)	Fat (grams)	Kilocalories (exchange)
1	Nonfat milk	1 cup	12	8	—	80
2	Vegetables	½ cup	5	2	—	25
3	Fruit	Varies with CHO concentration	10	—	—	40
4	Breads, cereals, and starchy vegetables	Varies with CHO concentration	15	2	—	70
5a	Lean meat	1 oz.	—	7	3	55
5b	Medium fat meat	1 oz.	—	7	5.5	78
5c	High fat meat	1 oz.	—	7	8	100
6	Fats	Varies according to source (1 tsp. butter, margarine)	—	—	5	45

1. Prescription: _____Ht _____Wt _____Sex _____Age
_____Calories _____g Protein _____g CHO _____g Fat
divided _____ .

2. Translation into food exchanges.

List	Exchange group	No. of exchanges	CHO g	Protein g	Fat g
1	Milk				
2	Vegetable				
3	Fruit				
	Total CHO from 1 + 2 + 3				
	_____g CHO in prescription				
minus	_____g from 1 + 2 + 3				
4	_____g ÷ 15 = no. of bread exchanges				
	Total protein from 1 + 2 + 3 + 4				
	_____g protein in prescription				
minus	_____g from 1 + 2 + 3 + 4				
5	_____g ÷ 7 = no. of meat exchanges				
	Total fat from 1 + 2 + 3 + 4 + 5				
	_____g fat in prescription				
minus	_____g from 1 + 2 + 3 + 4 + 5				
	_____g ÷ 5 = no. of fat exchanges				
	Total grams				

Figure 6.10 Worksheet for planning diabetic and weight control diets.

Summary of exchanges for the day

List	Exchanges	No. of Exchanges
1	Milk	
2	Vegetable	
3	Fruit	
4	Bread	
5	Meat	
6	Fat	

Meal plan for the day

Meal	Exchange	Number	CHO (g)	Pro (g)	Fat (g)
Breakfast	Milk				
	Fruit				
	Bread				
	Meat				
	Fat				
Total for meal					
Lunch	Milk				
	Veg.				
	Fruit				
	Bread				
	Meat				
	Fat				
Total for meal					
Dinner	Milk				
	Veg.				
	Fruit				
	Bread				
	Meat				
	Fat				
Total for meal					

Figure 6.11 Continued

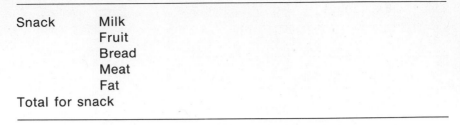

Snack	Milk
	Fruit
	Bread
	Meat
	Fat
Total for snack	

Figure 6.11 Worksheet for conversion of food exchanges into meal plans.

with one drink being equivalent to 15 to 20 grams fat. This kind of substitution has the further advantage of demonstrating to patients the high calorie content of alcohol.

Patients particularly need to be educated in the proper use of "dietetic" foods. Many of these foods are not sugar-free at all but are sweetened with sorbitol, which is actually glucitol or the reduced form of glucose. This alcohol is slowly absorbed, but nevertheless contains about the same number of calories as sucrose and is only 60 percent as sweet (7).

An excellent checklist with which every dietitian should become familiar is one devised by West to aid physicians and dietitians in appropriate individualization of diabetic diets:*

1. In order of priority what are the main general purposes (not strategies or methods) of this patient's prescription?
2. How much should the patient weigh? How much do the doctor, the dietitian, and the patient think the patient should weigh? How much would the patient *like* to weigh?
3. What is the appropriate level of caloric consumption for this patient?
4. Does the patient require insulin? If so, is the blood glucose relatively stable, moderately labile, or severely labile? What kind of insulin is to be given, at what time, in what amounts?
5. What and when and how much would the patient *like* to eat if he/she did not have diabetes? Are there any special considerations relating to economic factors or to family or cultural dietary propensities?
6. Is the level of carbohydrate to be fixed? To what level or range? To what extent and under what conditions, if any, are concentrated carbohydrates to be used?

* From "Diabetes Mellitus" by Kelly West. *Nutritional Support of Medical Practice*, edited by Schneider et al. Copyright 1977 by Harper and Row, Publishers, Inc. Reprinted by permission of publisher and author.

7. Are there any special requirements concerning levels of protein?
8. Are there any specific or general requirements with respect to levels of dietary fat, either saturated or unsaturated?
9. How much alcohol is to be permitted? Under what conditions? Should alcohol be exchanged for another food? If so, what kind and in what amounts?
10. If time distribution of food is of any importance, are there specific requirements concerning: (a) the relative size and timing of each of the three main meals (b) the timing, size, and characteristics of any extra feedings?
11. To what degree is day-to-day consistency required in: (a) total calories, (b) size and characteristics of specific feedings such as lunch?
12. Are dietary adjustments to be made for exercise or marked glycosuria? Of what nature?
13. Are there any special conditions unrelated to diabetes requiring special diet (e.g., gout, hyperlipidemia, renal or cardiac failure)?
14. Can all elements of the prescription be reconciled, and how should this be done? (For example, it is usually not feasible to construct a palatable diet for a lean diabetic if the prescription calls for a diet that restricts both carbohydrate and fat.)
15. What kinds and what degree of changes are to be made subsequently by the dietitian without consulting the physician?
16. What should this patient do if he/she finds it necessary to postpone or modify a meal (e.g., at a dinner meeting or social affair)? How should the patient adjust diet if his/her appetite fails (e.g., during illness)?
17. Tactical questions: (a) How much precision is required in the various elements of this prescription? (b) What foods can be freely allowed? (c) What foods, if any, are to be weighed or measured? (d) Are any modifications of the standard exchange system appropriate, such as simplification? (e) In general, is food to be unmeasured, estimated, measured, or weighed? (f) Is it necessary or desirable to teach this patient the carbohydrate, protein, and fat content of the common foods? (g) Under what circumstances are artificial sweeteners and diet drinks to be used?
18. Has this patient's understanding of dietary principles and methods been systematically evaluated?

The medical management of diabetes mellitus is determined by the severity, duration, and time of onset of the disease state. Two primary medicinal treatment modalities are presently utilized: insulin replacement and oral hypoglycemic agents. The role of dietary management has been previously discussed and its importance to the continuing management of diabetes cannot be overemphasized. However, for those patients who are not adequately controlled by diet alone, injectable insulin or oral hypoglycemic agents must be utilized in combination with dietary regulation. Insulin replacement therapy is primarily utilized in juvenile-onset diabetics and in all diabetics undergoing stressful situations. Oral hypoglycemic agents are limited to adult-onset diabetics who have some level of pancreatic function and in whom the condition cannot be controlled adequately by diet alone.

The pancreatic hormone insulin was discovered by Banting and Best who extracted it from the canine pancreas and demonstrated its effectiveness in humans (20). Knowledge of the chemistry of insulin has progressed from the crystallization of insulin by Abel in 1926 to the complete synthesis of bovine and human insulin molecules by Katsoyannis in 1966. Insulin is a polypeptide with a molecular weight of about 6,000. It is made up of two amino acid chains linked by three disulfide bridges. The beta cells of the islets of Langerhans of the pancreas form insulin from a single chain precursor called proinsulin which has only minimal biological activity and has been found as a contaminant in commercially produced insulin preparations.

The hormonal activity of various mammalian insulins is similar although chemically there are variations among species. Until recently, the procedures utilized in the preparation of insulin left significant amounts of proinsulin, and its incompletely converted products, as contaminants in commercially available products. The presence of these contaminants has been reported to produce dangerous local and systemic allergic responses. Since 1973, techniques have been developed to prepare more nearly pure preparations which have decreased the occurrence of such allergic responses. Two of these more nearly pure preparations presently available are single peak insulin (SPI) and single component insulin (SCI).

Single peak insulin has been purified of high molecular weight contaminants. It contains regular insulin and small amounts of incompletely converted proinsulin products—less than 0.1 percent proinsulin and 0.02 percent glucagon on a weight/weight basis (21). The required degree of purity for commercial insulin in the United States is now that of single peak insulin (99 percent) (22). Although SPI is more nearly purified than previous insulin preparations, Tantillo et al (23) have reported that some allergic responses are still occurring. Single component insulin is greater than 99 percent pure and contains only minute traces of higher molecular weight compounds. Thus, antibody production has been greatly reduced with the use of SCI and allergic reactions decreased.

Insulin preparations currently being utilized differ primarily in their onset of action and duration of activity. These insulin preparations are listed in Table 6.3 along with the division of food intake considered appropriate for those persons using any one of the specific preparations.

The oral hypoglycemic agents, as previously mentioned, are useful for the treatment of maturity-onset diabetes in the ketosis-resistant pa-

Table 6.3 Insulin Preparations and Suggested Division of Food Intake

Type	Preparation	Onset of action	Duration of action	Suggested division of food intake
Fast-acting	Regular insulin	1 hour	6 hours	1/3, 1/3, 1/3
	Regular insulin (made from zinc-insulin crystals) Semilente insulin (zinc suspension)	1 hour	8 hours	
Intermediate-acting	NPH insulin (Isophane insulin suspension)	1 hour 2 hours	14 hours 24 hours	1/5, 2/5, 2/5 with H.S. 2/7, 2/7, 2/7, 1/7 or 2/8, 2/8, 1/8, 2/8, 1/8
	Lente insulin (Insulin zinc suspension)	2 hours	24 hours	or 1/5, 2/5, 2/5 with H.S. or midafternoon snack 1/5, 2/5, 2/5 with afternoon or H.S. snack
	Globulin zinc insulin	2 hours	18 hours	
Long-acting	Protamine zinc insulin suspension	7 hours	36 hours	2/7, 2/7, 2/7, 1/7 or 2/8, 2/8, 1/8, 2/8, 1/8 or 1/5, 2/5, 2/5 with H.S.
	Ultralente insulin (Extended insulin zinc suspension)	7 hours	36 hours	

tient who does not respond to dietary control alone. Table 6.4 lists the criteria for the appropriate use of presently available oral hypoglycemic agents and Table 6.5 describes the duration of action and daily dosage of these agents. Oral hypoglycemic drugs are chemically classified as sulfonylurea compounds. They produce their therapeutic effects by stimulation of the islets of Langerhans to secrete insulin; therefore, a partially functioning pancreas is required for their effectiveness.

Side effects associated with the use of the sulfonylurea compounds can be hematological, cutaneous, gastrointestinal, and/or hepatic in nature. Hematological effects may include leukopenia, agranulocytosis, thrombocytopenia, pancytopenia and hemolytic anemia; cutaneous—rash and photosensitivity; gastrointestinal—nausea, vomiting, and occasionally hemorrhage; hepatic—elevated serum alkaline phosphatase and cholestatic jaundice. Other adverse reactions reported include hypoglycemic reactions, hyponatremia, and intolerance to alcohol. Hypoglycemic reactions have been most frequently reported in patients over the age of 50 who have impaired renal or hepatic function. Some reactions however may occur due to inadequate or irregular food intake.

In 1961, a cooperative clinical trial was undertaken by twelve university-based clinics (24) to determine whether the control of plasma glucose levels would help to delay or prevent vascular disease in diabetic patients who did not require insulin. Patients in the study were treated with diet and either placebo, tolbutamide, a standard or variable dose of insulin (or phenformin which is no longer marketed). The results of this study indicated that the combination of diet and either tolbutamide or phenformin was no more effective in prolonging life than was diet alone. Furthermore, the study provides suggestive evidence that diet in combination with either of the hypoglycemic agents is less effective than diet with insulin (or even diet alone) in preventing cardiovascular mortality (25). Since the publication of this report, further evidence has become available to indicate that the use of these hypoglycemic agents may indeed be detrimental to the health of the patient (26).

In the United States about one-fourth of the known diabetics are being treated with insulin, about one-half are receiving oral hypoglycemic

Table 6.4 Criteria for the Use of Oral Hypoglycemic Agents

1. Proven dietary failure
2. Nonketotic, maturity-onset diabetes
3. Patient age: 40 years or older
4. Blood sugar controllable on 40 units or less of insulin
5. Duration of diabetes: 10 years or less
6. Less than 20% overweight
7. Maximum whole blood sugar exceeds 150 mg/dl fasting and 175 mg/dl 2 hours p.c.

Table 6.5 Action Times and Dosages of Oral Hypoglycemic Agents

Drug	Duration of action (hours)	Usual daily dosage (mg)
Tolbutamide (Orinase®)	8	1000–3000
Acetohexamide (Dymelor®)	12–24	250–1500
Tolazamide (Tolinase®)	16–24	100–1000
Chlorpropamide (Diabenese®)	24–36	100–500

agents, and the rest are being treated by diet alone (7). The importance of division of meals and the exactness with which the diet prescription is followed will depend upon whether the patient is insulin-dependent. Typical diet prescriptions allow approximately 10 to 30 percent of calories at breakfast, 25 to 35 percent at lunch and at supper, with snacks making up as much as 25 percent of the calories in some cases and contributing no calories at all in others. Insulin-dependent patients appear to respond better to insulin therapy when they have two to three snacks and smaller meals. For the insulin-dependent patient receiving intermediate acting insulin, an afternoon snack is usually quite important and this snack should be appropriate for the circumstances under which the patient will be consuming it. Modifying the diet to fit into the patient's life-style is essential if adherence to the diet is to be expected.

Regularity of all activities, including the amount of food eaten at each meal and the time of these meals, is essential for a well-controlled insulin-dependent diabetic but may be regarded as desirable though not critical for the patient whose main concern is weight reduction. Education of the diabetic patient, including dietary instruction, should begin immediately upon diagnosis of the disorder. Again it must be emphasized that as much as possible the diabetic diet should be individualized to fit into the patient's life-style and former eating habits. Because this is a diet he/she will need to follow indefinitely, the patient needs to have meal patterns that are acceptable to him/her and are little different from those of the rest of the patient's family or friends. The diabetic child as well as the child's parents should be involved in the planning of dietary patterns. The child needs to understand the diet sufficiently well that he/she can manage food selections not only at home and at school but also in a variety of situations away from authoritarian figures.

Hypoglycemia. Hypoglycemia like hyperglycemia (diabetes mellitus) is a reflection of lack of balance between the physiological processes responsible for lowering blood sugar (i.e., tissue utilization and storage) and those required for elevation of circulating glucose (i.e., liver glycogenolysis and gluconeogenesis; absorption of carbohydrate from alimentary tract). The hormonal control of blood sugar has been described on pages

171–176. Because the lower normal limit of blood glucose is approximately 60 mg per 100 ml, anyone exhibiting on a day-to-day basis fasting blood sugar levels of 55 mg or less per deciliter for men and 35 mg per deciliter for women (27) *along with* various clinical symptoms of a precipitous onset such as tachycardia, tremulousness, sweating, weakness, anxiety, can be said to suffer from hypoglycemia (28). These symptoms can occur in the fasting state (spontaneous hypoglycemia) or can be "induced" by intake of specific foods and/or drugs (29).

Spontaneous hypoglycemia may be caused by hyperinsulinism, a condition often resulting from insulinoma, or by decreased gluconeogenesis. The inability of the liver to synthesize an adequate supply of glucose may be due to failure of tissues to release substrates in sufficient quantities for gluconeogenesis to occur or can be caused by a diseased liver. Induced hypoglycemia, on the other hand, occurs not in the fasting state but in response to some external stimuli.

The two most common forms of induced hypoglycemia are: (1) *functional,* the cause of which is undetermined but occurs about two hours after ingestion of a carbohydrate-containing meal and, (2) *alcohol-induced,* which develops when an excess of ethyl alcohol is consumed in a fasting or malnourished state.

Symptoms of functional hypoglycemia are found primarily in highly nervous women and it has been suggested that many patients diagnosed as having hypoglycemia actually may be suffering not from abnormally reduced blood sugar but from intense emotional disturbance. Symptoms associated with hypoglycemia are the same as those caused by excessive stimulation of the sympathetic nervous system and the consequent secretion of norepinephrine.

Functional hypoglycemia can be distinguished from that often accompanying mild diabetes by observing the glucose tolerance curve and carefully identifying the time at which blood sugar drops below fasting levels. The mild (noninsulin-dependent) diabetic has an elevated glucose that causes an excessive though belated secretion of insulin, the result of which is a precipitous drop in blood glucose three to five hours following ingestion of glucose. The functional hypoglycemic has a normal rise in blood sugar following an oral dose of glucose but blood glucose usually drops below fasting levels in about two hours (28) (Fig. 6.9).

Oxidation of alcohol in a liver containing no glycogen is the cause of alcohol-induced hypoglycemia. Oxidation of alcohol decreases gluconeogenesis because it keeps NAD in the reduced state, thereby inhibiting entrance into the gluconeogenic sequence of those substrates dependent upon NAD reactions for utilization (Fig. 8.6). Diabetics who are receiving hypoglycemic treatment must be particularly careful about overconsumption of alcohol because alcoholic hypoglycemia superimposed on some other cause of low blood sugar may cause irreversible damage to the central nervous system (6,29).

Other induced hypoglycemias of interest are those resulting from: (1) *leucine sensitivity,* in which the amino acid leucine elicits excessive production of insulin, (2) *fructose intolerance,* characterized by an accumulation of fructose metabolites which block glucose synthesis, and (3) *postgastrectomy "dumping,"* which promotes too-rapid absorption of carbohydrate and a consequent excessive insulin response.

Appropriate treatment of hypoglycemia is dependent upon the causative agent of the disorder. In the case of functional hypoglycemia, a low carbohydrate diet usually given in six small meals is the treatment of choice. Quickly absorbed carbohydrates, that is, refined sugars and monosaccharides, are avoided and total carbohydrate intake is limited to approximately 75 to 100 grams daily with most of the calories contributed by protein and fat. Keeping amounts of carbohydrate and protein constant in all meals is recommended (28).

Conversely, in treatment of leucine-induced hypoglycemia a diet containing only enough protein for growth and/or maintenance of body tissues is indicated with a high percentage of the calories coming from carbohydrate sources. Treatment for hypoglycemia due to fructose intolerance lies in removal of fructose from diet; dietary treatment for "dumping syndrome" is found on pages 146–147.

Obesity. Discussion of obesity is appropriate in association with pancreatic function because this disorder is commonly accompanied by hypertrophied islets of Langerhans and fasting hyperinsulinism with the level of insulin elevation paralleling the degree of obesity. In addition, glucose loading usually elicits an exaggerated insulin response in the obese because of their insulin resistance, and continued obesity may result in an impaired glucose tolerance and clinical manifestation of diabetes.

Obesity is a metabolic disorder distinguished by an excessively increased amount of body fat and is the number one health problem in the United States. The incidence of obesity has been estimated to occur in 15 to 40 percent of the population depending upon the criteria used to judge existence of the disorder and the techniques employed for its measurement (30). Almost twice as many women as men are estimated to be obese (31).

Accurate methods for measuring the degree of body fatness include densitometry and the various isotopic techniques. Such measurement techniques however, are not readily available to most clinicians; therefore, more practical but less accurate methods must be used in making determination of obesity. In the Ten-State Nutrition Survey, thickness of triceps skinfold was used to detect degree of body fatness and measurements greater than 18.6 mm for men and 25.1 mm for women indicated obesity (32). When relationship of weight to height is used to estimate body fatness, the best correlation is obtained by means of the Body-Mass Index (W/H^2).* A very simple method and the one most often used to measure obesity is *relative body weight* which is the percentage of actual weight to desirable weight. See Chap. 12 for quick method of calculating desirable weight. From the standpoint of health, any person with a relative body weight above 120 or a body-mass index greater than 30 is considered obese (32).

Classification of obesity is very difficult because it is so poorly understood, but for the purpose of discussion, two categories—obesity identified according to cellularity and obesity associated with etiological factors—will be used.

Obesity Identified According to Cellularity. Obesity can occur as a result of hypertrophy, that is, adipocytes that are normal in number have been engorged with stored fat. This type of obesity is common in persons who become excessively overweight as adults.

A seemingly more serious type of obesity is that due to *hyperplasia* of adipocytes, that is, abnormal proliferation of fat cells during periods of rapid body growth. Longitudinal studies of children have shown that there are no significant differences in weight between children who later become obese and those who remain at normal weight until after about 12 months of age. By two years, however, obese children have an increased body fat content due both to enlarged fat cells and increased fat cell number, while children of normal weight have decreased their fat stores to some extent. Studies suggest that obesity-prone children have a pattern of adipocyte development different from that of children of normal weight, which begins at about 12 months and continues until 14 to 16 years of age (33). In children of normal weight fat cells remain constant in number from age 2 to 10 years and proliferate only during the period of 10 to 16 years. Progressive childhood obesity may result in adult massive obesity characterized by hypertrophy and hyperplasia of adipocytes.

Obesity Associated with Etiological Factors. Numerous etiological factors are involved in development of obesity, none of which are unique to this condition (34). Some of the factors involved are cultural influences, emotional and psychological disturbances, socioeconomic strata, genetic influences, and hormonal imbalances.

Cultural influences. Some of the cultural influences potentiating the development of obesity include overfeeding of infants, improper distribution of food intake during the day, bad food habits, and decreased physical activity.

---

* Weight in kilograms; height in meters.

Overfeeding of infants is a common practice in the United States particularly among those mothers who bottle feed their babies. Not only do mothers want to be sure that the infants ingest every drop of formula but also they are likely to introduce solid foods into the baby's diet much earlier than is necessary. As a result of these practices numerous infants are receiving energy intakes well above the recommended dietary allowance. Chubbiness in infants seems to be desired by most parents despite the fact that babies who are breast fed, as intended by nature, are usually rather lean.

Distribution of food intake throughout the day has changed as society has moved from agrarian to industrial. The main meals of the day are no longer breakfast and midday dinner, but most of the food intake now occurs in the evening after the day's work is completed. Quite often the evening meal is preceded by a cocktail hour in which alcoholic beverages (and their accompaniments) not only provide a sizable energy intake in themselves but also stimulate flow of digestive juices, thereby increasing the appetite for a large, rather late repast. Leville and Rosmos (35) have demonstrated the enzyme adaptations in adipose tissue that occur in meal-eating rats and suggest that similar lipogenic adaptations are likely in man when most of his food is ingested at one time. An interesting study with humans has revealed that for both men and women the mean adiposity index gets smaller as the number of meals increase from two to six (36).

Bad food habits have developed with the proliferation of high caloric snack foods. These highly advertised foods are attractively packaged, easily accessible, and delicious to the palate. Snacking has become a way of life and is encouraged by the two or more "coffee breaks" that are provided for all blue collar and white collar workers. At home, snacks are usually considered a necessary component of an evening of TV watching and are a very important part of all spectator sport events. Most of these snacks are very high in fat and this fact has serious implications in regard to weight control. Bray (32) has demonstrated that a diet high in fat can cause failure in the regulatory mechanisms (whatever they may be) which normally maintain weight at a constant level. Animals are unable to compensate their food intake sufficiently to counteract the calorie effect of a high fat diet. In addition, the trend toward use of convenience foods at home and increased dining out at fast food chains increases fat intake among the population because most of the items consumed have a high fat content.

Decreased physical activity is another result of industrialized society, and this inactivity is further promoted by the proliferation of energy-saving devices, most prominent of which is the automobile. Furthermore, the possibility exists that obesity itself influences the energy required for performing physical activity. There is suggestive evidence that the obese develop a greater metabolic efficiency so that less than normal energy is used in work performance (6,37).

Psychological and emotional factors. These are often deeply interwoven into the development of obesity. A poor mother–child relationship originating early in childhood is sometimes responsible for the compulsive eating evidenced in some obese individuals. Also food is often associated with parental comfort and affection and, therefore, becomes a means by which to cope with various emotional stresses such as anxiety, depression, loneliness.

Socioeconomic strata. Adult fatness can be related to both the level of education and of income. As the level of education and income increases so does fatness in adult males. The opposite is true for females; they become leaner with increased education and wealth (38). An association also exists between race and obesity. Black women are fatter than white women, but white men are fatter than black ones. As blacks, however, move into a higher socioeconomic strata, women become leaner and men become fatter. Ethnicity may also affect development of obesity because Americans of Western European decent are not as prone to obesity as are those of Eastern European stock (39).

Genetic influences. Genetic factors may be involved in development of obesity either through direct transmission of a group of rare diseases in which excessive weight is characteristic or by providing a predisposition toward obesity, clinical evidence of which emerges upon interaction with critical environmental factors (32). Eighty percent of all obese individuals has been shown to have had at least one parent who was obese, with obese mothers being more common than obese fathers (37). Knittle et al. (33) suggest that if true genetic obesity does exist, it could be manifested in altered enzymatic activity, that is, a defect in the adenyl cyclase–cyclic AMP system or in synthesis of protein kinase. Because epinephrine stimulates lipolysis through these enzymes, a decreased activity of the enzymes could result in an insufficient release of fatty acids into circulation. Epinephrine, then, in order to overcome this deficiency of fatty acids needed for energy, might serve as the stimulus for development of a greater number of less responsive cells.

Hormonal imbalances. Hormones are rarely the primary cause of obesity but may constitute a necessary link in its development (37). Weight gain is augmented by an increased production of insulin and cortisol on one hand, but decreased by a secretion of growth hormone, thyroxin, and/or sex hormones on the other.

The consequences of true obesity are not all aesthetic in nature; there are many health consequences as well. When actual weight exceeds desirable weight by 25 to 30 percent or more, the mortality rate in this population group increases due to complications associated with diabetes, hypertension, and/or gall bladder disease. *Diabetes* may be unmasked by obesity because the islets of Langerhans are placed under stress by engorged adipocytes and excessive caloric intake. *Hypertension* may develop as a result of demand for increased circulation to carry nutrients to and remove wastes from expanded adipose tissue. Increased circulation demands may cause elevated blood pressure, a known risk factor in development of cardiovascular disease. *Gall bladder disease* is common in the obese because as body fat expands there is an increase in cholesterol turnover and in concentration of cholesterol in bile, thereby creating conditions favorable to formation of gall stones.

Therapies for Obesity. The number of existing treatments for obesity, particularly dietary treatments, attest to their lack of success. Studies have shown that of those persons attempting weight reduction, approximately 60 to 75 percent is able to take pounds off successfully but only about 5 to 20 percent can maintain weight loss (39,40). The foregoing statistics give support to the belief that the organism is constantly striving to maintain or to return to its equilibrium. Any weight reduction program, therefore, to be successful must cause a *permanent* change either in energy intake or energy expenditure.

The relative amounts of carbohydrate, protein, and fat in a reduction diet apparently have no effect on the actual decrease in adipose tissue. One advantage, however, in the diet that provides over half of its calories in the form of protein and fat is the satiety value of such a diet. A calorie restricted diet containing enough carbohydrate to prevent ketosis (approximately 100 g daily), but providing most of its remaining calories in protein and fat possesses a satiety value which may more nearly allow adherence to the lowered energy intake. Weight reduction and maintenance by dietary means is indeed a lifelong undertaking and involves a lifelong change in eating habits. The person undergoing dietary treatment for obesity must come to grips with the grim fact that he/she is faced with being hungry for the rest of his/her life. This is particularly true in the case of the person with hypercellular obesity because the amount of fat in cells can be reduced but the cell number remains constant. Furthermore, these reduced cells appear to be even more sensitive to the action of insulin than are cells of normal size (41). Therefore, the person attempting weight maintenance at a lower level is constantly fighting against enhanced lipogenesis and restoration of fat stores.

The dietitian working with obese patients must really care about these patients as persons if he/she is going to be successful in promoting weight loss and/or maintenance. When achievement of ideal weight can only be a remote possibility, the dietitian should encourage the patient to set short-range, modest goals, and to restrict moderately caloric intake. A reasonable caloric intake for weight reduction is approximately 20 kilocalories per kilogram body weight (7). Sometimes helping the patient to maintain his/her weight even at quite an elevated level is the greatest service that can be rendered.

Dietary counseling in weight reduction and maintenance should be geared around use of the Exchange Lists for Meal Planning with much emphasis placed on how to determine correct portion size. All too often obese patients underestimate the amounts of food they are consuming. The diet itself needs to be reviewed frequently so that any misconceptions can be cleared up quickly and the patient has a chance to ask any questions that may be of concern.

Obese persons need support and understanding as they undertake this arduous task of weight reduction, that is, they need a dietitian or another health professional who will rejoice with them in weight loss and commiserate with them (not condemn them) in failure to lose. All too often the obese person has a very poor self-image and needs badly to become aware of his/her innate worth. Health professionals have an opportunity to help the obese patient accept himself/herself even though they may not be successful in helping the patient to lose weight.

Encouraging exercise among the obese is extremely important, too. Although light to moderate exercise does not use up a great number of calories, it does help tremendously in weight control. Studies with rats and humans have shown not only that some calories are expended in exercise when activity is increased from a total sedentary state to one involving light exercise, but also that when this exercise lasts for only 30 minutes to an hour, food intake itself actually decreases (42).

Anyone attempting to reduce his/her stores of body fat should understand the dynamics of weight loss and realize that loss of weight depends on the relative amounts of fat and protein lost and, therefore, is not a good indicator of reduced energy stores (37). Adipose tissue has approximately 8 kilocalories per gram tissue because it is mostly fat with only a small amount of water and supporting tissue. Lean body mass, on the other hand, has only about 0.8 kilocalories per gram tissue because of its high percentage of water. In the first few days of caloric restriction, before conservation of nitrogen by the body is increased, weight loss is rapid because most of it results from destruction of lean body mass with its consequent release of large amounts of water. For every stored protein calorie lost, about 1.2 grams of tissue is destroyed; therefore, with a deficit of 500 kilocalories, a total weight loss of approximately 600 grams is possible. On the other hand, for every stored fat calorie lost, only about 0.12 grams of fat tissue is catabolized. A deficit of 500 kilocalories, therefore, could produce a weight loss of only about 60 grams were all the lost calories coming from adipose tissue.

The rapidity of weight loss experienced during the first few days of caloric restriction decreases as fatty acids increasingly replace carbohydrate as the primary source of energy. Decreased need for carbohydrate slows gluconeogenesis and as a consequence, protein catabolism is curtailed and so is weight loss.

When weight loss is achieved through fasting, the rapid weight gain that occurs with refeeding and is so discouraging to the dieter, is due to the retention of nitrogen and its large accompaniment of water necessary for protein synthesis. In addition, carbohydrate ingestion increases reabsorption of sodium with a consequent retention of water.

Regulation of food intake is a very complex and poorly understood mechanism but various studies have suggested that food intake by obese individuals is dictated more by external clues than by the internal ones that should regulate food consumption. Based upon the assumption that obesity is caused by a learned behavior (overeating), much research has been directed toward behavior modification in the hope that the obese may learn appropriate eating behavior and eliminate inappropriate behavior (40). The treatment is essentially a reeducation process and in its simplest form includes:

1. Identification of specific eating problems through detailed record keeping of food intake, including amount of food eaten, where, when, and with whom. Also is recorded the mood of the person when eating occurred.
2. Delineating techniques with which to combat identified problems, for example:
   a. Formulation of specific plans with built-in rewards for correcting fast eating, for curtailment of constant snacking, for modifying moods and/or emotions.
   b. Setting a realistic goal for weight reduction and planning an adequate diet that is not too restrictive to permit compliance.
   c. Statement of policies to be followed in purchase of food for home preparation or for consumption away from home.
   d. Obtaining support from family and friends in implementation of planned relearning experiences.
   e. Participation regularly in planned physical activities.

In the behavioral approach to obesity weight reduction becomes a positive activity rather than one of deprivation. Although the dieter is decreasing the enjoyable activity of eating, at the same time he/she is striving for a number of rewards that he/she has promised himself/herself upon attainment of a certain weight loss (43).

Education of the patient regarding a change in behavior toward food is best accomplished by a team of professionals, that is, the social worker with expertise in psychology and counseling, and the dietitian or nutritionist (44).

The effectiveness of behavior modification in the treatment of obesity is being scrutinized carefully because many researchers believe that no characteristic eating style can be identified for the obese (39).

Drug therapy for the treatment of obesity should logically be directed toward the etiology of the condition, although this concept is not necessarily always practiced by the physician. For example, patients made obese because of excessive food intake due to stressful situations or emotional instability may be treated with drugs that decrease anxiety or help to normalize the emotional state.

By far the most frequently used drugs for the treatment of obesity are those agents that decrease appetite, the anorexiant agents. These agents suppress appetite by either increasing bulk in the gastrointestinal tract and producing a sense of fullness or by stimulating the satiety center located in the hypothalamus of the central nervous system (CNS). The primary agents used as bulk producers are methylcellulose and carboxy-methyl-cellulose.

Drugs that produce anorexia by stimulation of the hypothalamic satiety center include caffeine, amphetamines, and other agents listed in Table 6.6. All of these agents with the exception of fenfluramine significantly affect other areas of the CNS as well as the satiety center; therefore, their side effects may include insomnia, mood elevation, excessive CNS stimulation, and hypertension. Agents in this category should not be used for more than four to eight weeks and only then with appropriate caloric restrictions.

For some patients with massive refractory obesity, various drastic methods for weight reduction have been employed: total fast or protein-sparing fast for varying periods of time, jejunoileal bypass surgery, and the most recent of all, gastric bypass surgery. The metabolic conse-

Table 6.6 Anorexiant Agents

Generic name	Trade name
Amphetamine sulfate	Benzedrine®
Benzphetamine	Didrex™
Chlorphentermine	Pre-Sate®
Dextroamphetamine	Dexedrine®
Diethylpropion	Tenuate®, Tepanil®
Fenfluramine	Pondimin®
Mazindol	Sanorex®
Methamphetamine	Desoxyn®
Methylphenidate	Ritalin®
Phendimetrazine	Plegine®
Phenmetrazine	Preludin®
Phentermine	Ionamin®, Fastin®
Clortermine	Voranil®

quences of these procedures are suspect but they all can produce rapid weight loss.

Because of the decreased secretion of insulin, a total fast can have some consequences similar to those of uncontrolled diabetes (see Figs. 6.7 and 6.8). Patients can be maintained on a total fast for rather extended time spans because elevation of serum ketone bodies decreases hunger and after a period of adaptation, these ketone bodies can nourish the brain. Ketones, therefore, reduce the requirement of the central nervous system for glucose, thereby acting to spare lean body mass which otherwise would be the main source of the amino acids used in gluconeogenesis. Conditions accompanying this elevation in ketones, however, include a decreased creatinine clearance, an increased serum uric acid level, and increased retention of bilirubin and bromsulphalein.

The protein-sparing fast can cause extensive weight loss but when used *properly* can prevent some of the untoward consequences of a total fast. Ketogenesis still occurs because of the absence of carbohydrate in the diet, but the addition of approximately 1.5 grams protein per kilogram IBW* per day (about 6 to 9 ounces cooked weight of *meat*) acts to spare much of the lean body mass lost in a total fast. The RDA of vitamins and minerals plus 25 milliequivalents of potassium and some additional calcium are administered daily. A potassium supplement is needed in the protein-sparing fast because unlike the total fast, serum potassium is not being maintained by the breakdown of lean body mass with its consequent release of potassium (45).

The discouraging aspect of total fast and protein-sparing fast is the inability of persons reduced by these methods to maintain their weight loss. When they return to eating in a normal fashion, all too often the weight is rapidly regained. Some programs, in order to avoid this, have employed behavior modification techniques throughout the fast.

The jejunoileal bypass surgery has been the therapy of choice for many patients with morbid obesity. This operation so reduces the absorptive area of the small intestine that weight loss can be achieved without curtailment of caloric intake. The operative and postoperative risks of this procedure are quite hazardous and lifelong follow-up is essential; however, the improved psychological state of many patients who have lost weight by this method suggests that bypass surgery with all its undersirable side effects still has value as a therapeutic tool for persons with obesity extreme enough to be life-threatening in itself (46,47).

Follow-up of the patient undergoing bypass surgery is divided into three phases: crucial phase which includes the first six months after surgery; early adaptive phase extending from six to eight months after surgery to about 18 months postsurgery; late adaptive phase beginning 18 months postoperatively and extending indefinitely (48). During the crucial

---

* Ideal body weight.

phase, malabsorption causes extensive diarrhea with large losses of fat, protein, minerals, and vitamins. Very careful counseling by the dietitian is necessary during these first six months because weight loss should not exceed seven to 10 pounds per month. The daily diet prescribed usually includes: 3000 or more calories, a high protein intake of 120 to 150 grams, low fat intake of not more than 80 to 100 grams, at least 4000 mg potassium, approximately 1600 mg calcium, about 600 mg magnesium, and a restricted oxalate intake of 50 mg or less. Also, care must be taken to omit gaseous foods and to assess the effect of lactose on gastrointestinal function.

A high potassium intake helps protect against hypokalemia which can result from excessive diarrhea. Restricted oxalate is aimed at reducing the amount of oxalate that will be absorbed and consequently excreted in the urine because increased urinary oxalate promotes formation of kidney stones (see pp. 388–389). Ordinarily oxalate is held in the gastrointestinal tract as an insoluble calcium salt. When, however, unabsorbed fatty acids have already bound the calcium in formation of soaps, oxalate remains in the gut as a soluble salt and is easily absorbed.

Fluid intake is carefully controlled with nothing being drunk immediately before a meal or for an hour thereafter. In order to retard peristalsis only small amounts of fluids (4 to 6 oz.) are allowed at any one time and these should never be iced. Alcohol in any form is forbidden for the same reason.

During the early adaptive phase the dietary treatment is much the same as that for the crucial phase except that some relaxation of restrictions may be possible according to individual response. In the late adaptive phase, dietary treatment is individualized to provide good nutrition at a calorie level appropriate for desired weight loss or maintenance. Bray et al. (49) have found that food intake by patients undergoing jejunoileal bypass surgery decreases and remains below preoperative levels for as long as three years.

As mentioned earlier, the most recent treatment for massive obesity is gastric bypass surgery in which the small proximal compartment of the stomach is separated from the rest of the organ and anastamosed to the jejunum (50). Because this technique has been in use for a relatively short time, its possible long range problems have not been determined. Nevertheless, present indications are that although the surgery itself is more complicated than the jejunoileal bypass, the postsurgical results may hold fewer hazards and provide more success in weight control.

Recent studies with (−) hydroxycitrate suggest that in the future an additional method of weight control may be operative, that is, metabolic regulation of obesity (51). In rodents (−) hydroxycitrate not only decreased caloric intake, but also inhibited ATP citrate lyase, thereby reducing the pool of acetyl CoA and decreasing lipogenesis. Rats showed a significant decrease in total body fat but no change in protein levels. The effect of $(-)$ hydroxycitrate on metabolite flux (decreased lipid synthesis and increased glycogen synthesis) and on appetite is interpreted by investigators in the context of a peripheral factor that influences the regulation of food intake.

Regulation of food intake has been a subject for extensive research during the last several years but the regulatory mechanisms that allow individuals to maintain a relatively constant weight is unknown. It is believed, however, that both central and peripheral influences are involved in control of caloric intake. Apparently in regulation of food intake there is a short-term component that varies in relation to the nature and quantity of foods consumed and a long-term component that is dependent upon the nutritional status of the animal. Normally these two components interact reciprocally and maintain body weight within narrow limits. A basic cause of obesity is believed to be a derangement of these mechanisms so that more food than needed is consumed (32,52).

Central influences in food behavior appear to be exerted by the hypothalamus, with the ventromedial area regulating long-term eating behavior and the lateral area controlling short-term food intake. Certain signals from the periphery come to the hypothalamus control centers and influence the onset, duration, and cessation of eating. These signals, however, are subject to modulation by corrective signals that reflect the nutritional state of the organism (53,54). The signals from the periphery that influence eating behavior may include among others: the size of the stomach, caloric content of food, circulating levels of amino acids, glucose, fatty acids and glycerol, and circulating levels of certain hormones, for example, insulin. Feeding behavior is also influenced by certain environmental cues such as the sight, smell, and taste of food. Human eating behavior is poorly understood and its complexities are the subject of much current research (24).

The fact that regulation of food intake appears to be deranged in the obese makes it very important to try to prevent obesity in infancy and childhood. Investigators agree that prevention, not treatment, is the ultimate solution to the problem of obesity because its causes and correct mode of treatment are unknown. Prevention should begin at birth and the dietitian has a real challenge in educating the young mother about the correct feeding of her infant. The mother needs to realize that the lean breast-fed baby is the ideal rather than the chubby baby being fed excess amounts of formula and supplementary foods (55). Education regarding normal nutrition for the entire family is exceedingly important and emphasis should be placed on avoidance of all excesses as well as on securing an adequacy of the essential nutrients.

Careful records of weight gains in relation to increase in length or height need to be maintained on children all through their growing years in order that early preventive measures may be instituted for those children gaining too rapidly. Similarly, monitoring of weights and activity patterns is important in mature adults. Much obesity in later years is caused by the individual's failure to adjust food intake to decreased activity. Health professionals should emphasize to all clients the importance of careful food selection along with a consciously increased level of activity. Prevention of obesity, no matter how difficult, is bound to be easier than its cure!

EXOCRINE FUNCTIONS OF THE PANCREAS

The importance of the pancreatic enzymes in the digestive process was briefly mentioned on page 125 and Table 5.1 lists all enzymes involved in digestion. However, because proper digestion of carbohydrate, protein, and fat are all dependent on the presence in the small intestine of adequate amounts of pancreatic enzymes, the physiology of normally functioning pancreatic exocrine tissue needs to be reviewed.

On a per gram tissue basis the exocrine tissue of the human pancreas synthesizes and secretes more protein than any other organ (56). The digestive enzymes produced in the pancreas include an *amylase* which reduces starch and dextrins to maltose; a *lipase* which together with bile allows triglycerides to be hydrolyzed into fatty acids and glycerol; five proteolytic enzymes; trypsin, chymotrypsin, carboxypeptidases A and B, and elastase which reduce proteins and large peptides to tripeptides, dipeptides, and amino acids. In addition, the pancreas secretes ribonuclease and deoxyribonuclease; phospholipases A and B which with bile selectively remove the fatty acids from lecithin, and cholesterol esterase.

All the proteolytic enzymes are synthesized and stored in their inactive forms so as to prevent autodigestion of the pancreas. Also, the cells that secrete the proteolytic enzymes simultaneously produce trypsin inhibitors which prevent activation of trypsin until the enzyme-containing pancreatic juice has reached the duodenum. Although pancreatic enzymes are secreted by zymogen cells in response to vagal stimulation, production of the enzyme-containing pancreatic juice is stimulated primarily by the hormone CCK–PZ, released into circulation from mucosal cells of the duodenum. Another hormone, secretin, enters circulation from the duodenum and causes production of the enzyme-poor, bicarbonate-rich pancreatic juice. As chyme passes from the stomach into the duodenum, this bicarbonate-rich pancreatic juice pours into the small intestine in order to raise the pH of the duodenal contents. The enzyme-containing pancreatic juice is then delivered into the duodenum where the pH has been elevated to approximately 8, the optimal level for pancreatic enzyme activity.

Upon reaching the duodenum, the inactive form of trypsin (trypsinogen) is activated by the duodenal enzyme, enterokinase, through the cleavage of one leucine–isoleucine bond. This cleavage allows the molecule to fold into the structure necessary for forming its active site. A small amount of active trypsin can then activate more trypsinogen as well as converting the other proteolytic proenzymes into their active forms.

DIAGNOSIS AND THERAPY OF DISEASE STATES ASSOCIATED WITH PANCREATIC EXOCRINE TISSUE

Pancreatitis

Inflammation of the pancreas rarely appears in children but can affect adults of any age and is found equally in both sexes. Although pancreatitis is not a prevalent disorder, its development is most often associated with biliary disease or chronic alcoholism. The exact relationship between these disorders and the initiation of pancreatitis is not known. When, however, extensive damage occurs in the pancreas or the ducts become blocked, large quantities of pancreatic secretions are held in contact with the pancreas. The proteolytic enzymes penetrate their lipoprotein membranes, become activated and begin digestion of the pancreas. The result is acute pancreatitis. Some of the enzymes pooled in the pancreas are picked up by the capillaries and carried into the blood stream.

The exact method by which trypsinogen is activated is unknown. Some researchers believe that the trypsin inhibitors are overcome by the presence of large amounts of enzymes that must be held in check; others hypothesize that a duodenal reflux into the pancreas causes activation of trypsin (57). Once trypsin is activated, all other proteolytic enzymes are quickly activated also.

An elevated serum amylase in a patient presenting symptoms of severe pain and tenderness in the upper abdomen along with possible vomiting, fever, and leukocytosis is considered good evidence of acute pancreatitis.

Major therapy for acute pancreatitis is removal of all stimuli to pancreatic function. Continual gastric suction is employed in order to prevent a lowered pH in the duodenum and its consequent secretion of secretin. Nutrition is provided parenterally until the acute attack is over. No special diet is indicated for the recovered patient, but he/she should be warned against the apparently precipitating factors of overeating and overindulgence in alcohol. Furthermore, if the patient is overweight, he/she should be encouraged to lose weight in order to lessen the burden on the islets of Langerhans (57,58).

Chronic pancreatitis results when acute attacks are superimposed on a previously injured pancreas. This chronic disorder is due in most instances to alcoholism of long duration and is characterized by a gradual replacement of the pancreatic parenchyma with fibrotic tissue and calcium deposits (57,58). The pancreas has great reserve capacity, however, and approximately 90 percent of its tissue can be destroyed before digestion and carbohydrate metabolism are severely impaired.

An x-ray revealing the presence of calcified areas in the pancreas is considered positive evidence of chronic pancreatitis. In advanced cases of the disease, excess excretion of fat and nitrogen will be found in stools due to the insufficiency of digestive enzymes. Diabetes develops in about 10 percent of the patients with chronic pancreatitis and is a sign of advanced disease (56).

Little can be done medically to halt progression of the disease but measures employed include a bland, low fat diet. The patient must avoid any substance that would stimulate hydrochloric acid production such as caffeine-containing beverages, pepper, and meat extractives and consequently cause excessive secretion of secretin. Because ordinary triglycerides cannot be digested and therefore cause malabsorption of other nutrients, dietary fat is restricted to approximately 70 grams daily. To assure adequate caloric intake, increased amounts of carbohydrate and protein must be consumed. The use of medium chain triglycerides may be desirable when weight gain is needed. Along with meals is given a replacement pancreatic enzyme preparation. Alcoholic beverages are forbidden and overeating strongly discouraged (58).

Emergency drug therapy for acute pancreatitis may include anticholinergic drugs (e.g., atropine) to decrease gastric acid secretion and meperidine (Demerol®) or pentazocine (Talwin®) for severe pain. Various electrolytes and intravenous fluids may be used to restore fluids lost due to vomiting. Insulin is utilized only if hyperglycemia is detected. The treatment of chronic pancreatitis not only may include the use of analgesics and anticholinergic drugs, but also will include antacids, vitamin supplements, and replacement pancreatic enzymes. These pancreatic enzymes are extracted from porcine pancreas and are administered in doses of 1.8 to 2.7 g with each meal. Recent clinical research indicates that the administration of cimetidine (Tagamet®) along with the enzyme extract may increase the efficacy of the enzyme by decreasing gastric acid secretion (59,60).

Cystic Fibrosis

Although the effects of cystic fibrosis (CF) are not limited to the pancreas, it was the clinical manifestations of pancreatic insufficiency that allowed identification of the disease some 40 years ago (61,62,63). Today cystic fibrosis is known to affect not only the enzyme-producing portion of the pancreas but also the exocrine glands throughout the entire body (64).

Despite the lack of identification of the basic defect in the disease, cystic fibrosis is thought to be transmitted as a Mendelian recessive trait (65). Heterozygotes show no clinical symptoms and are detected as carriers of the trait only when a child with cystic fibrosis is born to them. In the overall American population, one in every 20 people carries the gene for cystic fibrosis and the disease is manifested in one per 1000 to 2000 live Caucasian births. Other racial groups are also affected but to a lesser degree (66). Cystic fibrosis is now recognized as the most common of the eventually fatal genetic diseases.

Most of the clinical symptoms of cystic fibrosis are thought to be secondary to obstruction of normal function of an organ by abnormally thick and viscous mucus produced by glands throughout the body. The classic triad of symptoms include pancreatic deficiency, chronic pulmonary disease, and abnormal sweat electrolytes. Other organs or systems including the liver, heart, gall bladder, and small intestine may also be affected (65,66,67,68). The course of the disease is highly variable and is dependent not only on the organs involved but also on the extent of the involvement. Manifestations of the disease for children in the same sibship may even be strikingly different. Pancreatic involvement is not universal among cystic fibrotics but occurs in 80 to 85 percent of affected individuals as a consequence of the obstruction of the pancreatic ducts resulting in dilatation of the secretory acini and eventual degeneration and infiltration of the exocrine parenchyma by adipose tissue (65). Diagnosis of pancreatic achylia is made by analyzing duodenal fluid for pancreatic enzymes or more commonly by analyzing the stool for trypsin.

When the endogenous production of pancreatic enzymes is absent, commercially available preparations of hog or beef pancreas are administered. However, pancreatic enzyme replacement therapy only partially corrects the impairment in digestion (69,70,71,72,73,74). Steatorrhea and azotorrhea persist despite aggressive therapeutic regimens. Pancreatic enzymes taken orally are partially denatured in their route to the small intestine by the hydrochloric acid and proteolytic enzymes secreted in the stomach. Moreover, a reduction occurs in the bicarbonate-rich secretion which is normally delivered from the pancreas for the buffering of acid chyme as it passes into the duodenum (66). This decrease in buffering activity further compromises the digestive and absorptive processes in the small intestine of individuals with cystic fibrosis.

Mucus eventually obstructs normal function of lungs in 99 percent of individuals with cystic fibrosis. Pulmonary disease and its complications account for most of the mortality associated with this disease. Clinically, pulmonary disease is characterized by a dry hacking cough that eventually becomes productive. Although progressive, lung involvement can be influenced by therapy.

The primary objectives of therapy are to liquefy mucus and minimize its formation, prevent pulmonary obstruction, and control infection. Oral potassium iodide may be useful in liquefying mucus in milder cases, while in more severe cases mist tents may be helpful. Patients in an advanced state of the disease who require liquefaction of very thick secretions may benefit from the aerosol administration of a 10 percent solution of acety-cysteine, a mucolytic agent. To relieve pulmonary obstruction, broncho-dilators such as isoproterenol may also be administered by aerosol (75). Acute or chronic pulmonary infections are treated with oral or aerosol-ized antibiotics. Broad spectrum antibiotics such as tetracycline may be used safely for prolonged periods in most patients but their prophylactic use is not recommended (76). A most undesirable side effect of tetracy-cline is the discoloration of teeth in children. Instead, sputum cultures and drug susceptibility tests should be used to determine the most appropriate drug for the specific microbe. The major microbes cultured are penicillin-ase-producing staphylococci; therefore antibotics such as sodium cloxa-cillin and sodium methicillin are generally used in infection control (76).

The inability of persons suffering with cystic fibrosis to clear their lungs of mucus increases their susceptibility to infection. Unless the vi-cious cycle of obstruction, chronic infection, and tissue damage can be effectively arrested, the progressive loss of pulmonary function results. As pulmonary function becomes more compromised, respiratory rate and heart rate increase.

Abnormal concentration of sweat electrolytes (sodium and chloride) is the most universal symptom of cystic fibrosis affecting almost 100 per-cent of these individuals (65). Histologically no abnormality of the sweat gland has been identified. Although elevation in sweat electrolytes is unrelated to the severity of cystic fibrosis for an individual child, it is ex-tremely useful in diagnosis. Sweat chloride in excess of 60 mEq per liter together with evidence either of pancreatic deficiency, chronic pulmonary disease, or positive family history is sufficient to warrant a diagnosis of CF. However, sweat tests are unreliable in the first month of life and in extremely malnourished individuals. From a management perspective, the sweat electrolyte defect can result in massive salt depletion in hot weather or in the hospitalized patient receiving hyperalimentation fluids unless adequate salt replacement occurs.

The objective of diet therapy for individuals with cystic fibrosis is to provide a diet that supports normal growth and development. The diet should be nutritionally balanced. No food or food groups should be rou-tinely restricted or omitted from the diet because a child has cystic fi-brosis. The foods that children with CF cannot tolerate are highly variable and thus should be eliminated from the diet on an individual basis (77).

Food energy requirements for an individual with cystic fibrosis are generally two to three times the levels required by their healthy peers. Factors that contribute to the increased requirements for food energy include:

1. Malabsorption that persists despite adequate pancreatic enzyme replacement therapy.
2. Increased basal metabolism secondary to the increased respiratory and heart rates.
3. Chronic cough.
4. Chronic infection.

The best method for determining whether a child's diet is supplying his/her requirement for food energy is to weigh and measure the child accurately at regular intervals and to plot the measurements on acceptable growth charts. When a child's height or weight begins to deviate from the previous pattern of growth or when there are two percentile levels difference between height and weight, the food energy content of the diet should be increased.

Most pediatric texts describe the appetite of children with cystic fibrosis as "voracious." This classic description probably most aptly describes the appetite of the undiagnosed, untreated child who is virtually starving despite a ravenous appetite because of the pancreatic achylia. Appetites of children receiving treatment are more variable. Although some children continue to have good appetites, far more affected children are very picky eaters. Moreover, episodes of infection are associated with periods of anorexia for all children. These factors make providing diets with adequate food energy more difficult. For some children providing small but more frequent meals will meet their needs. For other children providing nutrition supplements that are more calorically concentrated will be required. For all children, a diet high in protein, carbohydrate, and fat will be necessary if their food energy requirements are to be met.

Diets for individuals with cystic fibrosis have traditionally been restricted in fat (78). No research thus far reported documents acceptable growth patterns when low fat diets are prescribed. In general, the fat content of the diet should be reduced when:

1. Abdominal pain is associated with fat intake.
2. Excessive steatorrhea persists despite adequate enzyme supplementation.
3. Rectal prolapse is a problem.

Pancreatic achylia results in malabsorption of fat-soluble vitamins which if untreated may result in vitamin deficiency syndromes. As prophylaxis, individuals with CF should take a multiple vitamin twice a day throughout their life.

CASE STUDY: CYSTIC FIBROSIS

A white male, aged 15 months, was admitted to the hospital for a complete evaluation because of his failure to gain weight. The child had appeared normal to his pediatrician until two months previous to hospitalization. At this time, during a routine physical examination, the pediatrician noted the child's slow growth rate and upon questioning the mother learned that her son was eating greedily but not enjoying his food. She also reported that the child was having four to five frothy, foul-smelling stools daily. The pediatrician instructed the mother to try feeding her son a gluten-free diet which she had been doing for approximately seven weeks. At the time of the child's admission to the hospital, the mother described the child's stools as still being frequent and foul-smelling although he seemed to be enjoying his food more than he had before he was started on the gluten-free diet.

A medical history obtained from the mother revealed that the child had frequent colds and had suffered from bronchitis on two occasions. Pertinent information obtained from the physical examination was as follows: weight $18\frac{1}{4}$ lbs.; height 29 in.; temperature 100 °F; pulse 100; respiration 35.

The admitting physician ordered laboratory tests aimed at determining the cause for the evident malabsorption. Lab values of particular importance included:

Stool neutral fat: 15% dry matter (normal 1 to 5% dry matter)

Stool trypsin activity: 0 (normal positive 2+ to 4+)

Sweat chloride: 111 mEq/liter (normal 4 to 60 mEq/liter).

Based upon the history, physical examination and laboratory data, a diagnosis of cystic fibrosis was made. Immediately upon diagnosis, the child was started on Cotazym 2® capsules with each meal. In addition, aerosol therapy with propylene glycol and Neo-Synephrine® was instituted twice daily and postural drainage in mist tent during the night was begun.

Questions

1. Why had the patient been placed on a gluten-free diet two months before his admission to the hospital?
2. What laboratory findings gave strong indication that the patient's malabsorption was caued by cystic fibrosis?
3. What is the purpose of Cotazym 2 capsules?
4. Why is respiratory therapy so important in the treatment of cystic fibrosis?

5. What dietary instructions will the dietitian need to give the mother regarding the proper feeding of the child?

Discussion

When the pediatrician discovered that this child was not growing properly (length and weight both below fifth percentile—see Chart 6.1) and that he gave evidence of malabsorption, his first thought was the possibility of celiac disease (nontropical sprue or gluten-sensitivity enteropathy) which is not uncommon among children. Since the treatment for celiac disease is a gluten-free diet, the physician instructed the mother to feed her son only those foods that contained no gluten. Had such a diet been successful in relieving the malabsorption syndrome, a gluten-free diet would have been continued as the mode of treatment for the child. When the diet had no effect on the child's bowel habits, however, the pediatrician referred him to a specialist for a complete evaluation.

Among the laboratory findings, the abnormally high level of stool neutral fat together with the absence of stool trypsin activity is suggestive of exocrine pancreas disorder. The enzyme lipase, which is responsible for the hydrolysis of neutral fats in the small intestine, and the proteolytic enzyme trypsin are both normally secreted by the pancreas. In the absence of active lipase, intact neutral fat is excreted in excessive amounts. The accumulation of mucus in the pancreas, a common pathologic finding in cystic fibrosis, causes the obstruction of organ ducts and, therefore, a cessation of normal secretions. Sweat glands show no morphological changes, but the chemical composition of the sweat becomes abnormal. In nearly all cystic fibrosis patients, the sweat chloride increases to two to five times normal, and for this reason the "sweat test" is considered to be the single most reliable diagnostic test for this disease.

Cotazym 2 (pancrelipase) is a pancreatic enzyme concentrate of porcine origin that possesses lipase, amylase, cellulase, and protease activity. This immediate therapy is essential in correcting the malabsorption syndrome associated with cystic fibrosis as it will replace the activity of those enzymes missing due to pancreatic insufficiency. This therapy is rational based on the laboratory findings of excessive neutral fat and a lack of trypsin activity in stools.

Pulmonary function is greatly compromised in the cystic fibrosis patient, with the formation of thick mucous plugs in the lungs being prominent. Neo-Synephrine (phenylephrine) is utilized as a decongestant because it stimulates alpha-adrenergic receptor sites, causing constriction of blood vessels of the respiratory mucosa. This effect will decrease congestion via decreased blood vessel size and enlarge the respiratory passages. Care must be exercised in dosing the patient with Neo-Synephrine because systemic absorption may lead to central nervous system stimu-

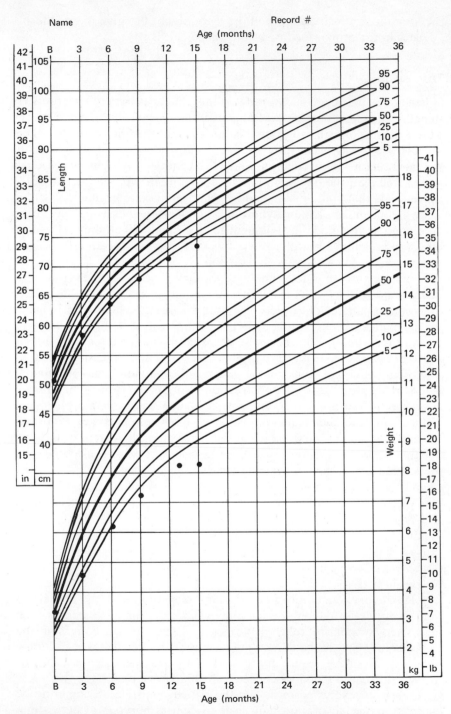

Chart 6.1 Growth curves for child with cystic fibrosis compared with those for children exhibiting normal growth. (Reproduced by permission of Ross Laboratories.)

lation. Propylene glycol is sometimes used with aerosolized medications to increase passage of the drug into the lungs.

The patient would also benefit from an agent such as acetylcysteine which will aid in breaking up the viscous mucus usually associated with cystic fibrosis. Mucus liquefies and can be expectorated more easily in the presence of an alkaline medium; therefore, bicarbonate might also be added to the aerosol to promote such an alkaline state.

From reading Chart 6.1 the dietitian is aware that the child is below the fifth percentile for height and weight. In order to catch up in growth the child will need to consume a high caloric, high protein diet, his requirements being two to three times as great as those of normal children his size. His desirable caloric intake, therefore, could approximate 1800 or more kilocalories daily. This young child's energy requirements are increased markedly because of persistent malabsorption, increased basal metabolism, chronic coughing and chronic infection, all of which usually accompany cystic fibrosis even when it is being treated vigorously.

Although a low fat diet has been ordered traditionally for the child with cystic fibrosis, such a diet will not supply the calories needed by the child. The dietitian, therefore, advises the mother to feed the child a nutritious diet and specific recommendations (e.g., finger foods) are based on the developmental needs of the child. The dietitian further encourages the mother to allow the child all the foods he likes unless by passage of excessive stools he demonstrates an intolerance to certain foods. Should an intolerance be demonstrated, the mother is instructed to try each high fat suspect food by itself in order to determine which one (or ones) is the offending item. The dietitian will see the patient whenever he returns for his outpatient clinic visits and will help the mother with any feeding problems she may encounter with her son. Should the child demonstrate an unsatisfactory weight gain, the dietitian will probably recommend increasing the number of meals served the child each day or suggest certain high caloric liquid supplements, for example, milk shakes and glucose-sweetened fruit juices, which the child can drink between meals.

REFERENCES

1. Gerich, J. E. Somatostatin. *Archives of Internal Medicine*. **137:** 659, May 1977.
2. Montgomery, R., R. L. Dryer, T. W. Conway, and A. A. Spector. *Biochemistry: A Case Oriented Approach*. 2nd ed. St. Louis: C.V. Mosby, 1977; pp. 308–311.
3. Guyton, A. C. *Textbook of Medical Physiology*. 5th ed. Philadelphia: W.B. Saunders, 1976; pp. 1036–1051.
4. Steinke, J. and J. S. Sceldner. Diabetes mellitus. In *Harrison's Principles of Internal Medicine*, G. W. Thorn et al., eds. 8th ed. New York: McGraw-Hill, 1977; pp. 563–583.

5. Cahill, G. F. Diabetes mellitus. In *Textbook of Medicine*, P. Bieson and W. McDermott, eds. 14th ed. Philadelphia: W.B. Saunders, 1975; pp. 1599–1619.

6. Bondy, P. K. and P. Felig. Disorders of carbohydrate metabolism. In *Duncan's Diseases of Metabolism*, Bondy, P. K. and L. E. Rosenberg, eds. 7th ed. Philadelphia: W.B. Saunders, 1976; pp. 221–340.

7. West, K. M. Diabetes mellitus. In *Nutritional Support of Medical Practice*, Schneider, Anderson, Coursin, eds. New York: Harper and Row, 1977; pp. 278–296.

8. Unger, R. H. Glucagon and insulin: Glucagon ratio in diabetes and other catabolic illnesses. *Diabetes* **20:** 834, Dec. 1971.

9. Felig, P., J. Wahren, R. Sherwin, and R. Hendler. Insulin, glucagon, and somatostatin in normal physiology and diabetes mellitus. *Diabetes* **25:** 1091, Dec. 1976.

10. Lacy, P. E. Research highlights: Present status, future hopes. *Dimensions in Diabetes*. Juvenile Diabetes Foundation, Winter 1976.

11. Maugh, T. H. Diabetes: Model systems indicate virus a cause. *Science* 188: 436, May 1975.

12. Rosenbloom, A. L. Nature and nurture in the expression of diabetes mellitus and its vascular manifestations. *Am. J. Dis. Child.* **131:** 1154, Oct. 1977.

13. Maugh, T. H. Diabetes: New hormones promise more effective therapy. *Science* **188:** 920, May 1975.

14. Maugh, T. H. Diabetic therapy: Can new techniques halt complications? *Science* **190:** 1281, Dec. 1975.

15. Clark, W. L., J. J. Perna, V. Lauris, D. Low, P. M. Galletti, G. Pavol, A. D. Whittemore, A. A. Like, C. K. Colton, and M. J. Lysaught. Artificial pancreas using live beta cells; effects on glucose homeostasis in diabetic rats. *Science* **197:** 780, Aug. 1977.

16. Anderson, J. W. Metabolic abnormalities contributing to diabetic complications—1. Glucose metabolism in insulin-insensitive pathways. *Am. J. Clin. Nutr.* **28:** 273, Mar. 1975.

17. Engerman, R. L. Animal models of diabetic retinopathy. *Tram. Acad. Ophth. and Atol.* **81:** 710, July/Aug. 1976.

18. Bunn, H. F., K. H. Gabbog, and P. M. Gallop. The glycosylation of hemoglobin: Relevance to diabetes mellitus. *Science* **200:** 21, Apr. 1978.

19. *Exchange Lists for Meal Planning, American Diabetes Association, Inc*. The American Dietetic Association, 1976.

20. Best, C. H. *Selected Papers of Charles H. Best*. Toronto: University Press, 1963.

21. Chance, R. E. Amino acid sequences of proinsulins and intermediates. *Diabetes* **21:** 461 (Supplement 2), 1972.

22. Larner, J. and R. C. Haynes, Jr. Insulin and oral hypoglycemic drugs; glucagon. In *The Pharmacological Basis of Therapeutics*, Goodman, L. S. and A. Gilman, eds. 5th ed., New York: Macmillan, 1975; pp. 1507–1533.

23. Tantillo, J. J., J. H. Karam, K. C. Burrill, M. A. Jones, G. M. Grodsky, and P. H. Forsham. Immunogenicity of "single-peak" beef–pork insulin in diabetic subjects. *Diabetes* **23:** 76, 1974.

24. University Group Diabetes Program. A study of the effects of hypoglycemic agents on vascular complications in patients with adult-onset diabetes. *Diabetes* **19:** 747 (Supplement 2), 1970.

25. Knatterud, G. L., C. L. Meinert, C. R. Klimt, R. K. Osborne, and D. B. Martin. Effects of hypoglycemic agents on vascular complications in patients with adult-onset diabetes. *J. Am. Med. Assoc.* **217:** 777, 1971.
26. Chalmers, T. C. Settling the UGDP controversy. *J. Am. Med. Assoc.* **231:** 624, 1975.
27. Ricketts, H. T. Hypoglycemia during fasting—editorial. *J. Am. Med. Assoc.* **234:** 186, Oct. 1975.
28. Fajans, S. S. Hyperinsulinism, hypoglycemia and glucagon secretion. In *Harrison's Principles of Internal Medicine*, Thorn et. al., eds. 8th ed., New York: McGraw-Hill, 1977; pp. 586–595.
29. Freinkel, N. Hypoglycemic disorders. In *Textbook of Medicine*, P. Bieson and W. McDermott, eds. 14th ed. Philadelphia: W.B. Saunders, 1975; pp. 1619–1624.
30. Current concepts of obesity. *Dairy Council Digest* **46:** 19, July/Aug. 1975.
31. McBride, G. Human appetite, eating behavior complexities tantalize scientists. Medical News, *J. Am. Med. Assoc.* **236:** 1433, Sept. 1976.
32. Bray, G. A. The overweight patient. *Advances in Internal Medicine* **21:** 267, 1976.
33. Knittle, J. L., F. Ginsberg-Fellner, and R. E. Brown. Adipose tissue development in man. *Am. J. Clin. Nutr.* **30:** 762, May 1977.
34. Committee on Nutrition of the Mother and Preschool Child, Food and Nutrition Board, National Academy of Sciences–National Research Council. Summary of a Workshop: Fetal and infant nutrition and susceptibility to obesity. *Nutr. R.* **36:** 122, Apr. 1978.
35. Leville, G. A. and O. R. Rosmos. Meal eating and obesity. *Nutrition Today* **9:** 4, Nov./Dec. 1974.
36. Metzner, J. L., D. E. Lamphiear, N. C. Wheeler, and F. A. Larkin. The relationship between frequency of eating and adiposity in adult men and women in Tucumseh Community Health Study. *Am. J. Clin. Nutr.* **30:** 712, May 1977.
37. Albrink, M. J. Obesity. In *Textbook of Medicine*, Bieson and McDermott, eds. 14th ed. Philadelphia: W.B. Saunders, 1975; pp. 1375–1376.
38. Garn, S. M., S. M. Bailey, P. E. Cole, and I. T. Higgins. Level of education, level of income and level of fitness in adults. *Am. J. Clin. Nutr.* **30:** 721, May 1977.
39. Kolata, G. B. Obesity—a growing problem. *Science* **198:** 905, Dec. 1977.
40. Tullis, I. F. and K. F. Tullis. Obesity. In *Nutritional Support of Medical Practice*, Schneider, Anderson, Coursin, eds. New York: Harper and Row, 1977; pp. 393–406.
41. Salans, L. B., J. L. Knittle, and J. Hirsch. The role of adipose cell size and adipose tissue sensitivity in the carbohydrate intolerance of human obesity. *J. Clin. Investigation.* **47:** 153, 1968.
42. Mayer, J. Why people get hungry. *Nutrition Today* **1:** 2, June 1966.
43. Leon, G. R. A behavioral approach to obesity. *Am. J. Clin. Nutr.* **30:** 785, May 1977.
44. Orkow, B. M. and J. L. Ross. Weight reduction through nutrition education and personal counseling. *J. Nutr. Ed.* **7:** 65, Apr.–June 1975.
45. Bristrain, B. R. Treatment of maturity onset diabetes with protein-sparing fast and hypocaloric diet treatment. Emory Medical School Television Network, Video Cassette #78-58, 1979.

46. Pi-Sunyer, F. X. Jejuno-ileal bypass surgery for obesity. *J. Am. Clin. Nutr.* **29:** 409, Apr. 1976.

47. Campbell, J. M., T. K. Hunt, J. H. Karam, and P. H. Forsham. Jejuno-ileal bypass as a treatment for obesity. *Arch. Int. Med.* **135:** 602, 1977.

48. Zachary, B. Dietary management of the jejuno-ileal bypass patient. *Nutrition and the M.D.* **8:** 2, June 1977.

49. Bray, G. A., B. Zachary, W. T. Dahms, R. L. Atkinson, and T. H. Oddie. Eating patterns of massively obese individuals. *J. Am. Diet. Assoc.* **72:** 24, Jan. 1978.

50. Cegielski, M. M. and J. A. Saporta. Surgical treatment of massive obesity: Current status of art. *Obesity/Bariatric Medicine* **7:** 156, 1978.

51. Sullivan, A. C. and J. Triscari. Metabolic regulation as a control for lipid disorders—I. influences of (−) hydroxycitrate on experimentally induced obesity in the rodent. *Am. J. Clin. Nutr.* **30:** 763, May 1977.

52. Thorn, G. W. and G. F. Cahill. Gain in weight, obesity. In *Harrison's Principles of Internal Medicine,* G. W. Thorn et. al., eds. 8th ed. New York: McGraw-Hill, 1977; pp. 228–233.

53. Van Itallie, T. B., N. S. Smith, and D. Quarterman. Short-term and long-term components in the regulation of food intake: Evidence for a modulatory role of carbohydrate status. *Am. J. Clin. Nutr.* **30:** 742, May 1977.

54. Keesey, R. E. and T. L. Powley. Hypothalmic regulation of body weight. *American Scientist* **63:** 558, Sept./Oct. 1975.

55. Overfeeding in the first year of life. *Nutr. R.* **31:** 116, Apr. 1973.

56. Snodgrass, P. J. Diseases of the pancreas. In *Harrison's Principles of Internal Medicine,* G. W. Thorn et. al., eds. 8th ed. New York: McGraw-Hill, 1977; pp. 1633–1645.

57. Dworken, H. J. *The Alimentary Tract.* Philadelphia: W.B. Saunders, 1974.

58. Kowlessar, O. D. Diseases of the pancreas. In *Textbook of Medicine,* Bieson and McDermott, eds. 14th ed. Philadelphia: W.B. Saunders, 1975; pp. 1243–1252.

59. Regan, P. T., J-R Malagelada, E. P. Dimagno, S. L. Glanzman, and V. L. W. Go. Comparative effects of antacids, cimetidine and enteric coating on the therapeutic response to oral enzymes in severe pancreatic insufficiency. *New Eng. J. Med.* **297:** 854, 1977.

60. Porro, G. B., R. Dolcini, E. Grossi, M. Petrillo, and A. Prada. Cimetidine in the treatment of pancreatic insufficiency. *The Lancet* **ii:** 878, 1977.

61. Andersen, D. Cystic fibrosis of the pancreas and its relation to celiac disease: A clinical and pathological study. *Am. J. Dis. Child* **56:** 344, 1938.

62. Blackfan, K. D. and C. D. May. Inspissation of secretion, dilation of the ducts and acini, atrophy and fibrosis of the pancreas in infants: A clinical note. *J. Pediatr.* **13:** 627, 1938.

63. Harper, M. H. Congenital steatorrhea due to pancreatic defect. *Arch. Dis. Childhood* **13:** 45, 1938.

64. Di Sant' Agnese, P. A. and R. C. Talamo. Pathogenesis and physiopathology of cystic fibrosis of the pancreas. *New Eng. J. Med.* **277:** 1287, 1967.

65. Di Sant' Agnese, P. A. The pancreas. In *Textbook of Pediatrics,* W. E. Nelson, V. C. Vaughan and R. J. McKay, eds. Philadelphia: W.B. Saunders, 1975.

66. Wood, R. E., T. F. Boat, and C. F. Doershuk. State of the art: Cystic fibrosis. *Am. Rev. Resp. Diseases* **113**: 833, 1976.
67. Feigelson, J., Y. Pecau, and J. Sauvergrain. Liver function studies and biliary tract investigations in mucoviscidosis. *Acta Paediat. Scand.* **59**: 539, 1970.
68. Esterly, J. R. and E. H. Oppenheimer. Observations in cystic fibrosis of the pancreas—I. The gallbladder. *Bull. Johns Hopkins Hosp.* **110**: 247, 1962.
69. Morin, C. L., C. C. Roy, R. Lasalle, and A. Bonin. Small bowel mucosal dysfunction in patients with cystic fibrosis. *J. Pediatr.* **88**: 213, 1976.
70. Haines, R. D., N. S. Hightower, W. A. Grozier, and J. M. Eiband. Pancreatic replacement therapy in fibrocystic disease. *J. Am. Med. Assoc.* **180**: 1000, 1962.
71. Harris, R., A. P. Norman, and W. W. Payne. The effect of pancreatin therapy on fat absorption and nitrogen retention in children with fibrocystic disease of the pancreas. *Arch. Dis. Child.* **30**: 424, 1955.
72. Mullinger, M. The effect of exogenous pancreatic enzymes on fat absorption. *Pediatrics* **42**: 523, 1968.
73. Lapey, A., J. Kattwinkel, P. A. di Sant' Agnese, and L. Laster. Steatorrhea and azotorrhea and their relation to growth and nutrition in adolescents and young adults with cystic fibrosis. *J. Pediatr.* **84**: 328, 1974.
74. Saunders, J. H. B. and K. G. Warmsley. Pancreatic extracts in the treatment of pancreatic exocrine insufficiency. *Gut.* **16**: 157, 1975.
75. R. Berkow, and J. H. Talbot, eds. The Merck Manual of Diagnosis and Therapy. 13th ed. Merck, Sharp and Dohme, Rahway, N.J.: 1977; pp. 595–597.
76. Kowlessar, O. D. Cystic fibrosis of the pancreas. In *Textbook of Medicine*, P. Bieson and W. McDermott, eds. 14th ed. Philadelphia: W.B. Saunders, 1975; pp. 1252–1254.
77. Weihofen, D. M. and D. J. Pringle. Dietary intake and food tolerances of children with cystic fibrosis. *J. Am. Diet. Assoc.* **54**: 206, 1969.
78. Harris, J. A., W. W. Waring, R. A. Langham, B. Judlin, M. Goins, B. C. Hilman, and G. Brouillette. Nutritional aspects of cystic fibrosis: Dietary recommendations. In *Mini-Guide to Lung Disease*. Atlanta: National Cystic Fibrosis Foundation, 1965.

RECOMMENDED READINGS

Anderson, J. W. and R. H. Herman. Effects of carbohydrate restriction on glucose tolerance of normal men and reactive hypoglycemic patients. *American Journal of Clinical Nutrition* **28**: 748, July 1975.

The authors present experimental evidence to suggest that the traditional low carbohydrate, high protein diet for treatment of hypoglycemia may not be the most appropriate therapeutic approach.

Berg, N. L., S. R. Williams, and B. Sutherland. Behavior modification in a weight-control program. *Family and Community Health* **1**: 41, Feb. 1979.

Behavior modification techniques are outlined and how these techniques can be used in promoting weight loss and maintenance is explained.

Bray, G. A. Endocrine factors in the modulation of food intake. *Proceedings of the Nutrition Society* **37**: 301, Dec. 1978.

This is one of the papers from a symposium on "Hormones and Food Utilization." The author identifies all the hormones that might influence food intake and describes their possible regulatory effect.

Brunzell, J. D. Use of fructose, sorbitol or xylitol as a sweetener in diabetes mellitus. *Journal of the American Dietetic Association* **73**: 499, Nov. 1978.

The author explains the effects of the various sweeteners on the blood glucose level of treated diabetics. Present evidence allows the conclusion that fructose, sorbitol, or xylitol can be used safely with the treated diabetic.

Elliott, J. Development of an artificial pancreas: The race is on. *Medical News, Journal of the American Medical Association* **241**: 223, Jan. 19, 1979.

Progress and problems in development of an open-loop and a totally implantable artificial pancreas are discussed.

Freinkel, N. The role of nutrition in medicine: Recent developments in fuel metabolism. *Journal of the American Medical Association* **239**: 1868, May 5, 1978.

Recent developments in understanding of fuel metabolism are discussed: acute hormonal effects, substrate interactions, modifications by way of exercise, and modulations by central nervous system. The importance of studying fuel economy in the various disease states is discussed.

Gunby, P. Research on the riddle of obesity gains new scientific insight. *Medical News, Journal of the American Medical Association* **239**: 1727, Apr. 28, 1978.

This is an excellent, concise review of papers presented at the Second International Congress on Obesity.

Hoffman, R. Starvation diets in the treatment of obesity. *Obesity and Bariatric Medicine* **7**: 10, Jan./Feb. 1978.

This is an excellent review of starvation diets in the treatment of obesity. Clinical course and weight loss patterns, possible hazards, long-range results, protein-sparing semistarvation regimens are all discussed and conclusions drawn as to the advisability of starvation as a means of weight loss.

Sims, L. S. The community nutritionist as change agent. *Family and Community Health* **1**: 83, Feb. 1979.

Functions and responsibilities of a change agent are described and determinants of success in accomplishing change are identified.

White, P. What it means to be female and diabetic. *Diabetes Forecast*, Part I, p. 10, Sept./Oct. 1975; Part II, p. 4, Nov./Dec. 1975; Part III, p. 12, Jan./Feb. 1976.

This three-part article is an excellent discussion of the development of the diabetic female, her adulthood, and the prospects for her offspring.

CHAPTER 7

The Cardiovascular System

Proper nourishment and oxygenation of all of the cells of the body are impossible without an adequately functioning cardiovascular system because it is only by means of this system, which is responsible for the circulation of blood, that nutrients and oxygen can reach cells and metabolic waste products can be transported from cells to various organs for excretion.

The cardiovascular system is composed of the heart, a muscular pump located in the thoracic cavity whose function is to force blood throughout the body, and blood vessels, which serve as conduits through which blood is carried to all cells of the body. Circulation of the blood is maintained by the pumping action of the heart which forces blood oxygenated in the lungs away from the heart through arteries and arterioles into capillaries and from these capillaries back to the heart through venules and veins. As the blood circulates through this complex system, nutrients absorbed from the gastrointestinal tract are carried throughout the body to all cells; waste products removed from cells are transported to the lungs, kidneys, or intestines for excretion; and secretions from specialized cells and glands are transported to their sites of action.

The complex functioning of the cardiovascular system is controlled by mechanisms that provide for the maintenance of a systemic blood pressure adequate to perfuse all body tissues at all times under highly variable physiologic conditions. Included among these mechanisms are the influence of both central and peripheral nervous systems; certain reflex mechanisms initiated by changes in blood pressure; and various endogenous regulators including renin, epinephrine, norepinephrine, and prostaglandins.

ANATOMY AND PHYSIOLOGY OF THE HEART AND BLOOD VESSELS

The organ that primarily controls the circulation of blood through the vascular system is the heart, a pump composed of four chambers (see Fig. 7.1). Although anatomically one organ, the heart performs as two separate pumps. The right side of the heart collects blood from the body and

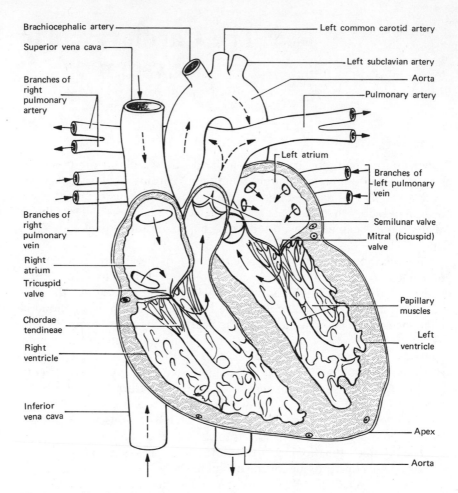

Figure 7.1 The heart in frontal section. (From *Human Anatomy and Physiology,* 2nd ed. by J. E. Crouch and J. R. McClintic. Copyright 1976 by John Wiley and Sons, Inc. Reprinted by permission of the publisher.)

sends it to the lungs for oxygenation while the left side receives oxygenated blood from the lungs and forces it throughout the body.

In the adult, the heart is located in the midportion of the thorax and measures about 12.5 cm long, 9 cm wide, and 5 cm deep with a total weight of approximately 300 gms (1). The upper chambers of the heart are the right and left atria, which are thin-walled and serve to collect blood. The lower chambers are the right and left ventricles, which possess thick muscular walls necessary for forceful propulsion of blood. The musculature of the left ventricle is even stronger than that of the right because whereas the right ventricle pumps blood into the rather low pressure pulmonary system, the left ventricle must exert sufficient force to move blood into the aorta, the great trunk artery responsible for distributing blood throughout the body.

The heart, which is essential to the nourishment of the body as a whole, must itself be well nourished. Nourishment of the heart is provided by the right and left coronary arteries which are located on top of the heart and arise from the aorta at a point where fresh, oxygenated blood leaves the left ventricle (see Fig. 7.2). Blood carried by the coronary arteries contains the highest level of oxygen and is under the greatest possible pressure. The vascular network of the heart is so extensive that some investigators believe that at least one capillary supplies nourishment to each muscle fiber (2). Blood carrying waste products from heart muscle fibers returns to the right atrium via the coronary veins. Nourishment of the heart is achieved only when the organ is at rest because blood cannot flow through the heart's system of arteries, capillaries, and veins when the myocardium (muscle of the heart) is contracted. Atherosclerotic heart disease results from the inability of diseased coronary arteries to nourish the heart adequately.

Cardiac contractions, which force blood through both the pulmonary and systemic circulations, are made possible because of the unique physiological properties of cardiac tissue. The actual contraction of cardiac muscle fibers occurs as a result of the passage of electrical impulses through specialized conducting tissues located throughout the heart. Certain areas of cardiac tissue are said to possess the property of automaticity because they have the ability to generate the electrical impulses necessary to produce the rhythmicity (chronotrophy of the heart). The primary area of automaticity is a specialized area of tissue located in the right atrium just below the opening of the superior vena cava which is termed the sinoatrial (S-A) node and is often referred to as the "pacemaker" of the heart. The S-A node generates electrical impulses at the rate of approximately 70 to 75 per minute under normal conditions, but this rate may be altered by intervening physiological or emotional conditions.

The electrical impulses generated by the S-A node first spread across the atrial tissue, which causes both atria to contract at the same time and allows blood to enter the ventricles. The electrical impulses that cause the atria to contract also stimulate or excite a second group of specialized cells located at the junction between the atria and the ventricles. This group of cells is called the atrioventricular (A-V) node. From the A-V node, electrical impulses descend into the atrioventricular bundle (bundle of His), which is located in the septum between the right and left ventricles. From the bundle of His, the electrical impulses are transported via the Purkinje fibers which spread the electrical impulses throughout the tissue of the ventricles.

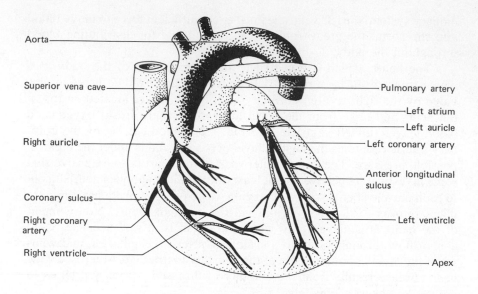

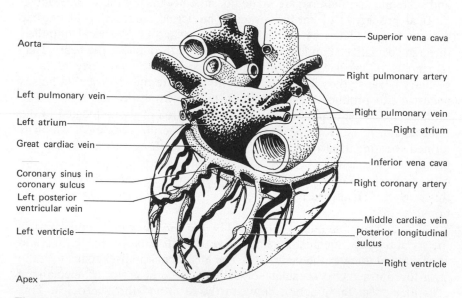

Figure 7.2 The coronary vessels. (*a*) Anterior view. (*b*) Posterior view. (From *Human Anatomy and Physiology,* 2nd ed. by J. E. Crouch and J. R. McClintic. Copyright 1976 by John Wiley and Sons, Inc.)

The orderly transport of electrical activity from the S-A node to all cardiac muscle fibers produces the sequence of contraction and relaxation events that pump blood throughout the body. Contraction of the ventricles (systole) forces blood into the pulmonary and systemic circulation while relaxation of the ventricles (diastole) allows for the ventricular chambers to be filled with blood from the atria. Obviously, the rhythmic contractions of the atria and ventricles must be well coordinated to assure that proper pumping of the blood in maintained.

Cardiac output (amount of fluid pumped by the left ventricle in one minute) equals the stroke volume (or amount pumped by one stroke) times the heart rate (or number of strokes per minute). Blood moves from the heart into the aorta, which forces blood through the arterial system into the capillaries. From the capillaries blood moves back toward the heart by means of venous return made possible by the venous valve system and by the action of muscles with which veins come in contact. Figure 7.3, depicts both pulmonary and systemic circulation. At any one time relatively more blood is found in the veins (60 percent) than in the arteries (30 percent), with approximately 10 percent in the capillaries. Blood enters the capillaries through an arteriole and leaves by way of a venule. Direction of blood flow is illustrated in Figure 7.4. Each arteriole is equipped with a strong muscular wall which can close off the vessel completely or allow its dilatation to several times its normal size. Because of their ability to contract and dilate, arterioles are very important in the regulation of blood pressure and control blood flow into the capillaries. It is through these capillaries that exchange of nutrients and other substances can be made between blood and the interstitial fluid, which surrounds the cells (see Fig. 7.5). Exchange occurs primarily through diffusion, with water and water-soluble substances of low molecular weight moving through the pores of the capillary membrane, and substances such as oxygen and carbon dioxide, which can be solubilized in fat, being exchanged through the capillary membrane itself. Endocytosis may be an important mechanism of exchange for substances of high molecular weight, for example, plasma proteins, glycoproteins, and large polysaccharides such as dextran. Filtration of fluid through the arterial end of the capillaries and reabsorption at the venous end is an important mechanism for transfer of fluid between the plasma and interstitial fluids. This transfer is regulated by capillary pressure, interstitial fluid pressure, plasma colloid osmotic pressure, and interstitial fluid colloid osmotic pressure (see Chapter 4).

Maintenance of an adequate systemic blood pressure (approximately 120 mm Hg during systole and 80 mm Hg during diastole) is under the control of a number of previously mentioned mechanisms. The S-A node is responsible for the control of heart rate under normal conditions, but this rate may be increased or decreased due to intervention by the auto-

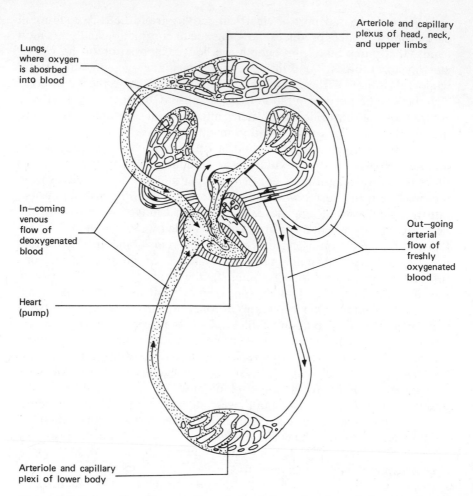

Figure 7.3 Schematic representation of circulation, showing relative distribution of blood between arterial and venous systems. (Adapted from *Textbook of Medical Physiology*, 5th ed. by Arthur C. Guyton. Copyright 1976 by W.B. Saunders Co.)

nomic nervous system (ANS), which is controlled by the hypothalamus, a structure located in the midbrain. The hypothalamus receives messages from blood pressure-sensitive receptors (baroreceptors) located in the arch of the aorta and in the carotid arteries that alert the hypothalamus to changes in blood pressure. In response the hypothalamus, via the ANS, makes appropriate modifications in the cardiovascular system to readjust the blood pressure to normal. The hypothalamus also receives messages from the limbic system (the area of the brain responsible for the control

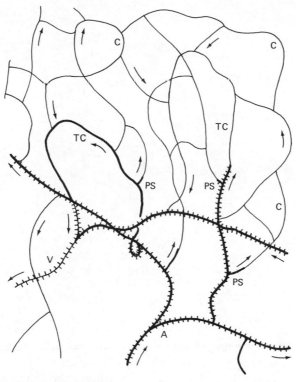

A = arteriole
V = venule
TC = thoroughfare channel
C = capillaries
PS = precapillary sphincter

Figure 7.4 Diagram of microcirculation—Note the thinning of the smooth muscle coat in the thoroughfare channels and its complete absence in the true capillaries. The black lines on the surface of the vessels are nerve fibers leading to smooth muscle cells. (Adapted from *Human Physiology—The Mechanisms of Body Function* by A. C. Vander, J. H. Sherman and D. S. Luciano. Copyright 1975 by McGraw-Hill Book Co. Reprinted by permission of the publisher.)

and display of emotions) and makes adjustments in cardiovascular function in order to meet emotional demands or combat stress situations.

The ANS is composed of two groups of nerve fibers. The parasympathetic (cholinergic) nerves for which the neurotransmitter is acetylcholine control most areas of the body during periods of relaxation or sleep. The sympathetic (adrenergic) nerves for which the neurotransmitter is norepinephrine exert their influence during periods of increased activity or during physical or mental stress situations. Stimulation of the vagus

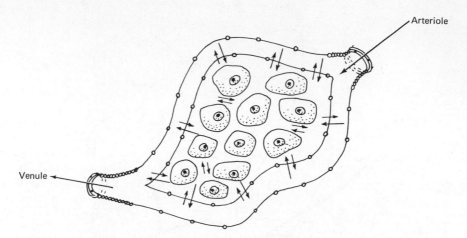

Figure 7.5 Diffusion of fluids through the capillaries and through interstitial spaces. (From *Textbook of Medical Physiology*, 5th ed. by Arthur C. Guyton. Copyright 1976 by W.B. Saunders Co. Reprinted by permission of the publisher and author.)

nerve, the parasympathetic nerve fiber leading to the heart, results in a decrease in heart rate and blood pressure, thereby decreasing the work of the heart during periods of low activity. Stimulation of the sympathetic nervous system, because of its neurotransmitter, norepinephrine, has two effects on the cardiovascular system. First, stimulation of the sympathetic nerves leading to the heart will increase the heart rate. Second, stimulation of sympathetic nerve fibers leading to arterioles will cause them to constrict. This combination of effects produces an increase in blood pressure and provides a more rapid movement of nutrients and oxygen throughout the body as well as permitting a more rapid removal of metabolic waste products from the cells.

The reflex control of blood pressure is also mediated via the ANS. When carotid or aortic blood pressure receptors detect change in systemic pressure, this information is relayed to the hypothalamus which, in turn, activates the ANS. When the pressure drops below normal, sympathetic nerve fibers are activated to increase heart rate and constrict arterioles. On the other hand, when blood pressure increases abnormally, stimulation of the vagus nerve decreases heart rate.

Hormones circulating in the blood also influence blood pressure. Norepinephrine and epinephrine are released from the adrenal medulla due to nervous system stimulation when the organism is under periods of physical or emotional stress. These hormones stimulate receptors of the sympathetic nervous system to increase blood flow throughout the body and thus provide the energy sources needed during the stress situation.

Another hormone, aldosterone, whose secretion is increased via the renin-angiotensin mechanism, also elevates blood pressure through an expansion of blood volume. Angiotensin not only causes an increase in blood pressure through its effect on aldosterone production but also acts as a potent vasonconstrictor itself (see Fig. 7.6).

Several other hormones, for example, kinins and prostaglandins, whose action is usually localized, also affect blood pressure and are released in response to specific physiological stimuli. Further discussion of these hormones is found in the section on hypertension.

Reflex control of blood pressure is important for changes in activity which occur minute by minute, while autonomic control is more important for gradual or long-term changes in activity.

HYPERTENSION

Increased pressure is required for the circulation of blood whenever: (1) the capacity of the vessels is decreased due to decreased elasticity of the arteries or to excessive contraction of the arterioles, or (2) the volume of

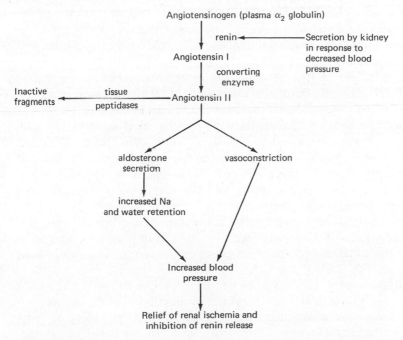

Figure 7.6 Renin-angiotensin-aldosterone mechanism in regulation of blood pressure.

circulating fluid is increased through excessive sodium and water retention.

Hypertension, or an arterial pressure of 160/95 mm Hg or higher in a resting supine adult (3), is one of the most common chronic diseases in the United States and affects approximately 24 million of the population. The onset of hypertension usually occurs between 25 and 55 years of age, is more common among women than men and is more prevalent among blacks than whites. Only 10 percent of patients with hypertension have elevated blood pressure because of known causes, which include: (1) kidney damage with narrowing of renal arteries so that arterial pressure always appears low to the kidneys; (2) excessive production of aldosterone (primary aldosteronism), perhaps as a result of a tumor of the adrenal cortex or ascites; (3) pheochromocytoma, a small tumor of the adrenal medulla which secretes epinephrine and norepinephrine. In order to assure proper therapy these possible causes of hypertension should be ruled out before any treatment is begun.

Aldosterone, along with other hormones of steroidal or protein structure, can be quantitated in a specimen of the patient's serum by the method of radioimmunoassay (RIA). The diagnosis of pheochromocytoma is based on the overproduction of the catecholamine neurotransmitters, epinephrine and norepinephrine, by the tumor. The presence of such a tumor causes elevated levels of the hormones and metabolites of the hormones in the urine of a patient. The major metabolites of the catecholamine hormones are vanillylmandelic acid (VMA), metanephrine, and normetanephrine.

The principle of RIA used for the determination of plasma aldosterone levels, and the methods commonly used to measure catecholamines and their metabolites are discussed briefly in Chapter 14.

Ninety percent of all patients with hypertension are afflicted with "essential" hypertension or hypertension of unknown causes. This fact has led to tremendous research resulting in the discovery that of essential hypertension patients, 16 percent have high renin activity in blood plasma, 27 percent have low renin activity, and the remaining 57 percent have apparently normal renin values (4).

The activity of renin, a proteolytic enzyme secreted by the juxtaglomerular apparatus of the kidney (see Fig. 10.4), is of particular interest in hypertensive patients because of its effect on vasoconstriction and blood volume (see Fig. 7.6).

In hypertensive patients with increased renin levels, an elevated blood pressure has failed to suppress the production of renin and as a result excessive vasoconstriction occurs. The increased incidence of heart attacks, strokes, and kidney failure in this group of hypertensive patients suggests that hypertension due to vasoconstriction is more serious than that resulting from increased blood volume, the apparent cause of elevated blood pressure in the group with low levels of renin. Hypertension in the group with apparently normal renin levels may be due to a combination of vasoconstriction *and* increased blood volume. Most researchers believe that the kidneys, because of their major role in the regulation of blood pressure, must be involved in the development of hypertension. It has been suggested that all hypertensive patients may have kidneys that are defective in their capacity to secrete sodium.

Also implicated in development of essential hypertension are: (1) stress, which may cause altered functioning of the central nervous system, resulting in increased activity of the sympathetic nervous system with concomitant release of excessive amounts of norepinephrine, a potent vasoconstrictor; (2) deficiency of the enzyme *kallikrein,* which splits an alpha globulin to form kinins, powerful vasodilators in themselves but also needed to cause release of the prostaglandin, PGE_2, another vasodilator, which antagonizes the vasoconstriction caused by angiotensin II and norepinephrine; (3) excessive sodium intake; and (4) excessive production of adrenal steroids or use of steroids in treatment of inflammation (1).

Almost all essential hypertensive patients are the descendants of one or more parents or grandparents who are hypertensive; therefore, a predisposition toward the disease appears to be inherited (4). Because experiments with rodents have demonstrated the effect of sodium on development of hypertension in genetically susceptible animals, sodium-controlled diets begun in infancy and continued throughout life are recommended as a means whereby development of hypertension may be prevented or at least somewhat impeded in humans with a familial tendency. Manufacturers of baby foods have complied with this recommendation and in the last few years have drastically reduced the sodium content of their products.

Therapy for Hypertension

Drug Therapy. Drug therapy for hypertension has advanced to such a degree in recent years that the disease is no longer considered the scourge that it once was. As is the case with many common disease states, primary therapy for essential hypertension is directed toward indirect methods of alleviating the presenting symptoms of the patient. For mild hypertension, drug therapy may not be necessary and the patient may be managed with a program of weight reduction, lowered sodium intake, and adequate periods of relaxation and sleep. When mild hypertension occurs as a response to tension, a mild sedative may be sufficient to prevent an increase in blood pressure. Some mild hypertension, however, will not respond to this type of therapy. In such cases, initial therapy usually consists of a diuretic agent. Diuretics increase the fluid loss, decrease edema, and, in general, decrease the work load placed on the heart. The mechanism by which diuretics lower blood pressure is not clear, but several theories have been developed to explain their actions:

1. Alteration of sodium and water content of arterial smooth muscle.
2. Reduction of vascular response to norepinephrine and epinephrine.
3. Reduction of blood volume and total extracellular fluid volume.
4. Direct vasodilator action independent of the diuretic effect (5).

Further information concerning these agents is included in Chapter 10.

For hypertension that does not respond to therapy with diuretic agents, more potent drugs are used, often in combination with diuretic agents. Included in the category of potent antihypertensive agents are adrenergic blocking agents, which antagonize the effects of the sympathetic nervous system, and vasodilators, which act via the central or peripheral nervous system to decrease peripheral resistance. These antihypertensive agents produce their therapeutic effects by two major methods: (1) by decreasing peripheral vascular resistance, that is, by dilating the arterioles so that there is less resistance to blood flow, or (2) by decreasing cardiac output. Some drugs act by both of these methods.

Adrenergic blocking agents such as guanethidine (Ismelin®) and reserpine produce their therapeutic effect by decreasing the amount of the neurotransmitter norepinephrine in the nerves that innervate the arterioles. These agents are nonspecific because they affect sympathetic nerves throughout the body and produce a number of side effects; therefore, their use is limited, in most cases, to patients who do not respond to the newer, more specific antihypertensive agents.

Methyldopa (Aldomet®) is an adrenergic blocking agent that acts as a false neurotransmitter and decreases the amount of norepinephrine in sympathetic nerves. Its primary action as an antihypertensive agent is due to its ability to depress the vasomotor centers of the medulla of the brain stem. This action decreases the activity of the sympathetic nervous system and decreases the tone (amount of constriction) of the arterioles. Methyldopa also inhibits the release of renin, an effect that may be of benefit to some hypertensive patients.

Clonidine (Catapres®) is similar in its actions to methyldopa in that it produces a decrease in blood pressure by a depressant effect on the medulla. It also increases activity of the vagus nerve. These actions result in a decrease in vascular resistance and a decrease in cardiac output.

Hydralazine (Apresoline®) and prazosin (Minipress®) are vasodilators that decrease peripheral resistance by a direct action on vascular smooth muscle. Hydralazine has been used for over 20 years as an antihypertensive agent, but is considered less useful than some other agents because a reflex increase in heart rate occurs along with the vasodilation. In order to decrease this reflex tachycardia, propranolol (Inderal®), a drug that decreases heart rate by blocking adrenergic receptors in cardiac tissue, is often used concomitantly. Prazosin differs from hydralazine in that it produces peripheral vasodilation but also prevents reflex tachycardia by blocking the response of cardiac tissue to adrenergic stimulation.

The side effects associated with the antihypertensive agents are primarily related to their effects on the cardiovascular system and the central nervous system. Guanethidine reduces cerebral blood flow which may result in lightheadedness. Fatigue occurs as a result of decreased perfusion of skeletal muscle. Orthostatic hypotension occurs with rapid change of positions due to depression of cardiovascular reflexes. Reserpine produces behavioral changes (depression which may lead to suicide) as well as increasing gastric acid secretion, gastrointestinal motility and tone. This drug should not be administered to patients with a past history of depression or peptic ulcers. Methyldopa produces sedation and sometimes depression (but to a lesser degree than reserpine) and causes some degree of orthostatic hypotension. Clonidine produces dry mouth and sedation. It may also produce impotence, constipation, and orthostatic hypotension. Hydralazine may produce headache, dizziness, and palpitations but does not produce orthostatic hypotension. Prazosin may initially produce orthostatic hypotension at high doses and also can cause headaches and palpitations (5).

Diet Therapy. Although hypertension can now be controlled by drugs, other principles, as listed below, including diet modification, are important for the management of elevated blood pressure and can augment the efficacy of the drugs (3):

1. Sodium intake restricted to approximately 2 gm (85 to 90 mEq) daily since kidneys of hypertensive patients are believed to be unable to secrete sodium efficiently. Some patients respond so well to a lowered sodium intake that drug therapy is not needed, and when drugs are necessary, the dosage required is usually reduced when accompanied by a sodium-restricted diet (6). An additional benefit of combination therapy is its potassium-sparing effect (see Chapter 10). Potassium supplements are often necessary in patients controlled by those diuretics that not only prevent reabsorption of sodium but also increase potassium loss.
2. Caloric restriction for the overweight person so that ideal weight may be reached and maintained. Weight reduction often is quite effective in reducing blood pressure.
3. Moderate restriction in intake of cholesterol and saturated fats. Because hypertension is a risk factor in development of atherosclerosis, such a diet may help in prevention of ischemic heart disease.
4. Regular exercise. An exercise program helps control weight, and physical conditioning itself seems beneficial in the lowering of blood pressure.

Dietitians who themselves have adhered to a 2 gm per day sodium diet will have found that it is not a difficult diet to follow and that the reduced use of salt allows discovery of the delicious natural flavor of the food itself. Furthermore, fruits and unprocessed vegetables, which are allowed in abundance because of their low sodium content, are high in potassium, and in experimental animals a simultaneous increase in potassium as sodium is decreased has been found quite beneficial in the lowering of blood pressure (7). Principles of the sodium restricted diet are found in the section on heart failure (pps. 255–256).

Prevention and/or control of hypertension is of particular importance because of the relationship between elevated blood pressure and development of sclerotic blood vessels throughout the body, the result of which can be coronary occlusion, cerebral hemorrage, and/or hemorrhage of renal vessels. After age 45 years, hypertension is the number one risk factor in the development of ischemic heart disease with the incidence among hypertensives being about two to three times as great as among the normal population.

CARDIOVASCULAR DISEASE

Atherosclerosis

Atherosclerosis is a disease of the medium and large arteries in which one of the wall layers—the intima—becomes thickened through the deposition of fibrous and fibrofatty plaques (8,9). Figure 7.7 shows a normal artery with its healthy three wall layers as well as the possible stages in the development of a fibrous plaque within the intima. The intimal layer is a single, continuous layer of endothelial cells, while the media is made up of smooth muscle cells. Extending from the basement membrane of the endothelial cells to the smooth muscle cells are fine elastic fibrils of collagen and elastin, which when considered as a whole are called the internal elastic lamina. With age the amount of collagen increases, thereby causing the lamina to thicken and become less elastic.

Various theories exist concerning the initiation and development of atherosclerotic lesions (9–12) but there is agreement regarding the components of a complicated lesion such as the one illustrated in Figure 7.7. The fibrous plaque is composed of connective tissue, smooth muscle cells, cell debris, and quantities of lipid deposits. Because atheromas contain such large quantities of lipids, much attention has been directed toward lipid metabolism not only in the arteries themselves but also throughout the body as a whole.

Coronary heart disease (CHD) or ischemic heart disease, which affects about five million Americans, ranks second to hypertension as the

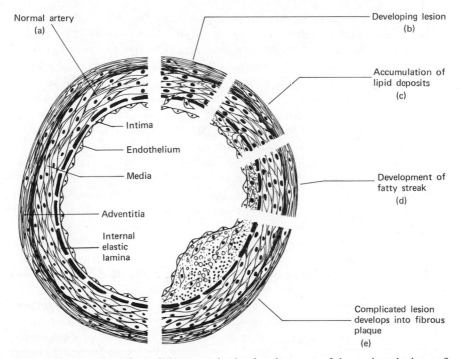

Normal artery
(a)

Developing lesion
(b)

Accumulation of
lipid deposits
(c)

Intima

Endothelium

Media

Adventitia

Internal
elastic
lamina

Development of
fatty streak
(d)

Complicated lesion
develops into fibrous
plaque
(e)

Figure 7.7 A series of possible stages in the development of the various lesions of atherosclerosis. (*a*) The appearance of a normal muscular artery and its component layers: the intima bounded by endothelium and internal elastic lamina, the media, and adventitia. In children and young adults the intima is thin and contains only an occasional smooth muscle cell; with age it slowly and uniformly increases in thickness and cell content. It is important to note that there are no fibroblasts present in either intima or the media of mammalian arteries. Fibroblasts are found only in the adventitia. (*b*) The first phase of a developing lesion in atherosclerosis: a focal thickening of the intima consists of an increase in smooth muscle cells and extracellular matrix. Smooth muscle cells are shown proliferating within the intima; two are in the process of migrating through fenestrae of the internal elastic lamina. Subsequent to or possibly concomitant with intimal smooth muscle proliferation, accumulation of intercellular lipid deposits (*c*) or extracellular lipid (*d*), or both, occur resulting in a fatty streak. A fibrous plaque (*e*) may result from a continued accumulation of a connective tissue cap covering increased numbers of smooth muscle cells laden with lipids, extracellular lipid, and cell debris overlying a deeper extracellular pool of lipid. A complicated lesion may form as a result of continuing cell degeneration, ingress of blood constituents, or calcification superimposed upon the elements present in the fibrous plaque. (From "Atherosclerosis and the arterial smooth muscle cell" by R. Ross and J. A. Glomset, *Science,* Vol. 180, pp. 1332–1339, June 9, 1973. Copyright 1973 by the American Association for the Advancement of Science. Reprinted by permission of publisher and author.)

most common disease of the cardiovascular system. Although coronary heart disease is the leading cause of death in males over 35 years of age and in all persons over 45, death rates from this disease have been decreasing since 1968. In 1975 the mortality rate from coronary heart disease fell by approximately 20 percent overall for persons 36 to 74 years of age and the trend continues to be downward (8,13). Most epidemiologists believe that this downward trend is real, but no concrete explanation can be given for it. There is evidence to suggest, however, that better control of certain risk factors such as hypertension, high levels of serum cholesterol, and cigarette smoking, may be contributing to the decrease in mortalities from atherosclerosis.

Atherosclerosis is a disease of aging, but premature atherosclerosis appears to be related to various risk factors which in addition to those listed above include diabetes mellitus, physical inactivity, obesity (because of its relationship to hypertension), emotional stress, and a positive family history of premature atherosclerosis (8). Of the various risk factors, *hypercholesterolemia* is of greatest significance until about age 45, after which time *hypertension* assumes the greatest importance in development of CHD in both men and women. The exact effect of hypertension on development of CHD is unknown, but a possible cause is pressure damage to the arterial walls, with subsequent deposition of cholesterol plaques (14). An *abnormal glucose tolerance,* characteristic of diabetes mellitus, increases twofold the incidence of myocardial infarction. Although body weight cannot be correlated with CHD, obesity presents a hazard to cardiovascular function and should be avoided as a preventive measure. There is no agreement among investigators concerning the etiologic relationship between *emotional stress* and incidence of CHD, but the general clinical impression is that a relationship does exist. Moreover, recent animal studies demonstrating the effect of electrical stimulation of the lateral hypothalamus in the development of aortic changes suggest that the human central nervous system has a role in the development of atherosclerotic lesions (15). *Genetic influences,* although very important in individual cases, appear to be less crucial than cultural ones in predicting the overall prevalence of CHD.

Control of those risk factors that can be manipulated appears extremely important in the maintenance of a healthy heart because in man there is no convincing evidence that atherosclerotic lesions, once developed, can be made to regress. In recent years, increased physical activity has received much attention as a possible deterrent to the development of heart disease. Although no precise mechanism has been delineated by which increased exercise can decrease the incidence of ischemic heart disease, steady physical activity is highly recommended as an important element of preventive hygiene. If exercise indeed does have a protective effect against development of CHD, this effect may be due to increased serum levels of alpha-lipoproteins (HDLs). Runners have been shown to have increased levels of HDL and levels of HDL have an inverse relationship with incidence of CHD (16–19).

Lipid Metabolism and Possible Interrelationship with Cardiovascular Disease

Because of the prominence of lipids in atheromas and the high correlation existing between hyperlipidemia and occurrence of coronary heart disease, most investigators believe that development of the disease is linked in some way to a disturbance of lipid metabolism. Consideration of the various hyperlipidemias and their relationship to nutrient intake will be made easier by a review of normal lipid metabolism (see Chapter 3).

Lipoproteins are the vehicles by which lipids are carried in the blood. These lipoproteins are characterized either by their density or by their movement in electrophoresis. When classified according to density, the ultracentrifuge has been used to separate sequentially: (1) chylomicrons, (2) very low density lipoproteins (VLDL), (3) intermediate lipoproteins (IL), (4) low density lipoproteins (LDL), and (5) high density lipoproteins (HDL). Electrophoresis allows separation of the lipoproteins by charge into (1) non-migrating particles (chylomicrons), (2) beta-migrating particles (LDL), (3) broad band, beta-migrating particles (IL), (4) pre–beta-migrating particles (VLDL), and (5) alpha-migrating particles (HDL). As indicated by use of parentheses, the nomenclature according to density is exchangeable with that relating to charge. The average lipid and protein composition of the most common plasma lipoproteins is found in Table 7.1.

Chylomicrons, the largest and lightest of the lipoproteins, are produced in the intestinal wall from triglycerides, cholesterol, and lipopro-

Table 7.1 Average Lipid and Protein Composition of Plasma Lipoproteins

Component	Average composition (%)			
	Chylomicrons	VLDL	LDL	HDL
Protein	2	9	21	50
Triglycerides	84	54	11	4
Cholesterol	2	7	8	2
Cholesteryl esters	5	12	37	20
Phospholipids	7	18	22	24

Source: From Montgomery, Rex, Dryer, R. L., Conway, Thomas W., and Spector, Arthur A.: *Biochemistry: A Case Oriented Approach,* 2nd ed. Copyright 1977 by the C. V. Mosby Co., St. Louis, Reprinted by permission of the publisher and authors.

teins provided by diet along with a phospholipid component synthesized by intestinal epithelial cells. The density of chylomicrons is extremely low (D < 0.94) due to their high percentage of triglycerides (approximately 84 percent). Chylomicrons travel via the lymphatics to the blood by which they are transported to adipose tissue and to the liver for removal from circulation. Whereas the degree of removal of chylomicrons from the blood is an indication of the body's handling of exogenous fat, the plasma composition of the other lipoproteins is a reflection of the metabolism of endogenous lipids. The interrelationship among the various lipoproteins is outlined in Figure 7.8 (20).

The VLDLs or pre–beta-migrating particles are also of very low density (D > 0.94–1.006) because of their high content of endogenous triglycerides (approximately 54 percent). The intermediate lipoproteins (D > 1.006–1.019) and low density lipoproteins (D > 1.019–1.063) are more dense because of their decreasing percentage composition of triglycerides. As the triglyceride content drops, there is a concomitant increase in other constituents, with cholesterol esters showing the greatest rise in the low density lipoproteins (37 percent as compared with 12 percent in the very low density lipoproteins).

The increased density of the HDLs or alpha-lipoproteins (D > 1.063–1.21) as compared with that of the LDLs is due to a decreased content of cholesterol and an accompanying rise in protein. Cholesterol drops by about 50 percent while protein more than doubles in amount.

The synthesis of the VLDLs occurs predominantly in the liver but the gastrointestinal tract also produces these lipoproteins. It is by means of the VLDLs that triglycerides are transported out of the liver and carried to other parts of the body, primarily to adipose tissue. Precursors of the fatty acids produced in the liver for synthesis of VLDLs are the circulating energy-producing nutrients, particularly carbohydrate, much of which is absorbed from the gastrointestinal tract. The VLDLs, like the chylomicrons, carry their load of triglycerides to the adipose cells for energy storage.

Fatty acids are removed from the VLDLs and from the chylomicrons by the action of the insulin-dependent lipoprotein lipase, which normally is found in abundant supply in adipose tissue. The mechanism proposed for removal of these lipoproteins from blood is that as the chylomicrons and VLDLs pass through the vessels of adipose tissue, lipoprotein lipase is released from tissues, enters capillaries, and causes rapid lysis of the triglycerides into fatty acids and glycerol. These fatty acids are lipid-soluble and therefore diffuse quickly through the capillary and cell membranes for resynthesis into triglycerides and storage in the adipocytes.

Remnants of degraded chylomicrons and VLDLs are designated as intermediate lipoproteins (IL) (20). These remnants are picked up by the liver and converted into LDLs, smaller and more dense lipoproteins

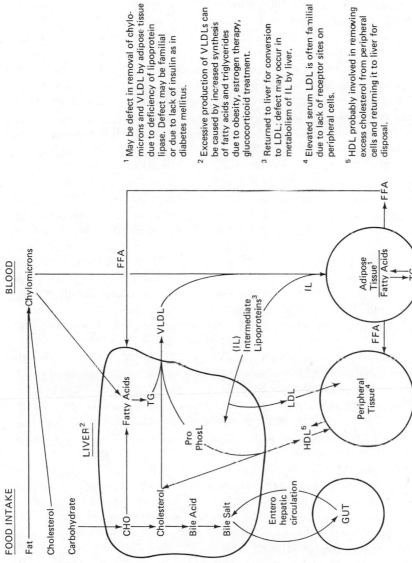

Figure 7.8 Proposed interrelationship among plasma lipiproteins. Possible defects that can cause hyper-lipidemia are identified.

[1] May be defect in removal of chylomicrons and VLDL by adipose tissue due to deficiency of lipoprotein lipase. Defect may be familial or due to lack of insulin as in diabetes mellitus.

[2] Excessive production of VLDLs can be caused by increased synthesis of fatty acids and triglycerides due to obesity, estrogen therapy, glucocorticoid treatment.

[3] Returned to liver for conversion to LDL; defect may occur in metabolism of IL by liver.

[4] Elevated serum LDL is often familial due to lack of receptor sites on peripheral cells.

[5] HDL probably involved in removing excess cholesterol from peripheral cells and returning it to liver for disposal.

characterized by their high cholesterol content. These LDLs are carried to the peripheral tissues where they are metabolized by the cells. Cholesterol in excess of that which can be metabolized by the peripheral cells may be picked up by the HDLs and returned to the liver for disposal. The exact function of these high density lipoproteins is unknown but evidence exists to support the theory of their role as scavengers. It is postulated that the HDLs pick up excess fractions of the various lipoproteins and perhaps remove unesterified cholesterol from peripheral tissues, carrying all of these back to the liver. Cholesterol returned thereby to the liver could be converted into bile salts, part of which could be excreted from the body (21).

The relationship among the various lipoproteins allows the recognition of how the different hyperlipidemias may occur. Hypertriglyceridemia can result from an overproduction of VLDLs in the liver and/or improper degradation of the VLDLs by adipose tissue; hypercholesterolemia can occur when peripheral tissues are unable to utilize the LDLs properly. Accumulation of ILs occurs when more remnants of chylomicrons and/or VLDLs are produced than can be catabolized by the liver at its normal rapid rate.

The body's handling of the LDLs appears to be dependent upon the ability of the fibroblasts to regulate on their surface the number of LDL receptor sites (22). An appropriate supply of LDL receptors allows the cell to bind the LDL at its surface and to ingest the lipoprotein by endocytosis. The lipoprotein is then hydrolyzed by action of the lysosomes and the resulting free cholesterol can be used by the cell in membrane synthesis. Accumulation of free cholesterol in the cell activates the various cellular mechanisms for cholesterol regulation, thereby preventing an overproduction of intracellular cholesterol. Cells lacking sufficient LDL receptors are unable to utilize circulating cholesterol and continue to produce the sterol regardless of the level of plasma cholesterol.

Although the exact role of the HDLs in fat metabolism is unclear, a high concentration of these lipoproteins in the plasma appears to exert protection against cardiovascular disease (18) (Chapter 3, p. 86). Of particular interest is the fact that familial alpha-lipoproteinemia can occur and as a consequence favors longevity. On the other hand, the various risk factors for CHD, for example, hypercholesterolemia, hypertriglyceridemia, obesity, and diabetes mellitus, are accompanied by reduced levels of alpha-lipoproteins, or HDLs (21).

The various hyperlipidemias—elevated chylomicrons, cholesterol, and/or triglycerides are diagnosed through laboratory analysis of plasma or serum samples. When an elevated plasma lipid (or lipids) cannot be explained in relation to some other extant disease state, the hyperlipidemia is usually classified in terms of an abnormal lipoprotein pattern. Six such patterns presently exist: Type I, characterized by elevated chylomicrons and indicative of the body's inability to clear dietary fat; Type IIa, often a familial disease, and characterized by elevated LDLs with cholesterol levels usually in the range of 300 to 600 mg per deciliter plasma; Type IIb in which both LDLs and VLDLs are elevated; Type III, an uncommon pattern characterized by an accumulation of the intermediate lipoproteins (often referred to as an abnormal form of LDL); Type IV, characterized by elevated VLDLs; and Type V in which a mixed hyperlipidemia is found.

Treatment of Hyperlipoproteinemia

Extensive information on dietary management of the various hyperlipoproteinemias is available in the DHEW Publication No. (NIH) 76–110 (23), a reference that all dietitians or dietetics students should have readily available. Also available from DHEW for use with patients are individual booklets, each dealing with the dietary treatment of one type of hyperlipoproteinemia. A summary of these diets is found in Table 7.2. As a word of caution however, the reader should note that as more is learned about the pathophysiology of the hyperlipidemias, the present nomenclature and treatment may be extensively revised (20).

Present dietary treatment of the various hyperlipoproteinemias is dictated by the source of the offending lipid. Excessive chylomicrons can be prevented by reduction of total fat intake, but reduction in endogenously produced lipoproteins requires different treatment. In most instances, elevated VLDLs (140 mg triglycerides/dl is the upper limit of normal) can be brought back to normal by attainment of ideal body weight, a process requiring reduced caloric intake. Occasionally special attention may have to be given also to the level of carbohydrate intake because of its rapid conversion to acetate. Usually, however, a sufficiently reduced energy consumption automatically will restrict effectively the ingestion of carbohydrate (24).

Reduction of elevated cholesterol (220 mg/dl is upper limit of normal) is a more difficult task. Severely abnormal levels of cholesterol appear to be heredity-related and seem to result from inability of peripheral cells to degrade the LDLs properly and regulate cholesterol synthesis because they have too few or defective LDL receptors (13). Familial hypercholesterolemia is inherited by an autosomal dominant mode (see Chapter 9) and the heterozygote frequency is estimated at one in every 200 to 500 persons (25,26). The frequency of homozygotes is more rare but the severity of the disease is much greater. Heterozygotes, although born with hypercholesterolemia, seldom develop other symptoms during the first decade of life and clinical symptoms of heart disease appear in the fourth decade (27). On the other hand, homozygotes, born with severe hypercholesterolemia and often with xanthomas, may die of myocardial infarc-

Table 7.2 Summary of Diets for Types I–V Hyperlipoproteinemia

	Type I	Type IIa
Diet prescription	Low fat 25–35 gm	Low cholesterol Polyunsaturated fat increased
Calories	Not restricted	Not restricted
Protein	Total protein intake is not limited	Total protein intake is not limited
Fat	Restricted to 25–35 gm Kind of fat not important	Saturated fat intake limited Polyunsaturated fat intake increased
Cholesterol	Not restricted	As low as possible; the only source of cholesterol is the meat in the diet
Carbohydrate	Not limited	Not limited
Alcohol	Not recommended	May be used with discretion

Source: From DHEW Publication No. (NIH) 76-110, U.S. Department of Health, Education and Welfare, Public Health Service, National Institute of Health.

tion before 30 years of age. Early diagnosis of this genetic disease is crucial; therefore, determination of serum cholesterol levels in suspect individuals is made early in infancy. An even more indisputable diagnosis than elevated serum cholesterol is measurement of low density lipoprotein receptor function in cultured skin fibroblasts (28).

Recommended therapy for familial hypercholesterolemia may include not only diet but also drugs, surgery, and/or plasma exchange (28).

Table 7.2 Continued

Type IIb & Type III	Type IV	Type V
Low cholesterol Approximately: 20% cal. pro. 40% cal. fat 40% cal. CHO	Controlled CHO Approximately 45% of calories Moderately restricted cholesterol	Restricted fat 30% of calories Controlled CHO 50% of calories Moderately restricted cholesterol
Achieve and maintain "ideal" weight, i.e., reduction diet if necessary	Achieve and maintain "ideal" weight, i.e., reduction diet if necessary	Achieve and maintain "ideal" weight, i.e., reduction diet if necessary
High protein	Not limited other than control of patient's weight	High protein
Controlled to 40% calories (polyunsaturated fats recommended in preference to saturated fats)	Not limited other than control of patient's weight (polyunsaturated fats recommended in preference to saturated fats)	Restricted to 30% of calories (polyunsaturated fats recommended in preference to saturated fats)
Less than 300 mg—the only source of cholesterol is the meat in the diet	Moderately restricted to 300–500 mg	Moderately restricted to 300–500 mg
Controlled—concentrated sweets are restricted	Controlled—concentrated sweets are restricted	Controlled—concentrated sweets are restricted
Limited to 2 servings (substituted for carbohydrate)	Limited to 2 servings (substituted for carbohydrate)	Not recommended

Dietary modifications consist of decreased fat intake to provide no more than 30 percent of energy, decreased saturated fat (<5 percent of total energy intake), and increased use of polyunsaturated fats (8 to 15 percent of total energy intake). Dietary cholesterol should be decreased to less than 250 mg/day in adults and less than 100 mg/day in children (28–30).

Reducing total fat and cholesterol intake as well as increasing the ratio of polyunsaturated to saturated fats (P/S ratio) is only partially successful in decreasing serum cholesterol in persons with familial hypercholesterolemia. Dietary modifications may lead to only a 10 to 15 percent decrease in plasma cholesterol levels (28) (see Chapter 3, p. 92). Consequently, more stringent methods, that is, drugs, surgery, and/or plasma exchange often must be employed to lower circulating cholesterol to acceptable levels.

One investigator (31) suggests that the recommended treatment for hypercholesterolemia should be based upon the level of serum cholesterol because the severity of elevation usually is indicative of its cause. Mild hypercholesterolemia (225 to 275 mg/dl) is often related to overindulgence and is responsive to dietary modification; moderate hypercholesterolemia (275 to 350 mg/dl) may be responsive to dietary modification but often requires drug therapy as well because the disorder is frequently heredity-related; severe hypercholesterolemia (>350 mg/dl) is most often heredity-related and requires drug therapy although treatment should also include dietary modification.

Many patients with elevated plasma lipid levels may not experience any definite physiological effects from this condition; therefore, it may be difficult to convince these patients that drug as well as diet therapy may be necessary to curtail or delay atherogenesis. All of the antihyperlipidemia agents produce some side effects and patients may fail to take their medication if such drugs make them feel less well instead of better.

Several categories of antihyperlipidemic agents are presently available. Their scope of action may be to reduce cholesterol levels, decrease triglyceride levels, or a combination of the two.

Clofibrate (Atromid-S®), one of the most widely used agents in this category, reduces plasma triglyceride concentration by lowering the levels of VLDL and, in most patients, plasma cholesterol and LDL also decrease. However, a large decrease in plasma VLDL may be accompanied by an increase in plasma LDL so that there may be little net change in plasma cholesterol levels. One recent clinical study indicated that in men treated with clofibrate (1.8 gm/day) on a continuing basis the plasma cholesterol concentration was decreased by only 6 percent while the reduction in plasma triglyceride was 22 percent (32). The mechanism of action of clofibrate is not well understood. It inhibits cholesterol synthesis and increases the excretion of neutral sterols. The effect on VLDL appears to be an enhancement of the rate of removal from the circulation (33). The clinical efficacy of clofibrate in decreasing or preventing cardiac mortality remains unproven at this time. The 1975 Coronary Drug Project, carried out over a period of five years with clofibrate therapy, showed increased incidence of thromboembolism, angina pectoris, and cardiac arrhythmia, and a two-fold increase in the incidence of gallstones without salutary effect on the preexisting coronary heart disease or reduction of total or coronary mortality (34).

Probucol (Lorelco®) lowers plasma cholesterol levels by an unknown mechanism. It is indicated as adjunctive therapy to diet for the reduction of elevated serum cholesterol in patients with elevated LDL. It is not indicated for patients with primary hypertriglyceridemia. The most commonly noted side effects associated with the use of probucol are diarrhea, flatulence, abdominal pain, nausea, and vomiting. Absorption from the gastrointestinal tract is most consistent when the drug is administered with food (35).

Bile acid-sequestering resins are a relatively new category of antihyperlipidemia agents and include cholestyramine (Questran®) and colestipol (Colestid®). They produce their cholesterol-lowering effect by combining with bile acids in the intestine to form insoluble complexes that are excreted in the feces. The result is a partial removal of bile acids from the enterohepatic circulation by preventing their reabsorption from the gastrointestinal tract. Because bile salts are required for the absorption of fat and lipids from the gastrointestinal tract, their removal results in a decreased absorption of these materials. The increased loss of bile acids leads to an increased conversion of cholesterol to bile acids (Chapter 3, p. 92) and thus a decrease in plasma LDL and cholesterol. Serum triglyceride levels are not affected by these agents.

Bile acid-sequestering agents are anion exchange resins and they may interfere with the absorption of concomitantly administered drugs or nutrients. They decrease the absorption of vitamins A, D, and K and supplemental amounts of these agents may be required by the patient. The most common side effect noted with these agents is constipation, which is usually transient. Other side effects may include abdominal pain, flatulence, nausea, vomiting, diarrhea, heartburn, anorexia, indigestion, and steatorrhea.

Sitosterols are antihyperlipidemia agents that lower elevated plasma cholesterol levels by interfering with the intestinal absorption of cholesterol. The mechanism for this action is unknown. Sitosterols (Cytellin®) are used as adjuncts to diet control and have variable effects on lowering cholesterol levels. The only primary side effect noted is a mild laxative effect.

Both nicotinic acid (niacin) and dextrothyroxine (Choloxin®) are also used in the reduction of elevated plasma lipid levels. Nicotinic acid, in large doses, reduces serum lipids by an unknown mechanism. The most frequently noted side effects include flushing, pruritus, and gastrointestinal distress. Dextrothyroxine reduces LDL and cholesterol and may also reduce elevated triglycerides. Its mechanism of action appears to be stimulation of hepatic catabolism and excretion of cholesterol. The use of dextrothyroxine in patients with known organic heart disease, hypertension, or advanced liver or kidney disease is contraindicated (35). Side effects associated with the use of dextrothyroxine include insomnia, anxiety, palpitations, weight loss, sweating, flushing, and other symptoms related to an increase in metabolism.

In considering these agents, it should be noted that "it has not been established whether the drug-induced lowering of serum cholesterol or lipid levels has a detrimental, beneficial or no effect on the morbidity or mortality due to atherosclerosis or coronary heart disease. Several years will be required before current investigations will yield an answer to this question" (35).

Whether reducing by whatever means a serum cholesterol that has been maintained at elevated levels for a period of years is of benefit in preventing heart disease is still questionable. Because of this doubt, much emphasis is being placed on the so-called "prudent diet", the purpose of which is to prevent occurrence of the dietary-related hyperlipidemias and to reduce the severity of those that are genetic in origin. The prudent diet had its origin in 1957 when the late Norman Jolliffe, M.D., of the Bureau of Nutrition, New York City, undertook the study of the effect of dietary manipulation in the incidence of coronary events among groups of men at risk. The results of this study begun by Dr. Jolliffe and continued by George Christakis, M. D., along with evidence from numerous epidemiologic studies, led the American Heart Association in 1973 to recommend this type of dietary modification for the entire American population. These studies also provided much of the impetus for the Dietary Goals for the United States proposed in 1977 (modified in 1978) by the Senate Select Committee on Nutrition and Human Needs. The main principles of the prudent diet include:

1. Reduction of dietary cholesterol to less than 300 mg per day.
2. Reduction of total dietary fat to approximately 30 to 35 percent of caloric intake with a P/S ratio of one or above.
3. Close attention to total caloric intake so that ideal body weight may be achieved and maintained.
4. Increased ingestion of complex carbohydrates, which would raise the level of total carbohydrate in the diet but would decrease sugar consumption.

Because doubts still persist concerning the relationship among diet, the hyperlipidemias, and atherosclerosis, support for such changes in the American diet is far from unanimous among health professionals (36–38) and particularly among pediatricians who are fearful that such dietary modifications may prove detrimental to the infant and rapidly growing child. Other pediatricians, however, feel that a change in life-style including diet should be instituted at birth and have presented experimental evidence of no detectable changes in growth and development among children maintained from birth through eight years of age on a low saturated fat, low cholesterol diet (39). The sum of evidence at present indicates little potential hazard from fat-modified, low cholesterol diets when fed to children after the first year of life. One possible problem in adulthood may be an increased incidence of gall bladder disease among those persons who begin consumption of a fat-modified diet in early childhood because gall stones have been reported to occur more commonly in persons whose diets have been characteristically rich in polyunsaturates and in plant sterols (40).

Other dietary factors that have been implicated theoretically or by limited experimental evidence as possible culprits in the development of heart disease are: (1) low dietary fiber, (2) excessive sucrose, (3) high zinc to copper ratios, (4) excessive ascorbic acid, (5) ingestion of xanthine oxidase, (6) intake of *trans*-fatty acids, and (7) consumption of protein from animal sources (41). All aspects of diet in relation to plasma lipids are reviewed by Truswell (19).

Myocardial Infarction

Regardless of the etiology of atherosclerosis the most common manifestations of advanced disease are angina and acute myocardial infarction. As mentioned earlier in the chapter, atherosclerosis is characterized by development of fibrous plaques which impede arterial blood flow. These atherosclerotic plaques often break through the intima of blood vessels and cause the surface of the vessels to become rough. This roughness can initiate the clotting process which in turn can cause entrapment of platelets and a continuation of clot formation. Narrowing of the coronary blood vessels will cause ischemia and pain (angina), possibly due to release by muscle fibers of pain-promoting products such as kinins or histamine which cannot be removed with sufficient rapidity by the impeded blood flow.

Myocardial infarction is a result of total ischemia and causes death of the affected muscle fibers. Death of muscle fibers begins within approximately one hour following insorption and is complete in about four or five hours. When arteries other than coronary arteries are occluded by blood clots, clinical manifestations are dictated by the location of the affected arteries. For example, arterial occlusion occurring in the neck and circle of Willis in the brain results in stroke; in the leg, claudication and/or gangrene is the outcome; in renal arteries, hypertension and poor renal function may be produced (7).

Following occlusion of the coronary arteries (or myocardial infarction), death can result from four major factors: (1) decreased cardiac output, (2) venous damming of blood resulting in severe edema, (3) fibrillation of the heart, and, occasionally, (4) rupture of the heart (14). Total rest is prescribed for the patient with myocardial infarct in order to protect the mildly ischemic areas that surround the dead muscle tissue. At rest collateral circulation can nourish the mildly ischemic area but with exercising, blood flow is diverted to the normally functioning muscle fibers, and the mildly ischemic area may die from lack of oxygen.

Diagnosis of Myocardial Infarction. In addition to electrocardiography, routine laboratory tests are available for the diagnosis of a recent myocardial infarction. As a result of the cellular damage within the ischemic tissue, cell-based enzymes are released into the general circulation, thereby elevating the serum level of these enzymes. The tests, which are designated to measure the activity of the enzymes and isoenzymes in the serum, for example, creatine kinase, lactate dehydrogenase, glyceraldehyde-3-PO_4 dehydrogenase, glutamic-oxaloacetic transaminase, are of diagnostic value if carried out during the time span of a few hours to more than two weeks following the episode. Such tests are described in Chapter 14.

Treatment Following Myocardial Infarction. Appropriate drug therapy (42) and nutritional management (43) following a myocardial infarct are as follows:

1. Nothing by mouth prior to evaluation by physician. The usual treatment during the first 24 hours is administration of intravenous solutions, which allow administration of drugs needed in case of shock or arrhythmia.

   Drugs used in the treatment of myocardial infarction patients are employed to increase the force of cardiac contractions in order to maintain blood pressure and renal function. Adrenergic agents such as norepinephrine and isoproterenol have been used in the past for this purpose but their use has been sharply curtailed because they increase heart rate as well as the force of cardiac contraction and thus increase tissue oxygen demand and consumption. This increased oxygen consumption may lead to further damage to the tissue around the infarct because oxygen supply to the area is already decreased. At the present time, two newer agents, dopamine (Intropin®) and dobutamine (Dobutrex®), are becoming the preferred agents for this situation because they selectively increase the force of cardiac contraction without significantly increasing heart rate. Dopamine increases cardiac tissue contractibility and dilatation of renal arteries, to maintain urine output. This effect occurs at low doses which do not produce peripheral vasoconstriction. Dobutamine increases cardiac tissue contractibility without dilatation of renal arteries, but renal function is maintained due to the increased perfusion of the kidney caused by improved blood circulation.

   Arrhythmias associated with myocardial infarction may be treated with antiarrhythmic agents such as propranolol (Inderal®) which decreases heart rate by blocking the adrenergic receptors in the heart when the heart rate is rapid and irregular. If the heart is beating too slowly, due to excessive cholinergic stimulation, atropine, an anticholinergic agent, may be employed to increase heart rate.

Other agents that may be used during this emergency therapy include vasodilators such as nitroprusside (Nipride®), trimethaphan (Arfonad®) and nitroglycerin to increase coronary blood flow; anticoagulants, such as heparin; and diuretics such as furosemide (Lasix®), which appear to act by dilatation of vascular beds rather than by producing diuresis.

2. Any nourishment given during the first 24 hours should be a liquid diet supplying approximately 500 to 800 kilocalories and given in only small quantities at any one time in order to minimize stress on the heart. Volume of liquids usually ranges from 1000 to 1500 ml and can include clear soups and broth (usually salt free), skim milk, fruit juices, tea, ginger ale, and water. At the end of the 24 hours, the patient is re-evaluated for dietetic progression.

3. When progression is appropriate, the caloric level of feeding is increased to about 1000 to 1200 kilocalories with approximately 20 percent of the calories coming from protein, 45 percent from carbohydrate, and 30 to 35 percent from fat. Polyunsaturates are the primary source of dietary fat and cholesterol is limited to 300 mg or less per day. Moderate sodium restriction is advisable and potassium content of the diet may need attention depending upon specific drug therapy and clinical status of the patient.

4. Beverages and liquids are served at body temperature and if coffee is served, only the decaffeinated product is allowed. Careful attention must be given to the patient's tolerance of milk, his/her intake volume of fruit juice and/or carbonated beverages in order to prevent abdominal distention and displacement of the diaphragm toward the heart.

5. Meals are small and frequent including only those foods that are easily digested, free of gastric irritants, soft and low in roughage in order to prevent gastrointestinal irritation, distention, or accumulation of excessive residue which must be excreted. Egg yolks are limited to three per week, with cholesterol-free egg substitutes being used as replacements for eggs in general.

6. After five to ten days, the patient's nutrition plan is individualized on the basis of his/her clinical status, and physiologic and psychologic needs. Modifications may be required for several of the following dietary components: carbohydrate, protein, fat, total calories, electrolytes, and/or fluids. Common modifications include (1) adjustment of caloric intake to maintain or achieve optimal weight, (2) restriction of sodium intake, and (3) continuation of a fat-controlled diet.

The dietitian should use the meals served the patient during his/her hospital stay as tools for educating the patient and his/her family concerning the principles of the patient's individualized diet. Once the patient becomes familiar with the diet, continuity of the diet should be maintained as he/she moves from the acute-care facility into the community or from the community back into the hospital. Such continuity is important in promoting an increased sense of security in the cardiac patient. Dietitians must be aware of the importance of diet continuity to the patient's sense of security and attempt to maintain this continuity even when patients are admitted to the hospital for coronary surgery. Obtaining a dietary history from all new admissions, including surgical admissions, as soon as possible or feasible cannot be overemphasized if optimal care of the total patient is to be achieved (44).

Congestive Heart Failure

Heart failure is a disorder of the cardiovascular system in which the heart is no longer able to pump the five liters of blood per minute required for normal kidney function (14). This disease state is often referred to as congestive heart failure because its clinical manifestations are related to fluid accumulation resulting from an inadequate renal blood flow. When the heart is so weakened that it cannot pump an adequate cardiac output, renal blood flow and blood pressure are decreased, thereby causing a release of renin. Renin release is an important mechanism by which blood pressure can be raised. Renin reacts with angiotensinogen to form angiotensin I and II, the latter of which stimulates increased adrenal secretion of aldosterone (see Fig. 7.6). The result of increased aldosterone production is an enhanced absorption of sodium from the renal tubules. Consequently, water absorption is increased and a vicious cycle is begun (7).

The failure of the heart as an effective pump most often occurs in the left ventricle as a result of myocardial infarction. When one side of the heart becomes weakened, be it right or left, the resulting sequence of events causes the other side of the heart to fail also.

Pulmonary edema is frequently a consequence of myocardial infarction of the left ventricle because the weakened muscle is unable to propel sufficient blood out of this chamber. This creates a "back pressure" as venous blood continues to flow into the heart but cannot be pumped out properly. The failing ventricle first increases back pressure in the left atrium, then in the pulmonary vessels, and finally in the right side of the heart. The right ventricle stretched by accumulation of excessive blood in the chamber increases its force of contraction, thus forcing more blood into the pulmonary artery. This increased hydrostatic pressure causes loss of fluid into the interstitial space around the alveolar sacs. The pressure of fluid in the lungs causes the clinical symptoms of dyspnea and orthopnea associated with heart failure because the diffusion of carbon dioxide and oxygen across the respiratory membrane is impaired.

With the failure of the right side of the heart there is a generalized fluid accumulation throughout the body particularly in the lower periphery. Above-normal blood volume caused by excessive secretion of aldosterone with subsequent increased absorption of sodium and water and an elevated venous pressure resulting from inadequate cardiac output cause fluid to leak out of capillary beds into all the tissue spaces. Fluid collects throughout the body; weight gain and peripheral congestion occur.

Drug and Diet Therapy in Congestive Heart Failure. Because the primary symptoms of congestive heart failure include edema due to increased volume of the circulatory fluids and decreased ability of the heart to circulate blood due to weakening of the cardiac muscle, *drug therapy* for this condition most often includes diuretics and cardiotonic agents. The diuretic agents are used to increase the excretion of fluids while the cardiotonic agents increase the integrity of cardiac tissue. The primary cardiotonic agents utilized are the digitalis glycosides. Several different preparations of these glycosides are available and are listed in Table 7.3. The digitalis glycosides are naturally occurring products found in various species of the foxglove plant (*Digitalis purpurea* and *Digitalis lanata*) and *Strophantus gratus*. They produce two effects on the heart: (1) increased contractility of the myocardium (positive inotropic effect), and (2) altered electrophysiological properties of the heart to restore normal rate and rhythm (positive chronotropic effect).

The positive inotropic effect of the digitalis glycosides on the heart is the primary action that makes these drugs beneficial in the treatment of congestive heart failure. The positive chronotropic effect of the glycosides also makes them useful in the treatment of cardiac arrhythmias. Improvement of the pumping ability of the heart allows the ventricles to empty themselves more completely, thereby improving circulation in both the pulmonary and systemic circulations. This improved circulation

Table 7.3   Digitalis Glycosides

Generic name	Trade name	Route of administration
Acetyldigitoxin	Acylanid®	oral
Deslanoside	Cedilanid®-D	IV
Digitalis, Powdered	Digifortis®, Digitura®, Pil-Digis®	oral
Digitalis, Tincture		oral
Digitoxin	Crystodigin® and others	oral, IV
Digoxin	Lanoxin®, Davoxin®	oral, IV
Gitalin	Gitaligin®	oral
Lanatoside C	Cedilanid®	oral, IV
Lanatoside A, B & C	Digilanid®	oral, IV
G-Strophanthin	Ouabain®	IV

results in a decrease of edema and an enhanced elimination of fluids via the kidney. The strengthening of cardiac contractions and elimination of excessive body fluids produce a dramatic improvement in the patient within a relatively short period of time.

The mechanism by which the cardiotonic agents produce their therapeutic effects is dependent on the ability of these agents to alter electrical conduction through cardiac tissue. The heart of the patient with congestive heart failure beats more rapidly than the normal heart in an attempt to "compensate" for its decreased ability to pump blood and in an effort to maintain cardiac output. The digitalis glycosides decrease heart rate by slowing conduction through myocardial tissue and by strengthening the force of contractions. As a result, the heart expends less energy and utilizes less oxygen.

Most of the side effects of the digitalis glycosides are related to their therapeutic effects on cardiac tissue. Toxic doses of these agents will result in an excessive decrease in heart rate and may even cause cessation of cardiac contractions. An excessive lowering of the heart rate may result in symtoms such as faintness, dizziness, weakness, and chest pains due to a decrease in blood flow to the brain and cardiac tissue. Gastrointestinal complaints such as nausea and vomiting, and ocular effects such as blurred vision or flashing colored lights are indicative of impending toxicity.

Control of the heart failure state includes decreasing the work load of the heart, strengthening myocardial contractibility and reducing fluid retention by the body (45). Although strengthening of the heart muscle must be accomplished through drug therapy, the achievement of a decreased work load for the heart and a reduction in fluid retention is extensively influenced by the appropriate nutritional management of the patient in heart failure.

The principles of the *diet,* which are aimed primarily at decreasing work load of the heart, are as follows:

1. Calories are restricted in order to reduce excessive weight (if such exists), thereby reducing bodily oxygen consumption and the work of the heart in circulating oxygen to metabolizing tissues.
2. Foods included in the diet should be nongas-forming, as nutritionally adequate as possible, and given in small feedings in order to prevent stomach distention. When the stomach is distended, the diaphragm is elevated and can push the heart upward. For patients with a severely weakened heart, the Karrell Diet which was prescribed as early as 1866 is still being ordered by some physicians in order to reduce work load of the heart. This diet consists of only 800 to 1000 ml of milk per 24 hours. Although not completely adequate nutritionally, the Karrell Diet represents a calorically restricted diet that is given in small feed-

ings. Because of its consistency this diet prevents any distention of the stomach but, of course, such a diet would be totally inappropriate for the patient with a lactase deficiency. Here again can be seen the necessity of obtaining a good diet history from the patient (or from the patient's family) as soon as possible after his/her admission.

3. Adequate protein (0.8 gm/kg/day) should be included in the diet but the amount should not be excessive because of the increased oxygen supply required for digestion of high protein meals.

Restricting the sodium content of the diet is the main dietary modification aimed at the reduction of fluid retention. A sodium-restricted diet is usually employed to augment diuretic therapy, but in some instances only the elimination of salt from the diet (for example in the early stages of heart failure) can be effective in reducing fluid retention. When the amount of sodium available to the body is considerably reduced, the extracellular fluid decreases in osmolarity and the osmoreceptor system in the hypothalamus is inhibited. As a result the secretion of antidiuretic hormone (ADH) decreases and extra quantities of water can be excreted as urine. Only in severe cases of decompensation is reduction of fluid intake necessary. Limiting fluid intake becomes necessary in those instances in which sodium restriction does not relieve edema.

The level of sodium restriction required for the patient with heart failure will depend upon the severity of his/her disease. If control of fluid retention in a patient with advanced disease is being accomplished solely by sodium restriction, the level of sodium intake may be quite low, that is, 250 to 500 mg per day. Diets restricted this severely in sodium content are rarely acceptable to patients and because keeping fluid retention under control is a long-term process, many physicians elect to treat heart failure with diuretic therapy accompanied by a diet containing approximately two grams sodium daily. A diet containing this amount of sodium can be palatable, relatively easy to obtain or prepare, and is much more likely to be adhered to by the patient.

Although the American Heart Association has available pamphlets that delineate the daily dietary patterns for the various sodium-restricted regimens (250 mg to mild restriction) (46), the dietitian often finds that patients are a bit overwhelmed by all the information found in these pamphlets. The publications are excellent reference materials and should be used as such by both patients and dietitians. The dietitian, however, has the responsibility of simplifying for the patient any necessary dietary modifications, including identification of foods that can be eaten generously and those that are suspect or must be eliminated. Because the sodium-restricted diet probably must become a way of life for the patient, the dietitian has a further responsibility of helping the patient see how flavorful such a diet can be if imagination is used in food preparation. For some patients whose cultural food patterns include many foods extremely high in sodium, change will be traumatic. To be good teachers, (or agents of change) dietitians must be enthusiastic about their subject matter, must possess sound knowledge concerning the general sodium content of foods, must have available various teaching tools, for example, the sodium content of specific foods, the list of spices allowable on a sodium-restricted diet, a listing of beverages and their approximate sodium content, information about where specialty products low in sodium can be obtained, and must be able to explain clearly to patients the general principles of a sodium-restricted diet:

1. Limit animal food sources because these are all high in sodium. Allowances usually include one pint milk daily (250 mg),* one egg (61 mg),* and 5 to 6 oz meat (approximately 135 mg).*
2. Prepare meat and vegetables without salt. Because canned vegetables are usually salted and frozen ones often contain salt also, read labels carefully, selecting only those foods without added salt.
3. Use fruits generously because of their low sodium content. Restriction would occur only when caloric reduction is necessary. Most fresh vegetables can be used generously also. Only those vegetables with a high natural content of sodium, namely, celery, carrots, spinach, beets and beet greens, swiss chard, kale, mustard greens, dandelion greens, artichoke, should be used sparingly.
4. Add no salt to foods at the table and avoid all foods that are obviously salted, for example, cured and processed meats, nuts, corn chips, canned soups, beef and chicken consomme cubes, sauerkraut, and so on.
5. Use allowed spices as needed in order to enhance the flavor of food, but make continuous attempts to learn the enjoyment of the food flavor itself. Helping the patient make the adjustment to the flavor of food without salt is the responsibility of the dietitian. During this adjustment period, salt substitutes may make foods more acceptable to the patient, but these substitutes should be used sparingly and only in accordance with the physician's orders. In most of these substitutes potassium has replaced sodium and if the kidneys are diseased, potassium intake is contraindicated.
6. Certain further modifications are necessary as sodium restriction becomes more severe. When sodium intake is reduced to 1 gm daily, sweet butter must be substituted for regular butter or margarine. With a 500 mg sodium diet, all bread must be salt free and when only 250 mg sodium is allowed, low sodium milk must be substituted for regular milk.

Careful reading of *all* labels must be stressed for those patients whose

---

* Sodium content of foods.

Table 7.4 Drugs Containing Greater than 50 mg Sodium per Unit Dose

Sodium (mg)	Name and unit dose
	Antihistamines
59	Corilin Infant Liquid, 5 ml
51	Phenergan Expectorant, 5 ml
	Antiinfectives
62	Amcill-S, 1 gm. inj.
81	Chloramphenicol, 1 gm inj.
52	Chloromycetin Sodium Succinate, 1 gm vial
400	Citrasulfas Improved Liquid, 30 ml
71	Compocillin Oral Sol., 400,000 units/5 ml
67	Dynapen, 63 mg/5 ml
70	Erythrocin Filmtab, 250 mg
136	Geopen, 1 gm
62	Keflin, 1 gm
65	Kesso-Pen Syrup, 400,000 u/5 ml
60	Kesso-Pen VK 250 mg/5 ml
55	Methacillin Sodium pwd, 1 gm
70	Mycifradin Oral Sol., 125 mg/5 ml
62	Omnipen-N, 1 gm
600	Pasna Pack granules, 6 gm packet
50	Pasna, 500 mg tab.
490	Pasna Tri-Pack 300 granules, 5.5 gm packet
66	Penbritin-S, 1 gm
233	Penicillin G Sodium, 5,000,000 units
68	Polycillin, 1 gm
70	Principen N, 1 gm
215	Sodium Sulfadiazine, 250 mg/ml, 10 ml amp.
61	Staphcillin, 4 gm vial
73	Unipen inj., 1 gm
	Analgesics and antipyretics
521	Alka-Seltzer, tab.
72	Alysine Elixir, 5 ml
673	Fizrin, packet
86	Pabalate, tab.
97	Sodium Salicylate, 10 gr enseal
	Antacids
1540	Bisodol Powder, 10 gm
717	Bromo Seltzer, 80 gr
543	Calcium Carbonate and Soda, tab.
738	Eno Salts, tsp.
53	Rolaids, tab.
1000	Sal Hepatica, rounded tsp.
	Antidiarrheals
75	Diaquel, 5 ml
75	Pektamalt liquid, 30 ml

Continued

Table 7.4   Continued

Sodium (mg)	Name and unit dose
	Cathartics
56	Casyllium, 1 oz.
5000	Fleet Enema, 4.5 oz.
250	Metamucil Instant Mix, Packet
55	Phospho-Soda, 5 ml
68	Saraka Granules, 1 oz.
157	Siblin, 1 oz.
185	Travad liquid, 5 ml
	Expectorants and cough preparations
62	Coldene Adult Syrup, 5 ml
59	Dristan Cough Formula, 5 ml
280	Mucomist 1%, 10 ml
282	Mucomist 20%, 30 ml vial
51	Phenergan Expectorant, plain, 5 ml
51	Phenergan V.C. Expectorant, 5 ml
156	Sodium Iodide inj., 1 gm/10 ml
54	Vicks Cough Syrup, 5 ml
68	Vicks Formula 44 Syrup, 5 ml
	Hormones
55	Cortef inj., 500 mg/5 ml
52	Enovid, 10 mg tab.
54	Formatrix, tab.
56	Nilevar, 10 mg tab.
322	Ovulen-28
	Sedative-Hypnotics
717	Bromo-Seltzer, 80 gr
53	Brevital Sodium, 500 mg inj.
65	Nervine, capsule
89	Nervine, liquid, 5 ml
544	Nervine Effervescent, tab.
434	Pentothal Sodium, 5 gm vial
53	Surital, 500 mg amp.
	Spasmolytics
85	Mudrane, tab.
85	Mudrane-GG, tab.

sodium intake is being restricted because many drugs, dentrifices, beverages, and so on, may contain significant amounts of sodium. Table 7.4 lists those medications that contain 50 mg or more sodium per dosage.

Although the appetite for salt is acquired, the average American is consuming at least twice as much sodium as is needed for normal physiological functions. Approximately two to two and one-half grams sodium per day is considered a desirable intake for healthy persons living in a temperate climate and maintaining a moderate level of activity (7). Educating the general population concerning the advisability of reducing sodium intake and the means by which this reduction may be accomplished with little sacrifice in food palatability should become a responsibility of dietitians.

An unusually good resource for dietitians and for patients on sodium-restricted diets is the booklet entitled *Sodium Controlled Diet,* which is distributed upon request by North Dakota State Wheat Commission, 1350 East Central Avenue, Bismarck, ND 58505.

CASE STUDY: MYOCARDIAL INFARCTION

A 49-year-old white male, 5 feet, 10 inches tall and weighing 205 pounds was first seen in the hospital emergency room complaining of a "crushing" type of chest pain. He reported that the pain had a sudden onset and had persisted intermittently for about six hours, up until the time of admission. A medical history showed a routine examination, performed five years previously, had resulted in the diagnosis of a type IIa hyperlipoproteinemia. At the time of that examination, the patient's serum cholesterol was found to be 380 mg/dl and he was placed on a fat-controlled diet (low cholesterol, increased polyunsaturated fat).

Physical examination at hospital admission revealed an anxious, middle-aged male in obvious distress. He was sweating profusely and had difficulty breathing. His temperature was 99°F and his blood pressure, 200/105 mm Hg. The attending physician ordered an immediate electrocardiogram (EKG), and a blood sample was drawn for an analysis of serum enzymes and other pertinent chemical tests. The EKG tracing was abnormal, and the patient was immediately transferred to the coronary care unit. The significant laboratory findings were as follows:

Cholesterol 370 mg/dl (normal, 140–240 mg/dl)

Potassium 5.9 mEq/l (normal, 3.5–5.3 mEq/l)

Creatine kinase (CK) 215 units/l (normal, 12–65 units/l)

Glutamic-oxaloacetic transaminase (GOT) 52 units/l (normal, 7–21 units/l)

Lactate dehydrogenase (LDH) 90 units/l (normal, 35–88 units/l)

On the basis of the abnormal EKG and the laboratory test results, a diagnosis of acute myocardial infarction (MI) was made, and appropriate cardiac care was begun.

Questions

1. Does a connection exist among this patient's hypercholesterolemia, hypertension, and his apparent susceptibility to myocardial infarcts?
2. Since CK, GOT, and LDH are all "cardiac" enzymes, why is the CK elevated to nearly four times normal while the LDH in only marginally elevated?
3. Which of the three enzyme tests would have been most clinically significant if the patient had delayed his examination until several days after the attack?
4. Is the hyperkalemia (elevated potassium) significant in this case?
5. What drug therapy would be appropriate initially for this patient?
6. Assuming that the patient makes a good recovery, that is, there is little or no residual damage of the cardiac muscle, will he have any need for medication upon discharge?
7. What is the appropriate dietary regimen in the treatment of this patient?
8. How can the dietitian best prepare this patient for discharge?

Discussion

Elevated plasma cholesterol concentrations, particulary the fraction associated with the low density lipoproteins (LDL-cholesterol), such as would be found in a type IIa hyperlipoproteinemia, somehow increases the tendency toward atherosclerosis. This condition results from the deposition of fatty material, primarily cholesterol esters, within the arterial intima forming what are called fatty streaks. As this lesion develops, collagen deposits at the site also, and a fibrous plaque results. Ultimately the plaque calcifies, with the deposition of calcium salts. The end result of the growing lesion is that the arterial lumen (the diameter of the channel through which the blood flows) narrows, and the arterial wall loses its flexibility due to the invasion of the plaque. This accounts for the associated hypertension. The roughened intimal surface and narrowed lumen predisposes to clot formation, which can result in occlusion of the blood flow, and if the occlusion persists, the cells that normally are supplied with oxygen by that vessel become anoxic and die. Such cells are said to be infarcted, and when this process occurs within the arteries of the heart itself, the regional cell death is called a myocardial infarction.

The cell death resulting from an infarction causes the release of cytoplasmic enzymes into the circulation, and their serum level therefore can indicate if a prior episode of pain had been caused by an infarct. Creatine kinase, lactase dehydrogenase, and glutamic-oxaloacetic transaminase are of value as "marker" enzymes in such diagnoses. It is interesting to note, however, that they are released at different rates from the damaged tissue. For example, CK begins to rise within three to six hours, peaks (maximum concentration) in 24 to 36 hours, and returns to normal within three days. GOT follows a time course similar to that of CK, although its increase does not begin until six to eight hours after the attack, and it takes about five days for the serum level to return to normal. LDH, on the other hand, begins its rise about 12 hours after the onset of pain, peaks in 48 to 72 hours, and requires about 11 days to return to normal levels. It would therefore be of little diagnostic value to determine serum CK several days after a suspected infarct, or, for that matter, to assay LDH 6 hours after an attack. Nevertheless, all three enzymes are customarily determined even in the case of recent (three to six hours) suspected infarcts because these values serve as "baseline" levels to which subsequent test values may be compared.

Ischemic cell death can also release cellular substances other than enzymes into the circulation. Increased serum concentration of any substance will be more pronounced the higher the concentration of that substance in the infarcted tissue. Potassium exemplifies this. It is found in high concentration in heart cells, and a myocardial infarction predictably elevates the serum level. It is not of value in MI diagnosis, however, because its serum elevation could reflect unrelated physiological problems such as hormonal imbalance, impairment of renal function, or disturbance in acid–base balance.

Once within the coronary care unit, the patient was immediately placed on IV fluids and began receiving morphine and nitroprusside intravenously. Treatment was aimed primarily at making the patient pain free (morphine) and at reducing his blood pressure (nitroprusside). After 24 hours the patient was relatively pain free and his blood pressure had returned to normal where it remained throughout his recovery period.

The patient's recovery was noneventful and no evidence of residual damage to the myocardium could be detected except for an occasional mild arrhythmia. The physician felt medications could be kept to the minimum; therefore, the only drug therapy the patient received was propranolol (Inderal®) which served to reduce the heart rate of the patient and control his arrhythmia. The patient was instructed to continue on propranolol after discharge, but no other medications were prescribed for him. The physician anticipated that the patient's cholesterol level and mildly elevated blood pressure could be controlled through dietary modifications.

During the first 24 hours, the patient was receiving IV fluids and required nothing by mouth except small sips of water. His physician ordered a low fat, low sodium liquid diet (total volume, 1200 ml) to be begun the following day. All liquids were to be given in small quantities and served at body temperature. After two days on this liquid diet, which supplied approximatley 800 kilocalories, the patient was advanced to solid foods and calories were increased to 1200 with only 30 percent of these calories being supplied by fat. The diet, designed to restrict daily intake of sodium and cholesterol to approximately 2 gm and 250 to 300 mg, respectively, was divided into three small meals and a bed time snack. All liquids continued to be served in small quantities at body temperature and no caffeine-containing beverages were allowed. The dietitian visited the patient regularly in order to determine his response to his diet (and increase its acceptability to whatever extent possible) and to assess his understanding and that of his wife of the therapeutic principles of the diet. Since the patient had been on a special diet for the past 5 years, it was important for the dietitian to inquire carefully into past adherence to dietary modifications. Any barriers to successful dietary management needed to be discovered so that a realistic educational plan could be developed.

After three weeks, as the patient was being readied for discharge, the dietitian weighed the patient and found that his weight had dropped from his admission weight of 205 pounds to 192 pounds. He was, however, still about 25 pounds above his ideal body weight and needed to be continued on a diet restricted in calories as well as cholesterol and sodium. In consultation with the physician, the dietitian determined that the appropriate discharge diet would be one providing approximately 1800 kilocalories with no more than 35 percent of these calories coming from fat. Daily intakes of sodium and cholesterol were continued at the same level of restriction: 2 gm and under 300 mg, respectively. The polyunsaturated to saturated fat ratio was set at 1.5. Both the patient and his wife were carefully instructed about the new diet. By time of discharge both the patient and his wife were able to plan appropriate meals for two days. A copy of the discharge diet was sent to the clinic dietitian who would see the patient when he returned to the cardiac clinic for a follow-up visit one month after his discharge from the hospital. During this visit the clinic dietitian not only can assess the patient's progress to date in following his diet but also can continue education of the patient through making various recommendations appropriate and specific to his needs.

REFERENCES

1. Crouch, J. E. and J. R. McClintic. *Human Anatomy and Physiology*. 2nd ed. New York; John Wiley & Sons, 1976; pp. 475–575.
2. Katch, F. I. and W. D. McArdle, *Nutrition, Weight Control and Exercise*. Boston; Houghton Mifflin, 1977; p. 222.
3. Jagger, P. I. and E. Braunwald. Hypertensive vascular disease. In *Harrison's Principles of Internal Medicine*. G. W. Thorn et al., eds. 8th ed. New York: McGraw-Hill, 1977; pp. 1307–1318.
4. Marx, J. L. Hypertension: A complex disease with complex causes. *Science* **194:** 821, Nov. 1976.

5. Onesti, G. Antihypertensives and their modes of action. *Drug Therapy* **8:** 35, 1978.
6. Improved treatment of hypertension after physician tutorials. *Nutr. R.* **34:** 334, Nov. 1976.
7. Bene, R. Cardiology. In *Nutritional Support of Medical Practice*, Schneider, Anderson, and Coursin, eds. New York: Harper and Row, 1977; pp. 236–262.
8. Frederickson, D. S. Atherosclerosis and other forms of arteriosclerosis. In *Harrison's Principles of Internal Medicine*, G. W. Thorn et al., eds. 8th ed. New York: McGraw-Hill, 1977; pp. 1299–1307.
9. Ross, R. and J. A. Glomset. Atherosclerosis and the arterial smooth muscle cell. *Science* **180:** 1332, June 1973.
10. Ross, R. and L. Harker. Hyperlipidemia and atherosclerosis. *Science* **193:** 1094, Sept. 1976.
11. Benditt, E. P. The origin of atherosclerosis. *Scientific American* **236:** 74, Feb. 1977.
12. Kolata, G. B. Atherosclerotic plaques: Competing theories guide research. *Science* **194:** 592, Nov. 1976.
13. Glueck, C. J., F. Mattson, and E. L. Bierman. Diet and coronary heart disease: Another view. *N. Eng. J. Med.* **298:** 1471, June 1978.
14. Guyton, A. C. *Textbook of Medical Physiology.* 5th ed. Philadelphia: W. B. Saunders, 1976; pp. 320–341.
15. Gutstein, W. H., J. Harrison, F. Parl, G. Keir, and M. Avitable. Neural factors contribute to atherogenesis. *Science* **199:** 449, Jan. 1978.
16. Wood, P. D., W. Haskell, H. Klein, S. Lewis, M. P. Stern, and J. W. Farquhan. The distribution of plasma lipoproteins in middle aged runners. *Metabolism* **25:** 1249, 1976.
17. Castelli, W. P., J. T. Doyle, T. Gordon, C. G. Hames, M. C. Hjortland, S. B. Hulley, A. Kagen, and W. J. Zukel. HDL cholesterol and other lipids in coronary heart disease: The Cooperative Lipoprotein Phenotyping Study. *Circulation* **55:** 767, 1977.
18. Miller, N. E., D. S. Thelle, O. H. Forde, and O. D. Majos. The Thromso Heart Study: High-density lipoprotein and coronary heart disease: A prospective case control study. *Lancet* **i:** 965, May 1977.
19. Truswell, A. S. Diet and plasma lipids—a reappraisal. *Am. J. Clin. Nutr.* **31:** 977, June 1978.
20. Brunzell, J. The pathophysiology and treatment of hyperlipidemia. Georgia Regional Television Network, Emory University School of Medicine, 1976.
21. Miller, G. J. and N. E. Miller. Plasma high-density lipoprotein concentration and development of ischemic heart disease. *Lancet* **i:** 16, Jan. 4, 1975.
22. Brown, M. S. and J. L. Goldstein. Human mutations affecting the low density lipoprotein pathway. *Am. J. Clin. Nutr.* **30:** 975, June 1977.
23. DHEW Publication No. (NIH) 76-110, U.S. Department of Health, Education and Welfare, Public Health Service, National Institute of Health.
24. Lees, R. S. and A. M. Lees. Therapy of hyperlipidemias. *Postgraduate Med.* **60:** 99, Sept. 1976.
25. Goldstein, J. L., H. G. Schrott, W. R. Hazard, E. L. Bierman, and A. G. Motulsky. Hyperlipidemia in coronary heart disease. II. Genetic analysis of lipid

levels in 176 families and delineation of a new inherited disorder, combined hyperlipidemia. *J. Clin. Invest.* **52:** 1544, 1973.

26. Carter, C. O., J. Slack, and N. B. Myant. Genetics of hyperlipoproteinaemias. *Lancet* **1:** 400, 1971.

27. Kwitervich, P. O., Jr., D. S. Frederickson, and R. I. Levy. Familial hypercholesterolemia (one form of familial type II hyperlipoproteinemia): A study of its biochemical, genetic and clinical presentation in childhood. J. Clin. Invest. **53:** 1237, 1974.

28. Stanbury, J. B., J. B. Wyngaarden, and D. S. Frederickson, eds. *The Metabolic Basis of Inherited Disease.* 4th ed. New York: McGraw-Hill, 1978.

29. Myant, N. B. and J. Slack. Type II hyperlipoproteinemia. *Clin. Endocrinol. Metab.* **2:** 81, 1973.

30. Levy, R. I., D. S. Frederickson, R. Shulman, D. W. Bilheimer, J. L. Breslow, N. J. Stone, S. E. Lux, H. R. Sloan, R. M. Krauss, and P. N. Herbert. Dietary and drug treatment of primary hyperlipoproteinemia. *Ann. Int. Med.* **77:** 267, 1972.

31. Grundy, S. M. Treatment of hypercholesterolemia. *Am. J. Clin. Nutr.* **30:** 985, June 1977.

32. Coronary Drug Project. Clofibrate and niacin in coronary heart disease. *J. Am. Med. Assoc.* **231:** 360, 1975.

33. Wolfe, B. M., J. P. Kane, R. J. Havel, and H. P. Brewster. Mechanism of the hypolipemic effect of clofibrate in postalisorptive man. *J. Clin. Invest.* **52:** 2146, 1973.

34. Eder, H. A. Drugs used in the prevention and treatment of atherosclerosis. In *The Pharmacological Basis of Therapeutics,* Goodman, L. S. and A. Gilman, eds. New York: Macmillan, 1975; pp. 744–752.

35. Kastrup, E. K., ed. *Facts and Comparisons,* St. Louis: Facts and Comparisons, Inc., 1978; pp. 508–511.

36. Khachadurien, A. K. Hyperlipoproteinemia. *Ross Timesaver—Dietetic Currents* July/Aug. 1977.

37. Glueck, D. J. and W. E. Connor. Diet-coronary heart disease relationships reconnoitered. *Am. J. Clin. Nutr.* **31:** 727, May 1978.

38. Williams, C. L. and E. L. Wynder. A blind spot in preventive medicine, *J. Am. Med. Assoc.* **236:** 2196, Nov. 1976.

39. Friedman, G. and S. J. Goldberg. An evaluation of the safety of a low-saturated fat, low-cholesterol diet beginning in infancy. *Pediatrics* **58:** 655, Nov. 1976.

40. Gotto, A. M. Statement in Diet Related to Killer Diseases, II. Hearings before the Select Committee on Nutrition and Human Needs in the U.S. Senate, Part I—Cardiovascular Disease. U.S. Government Printing Office, 1977.

41. Alfin-Slater, R. C. Other dietary risk factors and CHD. *Nutrition and the M.D.* **3:** 2, July 1977.

42. Klein, M. S. and B. E. Sobel. Medical management of myocardial infarction. *Annual Review of Medicine* **27:** 89, 1976.

43. Christakis, G. and M. Winston. Nutritional therapy in acute myocardial infarction. *J. Am. Diet. Assoc.* **63:** 233, Sept. 1973.

44. Paterson, C. R. Dietary counseling for patients admitted for coronary artery bypass graft. *J. Am. Diet. Assoc.* **68:** 158, Feb. 1976.

45. Braunwald, E. Heart failure. In *Harrison's Principles of Internal Medicine*, G. W. Thorn et al., eds. 8th ed. New York: McGraw-Hill, 1977; pp. 1178–1187.

RECOMMENDED READINGS

Diet and coronary heart disease. A statement for physicians and other health professionals prepared by the Nutrition Committee of the Steering Committee for Medical and Community Programs of the American Heart Association. American Heart Association, 1978.

This is a concise statement concerning the prudent diet recommended for lowering serum lipid concentrations.

Feeley, R. M., P. E. Criner, and B. K. Watt. Cholesterol content of foods. *Journal of the American Dietetic Association* **61:** 134, Aug. 1972.

This article provides figures on cholesterol content of a variety of foods. This is an excellent working tool for the dietitian confronted with calculating cholesterol-controlled diets or with educating patients about cholesterol content of foods.

Feldman, E. B., ed. *Nutrition and Cardiovascular Disease*. New York: Appleton-Century-Crofts, 1976.

The monograph covers a variety of topics ranging from basic epidemiology and lipid metabolism through interrelations of lipids, carbohydrates, alcohol, calories, vitamins, and minerals in the pathogenesis and management of specific cardiovascular diseases.

Fisher, W. R. and D. H. Truitt. The common hyperlipoproteinemias—an understanding of disease mechanisms and their control. *Annals of Internal Medicine* **85:** 497, 1976.

This review includes an excellent discussion of the structure and normal catabolism of VLDL and LDL along with the possible metabolic derangements in catabolism of LDLs.

Gavras, H., A. R. Riberio, I. Gavras, and H. R. Brunner. Reciprocal relation between renin dependency and sodium dependency in essential hypertension. *New England Journal of Medicine* **295:** 1278, December 2, 1976.

Authors present research that supports the view that in patients of all three renin subgroups sodium balance determines the degree of participation of the renin-angiotensin system in sustaining high blood pressure.

Glass, D. C. Stress, behavior patterns and coronary disease. *American Scientist* **65:** 177, Mar./Apr. 1977.

Author discusses the psychological risk factors in the development of coronary heart diesase. Methods of measuring A and B behavior patterns are discussed as are techniques for correcting the seemingly pathogenic life-style of behavior pattern A.

Hemzacek, K. Dietary protocol for the patient who has suffered a myocardial infarction. *Journal of the American Dietetic Association* **72:** 182, Feb. 1978.

The rationale for the cardiac diet used at Lutheran General Hospital, Park Ridge, Illinois is given. Each aspect of the diet is considered in light of physiologic responses of the cardiac patient.

Palumbo, P. J., E. R. Briones, R. A. Nelson, and B. A. Kottke. Sucrose sensitivity of patients with coronary artery disease. *American Journal of Clinical Nutrition* **30:** 394, Mar. 1977.

Authors present results of research which suggest that patients with coronary artery disease are much more sensitive to high intakes of simple carbohydrate (4 g/kg), as indicated by increase in serum triglycerides, than are normal controls.

Perry, H. M. Minerals in cardiovascular disease. *Journal of the American Dietetic Association* **62:** 631, June 1973.

The author reviews the relationship between soft-water regions and excessive cardiovascular disease. Also included in the article is a discussion of the possible relationship of cadmium to hypertension.

The value and safety of diet modification to control hyperlipidemia in childhood and adolescence. A statement for physicians and other health professionals prepared by an ad hoc committee of the Steering Committee for Medical and Community Programs of the American Heart Association. American Heart Association, 1978.

Statement contains the recommended dietary modification for children at high risk of developing cardiovascular disease. The rationale for these recommendations is also included.

Tzagournis, M. Triglycerides in clinical medicine. A review. *American Journal of Clinical Nutrition* **31:** 1437, Aug. 1978.

This review identifies all those hyperlipoproteinemias in which hypertriglyceridemia is likely to occur. Underlying causes of hypertriglyceridemia, its possible relationship to development of atherosclerosis and recommended therapy for its control are discussed.

CHAPTER 8

The Liver

ANATOMY AND PHYSIOLOGY

The liver, located in the upper right quadrant of the abdomen and weighing approximately 1500 grams in the adult, is the largest single internal organ in the body and from a metabolic standpoint is probably the most complex (1–3). The basic unit of the liver is the lobule and a human liver contains from 50,000 to 100,000 of these functional structures. Each lobule is constructed around a central vein and consists of cords of cells, usually two thick, which rotate out from the center (see Fig. 8.1). Between these cords of cells, commonly referred to as hepatic cellular plates, are the hepatic sinusoids which are capillaries possessing such extreme permeability that blood proteins may freely diffuse through them. This extreme permeability of the liver sinusoids allows the hepatic blood to come in very close contact with liver cells and thus promotes exchange of nutrients between the intravascular fluids and the hepatocytes. Afloat in the blood but delicately attached to the epithelial wall of the hepatic sinusoids are the star-shaped Kupffer cells, large phagocytes which by engorging bacteria cleanse the blood being brought to the liver lobules from the digestive tract.

Blood is supplied to the liver by both the hepatic artery (approximately 400 ml/min) and the portal vein (about 1000 ml/min), the terminal branches of which intercommunicate throughout the liver. The portal vein is formed by union of the intestinal vein bringing nutrient-rich blood from a large part of the intestine and the splenic vein carrying blood from the stomach, spleen, pancreas, and gall bladder. The blood reaching the liver by the portal vein flows through the hepatic sinusoids, coming in close contact with the hepatocytes, and then is carried by these capillaries to the central hepatic vein by which it leaves the liver and enters the inferior vena cava (see Fig. 8.2).

The hepatic cellular plates which make up the liver lobules radiate out from the central vein and are usually composed of two adjacent cells between which are located the small bile canaliculi which collect the bile secreted by liver cells and carry it to the terminal bile duct. This terminal bile duct along with portal blood vessels lies between adjacent liver lobules and is supported by fine connective tissue (see Fig. 8.3). The liver

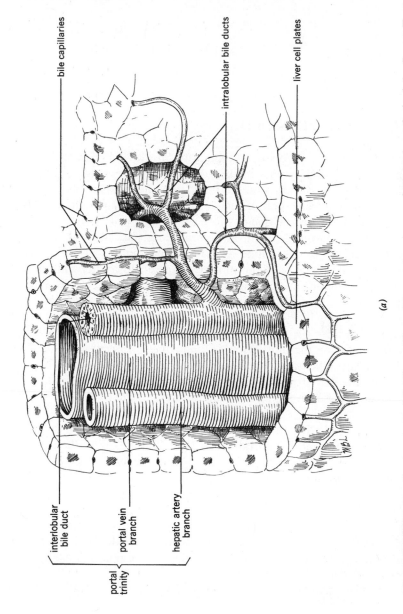

bile capillaries

intralobular bile ducts

liver cell plates

interlobular bile duct

portal vein branch

hepatic artery branch

portal trinity

(a)

Figure 8.1 Microscopic structure of the liver. (From *Human Anatomy and Physiology*, 2nd ed. by James E. Crouch and J. R. McClintic. Copyright 1976 by John Wiley and Sons, Inc. Reprinted by permission of the publisher.)

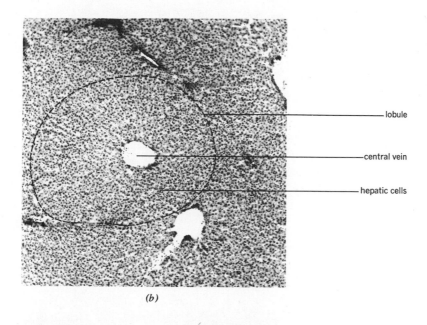

lobule

central vein

hepatic cells

(b)

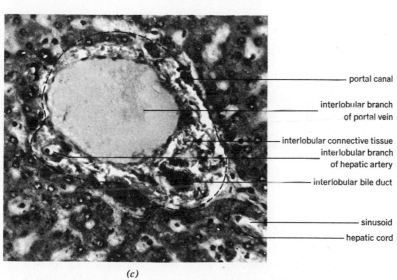

portal canal

interlobular branch
of portal vein

interlobular connective tissue
interlobular branch
of hepatic artery

interlobular bile duct

sinusoid

hepatic cord

(c)

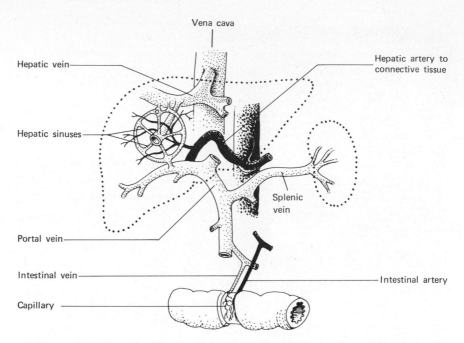

Figure 8.2 Blood circulation in the liver. (Adapted from *Textbook of Medical Physiology,* 5th ed., by Arthur C. Guyton. Copyright 1976 by W. B. Saunders Co. Reprinted by permission of the publisher and author.)

lobules with their rich blood supply and biliary canals are thus constructed to carry out the numerous functions of this very complex organ.

Primary Functions of Liver

Functions of the liver may be grouped into five major categories: circulatory, hematologic, protective and/or detoxifying, excretory, and metabolic (3).

Circulatory. The liver because it is so structured as to allow expansion or compression can serve as a reservoir for blood. Under normal circumstances the volume of blood held in the liver approximates 650 ml but every minute about 1400 ml of blood is flowing against little resistance through the liver into the systemic blood supply. When, however, disease states such as cardiac failure increase the pressure in the veins draining the liver, blood volume in the liver can be expanded to as much as a liter. Conversely, when large amounts of blood are lost from the systemic blood supply, the liver is able to help increase the level of circulating blood by reducing its blood volume below normal.

In addition, the liver is a very active site for production of lymph, the protein content of which is quite similar to that of blood plasma. The high protein content is due to the extreme permeability of hepatic sinusoids. It is estimated that the liver produces approximately ten times more lymph than can be produced by the same mass of skeletal tissue (2).

Hematologic. Blood coagulation to a large extent is regulated by the liver because hepatocytes not only synthesize most of the factors necessary for the clotting of blood—fibrinogen, prothrombin, and factors V, VII, IX, X, and XIII—but also produce components of the fibrinolytic system, namely plasminogen and heparin. The liver is also very important in embryonic hematopoiesis during the second trimester of gestation. After this time, however, normal red blood cell formation occurs in the bone marrow (2,4).

Protective and/or Detoxifying. The Kupffer cells, which are loosely attached to the epithelial cells of the sinusoids, are important protective devices for the body as a whole. Through their phagocytic activity they are able to remove foreign bodies from the blood entering the liver. They are particularly important in removing bacteria being brought by the portal vein from the digestive tract and in catabolizing worn out erythrocytes.

The detoxifying activity of the liver is of two distinct types: (1) removal from blood of ammonia and its conversion into urea by the hepatocytes (see urea cycle, Chapter 3), and (2) conversion of hydrophobic substances reaching the liver into water-soluble products, that may be excreted via urine or bile. This latter activity is accomplished by a mixed-function microsomal cytochrome P450 system. Lipophilic substances such as various drugs, pesticides, and endogenously occurring lipids (steroid hormones) for example, are made hydrophilic by oxidation, reduction, or hydrolysis and then are conjugated with some natural constituent of the body, for example, glucuronic acid, glycine, or glutathione, for excretion (5).

Excretory. The biliary function of the liver is of extreme importance not only in the production of bile salts which are necessary for absorption of lipids and fat-soluble substances but also in the provision of means by which these same bile salts and certain other waste products such as bilirubin and cholesterol can be removed from the body. In addition foreign substances, such as heavy metals and dyes, can be withdrawn from the blood by hepatic activity and excreted via the biliary tract (3,4).

Bile, consisting of water, bile salts, cholesterol, bilirubin, fatty acids, lecithin, and various electrolytes, is continually formed by the hepatocytes and secreted into the bile canaliculi (see Fig. 8.3). The bile flows through the liver until it reaches the hepatic duct and common bile duct

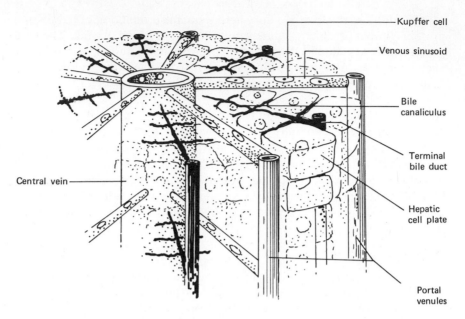

Kupffer cell

Venous sinusoid

Bile canaliculus

Terminal bile duct

Hepatic cell plate

Portal venules

Central vein

Figure 8.3 Structure of the liver lobule, showing relation of hepatic cell plates to blood vessels and bile ducts. (Adapted from *Textbook of Medical Physiology,* 5th ed. by Arthur C. Guyton. Copyright 1976 by W.B. Saunders Co.)

from which it may move into the upper small intestine or be carried to the gall bladder for concentration and storage. Bile salts are oxidation products of cholesterol conjugated with an amino acid, either glycine or taurine, and then combined with either sodium or potassium. About 80 percent of liver cholesterol is utilized in this manner (6). Although bile salts are regularly excreted into the small intestine, they are for the most part (approximately 94 percent) reabsorbed and carried by portal blood back to the hepatocytes where they again are incorporated into bile formation and recirculated. This recirculation is estimated to occur approximately 18 times before the bile salts are excreted in the feces. This recirculation is referred to as the *enterohepatic circulation.* In response to the small loss of bile salts from the body via the fecal route, the liver forms an approximate additional supply of one gram daily (6). The formation and excretion of bile salts from the body represent the primary route by which the body loses cholesterol (see Chapter 3).

The highly pigmented bilirubin becomes a constituent of bile after having been conjugated into a water-soluble compound by the action of the cytochrome P450 system. Bilirubin is the break-down product of heme originating from worn out erythrocytes. When for whatever reason an abnormal amount of bilirubin accumulates in the blood, the skin takes on a yellowish-green color, a condition referred to as "jaundice" (see Chapter 3).

Metabolic. Metabolic functions of the liver are those of most interest to the dietitian/nutritionist and these functions are legion. In addition to being an active site for metabolism of carbohydrate, lipids, and protein, the liver provides storage for many vitamins and minerals. Significant quantities of all fat-soluble vitamins, particularly vitamin A, are stored in the liver. It is estimated that maximum hepatic storage of vitamin A can be sufficient to prevent a deficiency of this nutrient for as long as two years (2,6). The liver is also very important in the metabolism of water-soluble vitamins as well. For example, it provides storage for large amounts of vitamin B_{12} and is the site for conversion of thiamine and pyridoxine into their metabolically active forms (7). Other B-complex vitamins as well as vitamin C are also found in considerable amounts in the liver.

Certain minerals such as iron and copper are found in large amounts in the liver. Aside from the iron incorporated into circulating hemoglobin, the greatest amount of iron found in the body is normally that stored as ferritin. An apoferritin–ferritin buffer system exists in the liver. Through this system iron is easily given up to circulation but also can be stored in large quantities when an excess exists. It is estimated that 60 percent excess body iron can be stored as either ferritin or hemosiderin in the liver (6,8).

Other minerals found in significant quantities in the liver are manganese, zinc, and magnesium.

Carbohydrate Metabolism (see Chapter 3). In the liver this is involved for the most part in the maintenance of a desirable level of blood glucose: glycolysis and glycogenesis in the fed state; glycogenolysis, and gluconeogenesis in the fasting state. Glycogen stores in the liver account for about five to seven percent of its weight (9). The hepatocytes also are responsible for the conversion of the monosaccharides, fructose and galactose, into glucose. The ability of the hepatocytes to convert galactose to glucose is particularly important because elevated serum galactose is toxic. In addition various mucopolysaccharides are synthesized in the liver.

Lipid Metabolism. Within the hepatocytes this includes very rapid beta-oxidation of fatty acids, production of ketone bodies, and synthesis of a number of lipid compounds such as cholesterol, phospholipids, and lipoproteins. Lipogenesis also occurs in the liver, with triglycerides being synthesized from the nonlipid nutrients, carbohydrate and protein (refer to Chapter 3 where lipid metabolism is discussed more fully). Approxi-

SOURCES

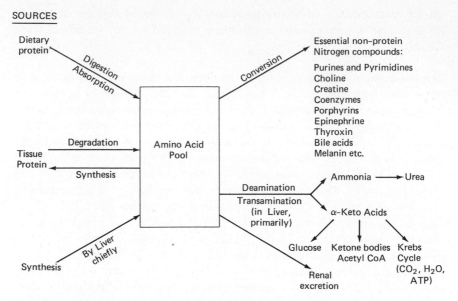

Figure 8.4 Scheme of protein and amino acid metabolism, illustrating role of the liver.

mately five percent of the weight of a normal liver can be attributed to its lipid stores.

Protein Metabolism (see Chapter 3). Despite the importance of the liver in the metabolism of carbohydrate and lipids, the body *might* be able to survive without the liver's participation in these activities. The same cannot be said, however, in regard to the liver's services in protein metabolism (see Fig. 8.4). Without the extensive functions of the liver in the metabolism of amino acids, the organism would die in only a few days (6). The most important of these protein-related metabolic functions include:

1. Oxidative deamination in which the amine group is removed from the amino acid and the resulting alpha-keto acid may serve as an energy source either by being oxidized to release energy or by being converted to glucose and/or fat.
2. Transamination in which the amine group from an amino acid is transferred to an existing alpha-keto acid, the result of which is creation of a new alpha-keto acid from the original amino acid and the formation of another amino acid from the former alpha-keto acid. Two major enzymes catalyzing the transamination reaction in the liver are glutamic-oxaloacetic acid transaminase (GOT) and the glutamic-pyruvic acid transaminase (GPT). Example of a typical reaction involving GPT is as follows:

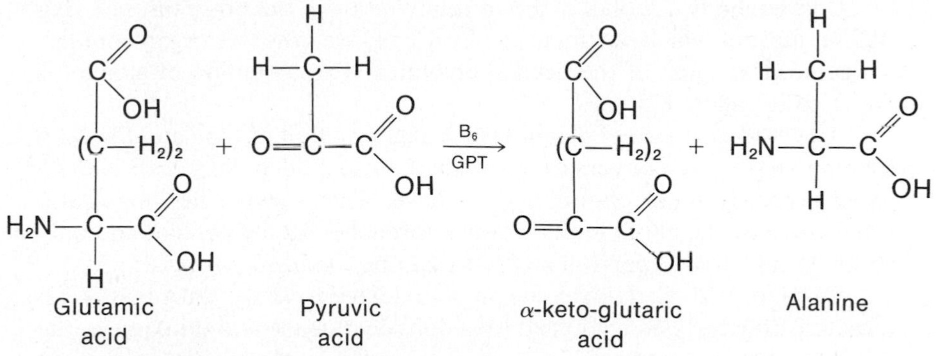

Glutamic acid + Pyruvic acid $\xrightarrow[\text{GPT}]{\text{B}_6}$ α-keto-glutaric acid + Alanine

The α-keto acids (or carbon skeletons) must receive amine groups through transamination in order to form nonessential amino acids. Therefore, protein synthesis in general is dependent on this process.

3. Synthesis of important nitrogenous chemical compounds from amino acids, for example, creatine, choline, purines and pyrimidines, coenzyme A, glutathione, porphyrins.

4. Urea synthesis in which the amino acids ornithine, citrulline, arginine, and aspartic acid participate. Through the urea cycle (outlined in Chapter 3) ammonia is rapidly removed from blood and detoxified by formation of the innocuous urea. Urea is then excreted from the body in urine. The amount of urea nitrogen in the urine is usually a good general indicator of the level of dietary protein.

5. Formation of plasma proteins, probably the most important of the liver functions in protein metabolism. The liver is responsible for the synthesis of more than 95 percent of all plasma proteins and the rate of production can be regulated by the body's need. A depletion of plasma proteins causes an increase of hepatic cell number and growth of the liver in order that the body can be replenished with the needed blood proteins. The only plasma proteins not synthesized by the liver are the immunoglobulins which make up about 20 percent of the globulins and are formed by the plasma cells themselves. Albumin, globulin, and fibrinogen are three major plasma proteins, with albumin existing in the greatest amount and being largely responsible for the colloid osmotic pressure of the plasma. Normally about 150 to 200 mgs albumin per kilogram body weight are synthesized daily (10). Although plasma proteins perform specific functions as components of the blood such as fibrinogen in blood clotting, and globulins in enzymatic activities and immune reactions, they also are valuable as a source of rapidly available amino acids for body tissues which may be protein-depleted. They also act as important transport mechanisms for many vitamins and minerals.

Alcohol Metabolism. Alcohol, although a source of calories (7.1 kcal/gm), cannot be stored for future use as can carbohydrate and fat. Consequently, alcohol must be removed from the body through oxidation, most of which occurs in the liver because only this organ contains a significant amount of the needed enzymes. The oxidation of alcohol is depicted in Figure 8.5.

The oxidation rate of alcohol is a linear function of time and the rate-limiting step is the conversion of ethanol to acetaldehyde which is catalyzed primarily by alcohol dehydrogenase. This enzyme becomes saturated when the level of blood alcohol approaches 10 mg percent and only about 15 mg alcohol per 100 ml blood can be oxidized per hour.

Once formed, acetaldehyde can be oxidized to acetyl CoA by two alternate pathways, one catalyzed by aldehyde oxidase and thiokinase, the other by pyruvate oxidase. In the former pathway the oxidation product of acetaldehyde is acetic acid which is converted to acetyl CoA by the action of ATP and thiokinase. Alternately, some acetaldehyde, catalyzed by pyruvate oxidase, may become acetyl CoA via an intermediary product, hydroxyethylthiamin pyrophosphate. This intermediate metabolite is probably identical to that formed when pyruvate is converted to acetyl CoA.

When alcoholic beverages are consumed in large amounts, the obligatory oxidation of the hydrogen-rich ethanol by the liver results in a decreased utilization of fat and an increased ratio of NADH:NAD. Because NAD is essential to so many metabolic pathways in the liver, reactions that are coupled with oxidation of NADH must increase (11,12). Consequences of such increased reactions are depicted in Figure 8.6 and briefly explained below:

1. Pyruvic acid is reduced to lactic acid. Lactic acid, unlike pyruvic acid, cannot pass through the mitochondrial membranes and therefore accumulates. Increased amounts of lactic acid cause a lowering of the plasma pH which in turn interferes with the kidneys' excretion of uric acid and increases the possibility of gout in susceptible individuals. Decreased availability of pyruvate for glucose synthesis can cause hypoglycemia (see section on hypoglycemia, Chapter 6).
2. Acetyl CoA, instead of being oxidized via the Krebs cycle (Fig. 3.9) is used preferentially in synthesis of fatty acids and cholesterol (Figs. 3.12, 3.15) or is condensed into ketone bodies.
3. Dihydroxyacetone phosphate is reduced to glycerol phosphate, a reaction which allows shuttling of hydrogen ions across mitochondrial membranes into the respiratory chain but primarily promotes triglyceride synthesis.
4. Existing fatty acids are made more saturated and are elongated.

It is postulated that the liver adapts to its oversupply of fat by proliferation of those organelles (endoplasmic reticulum) that synthesize and secrete lipoproteins. Lipoproteins allow mobilization of liver lipids and

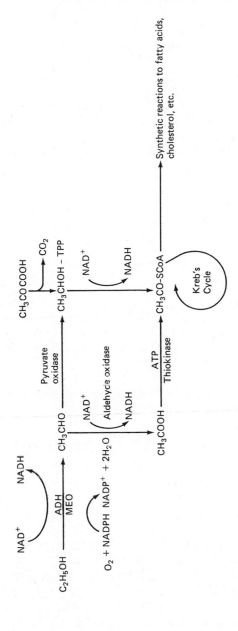

Overall reaction for complete
oxidation of ethanol:

$$C_2H_5OH + 3\,O_2 \longrightarrow 2CO_2 + 3H_2O + (18ATP)$$

ADH = Alcohol dehydrogenase
MEO = Microsomal ethanol oxidase
TPP = Thiamin pyrophospate

Figure 8.5 Metabolic pathways of ethanol.

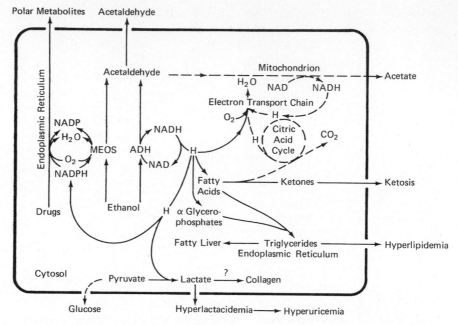

Figure 8.6 Metabolism of ethanol in hepatocyte and schematic representation of its link to fatty liver, hyperlipidemia, hyperuricemia, hyperlactacidemia, ketosis, and hypoglycemia. (ADH indicates alcohol dehydrogenase and MEOS, microsomal-oxidizing system. Pathways decreased by ethanol are represented by dashed lines.) (From "Alcohol and malnutrition in the pathogenesis of liver disease" by Charles S. Lieber, *Journal of the American Medical Association,* Volume 233, pp. 1077–1082, September 8, 1975. Copyright 1975, American Medical Association. Reprinted by permission of publisher and author.)

their placement into circulation (11). In addition, the microsomes of the endoplasmic reticulum contain a mixed function cytochrome system (P450) which is capable of oxidizing ethanol. With proliferation of the endoplasmic reticulum, activity of this cytochrome system is increased so that alcohol may be more rapidly oxidized by the liver. None of the energy, however, produced by this route of alcohol oxidation is trapped as ATP and therefore is lost as heat from the body.

Overconsumption of alcohol in itself is often a serious problem physically, socially, and emotionally. (Reference 31 provides an excellent discussion on disease of alcoholism.) However, only its possible relationship to the development of liver disease will be considered here. Until the last several years, alcoholism was believed to exert its effect on the liver indirectly, that is, as a result of the malnutrition that is commonly associated with excessive intake of ethanol. Lieber and his coworkers (13,14) have been able to demonstrate, however, that alcohol in itself exerts a toxic effect on hepatocytes. Therefore, liver disease resulting from excessive alcohol ingestion is probably a consequence of malnutrition coupled with the direct toxic effect of alcohol. The first pathogenic change occurring in the liver is an excessive accumulation of lipids, a condition referred to as "fatty liver". Fatty liver is a reversible condition but, if uncorrected, can progress to alcoholic hepatitis and finally to irreversible cirrhosis (15,16). Successful treatment of alcoholic liver disease requires complete abstinence from alcohol. Those principles of dietary management will be discussed in conjunction with the specific diseases of hepatitis and cirrhosis. A detailed discussion of dietary management of alcoholism along with excellent references can be found in the March 1978 issue of *Nutrition in Disease* (17).

DIAGNOSIS AND TREATMENT OF COMMON DISEASE STATES

Diagnosis

Diagnosis of liver disease is made possible by a large battery of clinical tests that measure liver function. Collectively they are referred to as liver function tests and are based on the various metabolic responsibilities of the liver such as: (1) conjugation and excretion of bilirubin; (2) metabolism of carbohydrate, protein, and lipids; and (3) detoxification and excretion of potentially poisonous substances. In addition, the determination of metabolic enzymes released into the circulation from pathologically damaged liver cells has proven to be of great diagnostic value. Several representative tests and the clinical implications of their results are described below. Chemical principles of the tests will be discussed in Chapter 14.

Tests Based on Bilirubin Conjugation and Excretion. Bilirubin is a yellow pigment formed from the degradation of the heme moiety of hemoglobin through a complex series of reactions (Chapter 3). Cells of the reticuloendothelial system, particularly those of the spleen, bone marrow, and liver (Kupffer cells), phagocytize aged or damaged red blood cells and convert the released hemoglobin into bilirubin. A total of about six grams of hemoglobin is released each day from the disintegration of overaged cells (18), and the bilirubin thus formed is attached to albumin (unconjugated bilirubin) so that it may be transported to the liver for conjugation. This conjugation process involves attachment of two molecules of glucuronic acid to one mole of bilirubin, a reaction catalyzed by the enzyme, UDP-glucuronyl transferase, and producing the diglucuronide of bilirubin (conjugated bilirubin). Conjugation greatly enhances the water solubility of the bilirubin and is necessary for its excretion via the bile into the small intestine.

A small amount of conjugated bilirubin, however, enters the general circulation, thereby giving rise to both conjugated and unconjugated forms of the pigment in the serum. (It is bilirubin that imparts the characteristic straw color to the serum.) In the event of liver disease, such as viral hepatitis, cirrhosis, or obstruction of the biliary circulation, bilirubin may accumulate to high levels in the serum, producing the condition of jaundice. Furthermore, and more important from the clinical standpoint, the differential quantitation of the conjugated and unconjugated forms can be used to diagnose precisely the nature of the pathological process. For example, an obstructed common bile duct, due perhaps to a stricture, stones, or neoplasm, in an otherwise normal liver, would cause the release of elevated amounts of conjugated bilirubin into the bloodstream because its normal passage into the small intestine is impeded. In hepatic disease, such as advanced hepatitis or cirrhosis, on the other hand, the parenchymal liver cells may lose their ability to conjugate, and the serum level of the unconjugated form consequently increases. In clinical testing, the conjugated and unconjugated forms are commonly referred to as "direct" and "indirect" bilirubin, respectively. These are terms that derive from the methodology for their quantitative assay.

Tests Based on Nutrient Metabolism. The liver is involved in so many reactions concerned with carbohydrate metabolism, it is reasonable to expect that tests to detect abnormalities in this function would abound. Curiously, this is not the case and extensive impairment of cellular function is necessary before any interference with carbohydrate metabolism is noticeable. This curiosity is evidenced by the normal glucose tolerance curves occasionally seen in patients suffering with serious liver disease (18).

A normally functioning liver is essential for protein metabolism. As indicated previously in this chapter (pp. 274–275), deamination and transamination of amino acids, urea formation, and synthesis of many of the plasma proteins are dependent on normal liver function. Like carbohydrate metabolism, however, aberrant metabolism is not demonstrable until extensive cellular damage is incurred. There are, nevertheless, two liver function tests based on protein and amino acid metabolism that are sensitive enough to warrant mention: concentration of serum albumin and level of serum ammonia.

The basis for the test of *serum albumin concentration* is that albumin, along with other plasma proteins, is synthesized by the liver cells. In general, therefore, parenchymal liver disease is characterized by a decrease in albumin and an increase in the gamma globulins, which originate from the lymphocytes, and not the liver. Inadequate intake of protein even in a normally functioning liver can cause depressed synthesis of albumin. Therefore, a low serum albumin can alert the health professional to possible malnutrition as well as to a malfunctioning liver (see Chapter 12).

Determination of *serum ammonia* is important because in spite of the continuous processes of deamination and transamination of amino acids, the level of circulating ammonia is extremely low in normal persons. The reason for the low level is that ammonia is efficiently incorporated into urea by the liver and then excreted in the urine as such. The liver also uses small amounts of ammonia to synthesize glutamine from glutamate. In the kidneys glutamine gives rise to ammonium ions which are excreted in the urine (see Chapter 3). Hepatic coma and the terminal stages of cirrhosis are often marked by an increase in blood ammonia due to the failing liver's inability to remove the ammonia from systemic circulation. The test for serum ammonia may be of questionable importance, however, since in some instances normal levels of ammonia have been found in diagnosed cases of hepatic coma.

A test of liver function based on lipid metabolism has recently attracted interest. Pathologically damaged liver cells allow the seepage of bile salts and bile acids into the bloodstream, and determination of serum levels of these substances constitutes the test (19). Normally the bile acids and salts are formed from cholesterol and represent the excretory form of cholesterol via the bile.

Tests Based on Detoxification and Excretion. Bromsulphalein is a dye that is conjugated and excreted almost exclusively by the liver. A prolonged retention of this dye in the circulation following parenteral administration of the dye indicates faulty excretory function on the part of the liver.

Enzyme Tests for Liver Function. The determination of enzymes and isoenzymes released into the serum from the damaged liver cells represents a sensitive and reliable diagnostic tool. Isoenzymes are structurally different forms of the same enzyme and are produced at different sites in the body (see Chapter 1). For this reason, the elevation of the serum activity of a particular isoenzyme indicates a disease process in the organ or tissue responsible for its synthesis. The advantage of isoenzyme assays, therefore, is organ specificity. Some of the enzymes and isoenzymes routinely assayed as liver function tests include alkaline phosphatase isoenzyme, lactate dehydrogenase isoenzyme, 5-nucleotidase, gamma glutamyl-transferase, glutamic pyruvic transaminase (alanylamino transferase), and glyceraldehyde 3-phosphate dehydrogenase.

Common Disease States

Viral Hepatitis. Hepatitis, characterized by hepatic cell necrosis and inflammation, is a commonly occurring disorder, normally the result of an acute systemic infectious disease. Acute viral hepatitis can be caused by one of at least three different viruses, designated as virus A, B, or C, but its clinical manifestations are similar regardless of the causative agent

(20,21). In 1976, 60,000 cases of acute hepatitis were reported in the United States, with approximately 60 percent diagnosed as hepatitis A, 25 percent as hepatitis B, and 15 percent as unspecified.

Hepatitis A, or short incubation hepatitis, which occurs most frequently in children and young adults, usually can be traced to ingestion of fecally contaminated milk and/or water. Also consumption of raw clams and oysters taken from contaminated waters has been implicated in spread of this disease. On the other hand, the virus causing hepatitis B (or long incubation hepatitis) gains entrance into the body primarily by the parenteral route and can be traced to contaminated needles or syringes. Nevertheless, both viruses A and B can be transmitted by routes other than the ones most commonly implicated. The most recent type of hepatitis identified is that associated with blood transfusions and caused by virus C, so designated for sake of convenience. Hepatitis C, like hepatatis B, has a long incubation period.

Acute hepatitis, regardless of the infectious agent, exhibits the same three phases of disease: the *prodromal* period in which the patient experiences nonspecific symptoms of anorexia, nausea, and extreme fatigue; the stage of *clinical jaundice* (appearance of jaundice may be primary means of diagnosis) which may last six to eight weeks during which time the liver enlarges and becomes tender; and finally the *recovery* period which may range from two to 12 weeks (22). During this last phase, as soon as the jaundice has subsided, the patient usually feels quite well except that he/she fatigues easily. Abnormalities of hepatic function are likely to remain evident during the recovery phase but complete remission of the disease can be expected within three to four months from the onset of jaundice in about 75 percent of those patients suffering no complications. It is possible, however, for patients to develop chronic hepatitis following an acute attack and the risk of such a complication appears to be higher in persons suffering from hepatitis B (20,22).

An antigen designated as HB_sAg may be used to diagnose hepatitis B, because this specific protein is not found in the blood of patients suffering with the other types of hepatitis. Extensive study of antigen particles isolated from blood of patients with hepatitis B holds promise for development of a vaccine against this particular type of hepatitis (20). Discovery that more than one antigen specific for hepatitis B exists in the blood of patients with this infection has opened up much exciting research on this particular disease (20,23).

Symptoms of hepatitis may occur following administration of certain drugs, for example, isoniazid, methyldopa, p-aminosalicylic acid, sulfonamide antibiotics, erythromycin, phenothiazines, anabolic steroids, and halothane. Liver cell necrosis is the most serious consequence of drug-induced hepatitis, which has a high mortality rate. If symptoms of hepatitis such as nausea, vomiting, anorexia, and jaundice occur following administration of a drug, this medication should be discontinued immediately. The danger of drug-induced hepatitis is illustrated by the massive liver cell necrosis that can result from administration of halothane. Although a rare occurrence, persons thus affected have a mortality rate approaching 100 percent (24).

Fortunately, in most instances of drug-induced hepatitis, discontinuation of the problem drug will allow symptoms to disappear within a few days and the patient's liver function will return to normal.

There is no specific treatment for acute hepatitis except rest and the intake of a high caloric, well-balanced diet. Getting the patient with acute hepatitis to eat a high caloric diet is indeed a challenge for the dietetics practitioner because quite often the disease is accompanied by nausea and vomiting. The patient needs to be tempted with foods that he/she particularly likes or with those that he thinks he might enjoy on this particular day. Learning what might appeal to the patient means daily (or even more frequent) visits to the patient. Enticing him/her to eat means not only providing those foods for which the patient has indicated a desire but also making sure that meals and supplements are attractive in appearance and foods are served at the appropriate temperatures. Although in the past the level of fat intake has been a concern, present emphasis is on sufficient calories. The fluctuating appetite of the patient with acute hepatitis usually will preclude ingestion of excessive fat.

Cirrhosis. According to LaMont and Isselbacher (25) "cirrhosis is a generic term that includes all forms of chronic diffuse liver disease characterized by *significant loss of liver cells,* collapse and fibrosis of supporting reticulin network with distortion of the vascular bed, and nodular regeneration of the remaining liver cell masses". Death of significant numbers of hepatocytes throughout the liver causes the clinical and biological symptoms associated with this complex disease, such as jaundice, ascites, encephalopathy.

The etiology of cirrhosis is obscure. Out of 155 patients studied by Stone et al. (26), 75 were designated as suffering from "cryptogenic" cirrhosis. Although clear-cut causes for liver failure are difficult to identify, most cases of cirrhosis can be classified as (1) Laennec's, (2) postnecrotic, (3) biliary, (4) hemochromatosis, (5) cardiac or congestive, (6) rare and nonspecific (22). Of these six categories, the most commonly occurring type on a worldwide basis is the postnecrotic, the development of which seems related to a history of acute or chronic hepatitis. In North America the most prevalent type of cirrhosis is Laennec's which can usually be traced to chronic alcoholism.

The amount of liver damage that occurs due to alcoholism is correlated not only with the amount of ethanol consumed but also with the period of time over which it is consumed. Also, it is important to remember that all alcoholics do not develop Laennec's cirrhosis. The incidence is only 10 to 12 percent. The incidence of Laennec's cirrhosis is greater in men than in women but sex difference is decreasing as women increase their consumption of alcohol. The average onset of symptoms usually occurs around age 50 years but can be exhibited during the third or fourth decade of life (25,26).

Because under normal conditions approximately 1400 to 1500 ml blood flows each minute through the liver, determination of hepatic blood flow can be a good measure of hepatic function. This determination is made through injection of the dye, bromsulphalein (see p. 281), into the circulatory system and measurement of its disappearance. To be removed from circulation, the dye must move through the hepatocytes into the biliary tract. Therefore, its rate of disappearance is indicative of the health of the liver.

In cirrhosis the fibrotic condition of the liver and the presence of nodules of regenerating cells cause an increased resistance to the flow of blood through this organ into the inferior vena cava (systemic circulation). As a result the portal venous pressure may increase markedly (portal hypertension) with the following possible consequences (6,25):

1. Leakage of fluid which is almost pure plasma through the outer surface of the liver into the peritoneal cavity and increase in liver lymph flow.
2. Development of portal-systemic venous collaterals accompanied by dilated veins particularly in the esophagogastric region (esophageal varices).
3. Occurrence of congestive splenomegaly with hypersplenism.
4. Onset of hepatic encephalopathy (hepatic coma).

When portal pressures reach 10 to 15 mm Hg, fluid leakage from the surface of the liver can be sufficient to cause accumulation of large quantities of almost pure plasma in the abdominal cavity. This accumulation of fluid is called ascites, a complication found in 60 to 85 percent of patients with advanced cirrhosis. Ascites differs from the other types of edema because of its very high protein content and its localization in the abdominal area. As fluid increases in the peritoneal cavity, less blood reaches the kidney and as a result the secretion of aldosterone is increased. To further complicate matters impaired liver function prevents the normal metabolism of aldosterone and consequently, circulating aldosterone remains at a higher than normal level. The resulting increased retention of sodium by the kidney tubules promotes development of further edema in all body compartments.

In severe portal hypertension development of some portal-systemic shunts occurs and blood carried by this collateral circulation bypasses the liver. The esophagogastric area is one in which these shunts are likely to occur and as a result distended varices that can easily hemorrhage may be present. Such varices can be life-threatening to the cirrhotic patient and are responsible directly or indirectly for death in approximately one-third of patients with Laennec's cirrhosis.

Collateral circulation can present another problem to the cirrhotic patient—an increased danger of hepatic coma resulting from elevated plasma ammonia. Normally, the liver removes circulating ammonia from the blood and converts it into urea (see urea cycle, Chapter 3). In the patient with advanced cirrhosis, however, not only may the liver be inefficient in its removal of ammonia from the blood but also some of the blood is not even approaching the liver so that any of its circulating ammonia can be removed. Most of the plasma ammonia has been absorbed from the digestive tract and results from deamination by bacterial enzymes of amino acids derived from dietary protein or from blood lost into the gastrointestinal tract. Ammonia is also formed from the urea which has been excreted from the blood into the intestinal tract. Normally about 25 percent of blood urea is excreated into the intestinal tract and here it can be converted by bacterial ureases into ammonia. In addition, when hepatic failure is accompanied by metabolic alkalosis, the kidney may increase its production of ammonia from glutamine (see Chapter 10) and as a consequence, the ammonia content of the blood increases. LaMont and Isselbacher estimate that about 50 percent of the patients with cirrhosis die in coma (25).

Dietary Treatment of Liver Disease

In no disease is individualization of treatment more important than it is in liver disease, that is, cirrhosis. Therapy must be limited primarily to that obtainable through nutritional means because liver disease greatly limits type of medication administration. In general, only those medications that can be excreted unchanged by the kidney can be administered to patients with severely compromised liver function because most therapeutic agents are detoxified or converted to active agents by the liver (see p. 271).

For cirrhotic patients who must be medicated due to other coexisting disease states, dosage of drugs must be decreased to allow for the lessened efficiency of detoxification in the compromised liver. Drug dosage can be returned to usual levels only as liver function progresses toward normal.

Severity of cirrhosis varies greatly among individuals; therefore, nutrition therapy must be designed accordingly. Dietary modification should be considered in light of existing symptoms, and needs for each nutrient or class of nutrients should be examined individually. Nevertheless, one general principle does exist in the treatment of cirrhosis, namely, sparing of protein for regeneration of liver cells through the administration of a diet as high in calories as the patient can tolerate. No diet should supply less that 1600 kilocalories daily (27). Ordinarily a majority of these calories should be furnished by carbohydrate but occasionally impaired glucose tolerance occurs in cirrhosis. The diabetic state associated with liver disease apparently is caused by insulin resistance because levels of plasma insulin are found to be normal or even elevated (9).

Fat is usually supplied in moderate amounts. An abundance of normally occurring triglycerides, although an excellent source of calories, is inadvisable because of the dependence of fat digestion upon availability of bile. Also a high intake of fat may further complicate lipid infiltration of the liver. Too little fat on the other hand is just as undesirable because food palatability for the already anorectic patient is further decreased. The use of medium chain triglycerides may be helpful in supplying calories needed by cirrhotic patients, but they should be used with caution (28,29).

Protein is a crucial nutrient in the treatment of cirrhosis. On the one hand, sufficient protein is needed to promote hepatocyte regeneration and synthesis of albumin which may have been lost in ascitic fluid, while on the other hand, production of protein metabolites, such as ammonia, must be closely monitored in order to prevent encephalopathy.

Metabolic studies have indicated that in cirrhotic patients without hepatic coma a protein intake of approximately 50 grams daily (caloric limit of no less that 1600 kilocalories) is high enough for maintenance of nitrogen equilibrium and still low enough to prevent encephalopathy. Based upon these studies, Gabuzda and Shear (27) recommend the following protocol for determining the level of protein to be fed a cirrhotic patient:

1. Begin cirrhotic patient without evidence of encephalopathy on a diet containing 50 grams protein daily and providing no less than 1600 kilocalories.
2. If the patient remains free of neurological symptoms for approximately a week on an intake of 50 grams protein, increase the level of intake by 10 to 15 grams. After another week of no neurological symptoms, further increase the level of protein intake until the daily amount approaches 1 gram per kilogram of ideal body weight. Approximately 85 grams protein daily is considered the upper limit of a desirable intake because higher levels of protein may increase the risk/benefit ratio.
3. In the event of mild signs of hepatic encephalopathy, immediately drop the protein intake to approximately 35 grams, the lowest limit for achievement of nitrogen equilibrium. If neurological symptoms persist, neomycin may be administered in order to destroy those gut bacteria that produce ammonia either through deamination of amino acids or by breakdown of urea. If the patient is unable to tolerate the neomycin, then even further reduction of dietary protein may be necessary—20 grams or less daily. The principles of the low protein diet as proposed by Giordano, Giovannetti, and Maggiore for treatment of kidney failure

(Chapter 10) would apply in patients subject to hepatic encephalopathy. In liver failure the problem lies with the inability of the body to convert toxic ammonia to urea for excretion while in kidney failure the body is unable to excrete that urea which is formed. In both disease states, excessive deamination of amino acids is undesirable (see Chapter 3).

Another substance used to decrease ammonia absorption from the gastrointestinal tract is lactulose (marketed as Duphalac® or Cephulac®), a synthetic derivative of lactose that contains one molecule of galactose and one of fructose and cannot be metabolized by the body. Only a very small amount of the sugar is absorbed and whatever reaches the blood passes from the body unchanged via the kidneys within 24 hours. Although its exact mechanism of action is unclear, lactulose appears to exert its effect through acidifying bowel contents, thereby converting ammonia into ammonium ions. In addition, the fact that the colon contents are more acidic than is blood allows ammonia to diffuse from the blood into the colon where it is converted into the nondiffusible ammonium ion. The cathartic effect of lactulose also may be an important aspect of its action since the osmotic effect of the organic acids produced via bacterial metabolism (i.e., lactic acid and small amounts of acetic and formic acids) causes excretion of trapped ammonium ions and possibly other nitrogenous substances from the colon (30).

Providing sufficient high quality protein for hepatocyte regeneration without excessive production of ammonia is of extreme importance in the successful treatment of the cirrhotic patient. Consequently, the patient's tolerance for protein should be evaluated periodically and adjustments made whenever necessary or advisable.

Preformed ammonia has been found in considerable quantity in certain foods, such as cheeses, meats, and certain vegetables (32). Therefore, in the coma-prone cirrhotic patient some vegetables as well as high protein foods may need to be restricted. Amino acids also vary in their effect on blood ammonia concentration in patients with liver disease (33). Those amino acids whose amine groups must enter the urea cycle as free ammonia, for example, glycine, serine, threonine, glutamine, and histidine cause a much higher elevation of blood ammonia concentration than do those amino acids that through transamination feed their amine groups into the cycle via aspartic acid.

Some researchers, however, are not convinced that ammonia is the only culprit in the development of hepatic encephalopathy (34). They think that elevated serum ammonia may be a marker for detrimental deviations in protein metabolism, that is, reduced production of substances essential for normal brain metabolism. Because metabolism of central neurotransmitters has been shown to be controlled in part by certain amino acids, one suggested approach to prevention of hepatic encephalopathy is administration of parenteral amino acids in a pattern that would normalize plasma amino acids. Parenteral amino acids are administered in appropriate quantities so as to decrease plasma methionine and aromatic amino acids and to increase threonine, arginine, and the branch-chained amino acids. As much as 120 grams protein when administered as amino acids in the described pattern has been tolerated by patients with hepatic encephalopathy.

Another possible means by which protein nutriture may be improved in the patient with advanced liver disease is through the feeding of alpha-keto acids. Some of the excessive nitrogen that collects in hepatic failure possibly could be used via transamination to convert the alpha-keto acids into their corresponding alpha-amino acids.

Minerals (e.g., zinc, calcium, magnesium) are recommended in generous amounts for the patient with alcoholic liver disease (31). Nevertheless, the mineral of primary concern in the treatment of the cirrhotic patient with ascites is sodium. Hyperaldosteronism, which increases sodium reabsorption in the distal tubules of the kidneys, accompanies ascites. In addition, the proximal tubules as well become more permeable to sodium in the cirrhotic patient with ascites. How much sodium a particular patient can tolerate may be determined by charting his/her weight each morning. Rapid weight increase signifies fluid accumulation as a result of excessive sodium retention and mandates a reduced sodium intake. Sodium restriction because of its effect on food palatability should be no more severe than is necessary to prevent increased fluid retention. Most patients with ascites can tolerate approximately 500 mg sodium daily (35). Although fluid restriction is necessary only in patients who are oliguric or exhibit progressive hyponatremia, excessive fluid ingestion should be avoided. Generally fluid intake for the patient with ascites should approximate 1000 to 1500 ml daily or be equivalent to the fluid volume removed from the body through urinary excretion and insensible losses during the previous 24 hours.

Vitamins in amounts greater than the recommended dietary allowances are advisable for the patient with cirrhosis, particularly if the disease is a result of alcoholism. Excessive alcohol consumption usually precludes the ingestion of an adequate diet and also decreases absorption of many nutrients, including several vitamins, such as folic acid, thiamine, and vitamin B_{12}. Hepatic disease regardless of its etiology seriously affects vitamin metabolism because normally the liver serves as a storage depot for the fat-soluble vitamins and as the conversion site of thiamine and pyridoxine into their metabolically active forms and of vitamin D_3 into its more active metabolite, 25-hydroxycholecalciferol. Also the liver is the synthesis site for transport proteins necessary for the mobilization of vitamins from the liver to the cells.

The patient with a diseased liver who is unable to utilize vitamins efficiently will need a higher intake of the vitamins than is required by the normal person. Extra vitamins are also important for the protection of the existing healthy hepatocytes.

The consistency of the diet can be quite important when cirrhosis is complicated by gastroesophageal varices which are subject to rupture and consequently are life-threatening. For such patients the diet should be bland and low in fiber.

Getting the alcoholic or the patient with liver disease to eat a nourishing, high caloric diet is a very difficult task indeed. In the first place, the appetite of such patients is usually very poor and the appearance of a tray loaded with food is repugnant to them. Then, to make matters worse, cirrhotic patients with ascites are expected not only to consume large quantities of food but also to eat food made less palatable by sodium restriction.

The dietitian needs to visit these patients at least once every day in order to encourage them to take sufficient nourishment and to explain why any particular dietary restrictions are necessary. Also, dietary personnel should visit these patients before each meal in order to learn what allowable foods would be appetite-tempting and then to make sure that these foods are served attractively and at the appropriate temperature. The dietitian also should be sufficiently concerned about patients with liver disease to be sure that help is available during meal time should the patients be unable to feed themselves. Such concern is warranted for all patients but for patients who are anorectic yet need a high caloric diet, it is essential.

Getting all of the needed calories into the regularly scheduled meals is often an impossibility for patients with liver disease. High caloric supplements that are low in sodium are often necessary (see Table 12.4). Here again the supplements should be made as palatable as possible for the patient and whenever feasible the patient should be allowed his/her choice of supplements served. All members of the health team should be aware of the taste of all supplements prescribed for patients, and dietitians should know how *every* item of food tastes before it is served.

Total parenteral nutrition may prove of much benefit in future treatment of patients with hepatic failure (36). Sodium-controlled solutions have been formulated that can provide sufficient calories and nitrogen for protein synthesis in a volume appropriate for patients with hepatic failure. Also the pattern of the amino acids in the solutions is one that neither causes serum imbalanaces nor leads to encephalopathic symptoms as would occur were protein fed in an amount sufficient to supply an equivalent quantity of nitrogen (34).

Therapy for liver disease must of necessity rely primarily on supportive measures such as rest and appropriate diet in order to promote hepatic regeneration. Because most drugs are metabolized by enzymes located in the hepatic microsomes, few medications can be used safely in hepatic insufficiency.

Any drug therapy undertaken is used only for specific symptoms that would be subject to therapy, such as antibiotics for infections. Drug therapy must also be undertaken with caution for any disease state that might exist concomitantly in the patient with hepatic insufficiency because of possible alterations in hepatic function that might increase or decrease the metabolism of drugs. Among the categories of drugs the metabolism of which is altered by hepatic insufficiency are certain analgesics, antibiotics, anticonvulsants, cardiac agents, sedative-hypnotic, and some miscellaneous drugs. In some instances, these alterations in metabolism are predictable from laboratory tests while in others they are not. Examples of commonly used drugs the metabolism of which is altered by liver disease are given in the concluding paragraphs of this chapter and should alert the health professional to possible consequences of drug therapy that is not closely monitored in the patient with hepatic insufficiency.

The half-life of acetaminophen (Tylenol®) is increased from 2 hours to an average of 3.3 hours (37) while the half-life of meperidine (Demerol®) is doubled in patients with acute viral hepatitis and cirrhosis (38,39). With acetaminophen, a correlation exists between half-life and serum albumin levels (37) while with meperidine no correlation has been determined between liver function tests and half-life.

The plasma half-life of certain antibiotics is increased in the presence of liver dysfunction. The half-life of carbenicillin is almost doubled in patients with hepatic disease (39). The half-life of chloramphenicol has been reported by some investigators to increase (40,41) and by others to be unchanged (42). The increased half-life appears to correlate with elevated levels of albumin and bilirubin (40).

The anticonvulsant phenytoin has an unchanged half-life in patients with acute hepatitis (43). The reason for this effect is not well understood.

Cardiac agents used in the treatment of congestive heart failure are variably affected by hepatic disease. Digitoxin, which has a half-life of 8.1 days in normal subjects, has a half-life of 4.4 days in patients with chronic active hepatitis (44) while the half-life of digoxin is unchanged (45). A derivative of digoxin, methyldigoxin, has an increased half-life in patients with hepatitis suggesting that there is some alteration in demethylation pathways of the diseased liver (46). Propranolol (Inderal®) has a prolonged half-life in patients with hepatic dysfunction (47).

The half-life of most sedative-hypnotics is increased in patients with liver disease. In patients with chronic liver disease in which plasma albumin levels are less than 3.5 mg %, the half-life of amobarbital was increased from 21 hours to 39 hours (48). The rate of amobarbital metabolism can be correlated with the degree of bromsulphalein retention but not with other laboratory tests. Other barbiturates whose half-life are increased due to liver disease include hexobarbital (49), pentobarbital (50), and phenobarbital (51). Other sedative-hypnotics such as diazepam (Valium®) and meprobamate also have a prolonged half-life in patients with liver disease (52,53).

Miscellaneous agents whose half-life are prolonged by liver disease include theophylline (54), lidocaine (37,55), and prednisone (56). Agents whose half-life is not affected by liver disease include disulfiram (Antabuse®) (57), chlorpromazine (Thorazine®) (58), and oxazepam (59).

The inability of the patient with liver disease to metabolize normally many of the more commonly used drugs makes it imperative that all drugs be administered with extreme care to patients with active liver disease or chronic dysfunction. Although none of the above mentioned drugs are contraindicated in patients with liver disease, doses must be decreased or given at less frequent intervals in order to prevent the occurrence of toxic side effects.

CASE STUDY: LAENNEC'S CIRRHOSIS

A white male, aged 38 years, was admitted to the hospital emergency room in apparent alcohol withdrawal syndrome. The patient stood 5 feet 10 inches tall, weighed 148 lbs, and gave the general appearance of being malnourished. A medical history taken by the clinical pharmacist indicated that the patient had a 20-year history of alcohol consumption with periods of sobriety of a few months' duration scattered throughout the 20-year period. For the past four years his alcohol consumption had averaged one quart per day and he had been treated for alcohol withdrawal four times during the past two years. On admission, the patient stated that it had been 12 hours since his last drink. He was showing initial alcohol abstinence syndrome symptoms which included profuse sweating, cramping of the gastrointestinal tract, diarrhea, heart rate of 85 beats per minute, and blood pressure of 160/98. His respiration was rapid and shallow and his body temperature was 100.5° F. Tests made on blood drawn at time of admission revealed the following values:

Albumin: 2.2 (norm 4.0–5.5 gm/dl)

Total Bilirubin: 9.1 (norm 0.1–1.2 mg/dl)

LDH: 400 (norm 71–207 I.U./l)

Magnesium: 1.2 (norm 1.5–2.5 mEq/l)

Calcium: 4.1 (norm 4.5–5.3 mEq/l)

Potassium: 3.3 (norm 3.8–5.0 mEq/l)

Sodium: 130 (norm 136–142 mEq/l)

Treatment of this patient was undertaken by the interdisciplinary team consisting of the physician, clinical pharmacist, dietitian, and mental health counselor. Objectives for treatment of the patient, as outlined by the team, included immediate treatment of withdrawal symptoms and prevention of convulsions; further diagnostic tests, and complete physical examination to determine the extent of damage to the liver; dietary management to improve the general physical state of the patient; and counseling concerning alternatives to excessive alcohol consumption.

Due to the apparent serious symptoms of alcohol withdrawal, the patient immediately was placed on a therapeutic regimen that was directed toward the administration of a drug that substitutes for alcohol in the body and prevents the withdrawal symptoms from becoming too severe. This drug would be administered in decreasing dosage over a period of five to eight days, until the patient was drug free. The drug chosen for this purpose was diazepam (Valium®). Because this drug is metabolized by the liver, the dosage was carefully titrated to make sure that the patient was not overdosed. Ancillary drug therapy included multiple vitamins, vitamin B_{12} injection, thiamine, magnesium by injection and an intravenously administered 5% dextrose solution. In addition, a 120 gram protein, high caloric, sodium-restricted (2 gm Na) diet was ordered for the patient, to be begun immediately.

A more complete physical exmination of the patient on the following day revealed an enlarged liver, decreased renal function, and the presence of ascites. The skin and eyes had a very definite yellowish tint. Based on these findings, a diagnosis of Laennec's (alcoholic) cirrhosis was made by the physician.

Questions

1. Would decreased serum electrolytes be consistent with chronic alcoholism?
2. What connection exists among a high bilirubin, high LDH, and low albumin?
3. Should the intravenous dextrose solution have been administered to this patient initially?
4. Why were vitamin supplements included in this patient's therapy?
5. Why was a high protein diet prescribed for this patient? Was 120 grams protein an appropriate level before a complete physical examination had been made on the patient?
6. In light of the low serum sodium, was sodium restriction advisable?

Discussion

The modern clinical laboratory has at its disposal instruments that are capable of performing numerous tests in a much shorter period of time than it would take the technologists to conduct the tests manually. The tests that are usually selected to be "run" on such instruments have a broad clinical significance, meaning that they can be of importance in diagnosing a variety of systemically unrelated diseases. The physician, therefore, frequently requests a screening "profile" of such tests on admitted patients.

Chronic alcoholism, in addition to its well-known and profound effect on liver cells, also exerts renal manifestations as well. Ethanol-induced renal losses of serum electrolytes, commonly observed in such cases, is attributed to the alcohol's interference with the reabsorptive process in the kidney tubules.

Among the many important metabolic functions of the liver are the excretion of bilirubin, derived from the breakdown of heme, and the synthesis of serum albumin. Aged or defective red cells are normally trapped and degraded by the cells of the reticuloendothelial system, and the heme portion of the hemoglobin in the red cells is catabolized to bilirubin. The liver cells conjugate the bilirubin delivered to it with glucuronic acid, and then excrete the conjugate into the bile. The diseased cells of the cirrhotic liver lose this ability, resulting in the accumulation of bilirubin in the bloodstream and tissues, causing jaundice. The reduced synthesis of albumin, characteristic of the cirrhotic syndrome, compounds the bilirubin problem because serum bilirubin is transported via albumin. As the albumin level falls, the accumulating bilirubin divested of some of its serum "carrier," is deposited to a great extent in the tissues. As serum bilirubin concentration approaches 18 to 20 mg/dl, brain damage may result due to the excessive deposition of bilirubin in the brain cells. The enzyme, lactate dehydrogenase, is produced in numerous tissues throughout the body and therefore the determination of total LDH. An elevated LDH generally indicates damaged liver or heart tissue. In order to determine which organ is involved, it becomes necessary to separate and quantitate the isoenzymes of the LDH because the individual isoenzymes have a greater organ specificity than the total enzyme.

For this patient with severely compromised liver function, diazepam was used cautiously due to the possibility that the decreased rate of metabolism might lead to toxicity. It was appropriate that no other drugs were used in this patient's treatment. The use of the intravenous 5 percent dextrose solution should have been avoided in this patient until further evaluation had been completed because most alcoholics exhibiting withdrawal symptoms are overhydrated rather than dehydrated. The vitamin and magnesium therapy was appropriate because these body constituents are usually quite depleted in the alcoholic patient. However, the magnesium injections should be discontinued after two days because hypermagnesemia may be as deleterious as hypomagnesemia.

Because liver damage was suspected, the physician had ordered a high protein, high caloric diet so that liver cell regeneration would be promoted. The dietitian, however, had some concern about the level of protein ordered, particularly after the diagnosis of cirrhosis had been made. She suggested that the physician lower the protein content of the diet to

85 grams while keeping calories at a level that would allow tissue synthesis to occur. (The patient even with ascites was 18 lbs below his ideal body weight.) The dietitian's concern about the protein level was threefold: (1) a very high protein, moderate fat diet may have little appeal for the anorectic patient, (2) the risk of such a high protein diet might outweigh its benefit should the patient's liver be damaged to the point that urea production was compromised and/or (3) excessive protein metabolites might accumulate in the blood due to impaired renal excretion. So long as caloric intake is adequate to spare protein for tissue synthesis, little advantage appears to be gained by increasing protein intake beyond 85 grams daily. Even 85 grams may be too high a protein intake for many cirrhotic patients because of the danger of encephalopathy (see pps. 286–287). Tolerance to dietary protein should be closely monitored using appropriate laboratory tests, such as serum ammonia and SUN (Serum Urea Nitrogen). Although the patient had a low serum sodium, excessive fluid was being held in his body (ascites). In order to decrease fluid retention, sodium restriction is nearly always necessary. A sodium restriction more severe than 2 grams (85 to 90 mEq) daily might be more effective in decreasing fluid retention, but it also would make food less palatable. Knowing how difficult it is to get an alcoholic to eat, the dietitian wanted his food to be as attractive and palatable as possible and therefore was eager that sodium restriction remain at 2 grams daily.

After visiting the patient and learning his preferences, the dietitian decided to supplement his meals with chilled dried fruit compotes because the patient particularly liked fruits and the dried fruits could add extra calories. In order to encourage the patient to eat as much as possible, the dietitian had dietary personnel visit the patient each day to determine just what allowed foods and supplements he would find most tempting to his appetite. In addition, procedures were initiated to monitor protein/calorie intake on a daily basis in order to assess the patient's progress and begin to plan for the patient's management after discharge.

REFERENCES

1. Crouch, J. E. and J. R. McClintic. *Human Anatomy and Physiology*. 2nd ed. New York: John Wiley and Sons, 1976; pp. 617–621.
2. Bell, G. H., D. Emslie-Smith, and C. R. Paterson. *Textbook of Physiology and Biochemistry*. 9th ed. New York: Churchill Livingstone, 1976; pp. 232–238.
3. Harper, H. A. *Review of Physiological Chemistry*. 15th ed. Los Altos, CA: Lange Medical Publishers, 1975; pp. 394–403.
4. Guyton, A. G. *Textbook of Medical Physiology*. 5th ed. Philadelphia: W.B. Saunders, 1976; pp. 375–378.
5. Kappas, A. and A. P. Alvares. How the liver metabolizes foreign substances, *Scientific American* **232**: 22, June 1975.

6. Guyton, A. G. *Textbook of Medical Physiology.* 5th ed. Philadelphia: W.B. Saunders, 1976; pp. 936–944.

7. Leevy, C. M., A. Thompson, and H. Baker. Vitamins and liver injury. *Am. J. Clin. Nutr.* **23:** 493, Apr. 1970.

8. Guyton, A. G. *Textbook of Medical Physiology.* 5th ed. Philadelphia: W.B. Saunders, 1976; pp. 56–66.

9. Alpers, D. H. and K. J. Isselbacher. Derangements of hepatic metabolism. In *Harrison's Principles of Internal Medicine,* G. W. Thorn et al., eds. 8th ed. New York: McGraw-Hill, 1977; pp. 1576–1579.

10. Rothchild, M. A., M. Oratz, and S. S. Schneider. Abnormalities in serum protein metabolism and amino acid effects. In *Modern Nutrition in Health and Disease,* Goodhart and Shils, eds. 5th ed. Philadelphia: Lea and Febiger, 1973; pp. 89–98.

11. Lieber, C. S. Alcohol, nutrition and the liver. *Am. J. Clin. Nutr.* **26:** 1163, Nov. 1973.

12. Montgomery, R., R. L. Dryer, T. W. Conway, and A. A. Spector. *Biochemistry: A Case-Oriented Approach.* 2nd ed. St. Louis: C.V. Mosby, 1977; pp. 696–697.

13. Lieber, C. S., D. P. Jones, L. M. DeCarli. Effects of prolonged ethanol intake: Production of fatty liver despite adequate diets. *J. Clin. Inv.* **44:** 1009, 1965.

14. Lieber, C. S., L. M. DeCarli, and E. Rubin. Sequential production of fatty liver, hepatitis and cirrhosis in sub-human primates fed ethanol with adequate diets. *Proc. Nat. Acad. Sci. U.S.A.* **72:** 437, 1975.

15. Lieber, C. S. The metabolism of alcohol. *Sci. Am.* **234:** 25, Mar. 1976.

16. Lieber. C. S. Alcohol and nutrition. *Nutrition News* **39:** 9, Oct. 1976.

17. Shaw, S. and C. S. Lieber. Nutrition and alcoholic disease. *Nutrition in Disease.* Columbus: Ross Laboratories, Mar. 1978.

18. Tietz, N. W. *Fundamentals of Clinical Chemistry.* 2nd ed. Philadelphia: W.B. Saunders, 1976; p. 1028.

19. Skrede, S., H. E. Solberg, J. P. Blomhoff, and E. Gjone. Bile acids measured in serum during fasting as a test for liver disease. *Clin. Chem.* **24:** 1095, 1978.

20. Melnick, J. L., G. R. Dreesman, and F. B. Hollinger. Viral hepatitis. *Sci. Am.* **237:** 44, July 1977.

21. Grady, G. F. Transfusions and hepatitis: update in 1978. *N. Eng. J. Med.* **298:**1413, June 1978.

22. Wands, J. R., R. S. Koff, and K. J. Isselbacher. Acute hepatitis. In *Harrison's Principles of Internal Medicine,* G. W. Thorn et al., eds. 8th ed. New York: McGraw-Hill, 1977; pp. 1590–1600.

23. Hoofnagle, J. H., L. B. Seeff, Z. B. Bales, H. J. Zimmerman, and V. A. Zimmerman. Hepatitis Cooperative Study Group: Type B hepatitis after transfusion with blood containing antibody to hepatitis B core antigen. *N. Eng. J. Med.* **298:** 1379, June 1978.

24. Bank, S., S. J. Saunders, I. N. Marks, B. H. Novis, and G. O. Barbezat. Gastrointestinal and hepatic diseases. In *Drug Treatment Principles and Practice of Clinical Pharmacology and Therapeutics,* G. S. Avery, ed. Acton, MA: Publishing Sciences Group, Inc., 1977; pp. 506–561.

25. LaMont, J. T. and K. J. Isselbacher. Cirrhosis. In *Harrison's Principles of Internal Medicine,* G. W. Thorn, et al., eds. 8th ed. New York: McGraw-Hill, 1977; pp. 1604–1615.

26. Stone, W. D., N. R. K. Islam, and A. Paton. The natural history of cirrhosis. *Quarterly J. of Med.* **37:** 119, 1968.

27. Gabuzda, G. J. and L. Shear. Metabolism of dietary protein in hepatic cirrhosis. *Am. J. Clin. Nutr.* **23:** 479, 1970.

28. Malagelada, J. R., W. G. Linscheer, U. M. T. Houtsmuller, A. J. Vergrosen, M. Shab, and F. L. Iber. Effect of medium-chain triglycerides on fatty acid composition in alcoholics with or without cirrhosis. *Am. J. Clin. Nutr.* **26:** 738, July 1973.

29. Lincheer, W. G. Malabsorption in cirrhosis. *Am. J. Clin. Nutr.* **23:** 488, 1970.

30. Oddis, J. A., ed. American Hospital Formulary Service. Washington: Am. Soc. Hosp. Pharmacists, **2:** 40:10, 1978.

31. Shaw, S. and C. S. Lieber. Alcoholism. In *Nutritional Support of Medical Practice,* Schneider, Anderson and Coursin, eds. New York: Harper and Row, 1977; pp. 202–221.

32. Rudman, D., R. B. Smith, A. A. Salam, W. D. Warren, J. T. Galambos, and J. Wenger. Ammonia content of food. *Am. J. Clin. Nutr.* **26:** 487, May 1973.

33. Rudman, D., J. T. Galambos, R. B. Smith, A. A. Salam, and W. D. Warren. Comparison of the effect of various amino acids upon the blood ammonia concentration of patients with liver disease. *Am. J. Clin. Nutr.* **26:** 916, Sept. 1973.

34. Fischer, J. E. Amino acid infusion in hepatic encephalopathy. *Dietitic Currents—Ross Timesaver* **3:** 5, Mar./Apr. 1976.

35. Summerskill, W. H. J., D. E. Barnardo, and W. P. Baldus. Disorders of water and electrolyte metabolism in liver disease. *Am. J. Clin. Nutr.* **23:** 499, Apr. 1970.

36. Host, W. R. F., O. Serlin, and B. F. Rush. Hyperalimentation in cirrhotic patients, *Am. J. Surgery* **123:** 57, 1972.

37. Finlayson, N. D. C., et al. Antipyrine, lidocaine and para-acetamol metabolism in chronic liver diseas. *Gastroenterology* **67:** 790, 1974.

38. McHorse, T. S., et al. Effect of acute viral hepatitis in man on the disposition and elimination of meperidine. *Gastroenterology* **68:** 775, 1975.

39. Hoffman, T. A., et al. Pharmacodynamics of carbenicillin in hepatic and renal failure. *Ann. Int. Med.* **73:** 173, 1970.

40. Azzollini, F., et al. Elimination of chloramphenicol and thiamphenicol in subjects with cirrhosis of the liver. *Int. J. Clin. Pharmacol.* **6:** 130, 1972.

41. Kunin, C. M., et al. Persistence of antibiotics in blood of patients with acute renal failure, II. Chloramphenicol and its metabolic products in the blood of patients with severe renal disease or hepatic cirrhosis. *J. Clin. Invest.* **38:** 1498, 1959.

42. Held, H., et al. Drug metabolism in acute and chronic liver disease. *Digestion* **4:** 151, 1971.

43. Blaschke, T. F., et al. Influence of acute viral hepatitis on phenytoin kinetics and protein binding. *Clin. Pharmacol. Ther.* **17:** 685, 1975.

44. Storstein, L., et al. Digitoxin pharmacokinetics in chronic active hepatitis. *Digestion* **12:** 353, 1975.

45. Marcus, F. L., et al. The metabolism of tritiated digoxin in cirrhotic patients. *Gastroenterology* **47:** 517, 1964.

46. Zilly, W., et al. Pharmacokinetics and metabolism of digoxin and b-methyldi-

goxin-12a-³H in patients with acute hepatitis. *Clin. Pharmacol. Ther.* **17:** 302, 1975.

47. Branch, R. A., et al. The pharmacokinetics of (+)-propranolol in normal subjects and patients with chronic liver disease. *Brit. J. Clin. Pharm.* **2:** 183P, 1975.

48. Mawer, G. E., et al. Metabolism of amylobarbitone in patients with chronic liver disease. *Brit. J. Pharmacol.* **44:** 549, 1972.

49. Breimer, D. D., et al. Pharmacokinetics of hexobarbital in acute hepatitis and after apparent recovery. *Clin. Pharmacol. Ther.* **18:** 433, 1975.

50. Ossenberg, F. W., et al. Pentobarbital pharmacokinetics in cirrhosis. *Digestion* **8:** 448, 1973.

51. Alvin, J., et al. The effect of liver disease in man of the disposition phenobarbital. *J. Pharmacol. Exp. Ther.* **192:** 224, 1975.

52. Klotz, U. et al. The effects of age and liver disease on the disposition and elimination of diazepam in adult man. *J. Clin. Invest.* **55:** 347, 1975.

53. Closson, R. G. and L. Y. Young. Diseases of the liver. In *Applied Therapeutics for Clinical Pharmacists,* M. A. Koda-Kimble, B. S. Katcher, and L. Y. Young, eds. 2nd ed. San Francisco: Applied Therapeutics, Inc., 1978; pp. 323 –346.

54. Piafsky, K. M., et al. Disposition of theophylline in chronic liver disease. *Clin. Pharmacol. Ther.* **17:** 241, 1975..

55. Thompson, P. D., et al. Lidocaine pharmacokinetics in advanced heart failure, liver disease and renal failure in humans. *Ann. Int. Med.* **78:** 499, 1973.

56. Powell, L. W., et al. Corticosteroids in liver disease: Studies on the biological conversion of prednisone to prednisolone and plasma protein binding. *Gut.* **13:** 690, 1972.

57. Shamszad, M., et al. Metabolism of ³⁵S-disulfiram in normals and in patients with liver disease. *Gastroenterology* **68:** 983, 1975.

58. Maxwell, J. D., et al. Plasma disappearance and cerebral effects of chlorpromazine in cirrhotics. *Clin. Sci.* **43:** 143, 1972.

59. Shull, H. J., et al. Normal disposition of oxazepam in acute viral hepatitis and cirrhosis. *Ann. Int. Med.* **4:** 420, 1976.

RECOMMENDED READINGS

Rosen, H. M., N. Yoshimura, J. M. Hodgman, and J. E. Fischer. Plasma amino acid patterns in hepatic encephalopathy of differing etiology. *Gastroenterology* **72:** 483, 1977.

Results of a study of plasma aminograms in patients with hepatic encephalopathy suggest that amino acid patterns vary according to etiology of the disease and, therefore, can help in determining effiacious therapy.

Soeters, P. B. and J. E. Fischer. Insulin, glucagon, amino acid imbalance and hepatic encephalopathy. *Lancet* **ii:** 880, 1976.

A possible explanation for development of hepatic encephalopathy is a decreased insulin/glucagon ratio resulting in an elevation of circulating aromatic amino acids.

CHAPTER 9

Nutrition in
Inherited Disease*

In inherited metabolic disorders treatment is so specific and outcomes so dependent on individualized therapy that attention to detail is exceedingly important. Because of this specificity, concepts in management have been described and illustrations given in various sections of this chapter. General principles such as appropriateness of timing for introduction of solid foods, infection-related catabolism, and osmolality of formula have been described in relation to one disease but are applicable to other diseases as well. In fact, in no other group of disorders are the science and art of nutrition so intertwined as in inherited metabolic diseases. A firm foundation in the science of nutrition is required in order to treat artfully those infants and children with inherited metabolic disorders because lack of knowledge may lead to mental retardation or even death.

CONCEPTS OF HUMAN GENETICS

Biochemical differences in individuals are due to differences in proteins and to types and amounts of substances made under the direction of certain of these proteins (enzymes). Protein (enzyme) synthesis is under the direction of genes. Genes reside in the chromosomes and are made up of deoxyribonucleic acid (DNA). DNA consists of phosphoric acid, deoxyribose, and purine and pyrimidine bases in repeating units. The sequence of these purine and pyrimidine bases in DNA determines the sequence of amino acids in a protein by directing the sequence of bases in messenger ribonucleic acid (mRNA). The bases in mRNA are the template for protein (enzyme) synthesis. Three bases in a particular sequence are required to direct the placement of one specific amino acid in a polypeptide chain (1) (see Chapter 1, pps. 10–11).

* This chapter was written by Phyllis B. Acosta, Dr. P.H., R.D., Associate Professor, Emory University School of Medicine, and Nutrition Consultant for Collaborative Study of Children treated for Phenylketonuria, Children's Hospital, Los Angeles, California, and was supported in part by Grant No. MCT000466, Bureau of Community Health Services, Health Services Administration, Department of Health, Education and Welfare, Rockville, Maryland.

One gene directs the synthesis of one polypeptide. Structural genes determine the primary structure of a polypeptide while *control* genes govern the expression of structural genes. Control genes are of two types: operator and regulator. Operator genes initiate the synthesis of mRNA while regulator genes control activity of operator genes (1).

Inborn errors of metabolism may arise via two major mechanisms. The first is through mutations in control genes (operator or regulator) and leads to synthesis of no protein (enzyme). The second is through mutations in structural genes and may lead to synthesis of no protein (enzyme) or synthesis of a protein with altered structure. Base replacement, deletion, insertion, or inversion account for the changes in the structural genes leading to synthesis of no enzymes or to synthesis of enzymes that may be fully or partially active or perhaps totally inactive (1).

Genes reside in chromosomes. *Somatic* (body) cells have two of each type of chromosome and are called *diploid. Gametes* (germ cells) which have one of each type of chromosome are called *haploid*. The normal diploid chromosome number of man is 46. The sex chromosome constitution of the male is designated as XY; of the female as XX. In addition, there are 22 pairs of autosomes. Genes residing on the X or Y chromosome are said to be sex-linked. Genes residing on autosomes are said to be autosomal or nonsex-linked. Genes determine an individual's *genotype,* while his/her *phenotype* is an expression of genotype as influenced by environment (1).

The three major modes of inheritance are autosomal dominant, autosomal recessive, and sex-linked. A gene that is fully expressed when in the heterozygous combination, if it occurs on other than the sex chromosome, is said to be *autosomal dominant*. With this mode of transmission at least one parent of an affected individual will carry the gene and if the gene has high *penetrance* that parent will also be affected. With autosomal dominant transmission the gene may be expressed in only one sex but it will be transmitted by either sex to children of either sex. Approximately one-half the children of an affected parent will be affected (1,2).

If the trait is only expressed in the homozygous combination it is *recessive*. For a rare gene the parents of an affected individual may be related more often than in the general population. The affected individuals in a family will nearly always be in a single sibship. Approximately one-fourth of the children born as a result of the mating of two heterozygotes (carriers) will be affected, about one-half will be carriers and about one-fourth will be normal. The probabilities are the same for *each* pregnancy. Homozygous males and females should occur in equal numbers (1,2).

In sex-linked inheritance, in males, a single mutant gene will be expressed because there is no normal allele to function. In females, the mutant gene usually must be present in both X chromosomes in order for the trait to be expressed. X-linked genes in heterozygous females have variable expression (1,2).

GENERAL PRINCIPLES OF GENETIC DISEASE MANAGEMENT

Individual enzymes, produced under the direction of individual genes, catalyze individual steps in metabolic sequences as noted in the following reaction sequence:

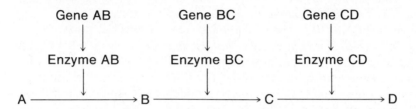

There are four possible effects resulting from nonfunctional enzyme CD in the above reaction sequence:

1. Lack of formation of D or some compound derived only from D. For example, in phenylketonuria (PKU) when phenylalanine cannot be catalyzed to tyrosine, melanin synthesis is depressed because of lack of tyrosine, a melanin precursor. If product D normally functions in feedback control, overproduction of another product may occur because D is not present in amounts necessary to function in feedback.
2. Accumulation of C, the immediate precursor of the blocked reaction. In PKU, blood phenylalanine levels increase because phenylalanine cannot be hydroxylated to form tyrosine (Fig. 9.1).
3. Accumulation of A or B, remote precursors of the blocked reaction. If the reactions preceding the block are freely reversible, a precursor other than that just proximal to the block may accumulate. This is illustrated by homocystinuria where not only homocystine but also methionine accumulate (Fig. 9.2).
4. Increased production of alternative normal products through little-used metabolic pathways. As illustrated in Figure 9.1, when phenylalanine is not hydroxylated to form tyrosine, phenylpyruvic, phenylacetic, and phenyllactic acids are produced in greater than normal amounts.

There are eight approaches to therapy of inherited metabolic disease and the appropriate approach is dependent on consequences resulting from the enzyme defect:

1. Correction of the biochemical abnormality. This correction often involves both a reduction of substrate and replacement of the missing metabolic product. In PKU for example, not only must substrate (phenylalanine) be limited, but the product (tyrosine) must also be provided in adequate amounts.
2. Depletion of stored substances. Treatment of gout with uricosuric agents leads to lower blood uric acid levels. The tissue deposits of uric acid salts are then mobilized.
3. Use of metabolic inhibitors. Allopurinol inhibits xanthine oxidase and decreases production of uric acid in gout.
4. Supplying the missing protein. In cystic fibrosis, the exocrine pancreas does not function in a normal manner to produce and secrete digestive enzymes. Administration of these pancreatic enzymes partially corrects the digestive defect in cystic fibrosis.
5. Artificial induction of enzyme production. If the structural gene is intact, but the control gene is not functional, it should be possible to "turn on" the structural gene. This has been done *in vitro* in cultured fibroblasts from a patient with orotic aciduria by treatment with 6-azauridine.
6. Induction of nonfunctional enzyme activity. Structural abnormalities in the apoenzyme impair its ability to bind with the coenzyme required for enzyme activity. Often, the binding defect is not absolute and the apoenzyme retains some binding capacity at abnormally high tissue levels of the coenzyme. It may be necessary to provide patients with this type of binding disorder up to 100 times the normal vitamin requirement for the apoenzyme to bind with the coenzyme. Vitamin B_6 dependency syndrome is illustrative because seizures occur without massive doses of pyridoxine.
7. Correction of the underlying defect in DNA so that body can manufacture its own functionally normal enzymes. This experimental approach has great possibility for the future, but has not been beneficial in any situations in humans in which it has been tested.
8. Limiting the frequency of undesirable genes through providing care to exclude consanguineous marriages and developing tests for the heterozygous or carrier states.

DISORDERS OF AMINO ACID AND NITROGEN METABOLISM

Aromatic Amino Acids

The essential amino acid, phenylalanine, may be utilized for two major purposes: tissue protein synthesis and hydroxylation to form tyrosine.

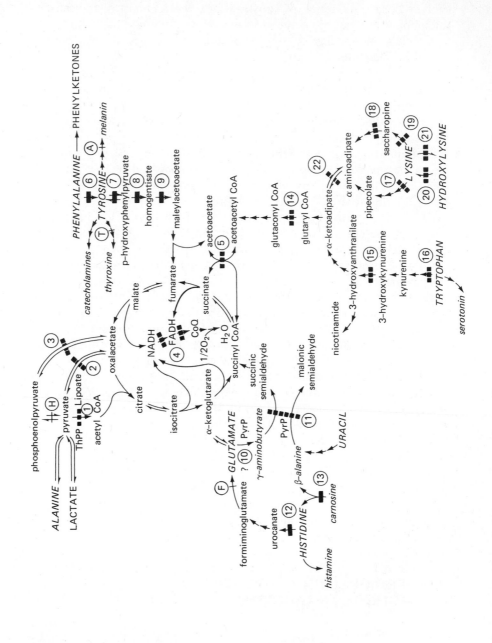

Figure 9.1 Metabolic map of citric acid metabolism and related pathways of catabolism of some amino acids. The conversion of triose phosphates via pyruvate to acetyl CoA is at the *top left* leading to the citric acid cycle. The glutamate cycle, with the important biogenic amine γ-aminobutyric acid is included, as well as β-alanine and its metabolism. The catabolism of phenylalanine and tyrosine are at the *top right* indicating pathways of pigment and hormone formation from tyrosine; that of tryptophan and lysine are at the *bottom,* including the relation of serotonin, 5-hydroxytryptamine, to tryptophan. Within the citric acid cycle is diagrammed the oxidative pathway of energy metabolism by which protons are transferred from NADH to molecular oxygen. Disorders of glycine and proline catabolism have been omitted.

Solid bars indicate the sites of enzyme defects; interrupted bars designate postulated blocks. The sites of metabolic blocks causing albinism are labeled A, and defects of thyroid hormone synthesis are labeled T. The symbol F locates the site of action of formiminofolate transferase on histidine catabolism. (Reprinted by permission of Y. Edward Hsia, M.D.)

	Enzyme	Deficient in
1.	Pyruvate dehydrogenase complex	? Lactic acidosis ? Thiamine responsive hyperalaninemic hyperpyruvicacidemia ? Leigh's subacute necrotizing encephalopathy
2.	Pyruvate carboxylase	? Leigh's subacute necrotizing encephalopathy
3.	Phosphoenolpyruvate carboxykinase	Phosphoenolpyruvate carboxykinase deficiency
4.	Undetermined	Enzyme defects of the respiratory chain
5.	Succinyl CoA-3-ketoacid CoA transferase	Succinyl CoA-3-ketoacid CoA transferase deficiency
6.	Phenylalanine hydroxylase	Phenylketonuria and variants
7.	Cytosol tyrosineaminotransferase	Hypertyrosinemia
8.	p-Hydroxyphenylpyruvate oxidase	Hereditary tyrosinemia and variants
9.	Homogentisic acid oxidase	Alcaptonuria
10.	Glutamate decarboxylase	? Pyridoxine-dependent seizures
11.	? β-Alanine aminotransferase ? γ-Aminobutyric aminotransferase	β-Alaninemia
12.	Histidase	Histidinemia
13.	Carnosinase	Carnosinemia
14.	? Glutaryl CoA dehydrogenase	Glutaricacidemia

15. Kynureninase   Xanthurenicaciduria
                                                                 3-Hydroxykynureninuria
16. Undetermined   Tryptophanuria
17. Lysine dehydrogenase   Periodic hyperlysinemia
18. Undetermined   Saccharopinuria
19. Lysine α-ketoglutarate reduc-   Persistent lysinemia with pipecola-
    tase   temia
20. Undetermined   Hydroxylysinuria
21. Lysine hydroxylase   Ehlers-Danlos syndrome variant
22. ? δ-aminoadipate transami-   Aminoadipic aciduria
    nase

The hydroxylation reaction requires phenylalanine hydroxylase, tetrahydrobiopterin, dihydropteridine reductase, dihydrofolate reductase, and NADH + H$^+$ (Fig. 9.1). In the normal adult approximately 90 percent of phenylalanine is hydroxylated to form tyrosine. Mass spectrometry and study of patients with phenylketonuria (PKU) provided information on other pathways available for phenylalanine metabolism. These normal pathways, outlined in Figure 9.1, are utilized for metabolism of minimal amounts of phenylalanine in the normal individual but become of more importance when phenylalanine cannot be hydroxylated to tyrosine.

Tyrosine may be used in five ways. These include protein synthesis and synthesis of catecholamines, melanin pigment, and thyroid hormones. Tyrosine also provides energy when catabolized through para-hydroxyphenyl pyruvate to fumarate and acetoacetate. Enzymes required in tyrosine's degradative pathway include tyrosine aminotransferase, p-hydroxyphenyl-pyruvic acid oxidase and homogentisic acid oxidase (Fig. 9.1).

Phenylketonuria (PKU). This disorder, inherited by an autosomal recessive mode, was discovered in 1934 by Folling (3) and was found to be due to deficient or inactive phenylalanine hydroxylase (4). The classic form of PKU, which affects one person in every 12,000 to 15,000 live births in the United States, if untreated leads to severe mental retardation, abnormal electroencephalogram, eczema, musty odor, and hyperactivity. Nevertheless, the life span of noninstitutionalized PKU patients appears to be normal.

The cause for mental retardation is not known, but several theories have been postulated. Among these are deficient myelination, abnormalities in brain proteolipids (5) and/or proteins (6), and tyrosine deficiency (7). Protein synthesis in the brain was shown to be depressed (6), probably due to altered amino acid transport.

Screening procedures developed by Guthrie (8) for early detection of PKU led to an awareness of the heterogeneity in phenylalanine metabolism. Based on phenylalanine loading studies with natural protein, Blaskovics (9) reported eight types of hyperphenylalaninemia, several of which are benign and do not require treatment. Others, however, are often lethal and fail to respond to therapy for classical PKU (10–12). Data in Table 9.1 classify the hyperphenylalaninemias.

Treatment of the classic form of PKU requires a phenylalanine-restricted diet (13). In order that near-normal intelligence may be achieved, diet must be instituted and control of blood phenylalanine level attained by one month of age (14). Newborn screening in most of the 50 states, in conjunction with aggressive approaches to retrieval and diagnosis, has led to early institution of diet therapy. To be successful, state-mandated screening programs must allow for easy collection and rapid evaluation of specimens while providing an organized, efficient retrieval system of babies having positive screening tests. With the present early discharge from hospital and nursery of both mother and baby after delivery the phenylalanine level considered to be positive becomes exceedingly important. Patients with initial blood phenylalanine levels of 4 to 8 mg/dl should have the test repeated immediately. If the initial or follow-up screening test is greater than 8 mg/dl, diagnostic blood and urine studies should be conducted on a known phenylalanine intake (180 mg/kg/day) from natural protein sources for a two to three day period (15).

Patients with blood phenylalanine levels of greater than 20 mg/dl accompanied by urinary excretion of phenylpyruvic and orthohydroxyphenylacetic acid and phenylacetylglutamine require prompt treatment with a phenylalanine-restricted diet. In those patients requiring treatment, a "challenge" to diagnosis should be carried out at three months and again at one year of age. The same procedures are employed as those used at time of diagnosis (15).

Objectives of diet management in PKU are three-fold:

1. Normal mental development.
2. Normal physical development.
3. Prevention of hunger and associated problems.

The most rapid decline of blood phenylalanine levels can be achieved by feeding normal dilution Lofenalac® without an added phenylalanine source. This approach should be used only if the blood phenylalanine level is monitored daily because phenylalanine deficiency may occur rapidly. A safer approach to initial therapy is to provide phenylalanine to meet minimal requirements until blood phenylalanine levels of 2 to 10 mg/dl are reached. One hundred fifty to 200 mg phenylalanine daily should allow a rapid decline in blood phenylalanine without excessive danger of deficiency (16,17).

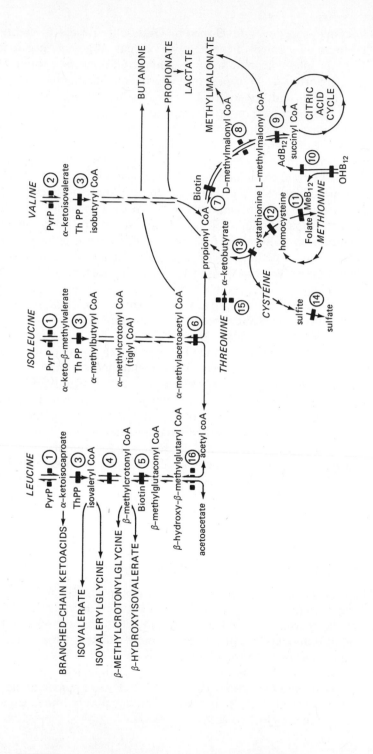

Figure 9.2 Metabolic map of branched-chain amino acid and sulfur amino acid catabolism. The catabolism of leucine, isoleucine, and valine descend to common intermediary metabolites from the *top*. Organic acids and other compounds excreted in these metabolic disorders are indicated on the left or right. The catabolism of threonine and methionine, with the pathways of vitamin B_{12} coenzyme synthesis, are *below*.

Metabolic blocks at six, seven, eight, nine, and ten have all produced the syndrome of ketotic hyperglycinemia. (Reprinted by permission of Y. Edward Hsia, M.D.)

Enzyme reaction	Deficient in
1. ? Branched-chain amino acid transaminase	Hyperleucine–isoleucinemia
2. ? Valine transaminase	Hypervalinemia
3. Branched-chain ketoacid decarboxylase complex	Maple syrup urine disease and variants
4. Isovaleryl CoA dehydrogenase	Isovalericacidemia
5. β-Methylcrotonyl CoA carboxylase	β-Methylcrotonylglycinuria ? biotin-responsive variant
6. β-Ketothiolase	β-Ketothiolase deficiency
7. Propionyl CoA carboxylase	Propionicacidemia and variants
8. ? Methylmalonyl CoA racemase	Methylmalonicacidemia
9. Methylmalonyl CoA carbonylmutase	Methylmalonicacidemia and variants
10. Steps in B_{12} coenzyme synthesis	B_{12}-dependent methylmalonic-acidemias
11. Homocysteine-methionine methyltransferase and steps in folate coenzyme turnover	Inborn errors of folate metabolism
12. Cystathionine synthase	Homocystinuria
13. Cystathionase	Cystathioninuria
14. Sulfite oxidase	Sulfite oxidase deficiency
15. ? Threonine deaminase	Threoninemia
16. β-Hydroxy-β-Methyl-glutaryl CoA lyase	β-Hydroxy-β-Methyl-glutaryl CoA lyase aciduria deficiency

Nutrient and energy requirements of infants and children with PKU are similar to those of normal children but there is one major exception. Tyrosine has become an essential amino acid. Protein sources therefore must be modified to provide adequate tyrosine and sufficient protein without exceeding phenylalanine requirements. Recommended phenylalanine, protein, and energy intakes for infants and children with PKU are

Table 9.1 Classification of Hyperphenylalaninemias

Type	Condition	Clinical aspects	Presumed defect	Blood Phe	Blood Tyr	Urine	Treatment
I	Phenylketonuria	Mental retardation and associated symptoms untreated	Phe hydroxylase absent	>20 mg/dl on regular diet	Normal–low	Elevation of Phe metabolites	Low Phe diet
II	Persistent hyper-phenylalaninemia	Normal	Decreased Phe hydroxylase	May be same as PKU early, later 4–20 mg/dl on regular diet	Normal–low	Normal or transiently increased	None or temporary diet therapy
III	Transient mild hyperphenylal-aninemia	Normal	Maturational delay of hydroxylase?	May be same as PKU early, progressively declines toward normal	Normal–low	Same as type II	Same as type II
IV	Transaminase deficiency	Normal	Phe transaminase deficiency	Varies with dietary protein intake	Normal	No Phe metabolites	Normal dietary protein

	Clinical features	Biochemical defect	Blood Phe	Blood Tyr	Urinary metabolites	Treatment
V Dihydropteridine reductase deficiency	Initially normal, seizures, abnormal development evident within first year of life	Deficiency of dihydropteridine reductase	Variable; may be as in type I	Normal	Variable, dependent on age and Phe concentration in blood	Dopa, 5-OH-tryptophan
VI Abnormal dihydropteridine reductase function	Myoclonus, uncontrolled movements, tetraplegia, greasy skin, recurrent hyperthermia	Unknown; functional abnormality dihydropteridine reductase	May be >20 mg/dl	Normal	Abnormal biopterin metabolites	Dopa, 5-OH-tryptophan and Carbidopa
VII ?	Progressive ataxia and seizures appearing between 12–18 mo. age	?	±10 mg/dl	Elevated	Phenylethylamine, mandelic acid, p-OH-mandelic acid	None known
VIII Transient neonatal tyrosinemia	Associated with low birth weight, high protein intake	p-hydroxyphenyl pyruvic oxidase inhibition	Transiently 4–12 mg/dl	Transiently elevated 5–50 mg/dl	Gross aminoaciduria, Tyr metabolites	Decrease protein to 1.8–2.2 g/kg
IX Hereditary tyrosinemia	Chronic liver disease	p-hydroxyphenyl pyruvic oxidase deficiency	2–8 mg/dl	4–12 mg/dl persistent	Gross aminoaciduria, Tyr metabolites	Symptomatic, low Phe and Tyr diet

Source: Modified from Blaskovics (9).
Phe = phenylalanine
Tyr = tyrosine

Table 9.2 Approximate Daily Requirements for Nutrients for Infants and Children with Various Inherited Metabolic Disorders

Nutrient	Unit	0–2 mo	2–5 mo	6–12 mo	1–2 yr	2–3 yr	3–4 yr	4–6 yr	6–8 yr	8–10 yr
Energy	kcal	120/kg	115/kg	105/kg	1100	1250	1400	1600	2000	2200
Volume (H_2O)	ml	120/kg	115/kg	105/kg	1100	1250	1400	1600	2000	2200
Carbohydrate	g	← Energy × 0.60 ÷ 4 →								
Protein										
Infants	g/kg	3.2–2.8	2.8–2.4	2.4–2.0						
Children	g/day	—	—	—	25	25	30	30	35	40
Fat	g	← Energy × 0.30 ÷ 9 →								
Sodium	mEq/kg	3	3	3	3	3	3	3	3	3
Potassium	mEq/kg	3	3	3	3	3	3	3	3	3
Calcium	mg	400	500	600	700	800	800	800	800	800
Phosphorus	mg	200	400	500	700	800	800	800	900	1000
Magnesium	mg	40	60	70	100	150	200	200	250	250
Iron	mg	6	10	15	15	15	10	10	10	10
Iodine	μg	25	40	45	55	60	70	80	100	110
Phenylalanine	mg/kg[a]	55 ± 16	36 ± 9	31 ± 9						
	mg/day[b]	—	—	—	200–500	200–500	200–500	200–500	200–500	200–500
Tyrosine	mg/kg[e]	60–80	60–80	42						
		—	—	—	25–85	25–85	8–50	8–50	8–50	25
Histidine[e]	mg/kg	16–34	16–34	16–34						
Leucine	mg/kg[c]	76–150	76–150	76–150						
	mg/day[d]	—	—	—	750–1000	750–1000	750–1000	750–1000	750–1000	750–1000
Isoleucine	mg/kg[c]	79–110	79–110	50–75						
	mg/day[d]	—	—	—	500–750	500–750	500–750	500–750	500–750	500–750
Valine	mg/kg[c]	65–105	65–105	50–80						
	mg/day[d]	—	—	—	400–600	400–600	400–600	400–600	400–600	400–600
Methionine	mg/kg[c]	20–45	20–45	20–45						
	mg/day[d]	—	—	—	400–800	400–800	400–800	400–800	400–800	400–800

Cyst(e)ine	mg/kg[c]	15–50	15–50	15–50	—	—	—	—	—	—
	mg/day[d]	—	—	—	400–800	400–800	400–800	400–800	400–800	400–800
Lysine	mg/kg[c]	90–120	90–120	90–120	—	—	—	—	—	—
	mg/day[d]	—	—	—	1200–1600	1200–1600	1200–1600	1200–1600	1200–1600	1200–1600
Threonine	mg/kg[c]	45–87	45–87	45–87	—	—	—	—	—	—
	mg/day[d]	—	—	—	800–1000	800–1000	800–1000	800–1000	800–1000	800–1000
Tryptophan	mg/kg[c]	13–22	13–22	13–22	—	—	—	—	—	—
	mg/day[d]	—	—	—	60–120	60–120	60–120	60–120	60–120	60–120
Vitamin B_1 (thiamine)	μg	200	400	500	600	600	700	800	1000	1100
Vitamin B_2 (riboflavin)	μg	400	500	600	600	700	800	900	1,100	1,200
Vitamin B_6 (pyridoxine)	μg	200	300	400	500	600	700	900	1,000	1,200
Vitamin B_{12}	μg	1.0	1.5	2.0	2.0	2.5	3.0	4.0	4.0	5.0
Folic acid	μg	50	50	100	100	200	200	200	200	300
Niacin	mg	5	7	8	8	8	9	11	13	15
Vitamin C	mg	35	35	35	40	40	40	40	40	40
Vitamin A	IU	1500	1500	1500	2000	2000	2500	2500	3500	3500
Vitamin D	IU	400	400	400	400	400	400	400	400	400
Vitamin E	IU	5	5	5	10	10	10	10	15	15

Source: Modified from American Academy of Pediatrics, Committee on Nutrition (59).

a. Mean ± standard deviation. Amounts found to maintain plasma phenylalanine levels between 2 and 10 mg/dl in PKU (18).

b. Estimate of requirements.

c. Based on studies of Snyderman, et al (121) on normal infants.

d. Based on studies of Nakagawa, et al. (122) in normal children from 8 to 14 years of age.

e. For infants and children with tyrosinosis (49). More tyrosine is required in normal children and children with PKU.

given in Table 9.2 (16,18). Because each child is an individual with specific requirements, intake for each affected child will need to be modified based on the indices of growth, blood phenylalanine, food intake, and appetite. During the first six months of life weekly diet changes may be required.

Protein sources available for use in the United States are Lofenalac® and Phenyl-Free™. Lofenalac, a casein hydrolysate with 95 percent of the phenylalanine removed, contains added L-methionine, tyrosine, tryptophan, carbohydrate, fat, vitamins, and minerals. Phenyl-Free is a phenylalanine free formula, consisting of pure L-amino acids, carbohydrates, lipids, vitamins, and minerals. Lofenalac is the product of choice for use with the child less than two years of age. Vitamin supplementation is unnecessary with either product if adequate amounts are given to meet protein needs. Fluoride will need to be supplied if the water is not fluoridated (Table 9.3).

Neither Lofenalac nor Phenyl-Free should be used alone as the sole diet of the child with PKU because both are deficient in phenylalanine and will lead to death if used in this fashion. In early infancy, evaporated milk or proprietary formula must be added in measured amounts to the Lofenalac to provide the required phenylalanine. As growth proceeds and solid foods are introduced, milk or formula should be proportionately decreased. Average phenylalanine, protein, and energy content of "serving lists" of solid foods are provided in Table 9.4. The lists are similar to diabetic exchange lists in that foods of similar phenylalanine content are grouped together and can be exchanged one for another within a list to give variety to the diet.

It is very important to maintain an adequate intake of protein and energy for the child with PKU even though phenylalanine must be restricted. Protein is obtained from Lofenalac or Phenyl-Free; therefore the amount of formula offered must be varied to provide protein needed. Nonprotein sources of energy such as Dextrimaltose®, corn syrup, sugar, and suitable foods from the "free-food list" (16) of nonprotein calories can be added to maintain energy intake and to satisfy the child's hunger without affecting blood phenylalanine levels. Solids should be prescribed in numbers of servings and introduced at the appropriate ages and in the usual textures as they would be for any child. It is important that children be given a variety of foods at the appropriate age so that these foods may be included in the diet later in life in order that increasing phenylalanine requirements may be met, jaw muscles needed for speech can be developed, and exercise for gums and teeth is provided.

A variety of factors may influence blood phenylalanine levels. Those that may produce an elevated blood phenylalanine include acute infection with concomitant tissue catabolism, excess or inadequate phenylalanine intake, and inadequate protein or energy intake. Wannemacher (19) described the effects of infection on plasma amino acids in normal adults. Similar increases in blood phenylalanine have been observed in treated PKU patients (20). Because of this, any infection should be promptly diagnosed and appropriately treated. The best approach to diet therapy during infection is to increase the intake of fluids and carbohydrates through use of fruit juices, Gatorade®, Koolaid®, Tang®, Start®, lemonade and noncaffeine-containing soft drinks.

Excess phenylalanine intake is the most common cause of elevated blood phenylalanine in the child with PKU. This may be due to overprescription, misunderstanding of the diet by the caretaker, or "snitching" of food by the child. Frequent blood tests with accompanying accurate diet records for calculation of intake provide data for determining whether or not phenylalanine prescription is excessive. Diet records are also useful in determining parental understanding. Misunderstanding of diet will require additional education of parents. "Snitching" of food by the child is the most difficult problem to handle. The first step is to make sure that energy intake is adequate. If the child is old enough, he should also be given sound reasons for avoiding foods not allowed on his diet. If neither of these approaches works, appropriate disciplinary measures should be applied by the parents.

Phenylalanine deficiency associated with inadequate phenylalanine intake has three specific stages of development (21). The first stage is characterized biochemically by decreased blood and urine phenylalanine. Clinically, the child may appear lethargic or anorectic. Vomiting, skin rashes, and fever of unknown origin may occur. In the second stage, blood phenylalanine is increased in conjunction with a generalized amino aciduria noted by two-dimensional paper chromatography. Normal infants fed formulas free of phenylalanine develop amino aciduria in six hours (22). In this stage, body protein stores are being catabolized. Eczema is common. In stage 3 of phenylalanine deficiency, blood phenylalanine is decreased below 1 mg/dl while urine phenylalanine is low. Accompanying clinical manifestations include failure to gain weight, bone changes, anemia, sparse hair, and finally death if the deficiency is not corrected by large supplements of dietary phenylalanine.

Inadequate protein intake results in an inadequate supply of essential amino acids and/or nitrogen for growth. When growth fails to proceed, phenylalanine that can no longer be used for growth accumulates in the blood. If catabolism occurs due to inadequate nitrogen and/or amino acid intake, blood phenylalanine increases because tissue protein contains some 5.5 percent phenylalanine. In case of protein insufficiency Lofenalac or Phenyl-Free intake should be increased to supply the required nitrogen and/or essential amino acids.

Energy, the first requirement of the body, is necessary for growth. When energy is provided as carbohydrate, and adequate nitrogen is avail-

Table 9.3 Approximate Nutritive Composition of Special Dietary Products Per 100 g Powder

Nutrient	*Lofenalac (MJ)	**PKU Aid (MS)I	*Low Methionine Isomil (RL)	*Phenyl-Free (MJ)	*3200-AB (MJ)	**MSUD Aid (MS)I	*MSUD Diet Powder (MJ)	**Methionaid (MS)I	*3200-K (MJ)	**Histinaid (MS)I	*80056 (MJ)
Energy (kcal)	454	240	516	406	460	248	476	242	464	240	486
Protein (g)	15	60	12.5	20.3	15	64.4	10.0	63.1	14	61.2	0
Fat (g)	18	0	28.1	6.8	18	0	20.1	0	19	0	22.5
CHO (g)	60	0	57.0	66	60	0	63.7	0	60	0	73.5
L-amino acids (g)											
Essential											
Isoleucine	0.75	2.6	0.56	1.08	0.86	0	0	2.4	0.67	2.5	0
Leucine	1.41	6.1	1.02	1.70	1.76	0	0	32	1.16	3.8	0
Lysine	1.57	6.1	0.77	1.85	1.91	7.1	0.80	6.0	0.87	5.8	0
Methionine	0.45	1.5	0.14	0.62	0.56	1.9	0.25	0.2	0.16	1.6	0
Phenylalanine	0.08	<0.07	0.6	0	<0.08	3.8	0.55	4.3	0.76	2.2	0
Threonine	0.77	4.8	0.51	0.93	0.65	3.3	0.55	3.2	0.52	3.1	0
Tryptophan	0.19	0.9	0.12	0.28	0.20	1.2	0.20	0.9	0.16	1.1	0
Valine	1.20	4.6	0.52	1.24	1.38	0	0	3.2	0.71	3.1	0
Histidine	0.39	1.8	0.28	0.46	0.40	2.7	0.25	2.8	0.34	0	0
Nonessential											
Arginine	0.34	3.1	0.83	0.68	0.39	5.1	0.50	4.4	0.96	4.6	0
Alanine	0.64	4.1	0.53	NL*	0.76	7.1	0.45	5.6	0.60	5.9	0
Aspartate	1.34	8.1	1.29	5.15	1.60	12.1	1.14	9.5	1.72	10.6	0
Cystine	0.025	1.5	0.15	0.34	0.042	2.1	0.25	3.7	0.107	1.8	0
Glutamate	3.78	9.3	2.48	1.85	4.31	13.3	2.09	11.0	2.76	12.3	0
Glycine	0.35	3.1	0.52	3.30	0.40	3.9	0.60	4.3	0.59	5.9	0
Proline	1.13	3.6	0.6	NL*	1.13	2.3	0.90	1.6	0.68	1.9	0
Serine	1.02	4.8	0.68	NL*	1.09	2.4	0.60	1.7	0.72	1.9	0
Tyrosine	0.81	6.0	0.40	0.93	<0.04	3.8	0.65	4.3	0.49	4.5	0
Glutamine	NL*	NL*	NL*	4.75	NL*	NL*	NL*	NL*	NL*	NL*	0

Vitamins											
Vitamin A (IU)	1160	0	2200	2030	1160	0	1190	0	1160	0	1440
Vitamin D (IU)	284	0	340	406	284	0	297	0	284	0	360
Vitamin E (IU)	7.2	0	12	10	7.2	0	7	0	7.2	0	0
Vitamin C (mg)	37	0	60	53	37	0	39	0	37	0	45
Thiamine (μg)	360	2000	0.5	609	360	2000	370	2000	360	2000	450
Riboflavin (μg)	430	2000	0.6	1015	430	2000	450	2000	430	2000	540
Vitamin B$_6$ (μg)	290	2000	0.5	508	290	2000	300	2000	290	2000	360
Vitamin B$_{12}$ (μg)	1.4	20	35	2.5	1.4	20	1.5	20	1.4	20	1.8
Niacin (μg)	5800	25000	9	8122	5800	25000	59000	25000	5800	25000	7200
Folic acid (μg)	72	400	0.12	100	72	400	74	400	72	400	90
Pantothenic acid (μg)	2200	20000	7	3046	2200	20000	2200	20000	2200	20000	2700
Choline (mg)	61	0	94	86	61	0	63	0	61	0	76
Biotin (μg)	36	600	0.13	30	36	600	40	600	36	600	45
Vitamin K (μg)	72	0	0.12	102	72	0	74	0	72	0	90
Inositol (mg)	22	0	0	30	22	250	22	100	22	100	90
Minerals											
Calcium (mg)	435	2500	650	609	435	2500	491	2500	435	700	540
Phosphorus (mg)	326	1500	440	457	326	1500	268	1500	326	1500	300
Magnesium (mg)	51	300	40	71	51	300	52	300	51	80	63
Iron (mg)	8.6	25	10	12	8.6	50	9	50	8.6	4	11
Iodine (μg)	32	150	120	66	32	150	33	150	32	60	41
Copper (μg)	430	2500	500	609	430	2500	400	2500	430	500	540
Manganese (mg)	0.7	3.5	0	1	0.7	3.5	0.7	3.5	0.7	0.5	0.9
Zinc (mg)	2.9	15	4	4.1	2.9	15	3.0	15	2.9	0.9	3.6
Sodium (mEq)	9	61	10.4	10	9	61	2.5	61	9	34	3
Potassium (mEq)	12	66	10.4	18	12	66	7.5	66	12	19	9
Chloride (mEq)	9	80	12.7	14	9	80	3.3	80	9	NL	4

Source: Modified from American Academy of Pediatrics, Committee on Nutrition (59).

*MJ = Mead Johnson Company; RL = Ross Laboratories; NL = not listed

**This product is manufactured by Milner Scientific and Medical Research Company, Liverpool, England.

Table 9.4   Average Nutrient and Energy of Serving Lists for
Phenylalanine-Restricted Diets

List	Phenylalanine (mg)	Protein (g)	Energy (kcal)
Vegetables, strained, and junior	15	0.5	20
table	15	0.5	10
Fruits, strained, and junior	15	0.6	150
table and juices	15	0.6	70
Breads and cereals	30	0.6	30
Fats	5	0.1	60

When analyses were not available, the phenylalanine content was calculated on the following basis:

Breads and cereals	Phenylalanine 5% of protein
Fat	Phenylalanine 5% of protein
Fruits	Phenylalanine 2.6% of protein
Vegetables	Phenylalanine 3.3% of protein

able, nonessential amino acids may be synthesized from the keto-acid metabolites. Further, carbohydrate ingestion leads to insulin secretion and insulin promotes amino acid transport into the cell where it can be used for protein synthesis. When energy intake is inadequate tissue catabolism occurs to meet energy needs. Such catabolism releases phenylalanine, leading to elevated blood phenylalanine. Providing sufficient energy through generous use of nonprotein and low protein foods (Table 9.5) is important in order to assure a normal growth rate.

Low blood phenylalanine (< 2 mg/dl) may lead to depressed appetite (23), decreased growth (24), and, if prolonged, to mental retardation (25). Low blood phenylalanine levels are most often due to inadequate prescription of phenylalanine or a capricious appetite in the affected child. In such cases the prescription for phenylalanine can be increased by addition of measured amounts of milk and/or solid foods. In some situations, formula volume may be too great for the child to consume in the allotted time period and formula volume will need to be decreased to the amount the child is able to ingest. Formulas as concentrated as one measure of Lofenalac to one ounce of water are frequently used without any untoward side effects. Lofenalac may also be mixed as a paste and spoon-fed, even to the young infant. When this method for feeding some of the prescribed Lofenalac is used, the practice should be begun at three to four months of age and extra fluid should be offered between feedings.

Along with frequent assessment of growth through measurement of height, weight, and head circumference and evaluation of development by appropriate developmental scales, the adequacy of phenylalanine intake is determined by frequent monitoring of the blood phenylalanine level. The first year is the period of most rapid growth and of greatest vulnera-

Table 9.5 Low Protein Energy-Containing Foods

Product	Source
Cellu Wheat Starch	Chicago Dietetic Supply, Inc.
Lo Pro Pastas	405 East Shawnut Avenue
Low Protein Baking Mix & Bread	LaGrange, Illinois 60525
Controlyte	D. M. Doyle Pharmaceutical Co.
	Highway 100 at West Twenty-Third Street
	Minneapolis, Minnesota 55416
Low Protein Bread & Mix	Ener-G-Foods, Inc.
Potato Mix	1526 Utah Avenue, South
Egg Replacer	Seattle, Washington 98134
Aproten Low Protein Cookies	General Mills Chemicals, Inc.
Aproten Low Protein Pastas, Rusks, Porridge	4620 W. 77th Street
Cal-Power Beverages	Minneapolis, Minnesota 55440
Dietetic Paygel Baking Mix	
Dietetic Paygel Wheat Starch	
Low Protein Canned Bread	
Prono	

bility to nutrition insult. Therefore, blood tests are suggested two times weekly during the first six months and weekly thereafter until the child is one year of age. After one year of age twice monthly blood tests are sufficient for monitoring diet. If, however, blood phenylalanine levels are greater than 10 mg/dl, more frequent determinations should be obtained. Where indicated, the prescription for phenylalanine is decreased and frequent blood tests are obtained until blood phenylalanine levels are between 2 and 10 mg/dl. In order for blood tests to be of use in adjusting the prescription they must be performed by the laboratory both accurately and promptly. Quantitative methods of phenylalanine determination using ion exchange chromatography or fluorometry are preferable but the microbiological (Guthrie) method may be acceptable for monitoring purposes if antibiotics are not being administered at the time the blood specimen is obtained (26). If properly instructed, parents may be given responsibility for obtaining the specimens and mailing them to the laboratory.

A record of food ingested prior to obtaining blood for phenylalanine measurement is essential and should be kept by the parents. The correlation between the child's intake of phenylalanine, protein and energy, his health status and the blood phenylalanine level should be considered before a diet change is prescribed.

The success of diet management rests with the parents and depends upon their understanding of the disease and their ability to cope with the diet and the child's understanding of the diet restrictions and his self-dis-cipline. These factors in turn are related to the help the parents receive from various professional members of the team. Roles and functions of some team members have been described (17).

Early diagnosis and prompt treatment of PKU with a nutritionally adequate phenylalanine-restricted diet have resulted in normal growth (27) and intelligence (14). Mean height, weight, and head circumference of 111 children treated from before 120 days of age were the same as those of normal children at four years of age (27). Assessment of mental develop-ment in these same children at four years of age provided a mean I.Q. of 93 on the Stanford Binet Intelligence Scale (14).

The semisynthetic nature of the phenylalanine-restricted diet has led to questions concerning its adequacy. Calculation of intake of major nutri-ents indicates that these are adequate (18) when compared to the RDAs. Balance studies of calcuim, phosphorus, magnesium, and iron in eight girls, six to eight years of age, on Lofenalac suggested that magnesium and iron may be inadequate to provide for optimal nutrition (28). Studies by the author of plasma zinc and copper, and hair zinc in 15 treated pa-tients one month to seven years of age on Lofenalac or Phenyl-Free imply that one-fourth to one-half the children may be suffering from zinc defi-ciency. Inadequate intake, poor absorption, or inefficient utilization may all be responsible. When Lofenalac is the protein source, the intake of vi-tamin E is sufficient to provide for normal plasma levels despite the high intake of polyunsaturated fatty acids (29). Adequacy of niacin status in children on Lofenalac is questionable because of limited tryptophan and niacin intake and disturbances in metabolism (30).

A number of clinicians have suggested that diet might be discontin-ued at four, six, or 12 years of age with no adverse effects (31–33). Inves-tigators have recently questioned this because controlled studies have shown significant differences in intelligence between children who go off diet at six years of age and those who remain on diet (34,35).

For the PKU female, diet discontinuation poses special problems. Few untreated PKU women who have carried the fetus to term have de-livered normal infants. Congenital malformations (36), microcephaly, and retarded physical and mental growth are associated with *in utero* eleva-tions of phenylalanine. Active transport of amino acids to the fetus leads to a fetal blood phenylalanine level two to three times that found in the maternal blood (37). Such elevated phenylalanine levels may interfere with brain development by one or more of the several previously described mechanisms. The theory of tyrosine deficiency, if proven, has far-reaching implications not only for the woman homozygous for PKU but also for the heterozygote as well (7). Bessman (7) has postulated that this and similar defects in amino acid metabolism may account for a large share of the nonspecific mental retardation seen in the United States.

Tyrosinemias. Several inherited disorders of tyrosine metabolism have been described. The designation, possible enzyme defect and clinical features are listed in Table 9.6.

Tyrosinemia, type I, is thought to be due to deficiency in activity of p-hydroxyphenylpyruvic acid oxidase, perhaps secondary to some other unknown defect (1,20). Gaull (38,39) has presented evidence for reduced activities of methionine-activating enzyme and cystathionine synthetase as well.

Clinically, type I tyrosinemia is characterized by liver failure leading to cirrhosis, generalized renal absorption defects (Fanconi syndrome and renal rickets), failure to thrive, vomiting, diarrhea, enlargement of the abdomen, dyspnea, hemorrhages, edema, ascites, hepatosplenomegaly, and in some patients mental retardation. Laboratory findings in type I tyrosinemia include: hyperphosphaturia, hypophosphatemia, glucosuria, proteinuria, and hyperaminoaciduria (Fanconi syndrome). Blood tyrosine is increased above normal levels and blood methionine may or may not be elevated. Moderate anemia, deficits in clotting factors produced in the liver, δ-aminolevulinic aciduria and intermittent porphyria may be found (38). Tyrosyluria occurs and urinary excretion of p-hydroxyphenolic acids is markedly increased, especially p-hydroxyphenyllactic acid (1,20).

There is a distinct aminoaciduria consisting of tyrosine, proline, threonine, alanine, glycine, phenylalanine, α-aminobutyric acid, isoleucine, serine, leucine, aspartic acid, methionine, and ethanolamine. Patients with this disorder seem prone to develop hepatoma (1,20).

Whatever the cause of this rare autosomal recessively inherited trait (with a carrier rate of one in every 20 to 30 persons in the Chicoutimi region of northeast Quebec), death occurs rapidly in a majority of cases particularly if untreated. Diet modification is the only known approach to therapy but there are many reports of poor response to phenylalanine- and tyrosine-restricted diets (40–46). A recent report (47) suggests that methionine restriction in addition to restriction of phenylalanine and tyrosine leads to a more positive outcome.

Objectives of therapy in tyrosinemia type I are:

1. normal mental development.
2. normal physical development.
3. prevention or alleviation of renal and liver damage.

Methods of achieving these objectives include utilization of phenylalanine-tyrosine- and possibly methionine-restricted diets, and if needed due to renal tubular defects, supplemental base, and vitamin D.

Suggested energy and nutrient intakes including phenylalanine, tyrosine, and methionine are given in Table 9.2. Natural proteins contain from 2.2 to 5.5 percent phenylalanine and tyrosine and from 0.60 to 3.50 percent methionine. Because of this, protein needs cannot be met from natu-

Table 9.6 Proteins and Amino Acids in Inborn Errors of Metabolism

Nutrient	Disorder	Defect	Disturbances	Diet treatment
Gluten (from wheat)	Celiac syndrome, nontropical sprue	Gluten sensitivity	Steatorrhea, growth failure	Exclude gluten
Nitrogen	Urea cycle defects	Carbamyl phosphate synthetase (Fig. 9.3:1)	Hyperammonemia	Restrict protein; ? synthetic diet
		Ornithine transcarbamyl-ase (Fig. 9.3:2)	Hyperammonemia	Restrict protein, ? synthetic diet
	Citrullinemia	Argininosuccinate synthetase (Fig. 9.3:3)	Hyperammonemia, liver damage	Restrict protein, supplement arginine, ? synthetic diet
	Argininosuccinic Aciduria	Argininosuccinase (Fig. 9.3:4)	Brain damage, growth failure, hyperammonemia	Restrict protein, supplement arginine
	Argininemia	Arginase (Fig. 9.3:5)	Brain damage	? Restrict protein
	Ornithinemia with homocitrullinemia	Transport defect of mitochondrial reentry of ornithine	Brain damage	? Restrict protein
Dibasic amino acids				
Lysine	Lysinuric familial protein intolerance	Transport of lysine	Abdominal cramps and distension, growth failure	Low protein, ? restrict lysine
	Other lysinemic syndromes	Enzyme defects of lysine and tryptophan (Fig. 9.1:16–19)	Variable brain damage and other features	Of doubtful value
Ornithine	Hyperornithinemia	? Ornithine transaminase (Fig. 9.3:6)	Seizures, hyperammonemia	Of doubtful value
Aromatic and heterocyclic amino acids				
Phenylalanine	Phenylketonuria	Hepatic phenylalanine hydroxylase (Fig. 9.1:6)	Brain damage, musty smell	Restrict phenylalanine, supplement tyrosine
	Variant	Dihydrobiopterine reductase	Brain damage	Of doubtful value
	Hyperphenylalaninemias	Reduced phenylalanine hydroxylase activity	Probably benign	Probably unnecessary

320

Amino acid	Disease	Enzyme defect	Clinical features	Protein restriction
Tyrosine	Tyrosinemia of prematurity	Immaturity of p-hydroxyphenylpyruvate oxidase (Fig. 9.1:8)	Perhaps mild mental retardation	
	Herediary tyrosinemia (Oregon type)	Cytosol tyrosine amino transferase (Fig. 9.1:7)	Brain damage, corneal ulcers, thickened skin	Restrict phenylalanine and tyrosine
	Hypertyrosinemia	? p-Hydroxyphenylpyruvate oxidase (Fig. 9.1:8)	Brain damage, liver damage, hypoglycemia	Restrict phenylalanine and tyrosine
Tryptophan	Blue diaper syndrome	Intestinal tryptophan transport	Fevers, irritability, brain damage, smell of stale cabbage	Restrict tryptophan
	Tryptophanemia	Undetermined (Fig. 9.1:16)	Brain damage, rashes, depigmentation	Restrict tryptophan
Histidine	Histidinemia	Histidase (Fig. 9.1:12)	? Brain damage, ? deafness	Of doubtful value
Proline	Hyperprolinemia type I	Proline oxidase	Kidney damage, ? brain damage	Exclude proline, may help
Branched-chain amino acids				
Leucine, valine, isoleucine	Maple syrup urine disease	Branched-chain ketoacid dehydrogenase (Fig. 9.2:3)	Metabolic acidosis, brain damage, smell of maple syrup	Restrict leucine, isoleucine, valine ? synthetic diet (plus thiamine in vitamin responsive variant)
Leucine	Leucine-sensitive hypoglycemia	Undetermined ? nonspecific	Postprandial hypoglycemia	Low protein, or reduce leucine
	Isovaleric acidemia	Isovaleryl CoA dehydrogenase (Fig. 9.2:4)	Metabolic aciduria, hypoglycemia	Restrict leucine, add glycine
	Methylcrotonyl-glycinemia	Methylcrotonyl CoA carboxylase (Fig. 9.2:5)	Metabolic acidosis, brain damage, smell of cats' urine	Restrict leucine (add biotin in vitamin responsive variant)
Isoleucine	Butanonemia	Ketothiolase (Fig. 9.2:6)	Metabolic ketoacidosis, hyperammonemia	Restrict isoleucine

Table 9.6 Continued

Nutrient	Disorder	Defect	Disturbance	Diet treatment
Isoleucine, valine, threonine, and methionine	Propionic acidemia	Propionyl CoA carboxylase (Fig. 9.2:7)	Metabolic ketoacidosis, hyperammonemia, brain damage	Restrict isoleucine, valine, threonine, methionine (add biotin in vitamin-responsive variants)
	Methylmalonic acidemia	Methylmalonyl CoA racemase or mutase (Fig. 9.2:8–10)	As above	As above (add vitamin B$_{12}$ in vitamin-responsive variants)
Sulfur amino acids				
All organic sulfur	Sulfite oxidase deficiency	Sulfite oxidase (Fig. 9.2:16)	Severe brain damage, dislocated lenses	Restricted methionine, cysteine may help
Methionine	Oast-House urine syndrome	Intestinal transport	Brain damage, white hair, smell of dried celery	? Restrict methionine
	Homocystinuria	Cystathionine synthetase	Lanky physique, dislocated lenses, thromboemboli, some retardation	Restricted methionine, may help (add pyridoxine in vitamin-responsive variant)
Other amino acids				
Glycine	Nonketotic hyperglycinemia	? Glycine cleavage enzyme	Severe brain damage	Of doubtful value
Glutamate	Monosodium glutamate	Excess artificial flavoring in infant foods	Brain damage	Avoid excess glutamate
Carnosine	Carnosinemia	Carnosinase deficiency (Fig. 9.1:13)	Brain damage	? Reduce carnosine intake

Source: Prepared by Dr. Y. E. Hsia.

ral sources. An investigational product, 3200 AB, available from Mead Johnson Laboratories, is low in phenylalanine (0.08%) and tyrosine (0.009%), but not methionine (Table 9.3). This product may be used if blood methionine is not elevated. When blood methionine is elevated along with phenylalanine and tyrosine, an amino acid mix based on the amino acid pattern in human milk, but free of these three offending amino acids may be used to provide nitrogen and amino acids. The three offending amino acids may be replaced with equal amounts of glycine, glutamine, or asparagine.

Both products will need to be supplemented with natural protein to meet phenylalanine, tyrosine, (and perhaps methionine) requirements in order to prevent their deficiency (48). In the young infant the amino acids may be added as a measured amount of evaporated milk or proprietary formula. As growth and development proceed, cereal products, fruits and vegetables should be added in amounts necessary to provide requirements. Table 9.7 gives the average composition of "serving lists" for the phenylalanine–tyrosine-restricted diet (49).

When a phenylalanine–tyrosine–methionine-free L-amino acid mix is used to provide nitrogen and amino acids, it must be mixed with Product 80056 (Table 9.3). Product 80056 is a nitrogen-free mixture consisting of carbohydrate, fat, minerals, and vitamins. Sodium is the only mineral found in low amounts in Product 80056. Assessment of all sources of sodium intake must be made to determine whether sodium needs for growth are being met. If not, measured amounts of sodium chloride should be added to the formula.

Free amino acids mixed with Product 80056 containing sugar and minerals in essentially free form can lead to a mixture of high osmolality. Formulas of high osmolality (>600 mOsm/1) may lead to diarrhea, dehydration, and hyperosmolar coma. Laboratory evaluation of the osmolality of the formula should be carried out before feeding to the critically ill infant. If diarrhea is present prior to formula introduction, a formula with an osmolality below 300 mOsm/1 should be used.

Table 9.7 Average Composition of Serving Lists for Phenylalanine–Tyrosine-Restricted Diet[a]

List	Phenylalanine (mg)	Tyrosine (mg)	Protein (g)	Energy (kcal)
Vegetables	15	10	0.5	10
Fruits	10	5	0.4	55
Bread/cereal	18	12	0.4	15
Fats[a]	4	6	0.1	90

Source: Acosta and Elsas (49).
[a]Energy content of foods in fat list vary greatly. If any one fat is frequently used, figures for its energy content should be used in calculating energy intake.

The initial diet prescription for tyrosinemia type I should contain specific amounts of phenylalanine, tyrosine (or phenylalanine plus tyrosine), methionine, protein, energy, and fluid for the day (Table 9.2). Subsequent prescriptions depend on blood amino acid levels and the patient's clinical course.

Normal plasma levels of tyrosine (1.24 ± 0.53 mg/dl), phenylalanine (0.76 ± 0.26 mg/dl), and methionine (0.25 ± 0.15 mg/dl) (40) should be aimed for while providing adequate nutrients and energy for normal growth to proceed. Frequent assessments of plasma amino acid levels, nutrient intake, and growth are indicated. Other indices of nutrition status such as hemoglobin, hematocrit, plasma albumin, transferrin, vitamins, or minerals may be requested as indicated. Other disorders of aromatic and heterocyclic amino acids are described in Table 9.6.

Branched-chain Amino Acids

The branched-chain amino acids isoleucine, leucine, and valine are used primarily for protein synthesis. Those present in the body in excess of needs for synthetic purposes are degraded through three major steps to provide energy. These steps are transamination, requiring a specific transaminase and the coenzyme pyridoxal phosphate; oxidative decarboxylation utilizing the branched-chain α-ketoacid dehydrogenase complex located on the inner mitochondrial membrane (1,20) and requiring the coenzyme thiamine pyrophosphate; metabolism of the fatty acid produced. Figure 9.2 outlines major steps in degradation of these amino acids leading to the Krebs cycle.

Branched-chain Ketoaciduria. This disorder is also called maple syrup urine disease (MSUD) because of the urine odor. It is an inherited disorder of metabolism of the ketoacids of isoleucine, leucine, and valine. It is characterized by listlessness, difficulty in feeding, a high-pitched constant cry, and loss of Moro and tendon reflexes. There is an accumulation of branched-chain amino acids and their ketoacids in the cerebrospinal fluid, erythrocytes, plasma, and urine. Death or severe mental retardation occur without immediate therapy (1,20).

Infants with MSUD appear normal at birth and may be clinically well until after a protein-containing feed. Initial symptoms include poor feeding, apathy and a high-pitched, constant cry. Neurologic signs appear shortly and include loss of tendon and Moro reflexes, abnormal eye movements, alternating periods of flaccidity and hypertonicity, opisthotonic position, convulsions, and respiratory distress. The characteristic odor of maple syrup appears when the neurologic signs are noted. It may be found in perspiration, ear wax, and urine and is due to the accumulation of α-keto-β-methylvalerate (Fig. 9.2). Death occurs due to respiratory failure.

Few patients survive beyond the period of respiratory distress and those that do are usually severely mentally retarded (1,20).

According to Naylor and Guthrie (51), the incidence of MSUD is approximately one in every 200,000 live births. Incidence figures vary however, being one per 53,000 in Maryland, one in 50,000 in West Germany, and approximately one in 1,000,000 in Switzerland and Japan. MSUD has been found in all ethnic groups. MSUD appears to be transmitted through an autosomal recessive mode. It is found in both males and females and is more frequent in offspring of consanguineous marriages.

Plasma changes seen in untreated MSUD include increased levels of branched-chain amino and ketoacids and the presence of alloisoleucine; alanine may be one-third to one-fourth normal levels. Urinary excretion of abnormal amounts of branched-chain amino acids, branched-chain ketoacids and hydroxy acids of the branched-chain amino acids occurs (1,20).

If death occurs in the first few days of life, few abnormalities are seen in the brain. With prolonged survival, deficient myelination is thought to be due to a number of factors including enzyme inhibition, inhibition of amino acid transport, and decreased oxygen utilization (1,20).

Diagnosis of MSUD can be made by measuring plasma amino acids using ion exchange chromatography to quantitate valine, leucine, isoleucine, and alloisoleucine (52). Urinary branched-chain alpha-ketoacids can be quantitated by gas chromatography (53). Diagnosis should be confirmed by quantitative enzyme assay of cultured skin fibroblasts (54). Prenatal monitoring is available for parents who have previously had a child with MSUD (55).

Several variants of MSUD have been found with a spectrum of branched-chain alpha-ketoacid dehydrogenase activity (Table 9.8) (1).

Except during periods of illness protein restriction may be adequate therapy for those patients with 15 percent or more of enzyme activity. Patients responding to pharmacologic doses of thiamine (100 mg/day) with lower urinary excretion of branched-chain ketoacids and lower plasma levels of branched-chain amino acids have been reported (56,57). The mechanism of this response is suggested to be through prolongation of the half-life of the enzyme complex (58).

Therapy at the time of diagnosis and during acute infections may include exchange transfusions or peritoneal dialysis. Indications for use are convulsions or coma (20).

Chronic therapy for MSUD is by means of diet. Objectives of therapy are to supply adequate energy and nutrients (nitrogen, essential amino acids, minerals, vitamins, and fluid) for normal growth while restricting the branched-chain amino acids to intakes compatible with normal plasma levels. Data in Table 9.2 provide recommended nutrient and energy intakes for infants and children of various ages with MSUD (59).

Table 9.8 Classification of Variants of Branched-chain Ketoaciduria

Types	Onset	Course and symptoms	Enzyme	Leucine	Treatment
I	First week	Severe/lethal, metabolic acidosis, etc.	"0"	60 mg%	Exchange/dialysis/synthetic diet
II	First week	Severe/nonlethal, MR,* seizures, acidosis	<2%	25–40 mg%	Exchange/dialysis/synthetic diet
III	One to two weeks	Chronic-mild; neurological signs, MR,* metabolic problems, ataxia	2–5%	15–20 mg%	Synthetic diet
IV	First month	Mild-intermittent; not MR,* but may have acidosis	~5%	5–10 mg%	Low protein not effective; synthetic diet
V	May not have symptoms until 2–8 years	Intermittent; clinically normal except when ill. May be lethal; ataxia when ill	15–25%	Normal except when ill	None except during illness; low protein diet and appropriate therapy for severe symptoms
VI		Thiamine-sensitive	?~15%		Thiamine 100 mg/day, P.O.

Source: Prepared by M. E. Blaskovics.
* MR—Mental Retardation.

A synthetic formula must be used to provide nitrogen and amino acids. Composition of MSUDAid and MSUD Diet Powder are given in Tables 9.3 and 9.4. MSUD Diet Powder consisting of L-amino acids and Product 80056 is the formula of choice in managing MSUD because it requires the least supplementation. Isoleucine, leucine, and valine must be provided in amounts required for growth. These are usually given in the form of measured amounts of evaporated milk or proprietary formula. With age and the introduction of solid foods (Table 9.9), milk will be decreased in the formula (49).

When leucine needs are met by milk or solid foods, the amounts of isoleucine and valine provided are inadequate to meet needs for growth. It is necessary to supplement the formula with individual pure solutions of isoleucine and valine. Parents may be given vials of dry isoleucine and valine to mix to a specific quantity. These solutions should be stored in the freezer until required for formula preparation. Parents are provided with disposable 50 ml syringes so that they can accurately measure evaporated milk or proprietary formula and amino acid solutions.

Terminal sterilization should never be used for formulas containing free amino acids and mono- or disaccharides because of the occurrence of the Maillard reaction. Parents should be taught the aseptic technique for formula preparation.

Solid foods should displace the milk which has been added to the formula as rapidly as the developmental milestones indicate readiness. Speech, as noted earlier, is dependent on the appropriate development of jaw muscles and chewing is required for the development of these muscles.

Energy, mineral (except sodium), and vitamin needs are provided by MSUD Diet Powder used in appropriate amounts and later by wise choices of solid foods (Table 9.9) (49). MSUDAid will require mixing with Product 80056 (Table 9.3).

Diet therapy is usually initiated by using amino acid mix completely free of branched-chain amino acids (20). Plasma levels are monitored every 24 hours until normal levels (Table 9.10) are achieved. As the plasma level of each branched-chain amino acid approaches normal, sup-

Table 9.9 Average Composition of Serving Lists for Diets Restricted in
Isoleucine, Leucine, and Valine

List	Ile (mg)	Leu (mg)	Val (mg)	Pro (g)	Energy (kcal)
Vegetables	23	30	27	0.7	15
Fruits	15	25	25	0.6	90
Bread/cereal	15	35	20	0.4	20
Fats	7	10	8	0.1	70

Source: From Acosta and Elsas (49).

Table 9.10 Plasma Amino Acids in
Normal Children

Amino acid	Normal concentration[a] average ± 1 SD (mg per dl)
Isoleucine	0.93 ± 0.40
Leucine	1.53 ± 0.49
Lysine	1.67 ± 0.52
Methionine	0.25 ± 0.15
Phenylalanine	0.76 ± 0.26
Threonine	1.20 ± 0.40
Valine	2.88 ± 0.71
Cystine	0.70 ± 0.20
Tyrosine	1.24 ± 0.53
Alanine	1.89 ± 0.53
Arginine	0.77 ± 0.28
Asparagine	0.10 ± 0.01
Glycine	1.07 ± 0.27
Histidine	0.91 ± 0.35
Ornithine	0.67 ± 0.41
Proline	2.13 ± 1.06
Serine	1.20 ± 0.20
Taurine	0.91 ± 0.60

[a]From Holt et al. (50).

plementation is begun with that specific amino acid. According to Snyderman (20), isoleucine becomes normal first, within two to three days. Valine becomes normal next. Leucine may take eight to 10 days to become normal.

Monitoring of therapy should use three combined approaches. Ion exchange chromatography initially should be used daily to determine requirements for the individual branched-chain amino acids. Following establishment of requirements, ion exchange chromatography should be used approximately every two weeks to quantitate branched chain amino acids to make sure the child has not "grown out" of his prescription.

Daily testing of urine with dinitrophenylhydrazine (DNPH) should be carried out. If the results are positive, a blood sample may be collected on filter paper for assay of leucine with *B. subtilis 6051*. Urine DNPH does not become immediately positive or negative with increases or decreases in plasma ketoacids. Weekly Guthrie tests, in conjunction with daily urine DNPH tests and diet record are required for diet management. Frequent assessments of growth are also necessary to evaluate diet adequacy. Every effort should be made to maintain plasma branched-chain amino acids in the normal range (Table 9.10). Plasma leucine levels greater than 10 mg/dl are associated with α-ketoacidemia and the appearance of ataxia.

Episodes of infection bring about catabolism of tissue protein and a rise in branched-chain amino acids (BCAA). Snyderman uses the approach of eliminating BCAA completely until plasma levels approach normal (20). Waisman and associates (60) found that clinical improvement was more rapid if some BCAA were administered along with an amino acid mix that provided energy needs. Bicarbonate, potassium, and fluids must be administered to prevent acidosis.

There is no information as to the length of time children with MSUD must be treated. According to Snyderman in all probability treatment may have to be continued for life. The oldest child under treatment still manifests clinical symptoms when there is elevation of the plasma leucine level (20).

Other disorders of metabolism of the BCAA are described in Table 9.7.

Sulfur-containing Amino Acids

Natural protein contains from 0.6 to 3.5 percent methionine. Some methionine is used by the body for tissue protein synthesis but the majority is degraded through the transsulfuration pathway to form cystine (and its derivatives) and α-ketobutyrate (Fig. 9.2). Homocysteine is formed as an intermediary product in this pathway. Homocysteine has three possible pathways open to it. Normally, homocysteine reacts with serine in the presence of an enzyme (cystathionine synthase, Fig. 9.2:12) found in liver and brain to form cystathionine. Cystathionine synthase requires pyridoxal phosphate as a coenzyme. Homocysteine can also be remethylated to form methionine. Either of two enzymes can carry out this reaction and may require either N^5–methyltetrahydrofolate or methylcobalamin (MeB_{12}) as coenzyme (Fig. 9.2:11). The third pathway open to homocysteine is spontaneous oxidation to homocystine. This occurs only when homocysteine is present in tissue in abnormal amounts. It is essentially a dead-end path because it must be reduced back to homocysteine for further metabolism. Cystathionine forms cysteine and α-ketobutyrate. The enzyme cystathionase, which utilizes pyridoxal phosphate as a coenzyme, is required for this reaction (Fig. 9.2:13). A deficiency of cystathionase results in cystathioninuria. Alpha-ketobutyrate is catabolized through propionyl CoA to methylmalonyl CoA and evenutally to succinyl CoA, a Krebs cycle intermediate. This pathway will be described in more detail in a later section. L-Cysteine is catabolized to pyruvate, NH_3 and H_2S in the presence of cysteine desulfhydrase, a pyridoxal phosphate-requiring enzyme (1,20).

Homocystinuria. This disorder results from one of several genetically determined errors of methionine metabolism. Deficiencies of cystathionine synthase (Fig. 9.2:12), betaine homocysteine methyltransferase (Fig.

9.2:11) or their respective coenzymes (pyridoxal phosphate, methylcobalamin or N^5-methyltetrahydrofolate) all cause homocystinuria (1).

The most common form of homocystinuria, due to a defect in cystathionine synthase, is characterized by specific skeletal changes, dislocated lenses, intravascular thromboses, osteoporosis, malar flushing, and in some patients mental retardation. The skeletal changes and dislocated lenses are presumably due to a structural defect in collagen formation. Intravascular thromboses may occur at any age and have been found in coronary, renal, carotid, and intracranial arteries. Fifty percent of untreated patients die before 20 years, 95 percent before 50 years of age (52).

Cause of the variable mental retardation is not clear. In a series of 84 patients, one-half were of average intelligence, several were university graduates, and one held a Ph.D. (1).

Cystathionine synthesis deficiency is inherited in an autosomal recessive manner. Accurate estimates of incidence are not available, but in limited newborn screening figures varying from one per 36,000 to one per 162,000 have been found. Homocystinuria occurs in many ethnic groups, but is higher in persons of Irish extraction than in other ethnic groups (20).

A positive screen for methionine should be followed by assay of plasma amino acids using ion exchange chromatography. With a cystathionine synthase defect, homocystine, cysteine–homocysteine and methionine should all be elevated in the plasma. Normal or low plasma methionine is associated with homocystinuria from other causes (Fig. 9.2:11) (20).

Objectives of therapy in homocystinuria vary according to the age at which diagnosis is made. If homocystinuria due to cystathionine synthase is discovered in the newborn, the objectives are:

1. Prevent the development of skeletal and ocular abnormalities.
2. Prevent intravascular thromboses.
3. Assure normal intellectual development.

If diagnosis is delayed until late in childhood or in adult life the main objective of treatment will then be to prevent thromboembolisms.

Megadoses of pyridoxine should be tried as the first approach to therapy because about one-half the patients with homocystinuria have been found to respond to vitamin B_6 (20). Trials of 1 g of pyridoxine daily should be given to determine its effects on plasma methionine levels. Anywhere from a few days to one month may be required for a biochemical response to occur if the patient is responsive to pyridoxine (20). If the plasma methionine and the urinary homocystine levels are reduced the amount of pyridoxine should be gradually lowered until one reaches the minimum dose required to maintain biochemical normality. Doses of 25 to 750 mg per day have been required by some patients (20,62).

Those patients who do not respond to pyridoxine will require a methionine-restricted diet supplemented with cystine, which is essential in homocystinuria (Fig. 9.2:12) (20). If plasma folate levels are below normal due to excess use in remethylating homocystine to methionine, folate should be added as a supplement (20).

In prescribing and implementing nutrition care plans for infants and children with homocystinuria, energy, nitrogen, amino acid, mineral, vitamin, and fluid needs should all be considered. Data in Table 9.2 suggest ranges of methionine for beginning treatment. Younger infants have a greater methionine requirement on a body weight basis than older infants. Suggested methionine intakes range from 42 mg/kg in the young infant to 10 mg/kg in the 10-year-old. Suggested energy, protein, mineral, vitamin, and fluid intakes are given in Table 9.2. If the formula provides more than 20 kcal/oz, extra fluid should be offered between formula feeds (20,49).

Calcium cystinate, a more soluble form of L-cystine, should supplement the methionine-restricted diet at all ages. Three hundred milligrams per kilogram of body weight should be offered the young infant. This may be decreased to 200 mg/kg at six months of age and 100 mg/kg at three years and thereafter (20). The calcium cystinate should be mixed with the low methionine formula to provide for even distribution throughout the day.

Two formulas have been developed as protein sources for patients with homocystinuria. These are the investigational soy product 3200K* and Methionaid†. Composition of these products is given in Table 9.3. Product 3200K is the formula of choice because, except for its low methionine content (138 mg/100 g powder), it is a complete formulation. Methionaid™, a beef serum protein hydrolysate free of methionine, must be supplemented with fat-soluble vitamins, essential fatty acids, energy, and methionine.

Methionine may be provided the young infant through the addition of specified amounts of evaporated milk or proprietary formula to the low methionine formula. As growth and development proceed, solid foods should be added at the usual ages. Methionine requirement is small and most foods contain moderate amounts in relation to requirement. Because of this, the amount of solid food that can be ingested is small. To provide variety and utility to the methionine-restricted diet serving lists have been prepared (49). Average methionine, protein, and energy content of these lists are given in Table 9.11 (49).

Following introduction of diet and stabilization, plasma methionine levels should be monitored twice weekly until six months of age. Weekly

---

* Manufactured by Mead Johnson Laboratories, Evansville, Indiana.
† Manufactured by Milner Scientific, Liverpool, England.

Table 9.11   Average Composition of Serving Lists for
Methionine-restricted Diet

List	Methionine (mg)	Protein (g)	Energy (kcal)
Vegetables			
Group 1	10	0.7	10
Group 2	10	1.5	35
Fruits	5	0.8	75
Bread/cereal	20	1.5	55
Fats	2	0.1	65

Source: Acosta and Elsas (49).

monitoring is suggested until one year of age and twice monthly thereafter
if blood levels are stable. Following a diet change, plasma methionine
should be measured after three days have elapsed. A three-day diet record prior to each blood sample is necessary to evaluate plasma methionine. It is suggested that methionine be kept between 0.45 and 1.0 mg/dl
in fasting plasma (49).

   Most clinicians who treat patients with homocystinuria are of the
opinion that patients should be kept on diet indefinitely. Termination of
diet after growth is achieved may lead to thromboembolisms. Evaluation
of diet therapy is difficult because many untreated patients have normal
intelligence and some reach early adult life with only ectopic lens or
asymptomatic osteoporosis.

   Other disorders of sulfur-containing amino acids are described in
Table 9.6.

Propionic and Methylmalonic Acids

Propionic acid is derived from the metabolism of four amino acids (isoleucine, valine, methionine, and threonine), odd-chain fatty acids and the
side chain of cholesterol (1,20), (Fig. 9.2). Propionic acid is further catabolized to succinyl CoA (a Krebs cycle intermediate) through D-methyl-
malonyl CoA and L-methylmalonyl CoA. A racemase changes D-methyl-
malonyl CoA to the L-form (Fig. 9.2:8) which is then catalyzed to succinyl
CoA by methylmalonyl CoA carbonylmutase, an enzyme that requires as
coenzyme 5′ deoxyadenosylcobalamin (Ad-B$_{12}$) (Fig. 9.2:9).

Propionic Acidemia (PA). This is one of the ketotic hyperglycinemias that
presents early in life and is fatal unless treated with a low protein diet or
an amino acid mixture low in threonine, methionine, valine, and isoleucine and managed during acute episodes of ketosis. Normal growth and
development are possible if diet management is initiated early in the new-

born period (63). This disease is a rare genetic disorder inherited in an autosomal recessive pattern. Diagnosis can be made by detecting an increase in serum propionic acid or demonstrating the block in propionate oxidation in peripheral leukocytes or cultured skin fibroblasts (64). Organic acids, tiglyl CoA derivatives, or methylcitrate in the urine may further confirm the diagnosis.

Infants with PA appear normal at birth but become symptomatic after a protein load. The most striking features include recurrent episodes of ketoacidosis, vomiting, lethargy, and neutropenia aggravated by infections or a high protein intake (65–67). In addition, infants with PA may have intermittent hyperglycemia and hyperglycinemia, long-chain ketonuria, and hyperammonemia (68,69). Other complications associated with this disorder include seizures, thrombocytopenia, osteoporosis, and developmental retardation (70,71).

The unusual early onset of ketosis and its induction by ingestion of methionine, isoleucine, threonine, and valine resulted in knowledge of the biochemical characteristics of PA. The striking long-chain ketonuria seen in patients results from accumulation of butanone, pentanone, and hexanone during isoleucine oxidation (69,72). Other abnormal urine products include tiglic acid, tiglylglycine, propionic acid, propionyl glycine, and methylcitrate (69,72–74). Elevated levels of plasma propionic acid and the organic acids—butyric, isobutyric, and isovaleric—are also found in patients with PA (69). Plasma glycine concentrations may or may not increase above normal in this disorder (69). Exogenous odd-chain fatty acids, normally metabolized to propionyl CoA are used by the patient with PA to synthesize long odd-chain fatty acids (C15:0, C17:0, C17:1). These fatty acids may be found in liver cells of patients with PA and indicate the need to restrict exogenous sources of odd-chain fatty acids (70,75).

The enzyme defect in PA is the failure of propionyl-CoA carboxylase to carboxylate propionate to methylmalonate. Defective oxidation of propionate to CO_2 can be identified *in vitro* using peripheral leukocytes or cultured skin fibroblasts (64,73,75,76,).

Some children with PA may respond to treatment with biotin, the coenzyme for propionyl-CoA carboxylase. Barnes et al. (69) identified a child with PA and secondary ketotic hyperglycinemia who showed an improved biochemical response to isoleucine loading after treatment with 10 mg biotin daily. The authors postulated that biotin responsiveness occurred in situations in which there was a failure to attach biotin to propionyl-CoA carboxylase resulting from either an altered apoenzyme or ligase. Hillman et at. (77) studied leukocytes and fibroblasts in an infant with PA and found an increase in enzyme activity with biotin therapy. Activity of propionyl-CoA carboxylase in fibroblasts increased from 26 percent to 70 percent of control values when biotin (10 ug/dl) was added to the media. A sevenfold increase in enzyme activity in leukocytes was also observed, from 12 percent to 98 percent, respectively, when the diet was supplemented with biotin. Serum concentrations of propionic acid fell from 40 μM to within normal range (5 μM) after initiating diet (1.5 g protein/kg/day) and 10 mg biotin daily. Furthermore, propionate concentrations remained within the normal range after the child consumed a regular diet with biotin supplementation. The data also indicated a defect in biotin binding to propionyl-CoA carboxylase. Unfortunately, not all patients with propionyl-CoA carboxylase deficiency respond to biotin therapy (64,75).

Inherited *methylmalonic acidemia* (MMAE) occurs due to defects in the racemase (Fig. 9.2:8) or in the mutase (Fig. 9.2:9). Clinical features are indistinguishable from propionic acidemia. Urinary methylmalonic acid may be as high as 4.85 g/day (normal = 0). Plasma glycine may be as high as 10 mg/dl (normal = 2.2 mg/dl). (1,20).

This rare genetic disorder is inherited via an autosomal recessive mode. Prenatal diagnosis is available for both PA and MMAE and entails tissue culture of amniotic fluid cells to evaluate for appropriate enzyme activity early in pregnancy (78–80).

It is possible to treat propionic acidemia and methylmalonic acidemia effectively by protein restriction (1.0–1.5 g protein/kg/day) or by an amino acid mixture low in isoleucine, methionine, threonine, and valine (63,65,67,81). Plasma free amino acid levels can be normal in infants with PA while in good health (65,67). Even though a low protein diet reduces serum glycine levels and ketosis, growth may be retarded.

Some patients with PA respond to massive doses of biotin (10 mg/day) (69), while some patients with MMAE respond to large doses of vitamin B_{12} (1 mg intramuscularly every three to four days) (82). However, some protein restriction is still required even with response to vitamin therapy. In determining an adequate diet for individuals with PA or MMAE, the amount of nitrogen must be considered in relation to total nutrient requirements, energy intake and the distribution of protein. General approaches to managing the hyperammonemia that occurs with the organic aciduria are discussed with urea cycle disorders.

Other disorders of amino acid metabolism and the approach to diet therapy presented are described in Table 9.6.

Urea Cycle Disorders (1,20)

There are five major steps in the synthesis of urea from ammonia. These are outlined in Figure 9.3 and the enzyme involved in each metabolic

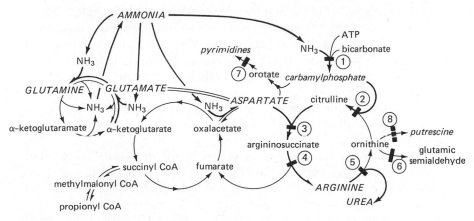

Figure 9.3 Metabolic map of ammonia metabolism. The important relationships among ammonia, glutamine, glutamate, and aspartate are emphasized. The purine nucleotide cycle which releases large amounts of ammonia from muscle has been omitted. The relationship of the Krebs cycle to the arginine cycle is shown, as is the synthesis of pyrimidines from aspartate and carbamyl phosphate. How disorders of propionate metabolism produce hyperammonemia is not clear. Alpha-ketoglutaramate, depicted on the left, has been found in the cerebrospinal fluid of patients with hepatic coma. A transport defect of ornithine reentry into the mitochondrion is the probable cause of hyperornithinemia with homocitrullinemia. (Reprinted by permission of Y. Edward Hsia, M.D.)

	Enzyme reaction	Deficient in
1.	Carbamylphosphate synthetase	Carbamylphosphate synthetase deficiency
2.	Ornithine transcarbamylase	Ornithine transcarbamylase deficiency
3.	Argininosuccinate synthetase	Citrullinemia
4.	Argininosuccinase	Argininosuccinicaciduria
5.	Arginase	Argininemia
6.	Ornithine transaminase	Gyrate atrophy of the retina One form of ornithinemia
7.	Orotidine-5′-phosphate pyrophosphorylase and orotidine-5′-phosphate decarboxylase	Oroticacidurias
8.	Ornithine decarboxylase	Hyperornithinemia

reaction is given. Urea synthesis is described in detail in Chapter 3. All the enzymes of the urea cycle have been found in the liver, brain, and kidney. Quantitatively, those in the liver appear to be of more importance than those found in the brain and kidney. The total quantities of urea cycle enzymes in the liver appear proportional to the daily protein intake.

Inherited defects have been found in all the urea cycle enzymes leading to one or the other of the first five disorders listed in Figure 9.3. There are many clinical manifestations common to all five of the disorders. These include early onset of hyperammonemia (except in ornithine transcarbamylase deficiency in females), vomiting, flaccidity, lethargy, coma, osteoporosis, mental retardation, and death due to respiratory and/or cardiac arrest (1,20).

The common biochemical feature of all urea cycle disorders is hyperammonemia. Other biochemical changes are characteristic of the individual disorder.

Patients with a deficiency of *carbamylphosphate synthetase* present hyperglycinemia, hyperglycinuria, ketosis, acidosis, and low plasma concentration of urea, arginine, pyruvate, and lactate. *Ornithine transcarbamylase deficiency* is associated with plasma elevations of glutamine, glutamic acid and alanine, and depression of plasma levels of citrulline, arginine, and urea.

There appear to be three forms of citrullinemia due to deficiency of *argininosuccinate synthetase* (Fig. 9.3:3). None of the infants with the acute neonatal form (type I) have survived beyond the newborn period. Biochemical characteristics include in addition to decreased plasma urea, increased citrulline in plasma, urine and cerebrospinal fluid with a general elevation in plasma of glutamine, glutamic acid, alanine, proline, lysine, methionine, and tyrosine. These latter elevations appear to be due to liver damage. With type II citrullinemia, symptoms begin during the first year of life. Elevations in blood ammonia are slight. Citrulline increases in plasma, urine, cerebrospinal fluid, and erythrocytes. There are increased plasma levels of glutamine, glutamic acid, alanine, proline, methionine, and lysine. Type III citrullinemia is a benign form and there is no increase in plasma ammonia although citrulline is increased in plasma, urine, and cerebrospinal fluid.

Argininosuccinic acidemia due to a deficiency of argininosuccinase (Fig. 9.3:4) is characterized by elevated levels of argininosuccinate in plasma, urine, and cerebrospinal fluid. Aspartate, glutamic acid, proline, and alanine are elevated in plasma. *Argininemia,* thought to be due to a deficiency of liver arginase (Fig. 9.3:5), is characterized by increased plasma arginine, SGOT and SGPT.

It is thought that all of the disorders of the urea cycle, except ornithine transcarbamylase deficiency are inherited by an autosomal recessive mode. Ornithine transcarbamylase deficiency is inherited as an X-linked dominant disease with full expression in the male who has only one X-chromosome. In the female with two X-chromosomes, expression of the disease will vary depending on the relative number of liver cells in which the normal X-chromosome is inactivated.

Treatment of urea cycle disorders must consider both the hyperammonemic crisis and ongoing chronic care. During a hyperammonemic crisis, dietary protein intake is stopped. Energy needs are met by intravenous glucose and Intralipid℠. Peritoneal dialysis or exchange transfusion may be necessary to remove excess ammonia.

The objective of chronic therapy is to reduce ammonia and thus prevent ammonia toxicity of the brain. Four general approaches are used to treat hyperammonemias. These are:

1. Restriction of nitrogen. In mildly affected patients it may be possible to give a low protein diet (1.5 to 2.0 g protein per kilogram of body weight per day). Restriction of protein below the minimum requirement may lead to body protein catabolism. Optimal protein sparing can be achieved by giving a diet that has ample fluids and energy and just enough protein to meet nitrogen and essential amino acid requirements. The amount will vary for each child. In acutely affected patients protein intake may have to be reduced below one-half gram per kilogram of body weight per day and supplements of ketoacid or hydroxyacid analogues given (83,84).
2. Detoxification. Excess ammonia stimulates respiration and can cause respiratory alkalosis. With alkalosis the equilibrium between the ammonia molecule and ammonium ion is shifted toward the ion that seems to be more toxic. Prevention of alkalosis and deliberate promotion of a little acidosis tends to render ammonia less toxic. The prescribing of glutamate, ornithine, or arginine to stimulate formation of glutamine or urea have not been as useful in practice as appeared to be in theory.
3. Excretion. Increased ammonia excretion can be accomplished through both the urine and the stools. In the colon, any urea in the feces is broken down by urease-containing organisms to release ammonia. This means that constipation can be very detrimental to a patient with hyperammonemia, because of increased ammonia absorption from the colon. Prevention begins with the use of nonconstipating diets. Interestingly, in patients with lactase deficiency, lactose-induced diarrhea promotes ammonia excretion because ammonium ions are trapped by the acid pH, and because the colonic contents are rushed out of the body. For the same reason, the prescription of lactulose, which in a nonassimilable disaccharide, helps hyperammonemia by producing an acid diarrhea. In the kidney, the more acidic the urine the more ammonia that is produced by the tubules to conserve other cations. Here again, acidosis would seem to be better than alkalosis, but the effect is indirect, because urinary ammonia is derived from blood glutamine and glutamate, not from blood ammonia. Nonetheless acidification will increase urinary nitrogen excretion.
4. Supplementation. In defects of the early urea cycle enzymes (Fig. 9.3), arginine becomes an essential amino acid because its pathway has been blocked, and these patients require arginine supplements to sustain growth. The newborn may require supplements of 250–500 mg/kg/day (85).

DISORDERS OF CARBOHYDRATE METABOLISM

Galactose and glycogen metabolism are linked in a complex fashion to the remainder of metabolism (Fig. 9.4). Prior to utilization, galactose must first be converted to glucose. This occurs primarily in the liver where through three enzymatic steps galactose becomes glucose. First, galactose is phosphorylated to galactose-1-phosphate by galactokinase (Fig. 9.4:8); then the hexose moiety is interchanged with the glucose moiety of uridyldiphosphoglucose by galactose-1-phosphate uridyl transferase (Fig. 9.4:9). Finally, the galactose moiety is rearranged to that of glucose by epimerase (Fig. 9.4:10). The glucose thus formed can be used for glycogen synthesis (Fig. 9.4:1) or for synthesis of glucose-1-phosphate (Fig. 9.4:5) (1).

Glycogen is formed by glycogen synthetase (Fig. 9.4:1) which strings together a chain of glucose moieties, each derived from uridyldiphosphoglucose. The branched structure of glycogen is determined by a brancher enzyme (Fig. 9.4:2) which starts a glucose side chain at approximately every eighth glucose. Glycogenolysis is the release of glucose-6-phosphate from glycogen by phosphorylase (Fig. 9.4:5) which is activated by phosphorylase kinase (Fig. 9.4:6). The branches of glycogen are hydrolyzed by amylo-1,6-glucosidase and oligo-1,4, 1,6-glucantransferase (Fig. 9.4:3) yielding free glucose. Glucose-6-phosphate must be acted on by glucose-6-phosphatase (Fig. 9.4:7) to release free glucose (1).

Galactosemia may occur because of deficient functioning either of two enzymes—galactokinase (Fig. 9.4:9) or galactose-1-phosphate uridyl transferase (Fig. 9.4:10). Patients with galactokinase deficiency accumulate galactose and galactitol and develop cataracts. However, they do not have the severe clinical manifestations nor the accumulation of galactose-1-phosphate seen with galactose-1-phosphate uridyl transferase deficiency (1,86).

Galactosemia due to deficiency of gal-1-P uridyl transferase leads to accumulation of galactose-1-phosphate which acts as a phosphate sink producing inaccessible intracellular phosphate. Progressive damage to the central nervous system, liver, renal tubule, and lens results if treatment is not instituted in the first few days of life (1,86).

Transferase deficiency is inherited by an autosomal recessive mode and each offspring resulting from the mating of heterozygotes has a 25 percent chance of being affected or normal and a 50 percent chance of being heterozygote. Estimates of the frequency of the transferase defect have increased with the improvement of screening and diagnostic procedures. Kelly and associates (87) identified four infants with transferase deficiency during analysis of blood samples from 141,402 infants in New

York providing an incidence of one in 35,000. Beutler (88) has estimated that the transferase defect occurs in one in 25,000 to one in 35,000 individuals while Hansen (89) has suggested a frequency from one in 18,000 to one in 70,000.

Clinical symptoms of the transferase defect appear early in infancy. Infants may appear normal at birth but some have been born with cataracts and cirrhosis (86). Symptoms generally appear with the onset of milk feedings.

Jaundice generally appears at four to ten days and outlasts the period of physiologic icterus. Jaundice may result from: retention of bilirubin secondary to toxic injury to liver cells by galactose-1-phosphate (86), delay or inhibition of maturation of glucuronyl transferase necessary for glucuronidation of bilirubin (86), or mild hemolysis. Anemia, the basis of which is unknown, occurs in about 40 percent of untreated cases (86). Lethargy, hypotonia, food refusal, vomiting, and diarrhea are common.

Retarded mental and physical growth occur in most of the untreated cases who survive. The basis for the mental retardation is unknown but several theories have been published. These include (86):

1. An altered UDP galactose:UDP glucose ratio which may influence oxidation in the brain.
2. A depression in brain protein synthesis related to the presence of high levels of galactose or galactose-1-phosphate.
3. Increased levels of galactitol in the brain; phosphatidyl inositol is an integral constituent of cell membranes; galactitol inhibits incorporation of inositol into lipids; inhibition of synthesis of nerve cell membrane could lead to permanantly altered function.

Retarded physical development may be due to food refusal, vomiting, diarrhea, proteinuria, aminoaciduria, loss of energy normally derived from galactose or altered oxidation related to UDP galactose:UDP glucose ratio (86). Depression of protein synthesis in the liver has been found and is thought to be due to decreased incorporation of leucine into protein resulting from the presence of high levels of galactose (86).

Cataracts occur in about 45 percent of untreated cases (86). They are thought to result from the formation and accumulation of galactitol in the lens of the eye leading to a loss of lens glutathione. When glutathione is lost glutathione peroxidase is inactivated and hydrogen peroxide accumulates to toxic levels. The hydrogen peroxide denatures lens protein causing production of lenticular cataracts (90).

Hepatomegaly occurs in nearly all cases of transferase deficiency and cirrhosis develops in untreated patients. The hepatomegaly appears to be due to the presence of abnormally large amounts of galactose-1-phosphate, UDP galactose, and glycogen in the liver. The inhibition of protein

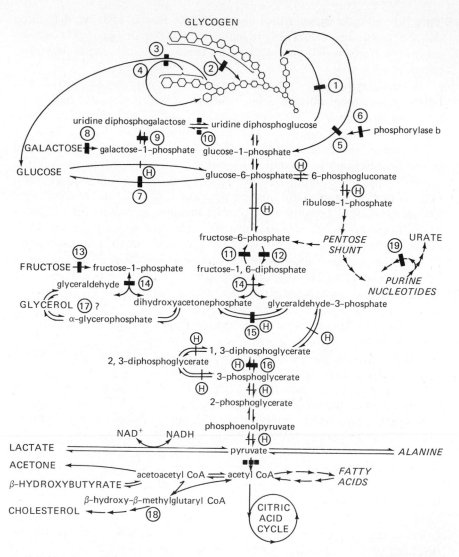

Figure 9.4 Disorders of carbohydrate metabolism. The branched polysaccharide structure of glycogen is represented by the hexagons at the top. The Embden-Meyerhof pathway of glycolysis descends down the center of the figure to the Krebs cycle. Glucose, other hexoses and glycerol enter this schema from the left, lactate, ketone bodies, and cholesterol are related to pyruvate and acetyl CoA as shown on the *lower left*. Purine nucleotide synthesis and fatty acid synthesis are related to carbohydrate metabolism as shown on the *right*.

Solid bars indicate the sites of enzyme defects; interrupted bars designate postulated blocks. Enzyme deficiencies causing hemolytic anemia are located by a circled H. (Reprinted by permission of Y. Edward Hsia, M.D.)

The following abbreviations are used for coenzymes, which are included only when relevant to the cause or treatment of an inborn error.

Ad-B$_{12}$	5'-Deoxyadenosyl-cobalamin	NAD	Nicotinamide adenine dinucleotide
ATP	Adenosine triphosphate	NAD+	Oxidized form of NAD
CoA	Coenzyme A	NADH	Reduced NAD
CoQ	Coenzyme Q	OH-B$_{12}$	Hydroxocobalamin
FAD	Flavine adenine dinucleotide	PyrP	Pyridoxal phosphate
FADH	Reduced FAD	ThPP	Thiamine pyrophosphate
Me-B$_{12}$	Methylcobalamin		

	Enzyme reaction	Deficient in
1.	Glycogen synthetase	Glycogenosis type O
2.	Brancher enzyme	Glycogenosis type IV
3.	Debrancher amylo-1,6 glucosidase	Glycogenosis type III
4.	Debrancher oligo-1,4→1,6-glucantransferase	Glycogenosis type III
5.	Phosphorylase	Glycogenosis type VI (also V-muscle)
6.	Phosphorylase kinase	Glycogenosis type VIII
7.	Glucose-6-phosphatase	Glycogenosis type I, von Gierke's
8.	Galactokinase	Galactokinase deficiency
9.	Galactose-1-phosphate uridylyl transferase	Galactosemia, variants
10.	Uridyldiphosphogalactose epimerase	Benign variants
11.	Fructose-1,6-diphosphatase	Fructose-1,6-diphosphatase deficiency
12.	Phosphofructokinase	Muscle glycogenosis type VII
13.	Fructokinase	Benign fructosuria
14.	Fructose-1-phosphate aldolase Fructose-1-6,-diphosphate aldolase	Fructose intolerance
15.	Triosephosphate isomerase	Triosephosphate isomerase deficiency
16.	Phosphoglycerate kinase	Phosphoglycerate kinase deficiency
17.	Undertermined	Glycerol intolerance
18.	3-hydroxy-3-methylglutaryl CoA reductase	Rate-limiting step in cholesterol biosynthesis
19.	Hypoxanthine-guanine phosphoribosyl-transferase	Hyperuricemia

synthesis that accompanies hepatomegaly results in fibrosis and decreased synthesis of prothrombin and albumin (86).

Because of decreased albumin synthesis and proteinuria, ascites and generalized edema occur in about 36 percent of cases (1,86). Untreated or poorly controlled patients are extremely susceptible to infection with gram-negative organisms (1,86). This is probably related to high circulating levels of galactose.

Galactose and its accumulated metabolites are toxic to the glomeruli and tubules of the kidney. Results of the toxic effects are proteinuria and aminoaciduria. Aminoaciduria is generalized with loss primarily of the neutral aliphatic amino acids such as glycine, alanine, serine, and threonine (1,86).

Extremely low blood glucose levels may be found in contrast to the high blood galactose levels. This hypoglycemia may result from the inability to convert glycogen to glucose because of inhibition of phosphorylase kinase (Fig. 9.4:5) by galactose-1-phosphate (1,86) or from excess insulin production due to high blood galactose (1,86).

Diagnosis of galactosemia is accomplished through measurement of activity of galactose-1-phosphate uridyl transferase. No activity occurs in individuals homozygous for the disease while heterozygotes have approximately one-half normal activity.

Objectives of therapy in galactosemia are to ameliorate or prevent symptoms while providing adequate energy and nutrients for normal growth and development. Treatment should begin as early in the first week of life as possible and consists of removal of all sources of lactose and galactose from the diet (Table 9.12).

Human milk contains 6 to 8 percent, cow's milk, 3 to 4 percent and many proprietary formulas 7 percent lactose. These milks must be replaced by formulas free of galactose (Isomil,® Nutramigen,® Pregestimil®, or Prosobee®). (See Tables 9.3 and 9.4 for formulation and composition.)

Formulas containing soy protein isolate contain about 14 mg of galactose per liter in the form of raffinose and stacchyose, oligosaccharides that contain galactose. At one time in was thought that these oligosaccharides yielded free galactose on hydrolysis in the intestine. It is now known that the human intestine has no enzymes to hydrolyze these oligosaccharides (91). Thus, they may be safely used for feeding infants with galactosemia.

When solid foods are added at appropriate ages (Table 9.2), careful label reading is required to make sure that neither galactose nor lactose has been added in food processing. Lactose is added to baked goods, dry mixes, ice cream, sherbets, confections and batter mixes, among others, to improve flavor, texture, body, viscosity, and mouth feel (92). Foods such as peas and organ meats that naturally contain galactose must also

Table 9.12 Foods to Exclude or Include in the Galactose-free Diet

Type of food	Foods included	Foods excluded
Milk and milk products	Soy milk substitutes Nutramigen Prosobee Meat base formula Cream substitutes free of milk or milk derivatives. Isomil	Breast milk Cows' milk or goats' milk or any other milk from an animal source in any form: Whole, nonfat, evaporated, condensed, whey, casein, dry milk solids, curds, lactose, Ovaltine and malted milk. Cream, butter, all cheeses, yogurt, ice cream, ice milk, sherbet, chocolate milk. All brands of "imitation" or "filled milk" Sodium and calcium caseinate
Legumes	All may be included if laboratory facilities are available for periodic testing of blood (erythrocyte galactose-1-phosphate).	
Meat	Plain meats, fish, poultry Eggs	Liver, pancreas, brain, or any organ meats. Creamed, breaded, processed meats, fish, poultry which may contain lactose.
Bread and cereal foods	Cooked and dry cereals without milk or lactose added *Bread or crackers without milk or lactose added; saltines, graham crackers. Macaroni, spaghetti, noodles, rice	Cereals, breads, crackers that have milk, milk products, or lactose added.
Fats	Vegetable oils, such as soybean, corn, cottonseed, safflower, olive, peanut oils. Shortening, lard, margarines that do not contain milk or milk products Olives, nuts, bacon.	Butter, cream Margarine unless free of lactose in any form.
Fruits and vegetables	Any fresh, frozen, canned or dried fruits, unless processed with lactose. Any vegetable unless excluded, or if processed with lactose. White potatoes, sweet potatoes, yams.	Fruits processed with lactose. Peas; vegetables processed with lactose Most brands of instant mashed potatoes.
Soups	Clear soups; vegetable soups that do not contain peas; cream soups made with milk substitutes listed.	Cream soups, chowders, commercially prepared soups containing lactose.

Table 9.12 Continued

Desserts	Water and fruit ices; gelatin, angel food cake, homemade cakes, pies and cookies made from acceptable ingredients; fruit-flavored cornstarch pudding made with water.	Ice cream, ice milk, sherbet, custard. Most commercial mixes for cakes and cookies
Miscellaneous	Unbuttered popcorn, marshmallows, sugar, corn syrup, molasses, honey, carbonated beverages, colas, root beer, instant coffee, unsweetened cocoa, unsweetened cooking chocolate, semisweet chocolate. Pure spices, punch base without lactose.	Caramels, toffee. Milk chocolate. Presweetened punch base with lactose. Sugar substitutes that contain lactose such as Equa and Sweet 'n Low.

Source: From Acosta and Elsas (49).
*Bread companies and markets should be contacted in each grographic area.

be excluded from the diet. The artificial sweeteners Sweet n' Low and Wee Cal and the proposed sweetener Equa contain lactose. Any products prepared with these sugar substitutes must be avoided. Some clinical centers treating patients with galactosemia have allowed fermented dairy products under the mistaken impression that all lactose has been converted to lactic acid. This is not the case (93), however, and these products should be excluded from the diet until 12 or 13 years of age when aged cheese may be allowed.

Drugs often contain lactose for a variety of purposes. A list of sugar-free drug preparations has been published (94) that should be updated frequently and scrutinized when galactosemic children require drug therapy.

Treatment, while lifesaving, has not resulted in complete freedom from intellectual impairment. Those infants diagnosed and treated early who maintain excellent dietary control have better intellectual function than those who have poor control or are diagnosed late (95,96). Control is defined on the basis of erythrocyte galactose-1-phosphate levels and is considered excellent if consistently below 3 mg/dl (97). However, even with excellent control children frequently have lower I.Q.s than their normal siblings. They may have difficulty with abstract thinking and visual perception. These deficits may be related to intrauterine brain damage from maternal blood galactose crossing the placenta into the vulnerable fetus. Prenatal diagnosis has been successfully used in one center to determine if the fetus is galactosemic, thus establishing the need for galactose restriction in the diet of the heterozygote mother (86,98).

The galactose-free diet may be liberalized to some extent in the patient with transferase deficiency at 12 or 13 years of age. However, it must not be abandoned because of damaging effects of galactose-1-phosphate and galactitol on the liver, kidney, and lens of the eye. Galactosemic females must be treated with strict exclusion of galactose during pregnancy to prevent *in utero* damage to the fetus (99,100).

Each of the enzymes in glycogen metabolism has been deficient in inborn errors of metabolism. The most destructive disorder is due to hepatic glucose-6-phosphatase deficiency (Fig. 9.4:7). This deficiency leads to *glycogenosis type I* or *von Gierke's disease*. Paradoxically, this enzyme is only indirectly related to glycogen metabolism. Its function is to hydrolyze phosphorylated glucose so that the free sugar can leave the liver cell to enter the bloodstream.

Ingested glucose, after absorption from the small intestine, is rapidly cleared from the blood by the liver. Following this, blood glucose concentrations are sustained by continual production of glucose by the liver. This endogenous glucose is derived initially from glycogen stores, and is also derived from amino acids and glycerol by gluconeogenesis (1).

The metabolic disturbances in type I glycogenosis have many ramifications. The primary consequence is that blood glucose levels plummet as soon as dietary glucose has been cleared from the circulation. This leads to the typical symptoms of hypoglycemia: irritability, obtundation, coma, and seizures. These are more likely to occur at night, are relieved promptly by ingested glucose and are associated with a voracious appetite (1).

The secondary disturbances in this condition require an appreciation of the intricacies of glucose metabolism illustrated in Figure 9.4. With deficiency of glucose-6-phosphatase and expansion of the pool of phosphorylated glucose inside the liver cell many pathways of glucose metabolism are accelerated (1):

1. Increased glycolysis leads to formation of more glycerol, lactate, and ketone bodies (Fig. 9.4, left column); only these can escape from the liver cell for utilization as energy by the rest of the body but at the cost of metabolic lactic acidosis, some ketosis, and triglyceridemia.
2. Increased glycogen synthesis probably explains the excessive liver (and kidney) glycogen in this disorder, with huge distension of these organs. An indirect benefit of glycogen excess is that this is a dynamic excess, with rapid turnover of glycogen. Since every eighth glucose moiety from glycogen is hydrolyzed by the debrancher enzyme system, some free glucose is released by the liver, although at low efficiency.
3. Increased pentose shunt activity leads to increased formation of ribose-5-phosphate and phosphoribosylpyrophosphate, which stimulates purine synthesis, resulting in high serum uric acid levels (Fig. 9.4, right margin).
4. Affected patients also tend to have chronic diarrhea and to have excess blood platelets with bleeding tendencies but the mechanisms for these complications are not understood.

All these metabolic complications are caused by disturbances of the hepatic homeostatic mechanisms for controlling glucose. A patient could be kept in biochemical equilibrium if only blood glucose could be sustained by dietary means alone. Treatment differs from that for other causes of hypoglycemia because the only usable dietary source of blood glucose is glucose and its multimers, maltose, starch, and glycogen. Galactose, fructose, or glucogenic amino acids will not help, because they can only be converted to glucose via glucose-6-phosphate.

The objective in diet management is to give enough glucose orally to prevent hypoglycemia while avoiding hyperglycemia which would stimulate reactive insulin release. At the same time, a balanced nutritious diet should be given without exceeding the normal energy needs, which would lead to obesity.

In practice, small frequent glucose-rich snacks, (as many as two per hour) judiciously mixed with protein and fat in order to retard gastric emptying, will suffice during waking hours. To allow normal uninterrupted sleep, an important recent advance is the use of an indwelling nasogastric tube overnight with constant infusion of a glucose solution (101). Effective dietary treatment has resulted in dramatic improvement in patients' metabolism, general health, and physical growth. Portacaval shunts that divert glucose-rich blood to peripheral tissues before it reaches the liver are being successfully used in an increasing number of patients (1). Other disorders of carbohydrate metabolism are described in Table 9.13.

Other hepatic glycogenoses due to deficiencies of the *debrancher* or *phosphorylase* enzyme systems are milder. These can be treated with diets containing any type of carbohydrate or glucogenic amino acids. *Brancher* deficiency is similar, but in addition, damage is caused to liver cells; hepatic scarring and fibrosis result from the abnormal unbranched glycogen molecules (1).

DISORDERS OF LIPID METABOLISM

Many of the inherited disorders of lipid metabolism are presented in Table 9.14. The most common of these disorders is familial hypercholesterolemia or type II hyperlipoproteinemia, which is discussed in Chapter 7.

DISORDERS OF MINERAL METABOLISM

Copper

Wilson's disease, inherited via the autosomal recessive mode, is characterized by progressive neurologic symptoms, corneal ring, hemo-

Table 9.13 Carbohydrates in Inborn Errors of Metabolism

Nutrient	Disorder	Defect	Disturbances	Diet treatment
Glucose and galactose	Glucose-galactose malabsorption	Specific transport	Explosive diarrhea, growth failure	Exclude glucose and galactose
Lactose	Lactase deficiency	Intestinal lactase	Acute diarrhea	Avoid lactose
Lactose and sucrose	Disaccharidase deficiency	Intestinal disaccharidase	Diarrhea, growth failure	Avoid lactose, sucrose
Galactose	Galactosemia	Galactokinase (Fig. 9.4:8)	Cataracts	Avoid galactose
		Gal-1-P uridyl transferase (Fig. 9.4:9)	Gastrointestinal, liver, and brain damage; cataracts	Exclude galactose
Fructose	Fructose intolerance	Fru-1-P aldose (Fig. 9.4:14)	Liver and brain damage	Exclude fructose
		Fru-1,6-diphosphatase (Fig. 9.4:11)	Hypoglycemia, ketosis, aggravated by fructose	Avoid fructose
	D-Glyceric acidemia	D-Glyceric dehydrogenase	Mental retardation	Avoid fructose
Glycerol	Glycerol intolerance	Undetermined (Fig. 9.4:17)	Hypoglycemia, ketosis	Exclude glycerol

Source: Prepared by Dr. Y. E. Hsia.

Table 9.14 Some Inherited Disorders of Lipid Metabolism

Disorder	Defect	Disturbances	Treatment
Abetalipoproteinemia	Not known	Absent CLM and VLDL, acanthocytes, retinitis, neurologic signs, malabsorption.	Restriction of triglycerides with long-chain fatty acids. Use of MCT and supplements of vitamins A, D, E (100 mg/day) and K
Hypobetalipoproteinemia	Not known	Low LDL, absent CLM and VLDL. Acanthocytes, retinitis, neurologic signs, malabsorption.	Supplementation with fat-soluble vitamins if indicated.
Tangier disease	Not known	HDL low and abnormal, corneal infiltration, abnormal tonsils, enlarged lymph nodes, hepatosplenomegaly, neuropathy, malabsorption.	? Fat restriction
Lecithin:Cholesterol Acyltransferase Deficiency (LCAT)	Absent or near absent LCAT activity in plasma	Abnormal plasma LP, anemia, proteinuria corneal opacities, renal failure.	Fat restriction
Hyperlipoproteinemia Type I	↓ Extrahepatic triglyceride lipase	Chylomicronemia; xanthomas, abdominal pain, pancreatitis, lipemia retinalis	Fat restriction, use of MCT to provide energy.

Type	Cause	Clinical features	Treatment
Type 2	↓ LDL receptors	Elevated plasma LDL, xanthomas, arcus cornea, premature atherosclerosis, polyarthritis, tenosynovitis	Fat and cholesterol restriction, increased PUFA; cholestyramine, nicotinic acid; ileal bypass, portacaval shunt; plasma exchange
Type 3	Unknown	Abnormal plasma LP containing B-VLDL with elevated cholesterol, palmar xanthomas, arteriosclerosis, hyperuricemia	Energy restriction to maintain ideal body weight. Decreased saturated fat; increased PUFA; Cholesterol <300 mg/day; alcohol restriction. Clofibrate, nicotinic acid D-thyroxine
Type 4	Unknown	Elevated plasma TG, moderate obesity, insulin resistance, fasting hyperinsulinemia, glucose intolerance, hyperuricemia, coronary artery disease	Weight reduction; carbohydrate restriction. Clofibrate
Type 5	Unknown	Elevated plasma TG, xanthomas, pancreatitis, coronary artery disease, obesity, hyperglycemia, hepatosplenomegaly Foam cells in bone marrow and other organs	Restriction of dietary fat and energy; elimination of alcohol. Nicotinic acid

lytic crises, cirrhosis, and storage of copper in several organs (1). Patients have decreased plasma concentrations of copper and ceruloplasmin, a copper containing enzyme (1). The relative amounts of copper bound by plasma amino acids and albumin are increased. Tissue copper content is increased, especially the lysosomal copper in the liver (1). The high copper content of the liver and brain are related to the dysfunction of these organs. The biliary and fecal copper excretion is decreased while renal copper excretion is increased. The pathogenesis of Wilson's disease is not known (1) although speculations are abundant.

Treatment for Wilson's disease is by reducing copper intake and promoting copper excretion. Shellfish, organ meats, chocolate, mushrooms, nuts, and certain cereals and spices are all high in copper and should be avoided in the diet of a patient with Wilson's disease. To reduce copper intake below 0.5 to 0.8 mg per day for an adult, however, requires an unappetizing stringent diet. Hence reduction of copper intake is only of limited utility by itself. Because promotion of copper excretion in the urine can be achieved very effectively with chelating agents such as penicillamine, this combination of a reduced copper intake with prescription of a chelating agent can sustain a negative copper balance in a patient with Wilson's disease until much of the excess copper has been eluted. Effective treatment can arrest the progression of this disease in symptomatic patients, and can prevent the appearance of any abnormalities in a brother or sister of an affected patient if the diagnosis is made presymptomatically. By a combination of drug and diet therapy it is possible to reduce the excess stores of copper and to improve the clinical state (1). Copper content of foods (102) and recipes low in copper have been published to provide variety to the diet (103).

Zinc

In 1973, a dramatic clinical improvement of the symptoms of acrodermatitis enteropathica (AE) by zinc sulphate therapy was observed by Moynahan and Barnes (104). This observation has been confirmed by others (105–107). AE is an autosomal recessive inherited disorder characterized by intermittent diarrhea, dermatitis, and alopecia. If untreated, the disease is usually, but not always, fatal. The symptoms start after weaning with perioral, acral, genital, and perianal dermatitis that consists of erythema and scaling during inactive phases and of vesicobullous lesions during active phases. Until 1973, the only treatment that controlled the symptoms to some extent was feeding with human milk and continuous oral medication of halogenated hydroxiquins. The long-term, high-dose use of these drugs produced optic nerve atrophy. Low serum zinc concentrations have been measured in these patients amounting to about 20 percent of the normal values. The zinc content of hair and the urinary excretion of zinc were also low (107). After oral zinc supplementation with 35 to 135 mg zinc/day, the serum zinc concentration rises to normal values, the skin lesions disappear within one week and the hair starts growing within four weeks. The patients remain free of symptoms during zinc therapy.

No toxic reactions have been reported using zinc sulphate, zinc aspartate or zinc gluconate other than occasional gastric distress caused by large doses. The therapeutic range corresponds to five to 20 times normal requirement.

The cause of the low serum zinc concentration in patients with AE was not clarified until 1974, when zinc absorption studies were performed in three patients with AE and then in one more in 1976 (108). The intestinal zinc absorption of the patients after oral administration of ^{65}Zn in the fasting state amounts to 16, 18, 30, and 42 percent of the ingested dose, whereas the absorption values of controls were in the range of 58 to 77 percent. The urinary zinc excretion was not increased in patients with AE nor did long-term measurements of zinc retention show increased losses of the absorbed zinc by any other way. Thus, in patients with AE a reduced intestinal absorption of zinc could be documented. The nature of this defect has not been defined. It could be a primary mucosal defect of zinc absorption or a secondary malabsorption due to other unknown factors impairing zinc uptake. In addition to these characteristics, inclusion bodies have been found in Paneth cells of the intestinal mucosa by ultrastructural examination of intestinal biopsies (109). Zinc deficiency leading to similar skin lesions and alopecia as in AE have been found in patients with adult celiac disease (108), in Crohn's disease (110), and in infants during prolonged parenteral nutrition (111). Zinc supplementation leads to a prompt rise of the serum zinc concentration and to healing of the skin lesions. Thus it is becoming more and more probable that the symptoms of AE are the real zinc deficiency symptoms of humans (112,113).

REFERENCES

1. Stanbury, J. B., J. B. Wyngaarden, and D. S. Fredickson, eds. *The Metabolic Basis of Inherited Disease.* 4th ed. New York: McGraw-Hill, 1978.
2. McKusick, V. A., and R. Claiborne, eds. *Medical Genetics.* New York: HP Publishing Co., 1973.
3. Folling, A. The original detection of phenylketonuria. In *Phenylketonuria,* H. Bickel, F. P. Hudson, and L. I. Woolf, eds. Stuttgart: Georg Thieme Verlag, 1971.
4. Jervis, G. A. Phenylpyruvic oligophrenia: Deficiency of phenylalanine oxidizing system. *Proc. Soc. Exp. Med.* **82:** 514, 1953.
5. Menkes, J. H. Cerebral proteolipids in phenylketonuria. *Neurol.* **18:** 1003, 1968.

6. Agrawal, H. C., A. H. Bone, and A. N. Davison. Hyperphenylalaninemia and the developing brain. In *Phenylketonuria,* H. Bickel, F. P. Hudson, and L. I. Woolf, eds. Stuttgart: Georg Thieme Verlag, 1971; pp. 121–125.

7. Bessman, S. P., M. L. Williamson, and R. Koch. Diet, genetics, and mental retardation: Interaction between phenylketonuria heterozygous mother and fetus to produce nonspecific diminution of IQ: Evidence in support of the justification hypothesis. *Proc. Natl. Acad. Sci.* **75:** 1562, 1978.

8. Guthrie, R. and A. Susi. A simple phenylalanine method for detection of phenylketonuria in large populations of newborns. *Pediat.* **32:** 338, 1963.

9. Blaskovics, M. E. Phenylketonuria and other phenylalaninemias. *Clinics in Endocrin. Metab.* **3:** 87, 1974.

10. Smith, I., B. E. Clayton, and O. H. Wolff. New variant of phenylketonuria with progressive neurological illness unresponsive to phenylalanine restriction. *Lancet* **1:** 1108, 1975.

11. Kaufman, S., N. A. Holtzman, S. Milstein, J. J. Butler, and A. Krumholz. Phenylketonuria due to a deficiency of dihydropteridine reductase. *N. Engl. J. Med.* **293:** 785, 1975.

12. Bartholome', K. and D. J. Byrd. L-DOPA and 5-hydroxytryptophan therapy in phenylketonuria with normal phenylalanine hydroxylase activity. *Lancet* **2:** 1042, 1975.

13. Bickel, H. The effects of a phenylalanine-free and phenylalanine-poor diet in phenylpyruvic oligophrenia. *Exp. Med. Surg.* **12:** 114, 1954.

14. Dobson, J. C., M. L. Williamson, C. Azen, and R. Koch. Intellectual assessment of 111 four-year-old children with phenylketonuria. *Pediat.* **60:** 822, 1977.

15. *Management of Newborn Infants with PKU.* U.S. Dept. of Health, Education and Welfare, PHS, HSA, Bureau of Community Health Services. DHEW Publ. No. (HSA) 78-5211, 1978.

16. Acosta, P. B., and E. Wenz. *Diet Management of PKU for Infants and Preschool Children.* U.S. Dept. of Health, Education and Welfare, PHS, HSA, Bureau of Community Health Services. DHEW Publ. No. (HSA) 77-5209, 1977.

17. Acosta, P. B., E. Wenz, and M. Williamson. Methods of dietary inception in infants with PKU. *J. Am. Diet. Assn.* **72:** 164, 1978

18. Acosta, P. B., E. Wenz, and M. Williamson. Nutrient intake of treated infants with phenylketonuria. *Am. J. Clin. Nutr.* **30:** 198, 1977.

19. Wannemacher, R. W. Key role of various individual amino acids in host response to infection. *Am. J. Clin. Nutr.* **30:** 1269, 1977.

20. Nyhan, W. L., ed. *Heritable Disorders of Amino Acid Metabolism: Patterns of Clinical Expression and Genetic Variation.* New York: John Wiley & Sons, 1974.

21. Umbarger, B., H. K. Berry, and B. S. Sutherland. Advances in the management of patients with phenylketonuria. *J. Am. Med. Assn.* **193:** 128, 1965.

22. Ingall, D., J. D. Sherman, and F. Cockburn. Immediate effects of phenylalanine deficient diet in young infants. *J. Pediat.* **65:** 1073, 1964 (Abstract).

23. Nakagawa, I., T. Takahashi, T. Suzuki, and K. Kobayashi. Amino acid requirements of children. Minimal needs of threonine, valine and phenylalanine based on nitrogen balance method. *J. Nutr.* **77:** 61, 1962.

24. Sibinga, M. S., C. J. Friedman, I. M. Steisel, and E. C. Baker. The depressing

effect of diet on physical growth in phenylketonuria. *Devpt. Med. Child. Neurol.* **13:** 63, 1971.

25. Hanley, W. B., L. Linsa., W. Davidson, and C. A. F. Moes. Malnutrition with early treatment of phenylketonuria. *Pediat. Res.* **4:** 318, 1970.

26. Lund, E., K. Vollmond, and B. Ovlisen. Phenylalanine levels in blood and urine in newborn infants, measured by Guthrie test. *Acta Path. et Microbiol. Scandinav.* **64:** 299, 1965.

27. Holm, V. A., R. A. Kronmal, M. Willanson, and A. F. Roche. Physical growth in phenylketonuria, II. Growth of children in the PKU Collaborative Study from birth to four years of age (In press).

28. Wong, R. G., P. B. Acosta, D. Jones, and R. Koch. Mineral balance in treated phenylketonuric children. *J. Am. Diet. Assn.* **57:** 229, 1970.

29. Lewis, J. S., A. K. Pian, M. T. Baer, P. B. Acosta, and G. A. Emerson. Effect of long-term ingestion of polyunsaturated fat, age, plasma cholesterol, diabetes mellitus and supplemented tocopherol upon plasma tocopherol. *Am. J. Clin. Nutr.* **26:** 136, 1973.

30. Lewis, J. S., S. Loskill, M. L. Bunker, P. B. Acosta, and R. Kim. N-methyl-nicotinamide excretion of phenylketonuric children and a child with Hartnup disease before and after phenylalanine and tryptophan loads. *Fed. Proc.* **33:** 666, 1974 (Abstract).

31. Hudson, F. P. Termination of dietary treatment of phenylketonuria. *Arch. Dis. Child.* **42:** 198, 1967.

32. Holtzman, N. A., D. W. Welcher, and E. D. Mellits. Termination of restricted diet in children with phenylketonuria: A randomized controlled study. *N. Engl. J. Med.* **293:** 1121, 1975.

33. Horner, F. A., C. W. Streamer, L. L. Alejandrino, L. H. Reed, and F. Ibbott. Termination of dietary treatment of phenylketonuria. *N. Engl. J. Med.* **266:** 79, 1962.

34. Cabalska, B., N. Duczynska, J. Borzmowska, K. Zorska, A. Koslacz-Folga, and K. Bozkowa. Termination of dietary treatment in phenylketonuria. *Europ. J. Pediat.* **126:** 253, 1977.

35. Smith, I., M. E. Lobascher, J. E. Stevenson, O. H. Wolff, H. Schmidt, S. Grubel-Kaiser, and H. Bickel. Effect of stopping low-phenylalanine diet on intellectual progress of children with phenylketonuria. *Brit. M. J.* **2:** 723, 1978.

36. Frankenburg, W. K., B. R. Duncan, R. W. Coffelt, R. Koch, J. G. Coldwell, and C. D. Son. Maternal phenylketonuria: Implications for growth and development. *J. Pediat.* **73:** 560, 1968.

37. Ghadimi, H. and P. Pecora. Free amino acids of cord plasma as compared with maternal plasma during pregnancy. *Pediat.* **33:** 500, 1964.

38. Gaull, G. E., D. K. Rassin, G. E. Solomon, R. C. Harris, and J. A. Sturman. Biochemical observations on so-called hereditary tyrosinemia. *Pediatr. Res.* **4:** 337, 1970.

39. Gaull, G. E., D. K. Rassin, and J. A. Sturman. Significance of hypermethion-inemia in acute tyrosinosis. *Lancet* **1:** 1318, 1968.

40. Scriver, C. R., J. Larochelle, and M. Silverberg. Hereditary tyrosinemia and tyrosyluria in a French Canadian geographic isolate. *Am. J. Dis. Child.* **113:** 41, 1967.

41. Halvorsen, S., and L. R. Gjessing. Studies on tyrosinosis. 1. Effect of low tyrosine and low phenylalanine diet. *Brit. Med. J.* **2:** 1171, 1964.
42. Halvorsen, S. Dietary treatment of tyrosinosis. *Am. J. Dis. Child.* **113:** 38, 1967.
43. Gentz, J., B. Lindblad, S. Lindstedt, L. Levy, W. Shasteen, and R. Zetterstrom. Dietary treatment in tyrosinemia. *Am. J. Dis. Child.* **113:** 31, 1967.
44. Kogut, M. D., K. N. Shaw, and G. N. Donnell. Tyrosinosis. *Am. J. Dis. Child.* **113:** 47, 1967.
45. Partington, M., C. R. Scriver, and A. Sass-Kortsak, eds. Conference on hereditary tyrosinemia. *Canad. Med. Assn. J.* **97:** 1047, 1967.
46. Bodegard, G., J. Gentz, B. Lindblad, S. Lindstedt, and R. Zetterstrom. Hereditary tyrosinemia. 3. On the differential diagnosis and the lack of effect of early dietary treatment. *Acta Paediatr. Scan.* **58:** 37, 1969.
47. Michals, K., R. Matalon, and P. W. K. Wong. Dietary treatment of tyrosinemia type I. *J. Am. Diet. Assn.* **73:** 507, 1978.
48. Cohn, M., M. Yudkoff, B. Yost, and S. Stanton. Phenylalanine tyrosine deficiency syndrome as a complication of the management of hereditary tyrosinemia. *Am. J. Clin. Nutr.* **30:** 209, 1977.
49. Acosta, P. B. and L. J. Elsas, II. *Dietary Management of Inherited Metabolic Disease: Phenylketonuria, Galactosemia, Tyrosinemia, Homocystinuria, Maple Syrup Urine Disease.* Atlanta: ACELMU Publ., 1976.
50. Holt, L. E., S. E. Snyderman, P. M. Norton, E. Roitman, and J. Finch. The plasma aminogram in kwashiorkor. *Lancet* **2:** 1343, 1963.
51. Naylor, R. and R. Guthrie. Personal communication.
52. Piez, K. A. and L. Morris. A modified procedure for the automatic analysis of amino acids. *Anal. Biochem.* **1:** 187, 1960.
53. Sternowsky, H. J., J. Roboz, F. Hutterer, and G. Gaull. Determination of alpha-ketoacids as silycated oximes in urine and serum by gas chromatography-mass spectrometry. *Clin. Chim. Acta.* **47:** 371, 1973.
54. Dancis, J., J. Hutzler, S. E. Snyderman, and R. P. Cox. Enzyme activity in classical and variant forms of maple syrup urine disease. *J. Pediatr.* **81:** 312, 1972.
55. Elsas, L. J., J. H. Priest, F. B. Wheeler, D. J. Danner, and B. A. Pask. Maple syrup urine disease: Coenzyme function and prenatal monitoring. *Metab.* **23:** 569, 1974.
56. Scriver, C. R., C. L. Clow, S. Mackenzie, and E. Delvin. Thiamine responsive maple syrup urine disease. *Lancet* **1:** 310, 1971.
57. Danner, D. J., F. B. Wheeler, S. K. Lemmon, and L. J. Elsas, II. In vivo and in vitro response of human branched chain L-ketoacid dehydrogenase to thiamine and thiamine pyrophosphate. *Pediat. Res.* **12:** 235, 1978.
58. Danner, D. J., S. K. Lemmon, L. J. Elsas, II. Substrate specificity and stabilization by thiamine pyrophosphate of rat liver branched chain L-ketoacid dehydrogenase. *Biochem. Med.* **19:** 27, 1978.
59. American Academy of Pediatrics, Committee on Nutrition. Special diets for infants with inborn errors of metabolism. *Pediat.* **57:** 783, 1976.
60. Waisman, H. A., B. A. Smith, E. S. Brown, and T. Gerritsen. Treatment of branched chain ketoaciduria (BCKA) during acute illness. *Clin. Pediat.* **11:** 360, 1974.

61. McKusick, V. A., J. G. Hall, and F. Char. The clinical and genetic characteristics of homocystinuria. In *Inherited Disorders of Sulfur Metabolism*, N. A. J. Carson and D. N. Raine, eds. Edinburgh: Churchill Livingstone, 1971.

62. Fernhoff, P. Personal communication.

63. Brandt, I. K., Y. E. Hsia, D. H. Clements, and S. Provence. Propionicacidemia (ketotic hyperglycinemia): Dietary treatment resulting in normal growth and development. *Pediat.* **53:** 391, 1974.

64. Hsia, Y. E., K. J. Scully, and L. E. Rosenberg. Inherited propionyl CoA carboxylase deficiency in patients with ketotic hyperglycinemia. *J. Clin. Invest.* **50:** 127, 1971.

65. Childs, B., W. L. Nyhan, M. Borden, L. Bard, and R. E. Cooke. Idiopathic hyperglycinemia: I. A new disorder of amino acid metabolism. *Pediat.* **27:** 522, 1961.

66. Nyhan, W. L., M. Borden, B. Childs. Idiopathic hyperglycinemia: a new disorder of amino acid metabolism. II. The concentrations of other amino acids in the plasma and their modifications by the administration of leucine. *Pediat.* **27:** 539, 1961.

67. Nyhan, W. L. Treatment of hyperglycinemia. *Am. J. Dis. Child.* **113:** 129, 1967.

68. Ando, T., K. Rasmussen, W. L. Nyhan, G. N. Donnell, and N. D. Barnes. Propionic acidemia in patients with ketotic hyperglycinemia. *J. Pediat.* **78:** 827, 1971.

69. Barnes, N. D., D. Hull, L. Balgobin, and D. Gompertz. Biotin-responsive propionic acidemia. *Lancet* **2:** 244, 1970.

70. Hommes, F. A., J. R. Kuipers, J. D. Elema, J. F. Jansen, and J. H. Jonxis. Propionicacidemia, a new inborn error of metabolism. *Pediat. Res.* **2:** 519, 1968.

71. Childs, B. and W. L. Nyhan, Further observations of a patient with hyperglycinemia. *Pediat.* **33:** 403, 1964.

72. Menkes, J. H. Idiopathic hyperglycinemia: Isolation and identification of three previously underscribed urinary ketones. *J. Pediat.* **69:** 413, 1966.

73. Rasmussen, K., T. Ando, and W. L. Nyhan. Excretion of tiglyglycine in propionic acidemia. *J. Pediat.* **81:** 970, 1972.

74. Ando, T., K. Rasmussen, J. M. Wright, and W. L. Nyhan. Isolation and identification of methylcitrate, a major metabolic product of propionate in patients with propionic acidemia. *J. Biol. Chem.* **247:** 2200, 1972.

75. Gompertz, D., D. C. Bau, C. N. Storrs, T. J. Peters, and E. Hughes. Localization of enzymatic defect in propionic acidemia. *Lancet* **1:** 1140, 1970.

76. Ando, T., W. L. Nyhan, J. D. Connor, K. Rasmussen, G. N. Donnell, N. Barnes, D. Cottom, and D. Hull. The oxidation of glycine and propionic acid in propionic acidemia with ketotic hyperglycinemia. *Pediatr. Res.* **6:** 576, 1972.

77. Hillman, R. E., J. P. Keating, and J. C. Williams. Biotin-responsive propionic acidemia presenting as the rumination syndrome. *J. Pediat.* **92:** 439, 1978.

78. Gompertz, D., P. A. Goodey, H. Thom, G. Russell, A. W. Johnston, D. H. Mellor, M. W. MacLean, M. E. Ferguson-Smith, and M. A. Ferguson-Smith. Prenatal diagnosis and family studies in a case of propionic acidemia. *Clin. Genet.* **8:** 244, 1975.

79. Mahoney, M. J., L. E. Rosenberg, B. Lindbald, J. Waldenstrom, and R. Zetterstrom. Prenatal diagnosis of methylmalonic aciduria. *Acta. Paediatr. Scand.* **64:** 44, 1975.

80. Ampola, M. G., M. J. Mahoney, E. Nakamura, and K. Tanaka. Prenatal therapy of a patient with vitamin B_{12} responsive methylmalonic acidemia. *N. Engl. J. Med.* **293:** 313, 1975.

81. Nyhan, W. L., N. Fawcett, T. Ando, O. M. Rennert, and R. L. Julius. Response to dietary therapy in B_{12} unresponsive methylmalonic acidemia. *Pediat.* **51:** 539, 1973.

82. Hsia, Y. E., K. Scully, A. Ch. Lilljeqvist, and L. E. Rosenberg. Vitamin B_{12} dependent methylmalonicaciduria. *Pediat.* **46:** 497, 1970.

83. Batshaw, M., S. Brusilow, M. Walser. Treatment of carbamyl phosphate synthetase deficiency with keto-analogues of essential amino acids. *N. Engl. J. Med.* **292:** 1085, 1975.

84. Thoene, J., M. Batshaw, E. Spector, S. Kulovich, S. Brusilow, M. Walser, and W. Nyhan. Neonatal citrullinemia: Treatment with keto-analogues of essential amino acids. *J. Pediat.* **90:** 218, 1977.

85. Hartlage, P. L., M. E. Coryell, W. K. Hall, and D. A. Hahn. Argininosuccinic aciduria: Prenatal diagnosis and early dietary management. *J. Pediat.* **85:** 86, 1974.

86. Hsia, D. Y. Y., ed. *Galactosemia*. Springfield: Charles C. Thomas, 1969.

87. Kelly, S., S. Katz, J. Bivens, and J. Boylan. Screening for galactosemia in New York State. *Publ. Health Reports* **85:** 575, 1970.

88. Beutler, E. Field test for galactosemia screening. Methods in newborn infants. *J. Am. Med. Assn.* **199:** 501, 1967.

89. Hansen, R. G., R. Bretthauer, J. Mayes, and J. H. Nordin. Estimation of frequency of occurrence of galactosemia in the population. *Proc. Soc. Exp. Biol. Med.* **115:** 560, 1964.

90. Cordes, F. C. Galactosemia cataracts: A review. *Am. J. Ophthal.* **50:** 1151, 1960.

91. Gitzelman, R. and S. Auricchio. The handling of soya alpha-galactosides by a normal and a galactosemic child. *Pediat.* **36:** 231, 1965.

92. Nickerson, T. A. Why use lactose and its derivatives in food? *Food Tech.* **32:** 40, 1978.

93. Fagen, J. H. The identification of reducing sugars in cheddar cheese during the early stages of ripening. *J. Dairy Sci.* **35:** 779, 1952.

94. Sugar-free liquid preparations. *Am. Drug.* :51, May 1975.

95. Fishler, K., G. N. Donnell, W. R. Bergren, and R. Koch. Intellectual and personality development in children with galactosemia. *Pediat.* **50:** 412, 1972.

96. Lee, D. H. Psychological aspects of galactosemia. *J. Ment. Def. Res.* **16:** 173, 1972.

97. Donnell, G. N., W. R. Bergren, G. Perry, and R. Koch. Galactose-1-phosphate in galactosemia. *Pediat.* **31:** 802, 1963.

98. Fensom, A. H. P., F. Benson, and S. Blunt. Prenatal diagnosis of galactosemia. *Brit. Med. J.* **4:** 386, 1974.

99. Roe, T. F., J. G. Hallatt, G. N. Donnell, and W. G. Ng. Childbearing by a galactosemic woman. *J. Pediat.* **78:** 1026, 1971.

100. Tedesco, T. A., G. Morrow, and W. J. Mellman. Normal pregnancy and childbirth in a galactosemic woman. *J. Pediat.* **81:** 1159, 1972.

101. Burr, I. M., J. A. O'Neill, D. T. Karzan, L. J. Howard and H. L. Greene. Comparison of effects of total parenteral nutrition, continuous intragastric feeding and portacaval shunt on a patient with type I glycogen storage disease. *J. Pediat.* **85:** 792, 1974.

102. Pennington, J. T., and D. H. Calloway. Copper content of foods: factors affecting reported values. *J. Am. Diet. Assn.* **63:** 143, 1973.

103. Lawler, M. R. and M. A. Jelenc. Recipes for low copper diets. *J. Am. Diet. Assn.* **57:** 420, 1970.

104. Moynahan, E. J., and P. M. Barnes. Zinc deficiency and a synthetic diet for lactose intolerance. *Lancet* **1:** 676, 1973.

105. Hirsh, F. S., B. Michel, W. H. Strain. Gluconate zinc in acrodermatitis enteropathica. *Arch. Derm.* **112:** 475, 1976.

106. Moynahan, E. J. Acrodermatitis enteropathica: A lethal inherited human zinc deficiency disorder. *Lancet* **2:** 395, 1974.

107. Nelder, K. H. and M. Hambridge. Zinc therapy of acrodermatitis enteropathica. *New Engl. J. Med.* **292:** 879, 1975.

108. Lombeck, I., and H. J. Bremer. Primary and secondary disturbances in trace element metabolism connected with genetic metabolic disorders. *Nutr. Metab.* **21:** 49, 1977.

109. Lombeck, I., D. B. Bassewitz, and K. Becker. Ultrastructural findings in acrodermatitis enteropathica. *Pediatr. Res.* **8:** 82, 1974.

110. MacMahon, R. A., M. L. Parker, and M. C. McKinnon. Zinc treatment in malabsorption. *Med. J. Aust.* **2:** 210, 1968.

111. Arakawa, T., T. Tamura, Y. Igarashi, H. Suzuki, and H. H. Sanstead. Zinc deficiency in two infants during total parenteral alimentation for diarrhea. *Am. J. Clin. Nutr.* **29:** 197, 1976.

112. Holt, L. E., Jr. and S. E. Snyderman. Protein and amino acid requirements of infants and children. Nutr. Abstr. Rev. **35:** 1, 1965.

113. Energy and Protein Requirements. Rome: Food and Agriculture Organization of the United Nations, 1973, p. 57.

CHAPTER 10

The Kidney

ANATOMY AND PHYSIOLOGY

Maintenance of the body's internal environment (i.e., homeostasis of body fluids and regulation of acid–base balance) is primarily the function of the kidneys, two bean-shaped organs located behind the lining of the abdominal cavity on either side of the spine just above the waist. These organs are held in position by tissue that anchors them to surrounding structures (Fig. 10.1). Each kidney measures approximately 11 to 13 cm long, 5 to 7.5 cm wide, 2.5 cm thick and weighs between 115 and 170 grams (1,2).

A longitudinal cross section of the kidney allows identification of its three distinct parts: the cortex, the medulla, and the renal pelvis. The renal pelvis is the upper portion of the ureter, a tube about 25 to 30 cm long that connects the kidney with the urinary bladder. At the entrance of the ureter into the bladder is a valvelike fold of epithelial tissue that prevents a back flow of urine. The urethra, a duct leading from the bladder, is the passageway through which urine is excreted from the body.

The functional units of the kidney are the nephrons, approximately 1 to 1.5 million of which are found in each kidney. The nephron is a tubule approximately 6 cm long, the component parts of which are designated according to specific physical and functional characteristics. The five components of the nephron are Bowman's capsule, proximal tubule, loop of Henle, distal tubule, and collecting duct. In actuality the collecting duct is not a part of every nephron but serves to collect fluid from several nephrons (Fig. 10.1).

The beginning of the tubule (nephron) is a dilated blind end (Bowman's capsule) into which invaginates a tuft of approximately 50 capillaries known as the glomerulus. The hydrostatic pressure in these capillaries is high and their permeability is about 25 times as great as that found in other capillaries. Of particular importance in the functioning of the kidneys is the rich blood supply reaching the glomeruli from the aorta via the renal arteries. Arteries entering the kidneys carry an average of 1200 ml of blood per minute, approximately 25 percent of the total cardiac output. In order to get a picture of how the kidneys perform their function of controlling the concentration of most body fluid constituents, it is necessary to consider blood circulation within the kidney (Fig. 10.2).

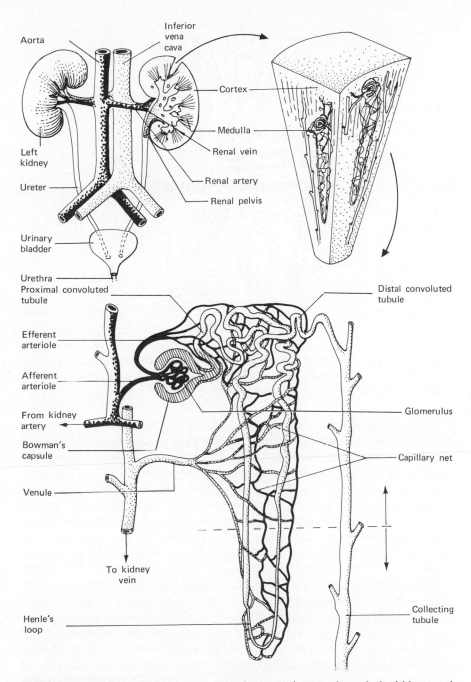

Figure 10.1 Human urinary system, showing a section cut through the kidney and a detailed view of a nephron. (From *The Biological World* by A. Nason and B. DeHaan. Copyright 1973 by John Wiley and Sons, Inc. Reprinted by permission of the publisher.)

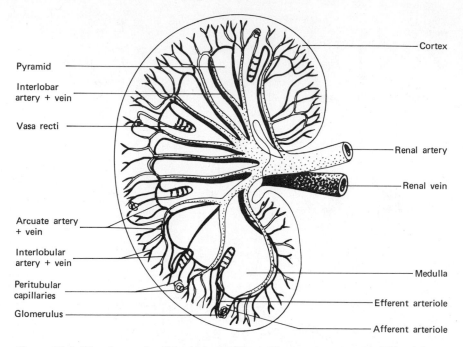

Cortex

Pyramid

Interlobar
artery + vein

Vasa recti

Renal artery

Renal vein

Arcuate artery
+ vein

Interlobular
artery + vein

Peritubular
capillaries

Medulla

Glomerulus

Efferent arteriole

Afferent arteriole

Figure 10.2 Blood vessels of the kidney. (From *Human Anatomy and Physiology,* 2nd ed. by J. E. Crouch and J. R. McClintic. Copyright 1976 by John Wiley and Sons, Inc. Reprinted by permission of the publisher.)

The renal artery upon reaching the kidney branches into many interlobar arteries. These vessels pass between the pyramids of the medulla which are composed primarily of collecting ducts, then form the arcuate arteries, so named because of their curved appearance. The plane of arcuate vessels forms a line of demarcation between the medulla and cortex of the kidney. The arcuate arteries branch into the interlobular arteries which run into the cortex of the kidney and give rise to the afferent arterioles. The afferent arterioles branch into the tufts of capillaries known as the glomeruli. These glomeruli are found almost exclusively in the kidney cortex.

Blood leaves the glomeruli by the efferent arterioles. This is the only place in the body where capillaries coalesce into another arteriole rather than a venule. These arterioles give rise to the peritubular capillary network that surrounds the nephron tubules and promotes their function of regulating concentration of the various constituents in body fluid. Hydrostatic pressure in the peritubular capillary network is low and the walls of the capillaries are very porous; therefore, quantities of fluids can be reabsorbed from the tubules into this capillary bed via the renal interstitial spaces (3).

The peritubular capillary network coaleses into the interlobular veins and blood flows from the kidneys successively via the arcuate veins, the interlobar veins, and finally through the single renal vein which empties into the inferior vena cava (Figs. 10.1, 10.2).

The kidneys in their formation of urine excrete metabolic waste products from the body, regulate fluid and electrolyte balance and acid–base balance and control the level of the various solid constituents in body fluids. The homeostatic function of the kidneys is made possible by the various mechanisms involved in urine production that occur along the length of the nephron, namely, filtration, reabsorption, secretion, and acidification.

Component Parts of the Nephron

Bowman's Capsule. That part of the nephron surrounding the glomerulus, this structure collects the filtrate forced by hydrostatic pressure through these capillaries. The glomerular filtration rate (GFR) refers to the amount of filtrate formed and averages approximately 120 ml/minute, a volume only about one-fifth the total plasma that arrives in the glomeruli. Nevertheless, this filtrate amounts to approximately 180 liters per 24 hours, about 12 times the total extracellular fluid in the body. The filtrate resembles plasma except for its lack of formed elements and its lower protein concentration. About 30 grams of protein, however, do move into the filtrate daily. Most of this protein is albumin but materials with molecular weights as high as 200,000 have the possibility of an occasional passage through the capillary membrane. Nevertheless, only substances with molecular weights of 70,000 or less are able to move easily through the glomeruli. That protein which is filtered through the glomeruli is not lost from the body normally, but instead is reabsorbed as the filtrate moves through the proximal convoluted tubule.

Proximal Convoluted Tubule. This is the primary site for selective reabsorption of filtrate substances and also is very active in secreting certain waste products from the blood that are not sufficiently removed by filtration. Rapid reabsorption and secretion of materials are facilitated by the microvilli which are found on the luminal side of the proximal tubule cells. These microvilli also provide the mechanism by which filtered protein (as mentioned above) can be reabsorbed. Protein is moved into the cell by endocytosis and then probably is digested into its constituent amino acids. These amino acids like those from the filtrate can be actively absorbed through the base of the cells into the interstitial fluids.

Materials in addition to amino acids that are actively reabsorbed include the physiologically useful solutes, for example, sodium, glucose, potassium, acetoacetate ions, vitamins, and many others. The average reabsorption of these solutes in the proximal tubule approximates 80 to 90 percent. Water movement accompanies the solute transport; therefore, the volume of the filtrate in the proximal tubule is reduced but the osmolality and pH of the filtrate are unaffected.

Filtrate composition also changes due to passive diffusion of substances along a concentration or electrical gradient from the filtrate into the peritubular fluid or from the peritubular fluid into the filtrate. The electrical gradient is particularly important in the absorption of the negatively charged chloride and bicarbonate ions because the peritubular fluid has been made positive (+) by absorption of sodium. The rate of absorption of nonactively absorbed solutes is determined: (1) by the amount of water reabsorbed osmotically as a result of the active transport of those materials particularly important to the body, and (2) by the permeability of the tubular cell membrane to these solutes. Solutes that are poorly reabsorbed represent metabolic waste products and include urea, uric acid, sulfates, phosphates, and nitrates. One solute not reabsorbed in *any* amount is creatinine. In fact, some creatinine is actually secreted by the proximal tubular cells into the filtrate. Other substances secreted by the proximal tubule are certain strong organic acids and bases, such as hippuric acid and histamine (2).

Loop of Henle. This is the section of the nephron with a descending and an ascending portion, an arrangement that allows the tubule to move from the cortex down into the medulla of the kidney and back up again. Because of conditions existing in the two portions of the loop, the isotonic filtrate (approximately 300 mOsmol/l) as it moves through this part of the nephron becomes hypotonic and the surrounding interstitium increases in sodium content. Included in conditions governing the change in tonicity of the filtrate and of the interstitium are: (1) the ascending portion possesses an active transport system that moves chloride ions (accompanied by sodium ions to preserve electrochemical neutrality) from its lumen into the descending part of the loop; (2) the ascending loop is impermeable to water; therefore, water does not osmotically follow the actively transported chloride ions; and (3) the descending portion of the loop allows free diffusion of materials; consequently, any changes occurring in the osmolality of its filtrate will be reflected in the surrounding interstitium.

Distal Convoluted Tubule. Like the proximal tubule, this is located in the cortex. The hypotonic filtrate (approximately 100 mOsmols/l) moves from the ascending portion of the loop of Henle into the distal tubule where the final modification of the filtrate occurs. By the time the filtrate reaches the distal tubule its volume is approximately one-eighth of its original amount. Modifications in the distal tubule include absorption, secretion, and acidification.

Aldosterone controls the distal tubular absorption of sodium (about 10 percent of the filtered load) and the simultaneous secretion of either potassium or hydrogen in exchange for the sodium absorbed. The antidiuretic hormone (ADH) also exerts its action in the distal tubule, dictating the amount of water to be removed from the filtrate. ADH promotes absorption of water in the distal tubule and also causes increased permeability of the collecting duct which passes down through the hypertonic interstitium of the medulla on its way to the ureter. Under the influence of ADH water passes osmotically from the collecting duct into the surrounding interstitium. The plasma concentration of ADH, therefore, determines whether urine will be concentrated or dilute. ADH is released from the posterior pituitary in response to stimuli reaching osmoreceptors in the hypothalamus. Stimuli causing increased release of ADH are dehydration, pain, diminished cardiac output, cigarette smoking (1).

The secretion of potassium by the distal tubule under the influence of aldosterone is a very important mechanism for controlling potassium concentration in body fluids. The amount secreted is in exchange for sodium absorbed and represents approximately 7 percent of the filtered load of potassium.

Hydrogen ions compete with potassium ions for secretion as sodium is reabsorbed. This secretion of hydrogen ions along with the production and release of ammonia is responsible for the acidification of the urine. Ordinarily over 25 mEq of hydrogen ions are excreted daily (4). Figure 10.3 depicts the secretion of ions and acidification of urine in the distal tubule as sodium and bicarbonate are conserved.

In summary, homeostasis of body fluids and regulation of acid–base balance are achieved by the kidney through (1) filtration of plasma; (2) reabsorption of physiologically necessary substances, that is, various electrolytes, bicarbonate, nutrient molecules, and water; (3) secretion of certain materials noxious to the body, namely, creatinine, strong acids and bases, and excess potassium; (4) acidification of urine. The variation in urine concentration (volume ranges from 600 to 2500 ml/daily; specific gravity from 1.003 to 1.030) and urine pH (range from 4.7 to 8.0, although urine is normally acid with a pH of about 6) is a result of the kidney's attempt to maintain a constant "internal environment" for the body's cells regardless of external conditions. Table 10.1 illustrates the tremendous absorptive capacity of normal kidneys.

The kidneys' ability to maintain a constant "internal environment" is due not only to their extraordinary excretory activities but also to their many metabolic and hormonal functions as described below.

Metabolic Functions of the Kidney

The metabolic activity of the kidney is second only to that of the liver. In fact, the oxygen consumption of the renal cortex is higher than that of any

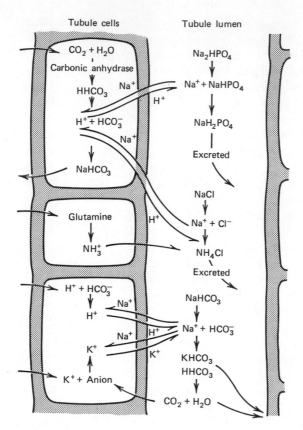

Figure 10.3 Ion exchanges in renal tubule. (From *Fluid and Electrolyte in Practice* by Harry Statland. Copyright 1963 by J. B. Lippincott Co. Reprinted by permission of the publisher.)

other tissue in the body, probably because of the energy required for active transport (5). Although the kidney is thought of primarily as an organ for the removal of nitrogenous wastes produced in other parts of the body, it is itself an active site for nitrogen metabolism. Amino acids may be deaminated in order to produce ammonia and to provide the carbon for glucose synthesis.

Ammonia Production. Renal cells with their many enzymes for breaking down glutamine have a great avidity for this circulating amino acid (6). Renal glutaminase hydrolyzes glutamine into ammonia and glutamate; the glutamate produced may be further deaminated by glutamate dehydrogenase to form another molecule of ammonia. The uncharged ammonia molecule diffuses freely through cell membranes of the distal tubules into the

Table 10.1 Filtration, Reabsorption and Excretion of Ions and Water by an Adult Man, with a Glomerular Filtration Rate of 180 l/24 hr.

	Plasma concentration	Amount filtered	Amount excreted	Amount reabsorbed	Percent reabsorbed
	(mmol/l)	(mmol/24 h)	(mmol/24 h)	(mmol/24 h)	
Sodium	142	25560	250	25310	99·0
Chloride	100	18000	250	17750	98·6
Bicarbonate	28	5040	2	5038	>99·9
Potassium	4	720	120	600	83
	kg/l	kg/24 h	kg/24 h	kg/24 h	
Water	0·93	167·4	1·5	165·9	99·1

Source: From *Textbook of Physiology and Biochemistry*, 9th ed., by G. H. Bell, D. Emslie-Smith, C. R. Paterson. Copyright 1976 by Churchill Livingstone. Reprinted by permission of the publisher.

urine where combination with a hydrogen ion may take place. The ammonium ion thus formed cannot pass freely through the cell membranes; therefore, it functions as a hydrogen ion sink and is very important in reducing body fluid acidity.

Other circulating amino acids—glutamic acid, aspartic acid, alanine, and glycine—also may be removed by renal cells and oxidatively deaminized to produce ammonia and alpha-keto acids. The alpha-keto acids thus produced may be used for energy in the kidney or may be converted into glucose.

Gluconeogenesis. Made possible by the deamination of amino acids, this is an important metabolic activity of the kidney, particularly during prolonged starvation and/or when acidosis exists, thereby necessitating production of ammonium ions. A study on obese humans showed that after subjects had been starved for 35 to 40 days, approximately 45 percent of the glucose secreted into the blood originated from the kidneys (7).

Condensation. Another major metabolic activity of the kidney (8), is condensation of a wide variety of toxic organic compounds with glycine, gluconate, sulfate, acetate, or glutamine into less toxic compounds that can be rapidly excreted.

Hormonal Functions of the Kidney

Hormonal functions of the kidney include: (1) conversion of a prohormone into its active metabolite; (2) synthesis of enzymes that act on certain plasma proteins to produce hormone-like substances; (3) degradation of excessive circulating hormones.

Conversion of a Prohormone into its Active Metabolite. The final conversion of vitamin D_3 into its active metabolite 1,25-dihydroxycholecalciferol occurs in the kidney. This metabolite acts like a hormone in the body and is much more active than its precursor, 25-hydroxycholecalciferol which is formed from vitamin D_3 in the liver. Along with the parathyroid hormone 1,25-dihydroxycholecalciferol is the primary regulator of calcium and phosphorus metabolism in the body.

Synthesis of Enzymes That Act on Certain Plasma Proteins to Produce Hormone-like Substances. Certain enzymes synthesized in the kidneys are very important in the regulation of blood pressure because their reaction with specific plasma proteins produces hormone-like substances. These substances may act as vasoconstrictors, vasodilators, or stimulants of the adrenal cortex for aldosterone secretion, depending upon the enzymes and plasma proteins involved. The renin–angiotensin–aldosterone mechanism in the regulation of blood pressure is well known and is depicted in Figure 7.6. Renin, a proteolytic enzyme, is produced by the juxtaglomerular cells (see Fig. 10.4) in response to decreases in blood pressure associated with a reduction in plasma volume and/or sodium ion concentration. A potent vasodilator is bradykinin, a substance resulting from the action of a renal enzyme, renal kallikrein, on a specific class of plasma proteins, the kininogens. Also, the kidney is the source of other vasodila-

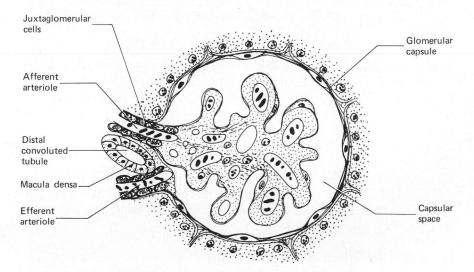

Figure 10.4 Cross section of a glomerulus to show the juxtaglomerular cells. (From *Textbook of Physiology and Biochemistry*, 9th ed. by G. H. Bell, D. Emslie-Smith, and C. R. Paterson. Copyright 1976 by Churchill Livingstone. Reprinted by permission of the publisher.)

tors and natriuretic substances thought to originate in the interstitial cells of the renal medulla in response to a rise in blood flow and blood pressure (1). Two of these substances are prostaglandins, PGA_2 and PGE_2. Since PGA_2, PGE_2, and bradykinin are all effective diuretic and natriuretic substances as well as vasodilators, they act in opposition to the renin–angiotensin–aldosterone mechanism.

Another enzyme believed to be produced in the kidney is a renal erythropoietic factor, which is secreted into the blood stream when the kidneys become hypoxic. This enzyme acts on a plasma globulin to split away the erythropoietin (a glycoprotein) molecule which then acts as a hormone by stimulating erythropoiesis in bone marrow (3). Sensitivity of the kidney to the body's need for oxygen apparently is due to the fact that the renal cortex (location of most of the glomeruli, proximal and distal tubules of nephrons) consumes more oxygen than any other tissue of the body.

Degradation of Excessive Circulating Hormones. Another important characteristic of the kidney in relation to hormone function is its ability along with that of the liver to degrade certain circulating peptide hormones, for example, insulin. Renal extraction of circulating insulin is approximately 40 percent of that entering the renal artery so that about 10 to 20 units are degraded daily (9). Other peptide hormones, elevated during renal failure, include parathyroid hormone, glucagon, growth hormone, thyrotropin, prolactin, leutinizing hormone, and gastrin (10). Their increased levels in the blood are probably due in part to a decreased ability of renal cells to metabolize circulating hormones.

DIAGNOSIS AND TREATMENT OF KIDNEY DISEASES

Because the kidneys are so active metabolically and hormonally and are primarily responsible for maintaining a constant "internal environment" for body cells, any condition that can cause an interference with the functioning of these organs is potentially life-threatening. There are many disease conditions, usually genetic or immunologic in origin, which fall within this life-threatening category. Complications associated with diseases of the kidney often result in chronic renal failure which is characterized by decreased functioning of the nephrons.

Diagnosis of Kidney Disease

As the functional capability of the nephrons decrease due to kidney disease, there is a consequent disturbance in the blood and urine chemistry.

Such chemical changes are determined by routine diagnostic tests referred to as renal function tests which can be broadly classified into two major groups: (1) those measuring glomerular filtration; and (2) those measuring tubular function. Several representative tests are mentioned because of their relevance to specific disease processes. The reader is referred to Chapter 14 for an explanation of the chemical basis for these tests.

Many of the earlier tests for evaluating the glomerular filtration function of the kidney are still widely used today. They are based on the retention in the plasma of certain nonprotein nitrogenous compounds which are removed from the plasma primarily by glomerular filtration. Among these compounds are urea, creatinine, and uric acid which are breakdown products of protein, creatine, and purines respectively. Impairment of glomerular filtration results in an accumulation of these substances in the plasma, and their plasma levels are easily determined. These are not considered sensitive tests, however, and kidney function may decrease to as little as 50 percent of normal before determination of these compounds would show abnormal results (11). Furthermore, these assays may be affected by prerenal effects such as diet. This is particularly true in the case of urea and uric acid, which are catabolic products of common nutrients, and it is established that a high protein diet can cause a marked elevation of the blood urea nitrogen (BUN) in spite of normal kidney function. For these reasons, the foregoing tests are employed mainly as screening tests for kidney function.

Clearance tests, on the other hand, are exceedingly useful in determining the ability of the kidney to eliminate certain substances from the plasma. Their sensitivity allows the detection of early disease. Furthermore, the tests can be made specific by selecting the type of clearance test that evaluates a certain aspect of kidney function. For example, to measure glomerular filtration, the clearance (removal) of creatinine or inulin from the plasma is determined (creatinine or inulin clearance tests) because these substances are removed almost exclusively by glomerular filtration, and they are not secreted by or reabsorbed by the tubules to any appreciable extent. Clearance tests may also be used to evaluate the tubular function of the kidney. For such tests, compounds that are eliminated from the plasma primarily by tubular secretion are measured. An example of such a compound is p-amino hippurate (PAH), and the PAH clearance test can provide valuable information on the functional integrity of the tubules. It should be pointed out that inulin and PAH clearance tests have the disadvantage that these compounds are not naturally occurring blood constituents and therefore must be continuously infused during the test procedure. The clearance of a substance is readily determined by quantitating the serum level and the urine level of the substance simultaneously and measuring the volume of urine voided per minute during the course of the testing period (usually 8 hours). The procedure and calculation for a creatinine clearance will be described in Chapter 14.

Other tubular function tests in use in the clinical laboratory include the phenolsulfophthalein (PSP) test, the urine specific gravity test, and the measurement of the osmolality of serum and urine simultaneously. The PSP test is based on the fact that intravenously injected PSP dye is removed from the plasma chiefly by tubular secretion. Following injection, the amount of dye excreted in the urine as a function of time is measured. The urine specific gravity and the osmolality tests determine the concentrating ability of the tubules, that is, the capability of the tubules to reabsorb water from the glomerular filtrate, a process regulated by ADH. The reabsorption of water results in an increase in the specific gravity and osmolality as the urine is formed from the glomerular filtrate.

Kidney Diseases and Their Treatment

Although diseases affecting the kidneys are legion, those most commonly implicated in renal failure include two disease states originating outside the kidney: *diabetes* and *hypertension*. The primary kidney disease often resulting in renal failure is *chronic glomerulonephritis* caused by the patient's failure to recover completely from the acute nephritic syndrome. The acute disease state usually follows a streptococcal infection which damages the glomerular basement membrane.

Other kidney diseases that may lead to renal insufficiency include:

1. *Pyelonephritis* caused by bacterial infections (usually *E. coli*). The pathogens originating in the colon reach the bladder via the urethra and then move upward into the pelvis of the kidney (12). Repeated attacks of bacterial infections can be dangerous, particularly in patients with urinary abnormalities, for example, obstruction or stones, or with diseases resulting in papillary injury, such as, diabetes mellitus, hypertension.
2. *Polycystic kidney disease* which is congenital in nature and characterized by the gradual replacement of normal kidney tissue by multiple cysts.

Chronic Renal Failure. On a yearly basis approximately 40 persons per million in the Western world develop chronic renal failure (13). It is estimated that the potential occurrence of the disease is much greater than that presently documented due to the high incidence of diabetes and hypertension among the population and the increasing number of elderly persons in our society.

As was mentioned under diagnosis, chronic renal failure is characterized by a decreased glomerular filtration rate (GFR). As the filtration rate falls, blood urea rises and the functioning nephrons which remain become hypertrophied (14). With an elevated blood urea level and increased filtration by the hypertrophied remaining nephrons, the solute load presented to each functioning tubule is greater than normal. One consequence of this condition is polyuria resulting from the inability of the tubular cells to concentrate the filtrate properly. This decrease in renal concentrating ability is probably caused by the increased amount of urea in the filtrate, the result of which is a solute diuresis.

As severe renal insufficiency approaches, the volume of urine no longer remains excessive but instead decreases below normal. When the GFR falls to 5 to 10 percent of normal, urine flow is so limited that ordinary intakes of sodium and water can no longer be excreted. At this point intake of sodium and water must be restricted or hypertension, edema, and congestive heart failure will result. It is clear, therefore, that renal insufficiency can exist at varying levels of severity and each diagnosed case of kidney failure must be treated according to individual clinical and biochemical indices.

Dietary manipulation is an important aspect of the treatment for renal disease and nutrients of special significance in this treatment can be grouped as follows: protein and other energy sources; sodium and water; vitamin D, calcium and phosphorus; potassium, and occasionally, magnesium. Dietary modifications will differ depending upon the degree of renal insufficiency and whether dialysis therapy is being utilized. To understand the basis for these dietary modifications, it is necessary to consider the interrelationship that exists among the various nutrients and between each nutrient and kidney function.

Protein and Other Energy Sources. Amino acids arising from digestion of dietary protein are absorbed and utilized according to the body's need and the biological value of the protein. The interrelationship between dietary protein and nitrogen metabolism is explained by the concept of the "amino acid pool," with the largest such pool being found in the blood (Figs. 3.16 and 10.5).

Deamination of amino acids provides the nitrogen found in ammonia and urea. Most of the alpha-ketoacids resulting from deamination will follow the metabolic pathway of either carbohydrate or fat and be used for energy. Other normally occurring nitrogenous wastes include: creatinine (break-down product of creatine), a constant amount of which is produced each day according to muscle mass size; and uric acid, metabolic product of the purines.

The only nitrogenous waste critically affected by protein intake is urea, the amount of which can fluctuate dramatically. The efficacy of a low protein, high caloric diet in the treatment of renal insufficiency as proposed by Giordano, Giovannetti, and Maggiore (15,16) was based on this

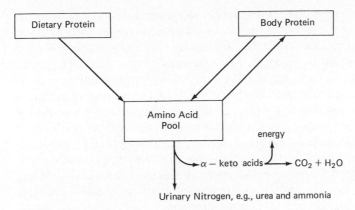

Figure 10.5 Central role of the "amino acid pool" in the relationship between dietary protein and nitrogen metabolism.

relationship between protein intake and urea production and on additional principles of nitrogen metabolism as listed below:

1. When the body is receiving no protein, it reaches a plateau of low endogenous nitrogen loss at which point there is a strong stimulus toward protein anabolism. In other words, although some wear and tear of body tissue is inevitable, the amino acids in the "pool" are being conserved as much as possible for body protein anabolism. With this strong stimulus toward protein anabolism, very little protein is needed to keep the body in nitrogen equilibrium provided the protein ingested is of high biological value, such as egg protein.
2. High caloric intake decreases tissue breakdown. If sufficient carbohydrate and fat can be ingested to meet the energy needs of the body, no body tissue need be broken down for energy.
3. Nonessential amino acids can be synthesized easily and efficiently provided sufficient energy and nitrogen are available to the body.

Giordano, Giovannetti, and Maggiore theorized, therefore, that urea that collects in the blood of uremic patients under the conditions listed above could serve as the source of nitrogen for the synthesis of the nonessential amino acids. This utilization of urea for synthesis of nonessential amino acids would promote nitrogen equilibrium while at the same time it would decrease the level of serum urea, thereby relieving some of the symptoms of uremic toxicity. Clinical trials with a high caloric diet, containing only 20 grams protein of high biologic value appeared to confirm this theory because selected uremic patients exhibited symptomatic improvement (16). Subsequently, however, utilization of endogenous urea in protein synthesis has been shown to be quite limited (17).

The necessity for protein restriction in patients with renal failure is directly related to the level of blood urea nitrogen (more recently referred to as serum urea nitrogen or SUN), since a level of over 90 mg/100 ml is usually accompanied by many of the symptoms of uremic toxicity, such as anorexia, nausea, vomiting, diarrhea, twitching. Although the exact relationship between an elevated BUN (or SUN) and symptoms of uremia is unclear, it is known that hydrolysis of urea to ammonia in the mouth is responsible for the uremic odor and bad taste associated with advanced renal failure. Also some of the characteristic gastrointestinal irritation associated with advanced uremia may be due to the hydrolysis of urea to ammonia by bacterial ureases in the stomach and the intestine (15). When blood urea is elevated it can find its way into all body secretions because it is readily diffusible through all cell membranes.

Although protein restriction is necessary in advanced renal failure, the degree of restriction needed to keep the BUN (or SUN) within limits compatible with minimal symptoms is debatable. Most investigators advocate a protein intake greater than the 20 grams recommended by Giovannetti because of the increased palatability of such a diet and the increased likelihood of achieving nitrogen and mineral equilibrium (18,19). A patient ingesting no more than 20 grams protein daily is likely to become malnourished.

An approach to a more nearly palatable low protein diet that encourages nitrogen equilibrium and reduces urea accumulation is the utilization of analogs of amino acids (20). In this experimental diet a low protein diet (15 to 20 grams protein, the source of which is not specified) is supplemented with four essential amino acids (tryptophan, lysine, threonine, and histidine) and the keto-analogs of the other five (valine, leucine, isoleucine, methionine, and phenylalanine). These keto analogs apparently reduce urea accumulation by promoting increased anabolism of body tissue. This accelerated anabolism is believed related to the effect of leucine (or its keto analog) which presumably has some regulatory effect on anabolic enzymes (20). Keto-acid therapy appears to hold much promise in the treatment of chronic renal failure (21).

Kopple and Coburn (22) studied the interrelationship between protein intake and serum urea nitrogen to serum creatinine ratios in chronically uremic men and discovered that this relationship allows determination of the specific intake of protein allowable for the maintenance of minimal clinical symptoms of uremia. Through use of this curve (Fig. 10.6), Kopple has estimated that in men with a serum creatinine of 15 mg/100 ml (normal, 0.6–1.2 mg/100 ml), an intake of 40 grams protein would be expected to cause a serum urea nitrogen of approximately 89 mg/100 ml. Because clinical symptoms of uremia do not usually appear in any severity until serum urea nitrogen approaches 100 mg/100 ml, a protein level lower than 40 grams daily seems unwarranted for a man of

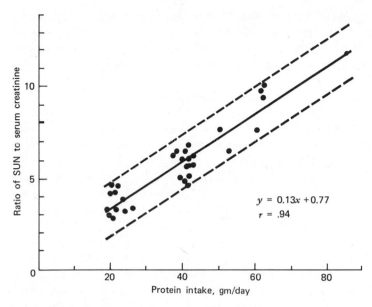

Figure 10.6 Serum urea nitrogen (SUN) to serum creatinine ratio versus protein intake in chronically uremic men. (From "Evaluation of chronic uremia: importance of serum urea nitrogen, serum creatinine and their ratio" by J. D. Kopple and J. W. Coburn. *Journal of the American Medical Association,* Volume 227, pp. 41–44, January 7, 1975. Copyright 1975, American Medical Association. Reprinted by permission of the publisher and authors.)

average size whose glomerular filtration rate (GFR) is above 4 ml/minute. These investigators further recommend that for even small men and for women the protein intake be at least 35 grams daily. Even with a higher level of protein intake, however, it is important that most of the protein be of high biological value. When the GFR decreases below 4 to 5 ml/minute, dietary manipulation can probably no longer adequately prevent progression of the uremic syndrome and dialysis therapy or renal transplantation becomes necessary (19).

Provision of sufficient calories from carbohydrate and fat sources is extremely important in uremic patients whose limited protein intake is needed for maintaining nitrogen equilibrium. In order to prevent oxidation of protein for energy production, a caloric intake of at least 35 kcal/kg body weight daily is recommended. The relative amount (and type) of carbohydrate and fat used to supply these calories may be quite important in the control of the hypertriglyceridemia that occurs in most patients with chronic renal disease. Lowering of serum triglycerides has been possible in renal patients through manipulation of diet: reduction of carbohydrate calories to only 30 to 50 percent of total calories and provision of as many calories as possible from polyunsaturated fats. Although a defect in triglyceride clearance rather than one of overproduction appears to be the problem in patients with chronic renal disease, decreasing the substrates for triglyceride synthesis promotes a lowering of these serum lipids (23,24).

Patients who receive maintenance hemodialysis or peritoneal dialysis therapy have approximately the same caloric requirements as do uremic patients who are managed by diet, that is, 35 kcalories per kilogram body weight. This level may be increased in the very active patient or be decreased in the obese. The intake of protein, however, is not as restricted for the patient on maintenance dialysis therapy as it is for patients treated by diet alone. Patients on dialysis therapy particularly those on peritoneal dialysis, lose some amino acids, peptides, and small proteins, which need to be replenished through diet. The recommended level of protein intake for adults undergoing dialysis treatments of 6 to 8 hours each, three times per week, is 65 to 85 grams daily depending on body size. Although at least 50 percent of this protein should be of high biological value, the allowance of approximately 20 grams unselected protein permits a much more acceptable diet for the patient (19).

Peritoneal dialysis is becoming more popular as the treatment of choice for certain patients with end-stage renal disease. This is a much cheaper method of dialysis and as techniques for its use are improved, more and more patients are expected to utilize this mode of treatment. Predictably, much research presently is being directed toward determining nutrient needs of patients maintained for long periods through peritoneal dialysis therapy (24).

Sodium and Water. As was mentioned earlier, one of the first symptoms of chronic renal failure is the inability of the remaining functioning nephrons to concentrate the glomerular filtrate properly and to regulate urinary sodium excretion. Patients who are likely to be "salt losers" are those affected by interstitial nephritis (e.g., pyelonephritis and analgesic nephropathies), hydronephrosis, medullary cystic disease, and polycystic kidney disease. On the other hand, as renal failure becomes progressively severe and the GFR falls to 10 percent or less of normal, urine flow is so minimal that ordinary intakes of water and sodium can no longer be tolerated. Consequently, the amount of water and sodium allowed the patient with kidney failure must be prescribed on an individual basis, depending upon the degree of renal function and basic disease process.

One approach for assuring sufficient sodium and water in the "salt loser" (13) is to increase slowly the patient's intake of sodium under controlled conditions until slight edema occurs. The patient can then be placed on a constant sodium intake and a determination of urinary sodium made. This determination can be used to make any necessary adjustments in the amount of sodium ingested because urinary and dietary sodium should approximate each other. It is very important to realize that azotemic patients without edema, hypertension, congestive heart failure, or oliguria need to be encouraged to ingest sufficient sodium rather than to restrict it. Bouillon which contains 2.5 grams sodium chloride per cube can be a valuable and palatable source of sodium for the "salt loser" kidney patient.

The patient's water requirement can be determined by measuring in a graduated cylinder his/her urinary output for 24 hours, then adding approximately 600 ml to the amount excreted. (This additional 600 ml represents the approximate 800 ml insensible water loss plus the estimated 200 ml fecal fluid loss less the water of metabolism which amounts to about 400 ml daily.) This amount of fluid lost from the body (urine volume + 600 ml) during 24 hours represents the amount of fluid the patient should receive the following day. Recording the patient's weight on a frequent and regular basis allows a good estimate of his/her state of hydration because one liter of water weighs one kilogram (or 2.2 pounds).

In the oliguric patient, attention must be given to possible fluid overload, sodium retention, and accompanying hypertension. Correction of excessive sodium and water retention must be accomplished through drug therapy (potent diuretics) and then the patient's intake of sodium should be regulated according to his/her urinary losses plus any additional losses from vomiting and/or diarrhea (13). Fluid intake should be regulated as outlined above.

Diuretics used to enhance elimination of fluids from the body via the kidneys are a diverse category of drugs, differing not only in their mechanism and site of action but also in their potency. Diuretics are used in a wide variety of conditions; therefore, their functions, effects, and side effects should be well understood by all members of the health care team.

Diuretics may be categorized according to their site of action in the kidney. These sites include the proximal and distal tubule, and the ascending limb of the loop of Henle or "diluting segment". Table 10.2 indicates the commonly used diuretics and their site of action. Diuretics that act on the proximal tubule are included in three groups: (1) osmotic agents which keep sodium and water in the tubular lumen so that they cannot be absorbed, thereby causing their excretion; (2) the carbonic anhydrase inhibitors which force sodium excretion by inhibiting hydrogen ion formation, thereby preventing the exchange of hydrogen ions for sodium ions; and (3) mercurial diuretics which probably inhibit enzymes in the proximal tubule cells that are responsible for absorbing sodium ions (25).

Diuretics that act on the distal tubule inhibit the exchange of sodium for potassium; consequently, sodium is excreted and potassium is reabsorbed. Two agents in this category are triamterene (Dyrenium®) and spironolactone (Aldactone®). Triamterene acts directly on the distal tu-

Table 10.2 Commonly Used Diuretics (selected agents)

Site of action	Category or mechanism	Drug
Proximal tubule	Osmotic	mannitol I.V.
		isorobide
		urea
		glycerol
	Carbonic anhydrase inhibitor	acetazolamide (Diamox®)
	Mercurial	mercaptomerin (Thiomerin®)
Loop of Henle	Inhibits sodium reabsorption	furosemide (Lasix®)
		ethacrynic acid (Edecrin®)
		chlorothiazide (Diuril®)
Distal tubule	Inhibits sodium reabsorption	triamterene (Dyrenium®)
	Inhibits aldosterone	spironolactone (Aldactone®)

bule to prevent the transport of sodium while spironolactone is an antagonist of aldosterone, the steroid hormone that enhances tubular reabsorption of sodium and chloride and increases the secretion of potassium (26).

The diuretic agents that act at the loop of Henle are considered to be very potent diuretics. They antagonize the mechanism by which sodium is reabsorbed from the ascending limb of the loop of Henle in the medullary area. Agents that act at this site are furosemide (Lasix®), ethacrynic acid (Edecrin®), and to a lesser extent the thiazide diuretics. The diuresis produced by these agents is great because 20 percent of sodium and chloride filtered by the glomeruli normally is reabsorbed by this segment of the nephron. Because these agents prevent reabsorption of sodium in the ascending limb of the loop of Henle, a larger fluid volume containing more than normal amounts of sodium reaches the distal tubule. As a consequence, more potassium is excreted by the distal tubule.

Diuretic agents that cause excessive potassium loss have the potential for producing electrolyte imbalance and must be monitored closely. For most patients who use these drugs on a chronic basis, a potassium supplement is administered concomitantly (see Table 11.5).

Although much emphasis usually is placed on educating patients concerning the sodium content of foods, quite often the fluid content of food may be overlooked. Patients for whom fluid intake must be severely restricted need to be aware that many apparently dry foods contain a certain amount of "hidden" water (Table 10.3). Free foods for patients with kidney failure are restricted indeed!

Once the patient's GFR has dropped to as low as 4 to 5 ml per minute, diuretics are no longer effective and dialysis therapy is usually instituted. Prevention of excessive sodium and fluid retention between dialysis treatments becomes a critical consideration. Fluid intake should be

Table 10.3 Water Content of Selected*
Popular Food Items

Food	Water content %
Fruits and vegetables	80–95
Meat, poultry, fish, eggs	50–75
Breads, cheese	25–35
Cooked cereal	60
Flour	12

*Additional water from foods is provided through the oxidation of their carbohydrate, protein, and fat. Water of oxidation for nutrients is calculated as follows: 0.56–0.60 g water/g CHO; 0.39–0.41 g water/g protein; and 1.07 g water/g lipid.

restricted sufficiently to prevent no more than one pound weight gain daily. Because of the high water content of most foods, no more than 300 to 500 ml of fluid per se should be consumed daily. A sodium allowance of 85 to 90 milliequivalents (approximately 2 grams) daily, although restrictive enough to prevent excessive thirst and to help in control of fluid retention and hypertension, is sufficient to permit a more palatable diet than would be possible with severe limitation. Since sodium (Na^+) exists as an electrolyte in body fluids, its measurement should be stated consistently in terms of milliequivalents. Measurement in milliequivalents allows sodium to be delineated as ions originating from a wide variety of sources rather than being considered as one and the same with table salt.

Calcium and Phosphorus. Because the amount of phosphorus in the body is regulated through urinary excretion, a fall in the GFR leads to retention of phosphate with the following results:

$$\uparrow \text{serum P} \longrightarrow \downarrow \text{serum Ca} \longrightarrow \uparrow \text{parathyroid hormone}$$
$$\uparrow \text{serum Ca} \longleftarrow \uparrow \text{P excretion}$$

When, however, the GFR falls to the point that creatinine clearance is less than 25 ml per minute, the increased parathyroid secretion is no longer effective in normalizing serum phosphorus and calcium levels. The resulting hypocalcemia is continuous and as a consequence the parathyroid hormone secretion remains elevated.

The parathyroid hormone normally regulates serum calcium through causing excretion of excess phosphorus, reabsorption of calcium from kidney tubules, and resorption of bone calcium. Bone resorption and decreased mineralization of newly formed bone are accelerated by the unavailability of the vitamin-hormone, 1,25-dihydroxycholecalciferol which normally increases serum calcium by enhancing calcium absorption from the gut. Under normal conditions 25-hydroxycholecalciferol (produced from vitamin D_3 in the liver) is converted into its more active form, 1,25-dihydroxycholecalciferol, by renal cells. In the chronically diseased kidney, however, this conversion is decreased or is entirely absent. Deficiency of this active metabolite of vitamin D causes rickets in children and osteomalacia in adults.

Improved absorption and utilization of calcium in the patient with renal failure can be achieved through administration of massive doses of vitamin D (50,000 to 200,000 I.U. daily) (14). Large doses of the vitamin can be given, however, only when serum phosphate has been controlled to normal levels; otherwise, metastic calcification is likely to occur (13). Microgram doses of 1,25-dihydroxycholecalciferol have the same effect on calcium metabolism as the large doses of vitamin D, are of short duration, and are not likely to be stored in the body. Only recently has 1,25-dihydroxycholecalciferol (calcitriol) been synthetically manufactured and become available commercially (Rocaltrol®). Much research continues to be devoted toward production of synthetic analogues of 1,25-dihydroxycholecalciferol which may have similar activity.

Hypocalcemia and its accompanying hyperphosphatemia can be treated through calcium supplementation and phosphorus restriction, respectively. Calcium intake should be no less than 2 grams daily and dietary calcium can be supplemented through administration of various calcium salts, for example, calcium carbonate, lactate, or gluconate. A fall in phosphorus intake occurs with a decreased intake of protein; therefore, ingestion of phosphorus may not be excessive in the patient receiving only 40 grams protein daily. Phosphorus available to the body can be reduced further through oral administration with meals of an aluminum hydroxide gel which binds ingested phosphate and prevents its absorption from the gut. Administration of this gel is particularly important in the patient on dialysis therapy who must consume a larger amount of protein in order to compensate for protein lost in the dialysate but whose means of disposing of excess serum phosphorus is limited to diffusion of phosphate into the dialysis fluid.

Patients suffering with hyperphosphatemia may also be required to limit foods particularly high in phosphorus, such as milk and milk products, organ meats, nuts, cocoa and chocolate, whole grain breads and cereals, dried beans, peas, and dried fruits.

Potassium. Serum potassium must be maintained within a narrow range (3.5 to 5 mEq/l) in order to prevent serious consequences to the cardiac muscle. Because of the life-threatening nature of either an elevated or depressed serum potassium level, monitoring this electrolyte becomes extremely important in the patient with renal failure. Although hypokalemia may be a problem in the patient receiving certain potassium-depleting diuretics, the main danger is from hyperkalemia, which develops in advanced renal failure or acute renal failure (14). Patients who are dependent upon dialysis therapy for removal of serum potassium must always be conscious that a potential for excessive serum potassium may exist.

The control of potassium in the diet of patients in advanced renal failure or those maintained on dialysis therapy may be a difficult aspect of dietary manipulation. Potassium is found in nearly all foods and particularly unfortunate for the renal patient is the fact that those foods that are excellent choices for a sodium- and protein-restricted diet, that is, fruits and most vegetables, must nonetheless be limited due to their high potassium content. When limitation of potassium intake becomes a necessity, the acceptability of the renal diet decreases tremendously. One means by which potassium can be restricted without excessively decreasing the acceptability of the diet is through leaching of vegetables. Much of the potassium can be removed from vegetables by soaking them in large amounts of water for extended periods and then after rinsing off the soaking water, cooking these vegetables in another large amount of water.*

Comparison of normal intake of nutrients with that recommended for patients in renal failure is given in Table 10.4.

Magnesium. Because magnesium excretion is impaired in renal failure, compounds with a high magnesium content such as antacids or laxatives should be avoided (13). Hypermagnesemia may result in hypotension and respiratory paralysis.

----

* Explicit directions for leaching vegetables are given in *The American J. Clin. Nutrition,* vol. 22, pp. 490–493, April, 1969.

Table 10.4 Approximate Nutrient Intakes by Renal Patients Compared to Those of Normal Persons

	Normal intake	Chronic renal failure	Dialysis
Calories	30 per kg	35–45 per kg	35–45 per kg
Protein	80–100 g	20–50 g	1 g per kg
Sodium	3–4 g	1–3 g	2 g
	120–170 mEq	40–120 mEq	90 mEq
Potassium	3–4 g	2–4 g	2–4 g
	75–100 mEq	50–100 mEq	50–100 mEq
Fluids	Ad lib	400–600 ml + output	300–500 m + output

Source: From "Dietary management of renal disorders: in chronic renal disease, during transplantation with dialysis and following transplantation" by Therese M. Beaudette, Cassette-a-Month 4, 1975, The American Dietetic Association.

Despite all the dietary manipulations that may be necessary in order to maintain fluid and electrolyte balance and to prevent excess accumulation of protein metabolites in the serum of the renal patient, as near an optimal intake of nutrients as possible and the maintenance of ideal body weight still should remain goals of nutritional management of the disease. Vitamin supplementation for the patient on dialysis therapy is nearly always indicated and those vitamins requiring particular attention are folic acid, ascorbic acid, and pyridoxine, with recommendations set at 1 mg, 100 mg, and 10 mg, respectively. A supplement supplying the recommended dietary allowance of the other water-soluble vitamins is also recommended (19,24). Iron supplementation is often a necessity for the renal patient on dialysis therapy because of the small blood loss associated with this therapy.

Anemia is usually a consequence of the disease for a variety of reasons: loss of blood as mentioned above; decreased production of erythropoietic factor necessary for formation of erythropoietin which in turn stimulates erythrocyte production; inhibition of erythrocyte production and shortened life span of erythrocytes due to circulating toxins which are associated with chronic renal disease.

Persons placed in stressful situations often find relief in going on eating "binges" or consuming certain favorite foods which can provide some degree of comfort. Oral gratification provides a release of sorts, but such a release is impossible for the patient in renal failure. Not only does he/she have to bear the stresses of possible loss of independence, decreased sexual activity, and even possible imminent death but also must be severely restricted in the kind and amount of food that can be eaten (27). There appears to be little or no source of comfort for the patient in renal failure! It is imperative, therefore, that all health professionals on the renal team share information and approaches aimed at supporting patients in the total management of their disease. The all-pervasive effect of the uremic syndrome is graphically depicted in Figure 10.7.

Individualization of dietary prescriptions and instructions is important in diet therapy for any disease state but in the case of renal disease it becomes a necessity because of the various degrees of renal insufficiency that may exist. The renal dietitian in order to be an effective member of the health team must be knowledgeable about the anatomy and physiology of the kidney and be able to interpret the significance of changes in pertinent lab values. He/she needs to be alert in noting changing lab values in order to determine what aspects of dietary management may require modification. Changing laboratory values also may serve as a guide for improved dietary counseling because from them the dietitian possibly can discern what facet (or facets) of dietary control needs special emphasis.

The dietitian has the responsibility of teaching the renal patient the

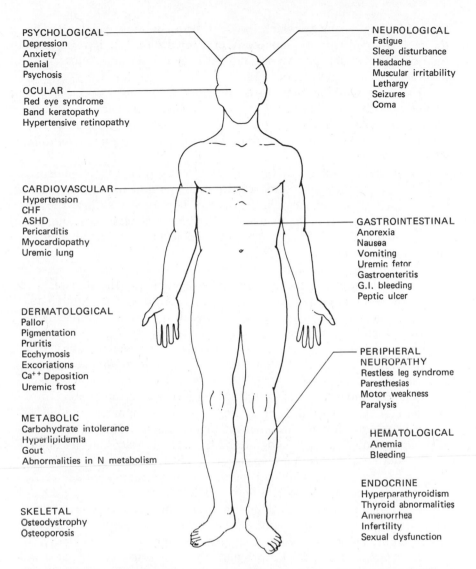

PSYCHOLOGICAL
Depression
Anxiety
Denial
Psychosis

OCULAR
Red eye syndrome
Band keratopathy
Hypertensive retinopathy

NEUROLOGICAL
Fatigue
Sleep disturbance
Headache
Muscular irritability
Lethargy
Seizures
Coma

CARDIOVASCULAR
Hypertension
CHF
ASHD
Pericarditis
Myocardiopathy
Uremic lung

GASTROINTESTINAL
Anorexia
Nausea
Vomiting
Uremic fetor
Gastroenteritis
G.I. bleeding
Peptic ulcer

DERMATOLOGICAL
Pallor
Pigmentation
Pruritis
Ecchymosis
Excoriations
Ca^{++} Deposition
Uremic frost

**PERIPHERAL
NEUROPATHY**
Restless leg syndrome
Paresthesias
Motor weakness
Paralysis

METABOLIC
Carbohydrate intolerance
Hyperlipidemia
Gout
Abnormalities in N metabolism

HEMATOLOGICAL
Anemia
Bleeding

ENDOCRINE
Hyperparathyroidism
Thyroid abnormalities
Amenorrhea
Infertility
Sexual dysfunction

SKELETAL
Osteodystrophy
Osteoporosis

Figure 10.7 The uremic syndrome. (From Brenner, Barry M. and Rector, Floyd C.: *The Kidney* © 1976 by the W.B. Saunders Co., Philadelphia. Reprinted by permission of the publisher and authors.)

principles of his/her rather complicated diet and the procedures by which an appropriate diet can be planned for the day. Equally important is educating the patient and his/her family about food selections and use of various spices and wines which can add variety to the diet and make it more nearly acceptable. The dietitian must listen with an understanding ear to the complaints of the patient about his/her food and continuously work toward finding means by which food can be made more palatable. Only the person faced with the monotony of a renal diet, low in protein and restricted in sodium, potassium, and fluids can describe adequately the frustration of such restrictions (28).

Excellent working tools for meal planning for the renal patient are provided by the Los Angeles District of the California Dietetic Association. Two booklets have been prepared, one entitled *A Guide to Protein Controlled Diets for Dietitians,* the other *A Guide to Protein Controlled Diets for Patients.* *

Maintenance dialysis therapy, although life-saving for the patient in renal failure can never be considered a really good substitute for actual kidney function, particularly in the area of hormonal function. For this reason renal transplantation is usually desirable whenever possible, particularly in the case of children. To many people a kidney transplant is the gift of a new life (28).

Renal transplantation, however, presents its own hazards because of the immunosuppressive therapy that must accompany the transplant in order to prevent the body's rejection of the new kidney. The required dosage of steroids may be massive and can result in various complications, many of which have implications for dietary management. Common complications resulting from steroid therapy are hypertension (due to excessive sodium and fluid retention), decreased glucose tolerance, obesity, hyperlipidemia, and gastric ulcer. Because of these possible complications, the recommended diet for the patient with a well-functioning transplanted kidney is one that is bland, low in sodium (approximately 85 to 90 mEq or 2 gm), low in carbohydrate (approximately 120 gm), but high in protein (about 2 gm per kilogram body weight). Also, calories should be adjusted so as to maintain weight or permit weight loss if necessary. The use of polyunsaturated fats is advised as is a generous intake of calcium (approximately 800 to 1200 mg daily) (29).

There also exists the possibility that the transplanted kidney will not operate perfectly and the patient will then require the same sort of dietary modifications as are necessary in patients with renal insufficiency. All health professionals need to keep in mind the numerous psychological and emotional problems as well as physical problems being faced by patients with severe renal disease (Fig. 10.7). Offering these patients and their families an understanding ear and emotional support may well be of more assistance than any kind of drug or diet therapy!

Other conditions in which dietary modification plays a part in management include acute renal failure, the nephrotic syndrome, and kidney stones.

---

* These may be obtained from Los Angeles District of Cal. Diet. Assoc., 1609 Westwood Blvd., Suite 101, Los Angeles, Cal., 90024.

Acute Renal Failure. Renal tubular degeneration resulting from insufficient renal blood flow or ingestion of nephrotoxins inhibits the kidneys from performing their normal excretory function. Sudden and acute loss of this excretory function is referred to as acute renal failure (ARF). This condition can occur in a variety of clinical settings. Individuals affected may include surgical patients, individuals with severe trauma, patients with various medical conditions, women with complications of pregnancy, and individuals having ingested various nephrotoxins (30).

Acute renal failure has been categorized (30) as: (1) prerenal, that is, extrarenal hemodynamic alterations which lead to decreased renal blood flow accompanied by a reduced GFR, an increased reabsorption by the proximal tubular cells and a decreased filtrate in the distal tubule; (2) postrenal, that is, obstructive uropathy which prevents excretion of urine; and (3) renal, or parenchymal renal diseases, the major types of which are glomerulonephritis and renal vasculitis. Because of the vast etiological differences that exist among the various types of acute renal failure, identification of etiology is essential before correct therapy can be instituted.

Although a variety of primary renal diseases can result in ARF, the most commonly occurring acute renal failure is caused not by renal disease but instead, either by drastically altered hemodynamics or by ingestion of nephrotoxins, both of which cause injury to the kidney. Here again the cause of renal failure must be clearly identified because the pathophysiology (and treatment) of these two types of kidney injury may be quite different (30).

Drastically altered hemodynamics resulting in renal failure may frequently occur following extensive burns, surgery associated with rapid hemorrhage, crushing injuries, etc., all of which can cause a severely decreased renal blood flow. On the other hand, decreased renal blood flow is not a necessary determinant of nephrotoxic acute renal failure. Instead, this syndrome can be caused by ingestion of heavy metals, organic solvents such as carbon tetrachloride or ethylene glycol, and various antibiotics such as amphotericin, gentamicin, kanamycin, and related compounds.

Investigators have used experimental animals to determine the mechanisms by which ARF is initiated and maintained. Although the picture is not totally clear, they have identified a variety of factors, including the status of extracellular volume, baseline renal resistance, and renal prostaglandins, all of which may influence the severity of the renal insult whether it be inflicted by altered hemodynamics or nephrotoxins. They also have found that a variety of other factors is involved in the maintenance of ARF and that their importance is related to the initiating cause. For example, persistent renal vasoconstriction and tubular obstruction are more related to the maintenance of the ARF caused by a hemodynamic insult while a decrease in glomerular permeability and backleakage of filtrate through damaged tubular cells maintain the ARF caused by nephrotoxins (30).

The possibility of preventing ARF, particularly that caused by hemodynamic insult, is improved through an understanding of its initiating and maintenance factors. For instance, the normalization of vascular fluid and relief of tubular obstruction (through use of certain diuretics) may allow restoration of kidney function. Once ARF is definitely established, however, therapy must be directed toward: (1) regulation of extracellular fluid volume and osmolality, and (2) maintenance of acceptable levels of serum urea nitrogen, creatinine, and potassium along with prevention of acidosis.

Regulation of extracellular fluid volume requires that fluid intake be rigidly controlled to prevent expansion of the extracellular fluid volume. The patient should receive only that amount of water and electrolytes excreted from the body in urine, feces, insensible losses, and expired air. Usually 400 to 600 ml of fluid plus that volume of fluid excreted in urine and feces is sufficient to provide normal hydration in the adult. Accurate daily weights can be extremely helpful in determining fluid balance. If proper management has been instituted, body weight should decrease by approximately one-half pound per day (14,30). Sodium intake is extremely important in the regulation of extracellular fluid osmolality and should be restricted to 30 to 60 mEq daily.

The aggressiveness of treatment for acute renal failure is determined by the degree of catabolic activity being experienced by the patient. Catabolic activity is indicated by the serum levels of urea nitrogen, creatinine, and electrolytes. These same values dictate the type of dietary management to be utilized. As long as the patient's serum urea nitrogen remains under 80 mg per 100 ml, dietary management is similar to that used in chronic renal failure, that is, high caloric intake accompanied by small amounts of protein of high biological value (usually a preparation of essential amino acids) and a multivitamin supplement (13). How the feedings are administered (orally or intravenously) depends upon the patient's ability to ingest foods without nausea. The aim of treatment is to supply sufficient calories and essential amino acids so that catabolism of body tissue is reduced to a minimum level. Accumulation of ketone bodies resulting from excessive utilization of body fat for energy contributes heavily to the acidosis associated with acute renal failure.

Patients exhibiting hypercatabolism as indicated by a serum urea nitrogen approaching 100 mg%, a creatinine level of 10 mg% or more, elevated serum potassium and acidosis usually require daily dialysis therapy and continuous monitoring of serum potassium levels. Patients who receive dialysis therapy daily should be given a high caloric diet (45 kilocalories or more per kilogram body weight) and approximately 1 gram protein per kilogram body weight. Potassium content of food becomes a critical consideration in feedings for patients in acute renal failure because hyperkalemia can cause sudden death due to cardiac arrhythmias or cardiac arrest. Although dialysis therapy reduces the danger of hyperkalemia, the amount of potassium allowed in the diet must be adjusted according to closely monitored serum potassium levels. Serum phosphate levels also need close monitoring in order that they may be kept as close to normal as possible.

An increase in urinary output to as much as 400 ml daily usually indicates that tubular recovery is occurring. Urine volume may increase very rapidly, reaching as high as 3000 ml daily (31). Although increased urine volume may signal restoration of kidney function, many of the complications of ARF can occur during this diuretic phase, for example, hyperkalemia, congestive heart failure, pyelonephritis.

The diuresis that may be associated with recovery of kidney function requires a careful monitoring of fluid and electrolyte balances and accurate recording of weight changes. It may be advisable to weigh the patient twice each day (13). A fact that muddies the water concerning polyuria in acute renal failure is that sometimes the disease is characterized by excessive urine output rather than oliguria (30); therefore, diuresis is not always a sign of improved tubular function.

Initially during excessively high urinary output, adjustments in quantities of fluid and electrolytes may be necessary as often as each half hour in order to prevent hypovolemia or electrolyte imbalances. As the diuretic phase progresses, however, the alert patient can usually satisfy fluid needs by using thirst as a guide for fluid consumption. Records of daily weights and urine outputs along with the closely monitored levels of serum urea nitrogen, creatinine, sodium, and potassium are used in order to help the patient progress toward a normal diet once more.

Total parenteral nutrition (TPN) appears to hold much promise in the treatment of acute tubular necrosis because a high caloric diet low in protein but supplying adequate amounts of essential amino acids can be given intravenously to patients who are hypercatabolic and unable to eat. The essential L-amino acids in the amounts recommended by Rose for attainment of nitrogen equilibrium (total nitrogen approximates 1.5 grams) are combined with a 70 percent dextrose solution so that about 1400 kilocalories from nonnitrogen sources are provided the patient in a volume of only 750 ml. Vitamins and electrolytes as needed are also added to the solution.

Investigators believe that success of total parenteral nutrition in the treatment of patients with acute renal failure may be due to an earlier reversal of azotemia and hypercatabolism. This shortened time span of renal failure probably decreases the incidence of later complications that can lead to death (22,23).

Currently, extreme caution in the care and administration of parenteral fluids is essential to prevent infections and thrombosis in the patient receiving intravenous feedings. Once the possibilities of these complications have been sufficiently lessened, TPN will probably become part of the standard treatment for acute renal failure (13).

Nephrotic Syndrome. The nephrotic syndrome is a group of biochemical and clinical symptoms related to the pathologic permeability of glomerular capillaries that allows filtration of plasma proteins. Normally only proteins of low molecular weight are filtered through the glomeruli and most of these are completely reabsorbed by the tubular cells. In nephrosis, however, massive proteinuria occurs, thereby causing the production of other classical symptoms of the syndrome, that is, hypoalbuminemia and edema. Edema is the chief complaint of the nephrotic patient and in some patients edema fluid can exceed 20 liters. Figure 10.8 indicates the pathogenesis of edema. Additional symptoms of the nephrotic syndrome include hyperlipidemia and lipiduria.

Proteinuria exceeding 3.5 gm/m²/day indicates the existence of the nephrotic syndrome (34). Approximately 70 percent of the protein excreted in the urine is albumin but other important plasma proteins such as ceruloplasmin are also lost. Failure of the glomerular capillaries to inhibit filtration of plasma proteins is due most often in adults to existing glomerulonephritis but may also be caused by other intrinsic renal diseases

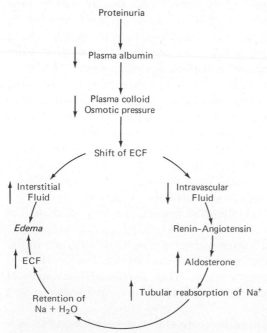

Figure 10.8 Pathogenesis of edema in the nephrotic syndrome. (From "Nephrotic syndrome" by R. W. Schrier and S. Griggenbeim *Harrison's Principles of Internal Medicine.* Copyright 1977 by McGraw Hill Book Co. Reprinted by permission of the publisher.)

such as lipoid nephrosis, membrane nephrotoxins, allergens, and drugs. In addition, systemic diseases affecting the glomerulus (e.g., diabetes mellitus) or diseases severely increasing the renal venous pressure (e.g., renal vein thrombosis) may produce the nephrotic syndrome.

The nephrotic syndrome carries with it the potential for many complications including hypotension, renal failure, accelerated atherosclerosis, thromboembolic vascular occlusion and infections. In children particularly, an increased susceptibility to infections commonly accompanies the nephrotic syndrome.

Renal failure is the expected outcome in nephrotic patients whose condition is due to chronic progressive glomerular diseases. A severely compromised GFR will eventually result in azotemia and uremia-related symptoms.

The increased incidence of atherosclerosis in nephrotic patients apparently is related to the elevated levels of serum lipids that accompany the nephrotic syndrome. The cause for nephrotic hyperlipidemia has not been clearly delineated.

To a large degree prognosis depends on the underlying cause of the nephrotic syndrome; therefore, optimal therapy can be delivered only after the cause of nephrosis is identified. Often identification of specific etiologic factors is impossible and treatment must of necessity be directed toward alleviation of symptoms and correction of malnutrition.

Diet therapy is very important in treatment of the nephrotic syndrome and principles involved are as follows:

1. High intake of protein to replace that lost from tissues and to provide the liver with sufficient amino acids for accelerated synthesis of albumin. When GFR is not compromised, only the patient's appetite restricts the limit of protein intake. For the average adult, however, approximately 120 grams protein daily is adequate for repleting body stores provided the overall caloric intake is sufficient.
2. Increased energy consumption approaching 50 to 60 kilocalories per kg body weight in order to promote positive nitrogen balance including increased synthesis of plasma proteins.
3. Restricted sodium intake in order to prevent further accumulation of fluid. A sodium intake of less than 10 mEq daily (230 mg) is quite effective in preventing further fluid accumulation but often is not prescribed because such severe restriction results in an unpalatable diet.

The edematous nephrotic patient whose treatment is partially diet-dependent presents a real challenge to the dietitian. The patient is probably already anorectic and yet is being counseled to consume a high protein, high caloric, sodium-restricted diet which under the best circumstances cannot be described as tempting. Whether the patient eats or not depends to a large extent upon: (1) the relationship existing between the patient and members of the health team, especially the dietitian; (2) the temperature of the foods and attractiveness of trays presented to the patient; and (3) the extent to which the dietitian, although severely restricted by dietary parameters, attempts to tempt the patient's appetite and encourages him/her to eat. The effectiveness of the dietitian in discovering foods that will tempt the patient's appetite requires a thorough knowledge of food composition as well as careful exploration of his/her food tolerances.

The nephrotic syndrome in 60 to 80 percent of affected children is caused by lipoid nephrosis, a disease of unknown pathogenesis and of spontaneous remission. Remission of the disease usually occurs in three to six months but may be hastened by administration of adrenal corticoids (34).

Nephrolithiasis. Although the pathogenetic mechanisms responsible for the occurrence of kidney stones are currently under much investigation and are gradually being recognized, nephrolithiasis as a total disease entity remains an enigma despite its long history of existence and its high incidence in the United States and many other parts of the world. In the United States alone 200,000 persons are estimated to be hospitalized each year because of kidney stones (35).

The underlying cause for nephrolithiasis in individual patients may often be determined by careful analysis of the stones being formed. According to their composition, stones may be categorized as follows: (1) calcium oxalate, (2) calcium oxalate mixed with calcium phosphate in form of hydroxyapatite, (3) calcium phosphate monohydrate, (4) magnesium ammonium phosphate, (5) uric acid, (6) cystine, and (7) those of miscellaneous composition (e.g., xanthine, silicates).

Although calcium phosphate monohydrate stones are very rare, the other calcium-containing stones are the most commonly occurring nephroliths and account for approximately 66 percent of the total. The next most common stone is that composed of magnesium ammonium phosphate (15 percent) which in turn, is followed in frequency of occurrence by uric acid and cystine stones (10 percent) and finally by those in the miscellaneous category (9 percent) (35).

Treatment of nephrolithiasis needs to be individualized and directed toward management of the underlying condition believed responsible for stone formation. Nevertheless, one principle of therapy common to treatment of all nephroliths is the pushing of fluid intake. All patients should drink at least 3 to 4 liters of fluid daily and have a urine output of not less than 2400 ml per 24 hours. Drinking water during the night needs to be emphasized because overnight urines are likely to be concentrated and therefore conducive to precipitation of salts and stone formation (13).

Brief consideration will be given to those stones for which there are some recommended dietary regimens.

Stones Composed of Calcium Oxalate Alone or Combined with Hydroxy-apatite. Stones of this type make up approximately two-thirds of all nephroliths and may be caused by a variety of diseases, the most common of which is idiopathic calcium stone disease. Idiopathic calcium stone disease in itself is rather complex because it may occur in patients with no apparent abnormality in calcium or oxalate metabolism as well as in those with hypercalcuria and/or hyperoxaluria. Other possible causes of calcium stones include hyperparathyroidism, hyperthyroidism, chronic small bowel disease, renal tubular acidosis, immobilization, excessive intake of calcium and/or vitamin D, urinary infection, and alkali abuse.

Because immobilization is a part of the clinical management of many disease states (e.g., trauma, paraplegia, stroke), it can represent a real problem in fostering stone formation. When a patient is immobilized, excessive mineral loss from the bones occurs, thereby raising serum mineral levels which then must be normalized via the kidney.

Whether dietary manipulation is of much value in treatment of calcium oxalate stones will depend upon the amount of calcium and/or oxalate being excreted in the urine. In the case of patients who exhibit hypercalcuria and hyperoxaluria, dietary modification appears warranted.

Because one reason for idiopathic hypercalcuria may be a defect in absorption of calcium from the gut, the nutritional regimen is reduction of calcium intake and avoidance of vitamin D supplements and of foods fortified with vitamin D. Calcium intake should not exceed 200 to 300 mg daily. Conversely, patients with hyperoxaluria secondary to small bowel disease should consume a diet high in calcium but low in fat and oxalate (see Table 10.5 for foods to be avoided in low oxalate diet). The presence of calcium in the gut depresses oxalate absorption by forming insoluble salts with it. Steatorrhea, which usually occurs in small bowel disease, increases the need for calcium because much of the calcium will form soaps with the unabsorbed fatty acids and be excreted as such.

Pyridoxine deficiency has been linked to the formation of calcium oxalate stones because of its function as a coenzyme in the transamination of glyoxalate to glycine. When sufficient vitamin B_6 is not present, glyoxalate can accumulate and subsequently be oxidized to oxalate. Treatment of patients with oxalate stones through administration of pyridoxine, however, has had questionable success, perhaps because a deficiency of this vitamin is not common (36,37). Magnesium, although not directly involved in oxalate synthesis, acts as an inhibitor of oxalate stone formation by allowing more oxalate to be held in solution.

Magnesium Ammonium Phosphate Stones. Approximately 15 percent of all renal calculi is due to a urine alkalinity that causes precipitation of

Table 10.5 Foods to be Avoided in Low
Oxalate Diet

Green and wax beans	Gooseberries
Beets and beet greens	Concord grapes
Dandelion greens*	Plums
Chard	Raspberries
Endive	Rhubarb*
Okra	Almonds*
Spinach*	Cashew nuts*
Sweet potatoes	Chocolate*
Currants	Cocoa*
Figs	Tea*

References: Robinson and Lawler, *Normal and Therapeutic Nutrition,* 15th ed., Macmillan, 1977; Howard and Herbold, *Nutrition in Clinical Care,* McGraw-Hill, 1978.
*Foods particularly high in oxalate.

magnesium ammonium phosphate crystals. These particular stones usually occur in patients whose urinary tracts are infected with urea-splitting organisms. The ammonia released by the action of these ureases produces the alkalinity responsible for the stone formation. Treatment is geared toward treatment of the infection and acidification of the urine toward its normal pH. Because acidifying agents such as methionine and ascorbic acid cannot be administered indefinitely because of their tendency to cause metabolic acidosis, the use of the acid ash diet* with these patients may prove helpful.

Uric Acid and Cystine Stones. Together these stones comprise about 10 percent of the renal stones found among the population; however, uric acid stones are more common than those caused by cystinuria.

Uric acid stones are not necessarily due to hyperuricosuria and an overproduction of uric acid (see purine metabolism, Chapter 3) but can be caused by a persistently acid urine which promotes crystal formation. Since urate solubility increases dramatically with rises in urinary pH, treatment is aimed toward alkalinizing the urine. A helpful adjunct to

---

* *Acid Ash Diet* increases the acidity of the urine and includes generous quantities of whole grain breads and cereals and foods high in protein. Fruit and vegetable intake is severely restricted with the exception of cranberries, plums, and prunes. Foods allowed on the acid ash diet provide strong inorganic acid anions (e.g., Cl^-, $HPO_4^=$ and $SO_4^=$), which must be balanced with cations, thereby reducing the amount of bicarbonate existing in body fluids. The unusual value of cranberries in lowering the urinary pH is due to their high content of benzoic acid which cannot be metabolized in the body but which is detoxified and excreted as hippuric acid.

Table 10.6   Foods to be Restricted in Low
Purine Diet

Meats, fish, poultry
Dried beans, peas, lentils
Spinach, asparagus, mushrooms
Anchovies and sardines*
Brains and organ meats*
Meat extracts*
Mincemeat*
Gravies*
Alcohol**

Reference: Robinson and Lawler, *Normal and Therapeutic Nutrition,* 15th ed., Macmillan, 1977.
*Foods particularly high in purines.
**Alcohol is contraindicated for patients with elevated
uric acid levels because it may cause increased acidity of
body fluids, thereby leading to increased precipitation of
uric acid crystals.

medication may be the alkaline ash diet.* In case of hyperuricosuria, reduction in consumption of high purine foods may be advisable (see Table
10.6).

   Cystinuria is an inherited condition characterized by a defect in the
renal transport of cystine, lysine, arginine, and ornithine and if untreated,
eventually leads to secondary interstitial nephritis and uremia (35). Treatment is augmented by an alkaline ash diet which automatically reduces
methionine intake due to its limited allowance of protein foods. D-penicil-
linamine is often used in the treatment of this disease to prevent cystine
from being secreted by the tubular cells.

Other Urinary Tract Problems. Infection of the urinary tract is a common
problem in the elderly and in patients with indwelling catheters. Attention
to fluid intake is critical as a preventive measure. Sometimes when the
urine is alkaline, and consequently more offensive in odor, cranberry
juice can be helpful because of its pH-lowering effect.

   Dietitians working with this population need to assess carefully the
fluid intake of patients and take steps to increase volume whenever appropriate.

   * *Alkaline Ash Diet* increases the alkalinity of the urine and is composed primarily of vegetables and fruits with the exception of cranberries, plums, and prunes. Milk is also allowed
as are breads prepared with baking soda and/or baking powder. Foods with a particularly
high alkaline ash include the various greens, beans, peas, and dried fruits. Alkaline ash foods
produce more cations (Na^+, K^+, Mg^{++}, Ca^{++}) than anions, thereby allowing increased retention of bicarbonate ions. Although many fruits contain organic acids which give them a sour
taste, these acids are quickly metabolized in the body to form carbon dioxide and water. As
a result, excess cations remain and are available for combination with bicarbonate ions.

CASE STUDY: RENAL FAILURE

A 61-year-old black female, 5 feet, 1 inch tall and weighing 88 lbs., was admitted to the hospital with complaints of extreme thirst, swelling of hands and legs, nausea and vomiting, insomnia, muscle cramping, and twitching. The patient had a history of hypertension and two years earlier had been diagnosed as having chronic renal disease. At this time she had been placed on a sodium-restricted (90 mEq), low protein diet (35 gm), and furosemide (Lasix®) had been prescribed for her. The patient, although scheduled for routine out-patient visits, had failed to keep many of her appointments through the intervening two years.

The present physical examination of the patient revealed a blood pressure of 220/110 mm Hg, a heart rate of 100 per minute, and rapid, shallow breathing. Her skin was dry, her breath had the odor of urine, and pitting edema was evident in her hands and legs. The physician requested hematologic and chemistry screening and a creatinine clearance test. The initial diet order for the patient remained the same as had been prescribed for her during the hospitalization two years earlier. The patient, however, was anorectic and refused any food offered her. She admitted to the dietitian that she had found the low protein, sodium-restricted diet unpalatable and even when she had a good appetite, she never really followed the diet prescription given her two years earlier.

Laboratory findings were as follows:

BUN	110 mg/dl (normal 8–18 mg/dl)
Creatinine	12 mg/dl (normal 0.6–1.2 mg/dl)
Hematocrit	20% (normal 38–47%)
Potassium	5.5 mEq/l (normal 3.8–5.0 mEq/l)
Calcium	7 mg/dl (normal 9.0–10.6 mg/dl)
Albumin	2.0 g/dl (normal 3.2–4.5 g/dl)
Creatinine Clearance	4 ml/min (normal 97–110 ml/min)

Upon examination of the laboratory results, the physician referred the patient to the dialysis center for treatment.

Questions

1. What laboratory findings indicated to the physician that dialysis therapy was an immediate need?
2. Why would the physician have expected the calcium and albumin levels to be below normal in chronic renal failure?

Discussion

The condition of renal failure is marked by the kidneys' inability to allow passage of water and solutes through the glomerulus. This can be due to a loss of structural integrity of the glomerulus itself and/or an inadequate blood supply to the kidneys. The result is that solutes that are normally removed by glomerular filtration from the blood accumulate in the bloodstream. Among the laboratory findings, the elevated BUN, creatinine, and potassium, and the low creatinine clearance value are all consistent with a severe impairment of glomerular filtration. The most serious consequence of solute retention in renal failure is the resultant hyperkalemia (elevated serum potassium) because of the profound effect of potassium on neuromuscular excitability, and most importantly on cardiac contractibility. Elevated serum potassium inhibits cardiac contraction by interfering with intraventricular conduction, and a sufficiently high (usually above 10 mEq/l) concentration of the ion results in cardiac arrest. In renal failure, therefore, the removal of accumulated potassium from the plasma is one of the most important reasons for initiating dialysis therapy.

The patient's low protein diet during the two years prior to admission may have accounted in part for the reduced serum albumin value, but the major contributing factor relates to the impairment of glomerular filtration. The retention of water increases the total blood volume, thereby reducing the serum protein concentration by the dilution effect. Approximately 50 percent of the total serum calcium is bound to protein, and it follows that as the protein level falls, the calcium concentration falls accordingly. Another factor accounting for the hypocalcemia is the deficiency of 1,25-dihydroxycholecalciferol (1,25-$(OH_2)D_3$), the compound necessary for efficient calcium absorption from the gut (pps. 377–378). The patient's hematocrit was low not only because of the dilution effect but also because of decreased production of the erythropietic factor, inhibition of erythrocyte synthesis, and shortened life span of erythrocytes (p. 380).

In the dialysis center a team composed of the physician, nurse, dietitian, clinical pharmacist, and social worker planned the medical management for the patient. She was placed on dialysis therapy three times per week and medications included (by category):

Diuretic:	Lasix® (furosemide)
Antihypertensive:	Catapres® (clonidine)
Antacid:	Amphojel® liquid
Laxative:	Colace® (dioctyl sodium sulfosuccinate)
Antianxicty agent:	Valium® (diazepam)
Vitamin and mineral supplements:	Neocalglucon®
	Rocaltrol® (calcitrol)
	multivitamins with folic acid
	iron sulfate

Questions

1. Why were the above listed medications prescribed?
2. What is the appropriate diet prescription for this patient receiving dialysis therapy three times a week?
3. What particular challenge does the dietitian have in the treatment of this patient?
4. Why is the social worker an important member of the team involved in management of the chronic renal patient?

Drug therapy for this patient, as recommended by the clinical pharmacist and prescribed by the physician, was planned around the specific problems of the patient; therefore, several medications were administered concurrently for optimal efficacy. Lasix (furosemide) and Catapres (clonidine) were used together to lower blood pressure effectively. The initial, rapid diuretic effect of Lasix reduces edema and helps lower blood pressure as total body fluid volume decreases; further lowering of blood pressure is accomplished through action of Catapres which, by means of a central nervous system depressant effect, decreases sympathetic tone of blood vessels. The increased heart rate seen in the patient is probably due to cardiac overload and likely will decrease as fluid volume is lowered. Should this not be the case, however, the use of a beta adrenergic blocking agent such as propranolol (Inderal®) may be necessary in order to decrease heart rate toward normal.

The antacid (Amphojel liquid) is utilized to bind and increase the gastrointestinal excretion of phosphate, thereby decreasing phosphate absorption and improving the ratio of calcium to phosphorus in serum. The use of this antacid, however, often leads to constipation. If increasing the fiber content of ingested food does not succeed in improving elimination, then Colace (dioctyl sodium sulfosuccinate) will be used for softening the feces.

Most patients undergoing dialysis suffer from anxiety and insomnia; therefore, the antianxiety agent Valium (diazepam) is prescribed in order to alleviate anxiety and to allow sleep. Valium, through its relief of anxiety, may also have beneficial effects on cardiac function because at least part of the etiology of the tachycardia seen in this patient may have been induced by stress.

Vitamin and mineral supplementation, as ordered for this patient, is nearly always necessary for a person undergoing chronic renal dialysis therapy. This supplementation must be carefully monitored, however, because the condition of the patient can change quickly. Neocalglucon (calcium) and Rocaltrol [1,25-$(OH_2)D_3$] are used to stabilize serum calcium while iron sulfate and folic acid may help relieve the anemia being experienced by this patient. The multivitamin preparation replaces vitamins lost through dialysis therapy.

The renal dietitian was given the responsibility of prescribing this patient's diet which was then countersigned by the physician. Based upon the patient's weight for height and other indices of poor nutritional status (e.g., hematocrit, serum albumin) the dietitian determined that the patient should receive no less than 1900 kcal daily. (Ideal body weight for a 61-inch woman approximates 105 lbs or 47.7 kg). See Chapter 12 for calculation of ideal body weight. Renal patients on dialysis therapy should receive 35 to 45 kcal per kg body weight. Since this patient was underweight (88 lbs) but had a very poor appetite, a caloric intake of 40 kcal/kg was considered appropriate. Protein level was placed at 48 g (approximately 1 gram per kg ideal body weight), sodium at 90 mEq (2 grams) and potassium at 50 mEq (2 grams). Fluid intake was restricted to 500 ml daily, an amount sufficient for the replacement of normal fecal and insensible fluid losses.

The dietitian, aware of the patient's failure to follow her diet during the past two years, is faced with the problem of making the diet as nearly acceptable as possible and of motivating the patient to follow the newly prescribed diet. The patient had found the sodium restriction the most difficult aspect of her previous diet; therefore, the dietitian knows she must begin immediately to experiment with various allowable spices and with wines which can improve the palatability of various foods served the patient. Getting the patient to consume 1900 kilocalories without exceeding her sodium, potassium, and fluid allowances will be a real challenge for the dietitian. Sodium intake of the patient is crucial because of its effect on thirst, particularly since the patient is allowed only 500 ml fluid daily.

The social worker with his/her expertise in psychology is an invaluable member of the health team selected to manage the patient with chronic renal failure. The patient is faced with so many major adjustments in her life that she needs all the psychological and emotional support available to her. The social worker not only supplies support herself/himself but also can help all other team members and the patient's family to be more supportive. In addition, the social worker may provide guidance to the dietitian in approaches that may prove effective in helping the patient adhere to the regimen. For example, some patients respond to a strict authoritarian approach while others like to be involved in decision-making. The social worker may be in a better position than would the dietitian to make this determination.

REFERENCES

1. Bell, G. H., D. Emslie-Smith, and C. R. Paterson. *Textbook of Physiology and Biochemistry*. 9th ed. New York: Churchill Livingstone, 1976; pp. 393–414.
2. Crouch, J. E. and J. R. McClintic. *Human Anatomy and Physiology*. 2nd ed. New York: John Wiley and Sons, 1976; pp. 663–691.
3. Guyton, A. C. *Textbook of Medical Physiology*. 5th ed. Philadelphia: W. B. Saunders, 1976; pp. 438–455.
4. Harper, H. A., V. W. Rodwell, and P. A. Mayes. *Review of Physiological Chemistry*. 16th ed. Langes Medical Publication, Los Altos, Calif., 1977; pp. 609–632.
5. Kark, R. M. and J. H. Oyama. Nutrition and Cardiovascular-Renal Diseases. In *Modern Nutrition in Health and Disease*, Goodhart and Shils, eds. 5th ed. Philadelphia: Lea and Febiger, 1973; pp. 852–894.
6. McMurray, W. C. *Essentials of Human Metabolism*. New York: Harper and Row, 1977; p. 258.
7. Levine, R. and D. E. Hoft. Carbohydrate homeostasis, Parts I and II. *N. Eng. J. Med.* **283:** 175;237, 1970.
8. Wesson, L. G. *Physiology of the Human Kidney*. New York: Grune and Stratton, 1969; pp. 37–39.
9. Westervelt, F. B. Part I. Carbohydrate Metabolism. In *Clinical Aspects of Uremia and Dialysis*. Massry and Sellers, eds. Springfield, IL: Charles C Thomas, 1976; pp. 212–229.
10. Kopple, J. D. Part III. Nitrogen Metabolism. In *Clinical Aspects of Uremia and Dialysis*. Massry and Sellers, eds. Springfield IL. Charles C Thomas, 1976; pp. 241–273.
11. Tietz, N. W. *Fundamentals of Clinical Chemistry*. 2nd ed. Philadelphia: W. B. Saunders, 1976; p. 984.
12. Freedman, L. R. and F. H. Epstein. Urinary tract infection, pyelonephritis and related conditions. In *Harrison's Principles of Internal Medicine*, G. W. Thorn et al., eds. 8th ed. New York: McGraw-Hill, 1977; pp. 1460–1467.
13. Ing, T. S. and R. M. Kark. Renal Disease. In *Nutritional Support of Medical Practice*, Schneider, Anderson, and Coursin, eds. New York: Harper and Row, 1977; pp. 367–383.
14. Epstein, F. H. and J. P. Merrill. Chronic renal failure. In *Harrison's Principles of Internal Medicine*, G. W. Thorn et al., eds. 8th ed. New York: McGraw-Hill, 1977; pp. 1428–1438.
15. Giordano, C. Use of exogenous and endogenous urea for protein synthesis in normal and uremic subjects. *J. Lab. Clin. Med.* **62:** 231, 1963.
16. Giovannetti, S. and Q. Maggiore. A low-protein diet with proteins of high biological value for severe chronic uremia. *Lancet* **i:** 1000, 1964.
17. Varcoe, A. R., D. Halliday, E. R. Carson, P. Richards, and A. S. Tavill. Anabolic role of urea in renal failure. *Am. J. Clin. Nut.* **31:** 1601, Sept. 1978.
18. Ford, J., M. E. Phillips, F. E. Toye, V. A. Luck and H. E. de Wardener. Nitrogen balance in patients with chronic renal failure on diets containing varying quantities of protein. *Brit. Med. J. No.* **5646:** 735, Mar. 22, 1969.
19. Kopple, J. D. Dietary requirements. In *Clinical Aspects of Uremia and Dialy-*

sis, Massry and Sellers, eds. Springfield, IL: Charles C Thomas, 1976; pp. 453–489.

20. Mitch, W. E. and M. Walser. Analogs of amino acids in renal failure. *Drug Therapy* **7:** 39, Feb. 1977.
21. Walser, M. Keto acid therapy in chronic renal failure. *Nephron* **21:** 57, 1978.
22. Kopple, J. D. and J. W. Coburn. Evaluation of chronic uremia—importance of serum urea nitrogen, serum creatinine and their ratio. *J. Am. Med. Assoc.* **227:** 41, 1974.
23. Sanfelippo, M. L., R. S. Swenson, and G. M. Reaven. Response of plasma triglycerides to dietary changes in patients on hemodialysis. *Kidney International* **14:** 180, 1978.
24. Blumenkrantz, M. J., C. E. Roberts, B. Card, J. W. Coburn, and J. D. Kopple. Nutritional management of the adult patient undergoing peritoneal dialysis. *J. Am. Diet. Assoc.* **73:** 251, 1978.
25. Tarazi, R. C. The diuretic antihypertensives. *Drug Therapy* **5:** 55, 1975.
26. Morgan, T. O. Diuretics: Basic clinical pharmacology and therapeutic use. *Drugs* **15:** 151, 1978.
27. Moore, G. L. Psychiatric aspects of chronic renal disease. *Postgraduate Med.* **60:** 140, Nov. 1976.
28. Biller, D. C. Patient's point of view: Diet in chronic renal failure. *J. Am. Diet. Assoc.* **71:** 633, Dec. 1977.
29. Liddle, V. R., P. J. Walker, H. K. Johnson, and H. E. Ginn. Diet in transplantation. *Dialysis and Transplantation* **6:** 9, May 1977.
30. Patak, R. V., M. D. Lifschitz, and J. H. Stein. Acute renal failure: Clinical aspects of pathophysiology. *Cardiovascular Med.* **4:** 19, Jan. 1979.
31. Epstein, F. H. Acute renal failure. In *Harrison's Principles of Internal Medicine,* G. W. Thorn et al., eds. 8th ed. New York: McGraw-Hill, 1977; pp. 1424–1428.
32. Abel, R. M., V. E. Shib, W. M. Abbott, C. H. Berk, and J. E. Fischer. Amino acid metabolism in acute renal failure: Influence of intravenous essential L-amino and hyperalimentation therapy. *Ann. Surgery* **180:** 350, 1974.
33. Abel, R. M., C. H. Beck, W. M. Abbott, J. A. Ryan, G. O. Barnett, and J. E. Fischer. Improved survival from acute renal failure after treatment with essential L-amino acids and glucose. *N. Eng. J. Med.* **288:** 695, Apr. 1973.
34. Schrier, R. W. and S. Guggenheim. Nephrotic syndrome. In *Harrison's Principles of Internal Medicine,* G. W. Thorn et al., eds. 8th ed. McGraw-Hill, New York: 1977; pp. 1450–1456.
35. Williams, H. E. Physiology in medicine: Nephrolithiasis. *N. Eng. J. Med.* **290:** 33, Jan. 1974.
36. Van Reen, R. Pyridoxine in urinary stone treatment. *Nutrition and the M.D.* **3:** 1, Aug. 1977.
37. Gershoff, S. N. Magnesium oxide as a treatment for renal stones. *Nutrition and the M.D.* **3:** 1, Aug. 1977.

RECOMMENDED READINGS

The American Journal of Clinical Nutrition, vol. 31, September and October issues, 1978.

These two issues carry the proceedings of the First International Congress on Nutrition in Renal Disease which was held in Wurzburg, Germany, 1977. A wealth of in-depth information on all nutrition-related aspects of kidney disease.

Forwell, E., J. W. T. Dickerson, J. M. Duckham, and H. A. Lee. The influence of energy source and intake on nitrogen metabolism in chronic renal failure: relevance to hyperlipoproteinaemia. *Journal of Human Nutrition* **32:** 87, 1978.

Authors emphasize the importance of energy source in control of various hyperlipoproteinemias which are likely to accompany chronic renal failure.

CHAPTER 11

Nutrient–Drug Interactions

While the beneficial effects of dietary modification as an essential mode of therapy for many disease states has long been recognized, the concept that nutrient intake, dietary habits, and therapeutic agents may interact on a specific level has only recently come under close clinical scrutiny. Changes in eating habits, various alterations in methods of food processing, food additives, and changes in the quality of nutrition in general have produced situations in which interactions between foods and drugs may occur that would not have been possible even 20 years ago. Over the past decade, sufficient clinical data have become available to demonstrate the significance of some specific interactions between certain nutrients and therapeutic agents and their impact on the efficacy of dietary and drug therapy. Other interactions, which have been documented over a longer period of time, occur as nonspecific nutrient–drug interactions that are also of clinical importance in specific circumstances and must be considered in the individual patient.

While the list of possible nutrient–drug interactions is increasing at a rapid rate, the level of significance of such interactions in clinical situations is often difficult to validate because of variables such as the quantity of nutrient or drug involved, the presence of chronic disease states, and the age, size, and general physical condition of the patient. Therefore, the probability of the occurrence as well as the clinical significance of many interactions must be evaluated in the individual patient rather than by the use of generalized rules. It is expected that in the future, knowledge of the clinical significance of nutrient–drug interactions will increase and become better understood, and therefore the purpose of this chapter will be not only to present those interactions that are already well documented, but also to prepare the reader to understand interactions that may be documented in the future.

Interactions that occur between nutrients and therapeutic agents may be of either a nonspecific or specific nature. Such interactions fall into two categories:

1. Interactions resulting from the presence of food in the gastrointestinal tract that may alter drug absorption.
2. Interactions resulting from the presence of drugs that may alter nutrient absorption or utilization.

NUTRIENT ALTERATION OF DRUG ABSORPTION

Nutrients in the gastrointestinal tract may alter the rate and/or the extent of drug absorption by:

1. Acting as a physical barrier and preventing drugs from reaching absorbing surfaces.
2. Altering gastric motility, emptying time, or pH.
3. Reacting chemically with certain therapeutic agents.

The effects of nutrients on the kinetics of drug absorption are well known and always considered when calculating dosages for oral drug therapy. The presence of food in the stomach may decrease the ability of drugs to reach absorbing surfaces and thus retard both the rate and extent of absorption to some degree. This nonspecific interaction is not usually of clinical significance because the drug dosage can be increased to make up for any decreased absorption. In fact, many drugs that are highly irritating to the gastric mucosa are administered with meals to prevent such irritation from occurring. Table 11.1 lists some of the more commonly used irritating drugs that should be administered with meals.

The rate of drug absorption becomes important clinically when drugs are administered on an "as needed" basis, such as a mild analgesic for headache, where a rapid achievement of therapeutic plasma levels is important. In such cases, the drug should be taken on an empty stomach, if it is not irritating, to achieve the most rapid rate of absorption. Drugs that are administered chronically may be absorbed more slowly but the extent of absorption is usually equivalent whether the drug is taken when the stomach is full or empty. Thus, therapeutic plasma levels may be maintained even though the rate of absorption is decreased.

There are some exceptions to the general effects of food on the rate and extent of drug absorption. The absorption of some drugs may actually

Table 11.1   Drugs Irritating to Gastric Mucosa

Aminophylline	Nitrofurantoin
Para-aminosalicylic acid	Phenylbutazone
APC	Potassium salts
Aspirin	Prednisone
Chlorpromazine	Procyclidine
Chlorpropamide	Reserpine
Ferrous sulfate, lactate, etc.	Salicyclazosulfapyridine
Hydrochlorothiazide	Tolbutamide
Indomethacin	Triamterene
Isoniazid	Trihexyphenidyl
Nalidixic acid	

be enhanced by the presence of specific food types. At the present time, clinical data are lacking except for a few cases. For example, the absorption of griseofulvin, a fungistatic agent, and tetrachloroethylene, an anthelmintic agent, is enhanced in the presence of fatty meals (1,2) and fat is necessary for a portion of calcium salt absorption (3). With the use of such drugs, care should be taken to limit the intake of excessive fat or to lower the dose of the drugs in question.

The absorption of most drugs is unrelated to the absorption of nutrients. While nutrient absorption is dependent on secretions of the digestive system, enzyme activity and gastrointestinal pH, that of drugs is dependent on characteristics of the individual agent such as lipid solubility, pKa, particle size, and physical state. In order for almost all drugs to be transported across the gastrointestinal mucosa, they must be either small enough to pass through membrane pores or be in an un-ionized, lipid-soluble state because most drugs are transported via passive rather than active transport processes. Drugs that are acidic in nature are un-ionized in the acid medium of the stomach and thus are best absorbed from this site while basic drugs are un-ionized in the alkaline environment of the small intestine and are best absorbed from that site.

Because the presence of food in the gastrointestinal tract increases motility and stimulates emptying of the stomach contents into the small intestine, food can alter the absorption of some drugs that would be best absorbed in the stomach. Food in the stomach causes the drugs to be rapidly emptied into the basic environment of the small intestine, which retards their absorption. At the same time, administering a drug that is best absorbed in the small intestine after a meal will hasten its absorption because it will reach this site more rapidly. Thus a drug that requires an acidic environment for best absorption should be taken shortly before or with meals when gastric acid secretion is stimulated. Drugs that are un-ionized in the basic medium of the small intestine should be taken two to three hours after meals so that the drug will be rapidly moved into the small intestine. Drugs that are acid labile and thus destroyed or inactivated in the acidic medium of the stomach should be taken one hour before meals or two to three hours after meals (4) (see Table 11.2). A common practice is to give drugs with fruit juice, particularly when unpleasant tasting drugs are being given to children. Most fruit juices, cola bever-

Table 11.2 Representative Acid-labile Drugs

Ampicillin	Penicillin G
Cloxacillin	Pentaerythritol tetranitrate
Erythromycin	Phenmetrazine
Lincomycin	Tetracycline (except doxycycline and minocycline)
Penicillamine	

Table 11.3 Acidic Liquids

Canned Juices	Wines
Cherry	Soda (Club, Cream, Cherry)
Cider	Cola
Cranberry	Ginger Ale
Grapefruit	Root beer
Grape	Sarsaparilla
Lemon	
Lime	
Pineapple	
Prune	
Tomato	

ages, and other nutrients listed in Table 11.3 will produce an acidic environment which interferes with the absorption of the acid-labile or basic drugs. Precautions should be taken to see that these particular drugs are administered only with water.

Some nutrients specifically alter the absorption or activity of therapeutic agents by mechanisms other than altering the environment of the gastrointestinal tract. Dairy products and foods containing iron decrease the absorption of tetracycline antibiotics except for doxycycline and minocycline. Calcium from dairy products and iron form a chemical complex with the antibiotics (chelation) which prevents their absorption (3). Dairy products may also produce an alkaline medium in the stomach which will cause the enteric coating of drugs to dissolve and allow the drug to be released in the stomach rather than in the small intestine. The enteric coating of drugs is utilized as a mechanism for preventing excessive gastric irritation, for example the laxative bosocodyl (Dulcolax®) and aspirin, or to prevent inactivation of the drug in the acidic stomach pH, for example, penicillin.

NUTRIENT ALTERATION OF DRUG RESPONSE

Nutrients may alter the response to or level of activity of a drug by:

1. Alteration of drug metabolism or excretion.
2. Introduction of a naturally occurring pharmacologically active substance in the food that increases or decreases the response to the drug.

The effects of nutrients on drug metabolism have mainly been limited in the clinical setting to the presence of food contaminants and to the chronic use of alcohol. Food contaminants such as pesticide residues

(DDT, lindane, and so on) are found in varying amounts throughout the food chain. They enter the food chain through diverse routes such as application to seeds or growing plants, absorption by plants from the soil, or through animals who have eaten contaminated plants. These contaminants are capable of inducing or increasing the number of the hepatic microsomal enzymes (5) which are responsible for the biotransformation of certain drugs (e.g., phenytoin and phenobarbital). The therapeutic implications of such an interaction have not yet been verified, but it seems highly possible with the wide variety of additives used in today's food processing techniques, that other interactions will be forthcoming.

Alcohol, which may broadly be considered as either a nutrient or a therapeutic agent, has been reported to affect adversely the absorption of a number of nutrients as well as to alter metabolism of drugs. Large, acute doses of alcohol inhibit hepatic microsomal enzymes and may thus decrease drug metabolism (6) while the chronic use of relatively large amounts of alcohol results in the induction of hepatic microsomal enzymes and thus accelerates the metabolism of drugs such as phenytoin, tolbutamide, and warfarin (7). Alcohol dependence is often treated with the therapeutic agent disulfiram (Antabuse®) which inhibits the metabolism of alcohol by blocking the enzyme aldehyde dehydrogenase which causes the conversion of acetaldehyde to inert products. When alcohol is consumed, even in amounts as small as 5 ml, in the presence of disulfiram, a typical reaction consisting of flushing and nausea occur due to elevated plasma acetaldehyde levels. Other agents that also produce a disulfiram-like reaction include chlorpropamide, tolbutamide (in high doses), furazolidone, quinacrine, griseofulvin, chloramphenicol, and metronidazole (8). Alcohol in any form should be strictly avoided, even in small amounts, in patients taking any of these drugs. In fact, as a general rule, the use of alcohol should be avoided in patients taking any form of medication.

The rate of excretion of drugs may be altered by nutrients that produce changes in urinary pH. A drug that is un-ionized will be reabsorbed from the renal tubules back into the blood while an ionized drug will be readily excreted with urine. The rate of excretion of acidic and basic drugs will thus be directly influenced by the pH of the urine.

An acid ash diet (p. 390) consisting of meat, fowl, seafood, eggs, cheese, nuts, baked goods, pasta, cranberries, plums, prunes, and their juices will produce an acidic urine. The lowered urinary pH will decrease the normal excretion of acidic drugs such as aspirin and phenobarbital. Alkaline ash diets (p. 391) consisting of dairy products, most vegetables and fruits except cranberries, plums, and prunes will produce an alkaline urine which will retard the excretion of basic drugs such as quinidine and amphetamine. The effects of alkaline ash diets on urinary pH may be further heightened by the concomitant use of antacids which are absorbed in small amounts. In such patients, supplementary urinary acidifiers may be added to achieve an acidic urine.

Some foods contain active substances that can cause a direct druglike effect or that can interact with a drug to increase or decrease the expected response. Probably the most dangerous interaction of this type occurs between monoamine oxidase (MAO) inhibitors (a group of drugs that are used in the treatment of depression and hypertension including pargyline, tranylcypromine, and phenelzine sulfate) and nutrients that contain tyramine. MAO is an enzyme found in the gastrointestinal tract, liver, and adrenergic nerve endings that metabolizes norepinephrine and chemically similar compounds. Tyramine is an agent that resembles norepinephrine pharmacologically and produces an elevation of blood pressure. Normally, it is metabolized in the gastrointestinal tract and liver and does not appear in plasma in significant amounts. MAO inhibitors prevent the normal metabolism of tyramine and large enough quantities may be absorbed to produce severe hypertension. The foods that contain tyramine are included in Table 11.4.

MAO inhibitors are also thought to produce adverse reactions when combined with cola beverages, coffee, chocolate, and raisins. Other drugs that also inhibit MAO include procarbazine and furazolidone. The foods listed in Table 11.4 should also be avoided in the presence of these drugs.

Natural licorice, ingested in large amounts, may produce hypokalemia, salt and water retention, hypertension, paresthesias, and alkalosis (9). While most American candy manufacturers now use a synthetic licorice flavoring agent that does not produce these effects, some imported candies are still flavored with the nautral licorice and should be avoided by patients with cardiovascular diseases.

Monosodium glutamate, a widely used food additive, has been found to produce a syndrome characterized by headache, facial pressure, chest

Table 11.4 Foods Containing Tyramine

Pickled herring	Beef and chicken livers
Fermented sausages	Broad beans, e.g., fava
Salami	Canned figs
Pepperoni	Bananas
Sharp or aged cheeses	Avocados
Camembert	Soy sauce
Stilton	Active yeast preparations
Brie	Beer
N.Y. State cheddar	Wines
Gruyère	Sherry
Processed American	Sauterne
Yogurt	Riesling
Sour cream	Chianti

pain, and burning sensations of the extremities in susceptible individuals. This syndrome, often termed the "Chinese restaurant syndrome" because of the frequent use of this agent in preparing Chinese foods, is thought to occur because of a transient hyponatremia. Patients on chronic diuretic therapy should be cautioned to refrain from the use of monosodium glutamate.

Certain foods such as brussel sprouts, cabbage, cauliflower, kale, turnips, rutabaga, and soybeans contain thiooxazolidine (a goiterogenic agent) which complexes with iodine and prevents the production of the thyroid hormone (1). In the individual with normal thyroid function, ingestion of these foods will have no adverse effects because there is enough iodine in the normal diet to counteract the goiterogenic effect. However, persons requiring thyroid medications should exercise caution in eating the above listed foods.

Many types of foods contain large amounts of electrolytes such as sodium and potassium which may produce detrimental effects to patients on restricted diets. Thiazide diuretics do not produce optimal effects without some degree of sodium restriction and these same agents normally produce some degree of hypokalemia. Unless foods high in sodium are restricted, the full therapeutic effects of these agents will not be realized. While oral potassium supplementation is often used to avoid the hypokalemia produced with these diuretics, dietary potassium is often preferable and more acceptable to some patients. A few foods high in potassium and low in sodium are potatoes, oranges, dried apricots, peaches, dates, figs, raisins, bananas, and prunes. Table 11.5 lists amounts of various foods that could substitute for oral potassium. Of interest in the treatment of patients who require a low sodium diet is finding that a relatively high carbohydrate intake has an inhibitory action on sodium excretion (10), that is, sodium retention is related to the level of carbohydrate intake. While the impact of this finding has yet to be determined, alteration of the diet to lower carbohydrate intake may prove to have beneficial effects on the efficacy of diuretic therapy.

The consumption of foods such as green leafy vegetables and liver which contain large amounts of vitamin K has been reported to alter the efficacy of anticoagulants such as warfarin (11). Ingestion of vitamin K will alter prothrombin time in the patient stabilized on anticoagulant therapy.

Another interaction which has been reported to occur is that between L-dopa and pyridoxine. L-dopa is used in the treatment of Parkinson's disease, a condition in which there is a decreased amount of dopamine in certain brain areas. Dopamine cannot cross the blood-brain barrier and therefore cannot be used in the treatment of this condition. L-dopa is useful because it will cross the blood-brain barrier and can be converted to dopamine after it enters the central nervous system. A large portion of

Table 11.5 Comparison of Foods and Supplements as Sources of Potassium

Potassium supplements	Dosage	Amount of K+		Foods	Serving size	Approximate Amount of K+	
		mEq	*mg*			*mEq*	*mg*
Liquid							
10% potassium chloride	15 ml (1 Tbsp)	10.4	405.6	Cooked dry apricots	½c. (125 g)	10.2	398
				Avocado	½ (125 g)	17.4	680
				Banana	1 med (175 g)	11.3	440
Powder							
K-Lor	1 packet	7.8	304	Cooked dry lima beans	½c. (95 g)	14.9	581
K-Lyte	1 packet	13.0	507	Cantaloupe	¼ melon (238 g)	8.7	341
				Orange	1 (180 g)	6.7	263
Tablets							
Potassium chloride	1 tablet	4.3	169	Orange juice	1c. (248 g)	12.7	496
Kaon-Cl	1 tablet	6.7	260	Peach	1 (175 g)	7.9	308
Slow-K	1 tablet	8.0	312	Potato	1 med (150 g)	14.3	556
				Prune juice	½c. (128 g)	7.7	301
				Cooked dried prunes	½c. (140 g)	11.8	460
				Spinach	½c. (90 g)	7.5	291
				Acorn squash	½c. (122 g)	8.4	329
				Sweet potato	1 med. (146 g)	8.8	342
				Tomato juice	½c. (121 g)	7.1	276

L-dopa is converted to dopamine in the plasma by the enzyme dopa decarboxylase which utilizes pyridoxine as a cofactor. In order to decrease this conversion, pyridoxine-containing foods should be eaten sparingly and multiple vitamins containing pyridoxine should be avoided. Instead, a multiple vitamin especially formulated without pyridoxine, such as Larobec®, should be used.

DRUG ALTERATION OF NUTRIENT ABSORPTION OR UTILIZATION

Therapeutic agents may alter nutrient absorption or utilization by a number of nonspecific or specific mechanisms. Probably the most frequently documented interactions are malabsorption syndromes produced by specific mechanisms which may include: (1) a direct toxic effect causing morphologic changes in the mucosa of the small intestine; (2) inhibition of mucosal enzymes with or without mucosal damage; (3) binding of bile acids and fatty acids; (4) alteration of the physiochemical state of a dietary ion (12). While many drugs have been suspected of altering nutrient absorption or utilization, there is still a lack of clinical evidence for more than a few therapeutic categories. Table 11.6 summarizes those agents whose interactions with food have been well documented.

A number of antimicrobial and antiinfective agents including neomycin, cycloserine, erythromycin, sulfonamides, tetracyclines, penicillin, isoniazid and para-aminosalicylic acid (PAS) have been reported to specifically alter absorption and/or utilization of various nutrients. Examples of effects produced by the different agents include a decrease in vitamin K synthesis and folic acid utilization; a decrease in the absorption of calcium, magnesium, sodium, potassium, iron, fat, lactose, sucrose, and vitamin B_{12}; inactivation of pyridoxine and impairment of amino acid trans fer in protein synthesis (13–15). While the mechanisms involved in these effects are varied and often not completely elucidated, several drug effects have been extensively studied. Neomycin appears to decrease gastrointestinal absorption by three mechanisms: (1) by producing direct toxicity to mucosal cells, (2) by decreasing activity of pancreatic lipase, and (3) by binding of bile salts (16). PAS decreases fat absorption only at high doses (12g/day) (17) by an unknown mechanism. Palva and Heinivaara (18) have demonstrated that malabsorption of vitamin B_{12} produced by PAS occurs due to a mucosal blocking effect. Fortunately, these drug-induced malabsorption phenomena occur only with chronic use and are reversible when drug administration is stopped.

Laxatives, when taken on an occasional basis, have not been reported to produce malabsorption syndromes. However, when laxatives

Table 11.6 Drugs that Alter Nutrient Absorption

Drug	Effect	Mechanism
Antimicrobial or antiinfective agents	Decrease absorption of fat, fat-soluble vitamins, iron, B_{12}, sugars, cholesterol, Na, K, Ca, Mg	Toxicity to intestinal mucosa Binding of fatty acids and bile salts
	Decrease vitamin K synthesis	Decrease pancreatic lipase
	Decrease folic acid utilization	
Laxatives phenolphthalein cascara bisacodyl	Decrease absorption of vitamin D, Ca, xylose, glucose, protein, K, carotene, fat-soluble vitamins	Loss of structural integrity Irritation Increase motility
mineral oil	Decrease absorption of carotene, fat-soluble vitamins	Physical barrier Decrease micelle formation Solubilize vitamins
Hypocholesteremic agents cholestyramine clofibrate	Decrease absorption of vitamin B_{12}, xylose, iron, glucose, fat, fat-soluble vitamins	Bind bile acids and ions Decrease pH of small intestine
Antiinflammatory agents colchicine salicylazosulfapyridine	Decrease absorption of fat, carotene, Na, K, B_{12}, lactose, and folate	Structural defect Enzyme damage Mucosal blockade of folate uptake
Oral contraceptives	Decrease folic acid absorption	Interference with polyglutamate conjugase (?)
Anticonvulsant agents phenytoin	Decrease folic acid absorption	Interference with polyglutamate conjugase (?)
Potassium chloride	Decrease absorption of vitamin B_{12}	Decrease pH of small intestine
Antacids	Decrease absorption of phosphate, vitamin A, Fe	Chelation Decrease pH of small intestine

are taken on a chronic basis and especially when laxative dependency has developed, decreased absorption of vitamin D, calcium, xylose, glucose, protein, potassium, carotene, and fat-soluble vitamins has been reported. Irritant laxatives such as phenolphthalein, cascara, and bisacodyl produce malabsorption by causing a loss of structural integrity of the small intestine and by increasing intestinal motility while mineral oil acts as a physical barrier against absorption, decreases micelle formation and solubilizes vitamins A, D, E, and K (15). Rickets and osteomalacia from excessive mineral oil intake have been documented (19).

Hypocholesteremic agents (see pp. 246–247) such as cholstyramine and clofibrate may decrease the absorption of vitamin B_{12}, fat-soluble vitamins, xylose, glucose, iron, and fat by decreasing the pH of the small intestine and also by binding with bile salts and acids (15). Thirty grams/day of cholestyramine will produce frank steatorrhea (20) and therapeutic doses have also been reported to produce osteomalacia due to vitamin D deficiency (21). In addition, prolonged dosage with cholestyramine has been reported to produce vitamin K deficiency which is reversible following parenteral vitamin K administration (22).

Antiinflammatory agents such as colchicine, used in the treatment of gout, and salicylazosulfapyridine (Azulfidine®) may decrease the absorption of fat, carotene, sodium, potassium, vitamin B_{12}, lactose, and folic acid (15). Colchicine, an antimitotic agent, produces these actions by toxicity to the mucosal lining of the intestine and by producing enzyme damage while Azulfidine apparently produces a mucosal blockade of folate uptake (15).

Both oral contraceptives and anticonvulsant agents decrease the absorption of folic acid by interference with polyglutamate conjugase, the enzyme responsible for conversion of folate polyglutamate to free folic acid which can be absorbed (12). Some authorities argue that the relationship between decreased folate absorption and oral contraceptives is not a true drug-induced effect and that the decreased folate absorption cases that have been reported were actually due to undiagnosed causes unrelated to the use of oral contraceptives (23,24). The interaction between phenytoin and polyglutamate conjugase has also been questioned with some researchers believing that accelerated metabolism due to the induction of hepatic microsomal enzymes by phenytoin causes the apparent decrease in folic acid (25). Another effect of anticonvulsant agents is the blocking of the 25-hydroxylation of vitamin D by hepatic enzymes. The significance of this interaction is that patients treated for prolonged periods (more than two years) may show evidence of bone disease including elevated alkaline phosphatase and decreased bone density. For these patients treatment with supplemental vitamin D may be necessary.

The administration of potassium chloride as an adjunct to potassium-depleting diuretics has been reported to produce vitamin B_{12} malabsorption by lowering the pH of the small intestine to a level at which absorption cannot occur. Because the body contains large stores of this vitamin in the liver, it takes prolonged use of potassium chloride to produce a deficiency (1).

Commonly used antacids such as aluminum hydroxide have been shown to decrease the absorption of phosphate; therefore, they are used as phosphate binders in the treatment of renal disease. These components also decrease absorption of vitamin A and iron through chelation and increased pH of the small intestine (15). Aluminum hydroxide combines with phosphates in the intestine and the aluminum phosphate formed is excreted in the feces. It would be expected that these malabsorption effects would be seen only after high dose, chronic therapy, and only very rarely. However, cases of osteomalacia due to antacid therapy have been reported (26).

Alcohol ingested on a chronic basis will decrease the absorption of folic acid and water-soluble vitamins and will increase the excretion of magnesium and other electrolytes. Depletion of the vitamin B complex may be severe enough to produce neurological syndromes of a permanent nature. Excessive magnesium loss may lead to overt seizures (2).

Certain drugs may also affect taste and/or appetite. Recent reports have indicated that griseofulvin, penicillamine, clofibrate, lincomycin, and some tranquilizers are associated with decreased taste acuity and altered or unpleasant taste sensation (27). The precise mechanism for these effects is not known at this time, but the effects seem to be mediated by a systemic mechanism rather than related directly to specific foods.

Many unpleasant-tasting drugs such as chloral hydrate, paraldehyde, vitamin B complex, and penicillin leave an aftertaste or produce transient states of altered taste sensation. These effects usually are noted especially when the drugs are administered with food and should be taken at times other than with meals.

Some drugs such as the amphetamines and other stimulants of the central nervous system are used therapeutically to decrease appetite (anorexia). While this use is no longer considered to be appropriate, these agents significantly decrease appetite even in the presence of normal appetite stimuli such as gastric acid secretion. Some drugs, such as the antipsychotic drugs, antianxiety and antidepressant agents have been reported to stimulate appetite. This effect may be secondary to altered mental status and the resulting appetite improvement.

The foregoing examples of interactions between nutrients and therapeutic agents are probably only a few of those that occur on a relatively frequent basis. Care should be exercised in planning the overall therapy for a patient by all members of the health care team to ensure not only that such interactions do not continue to occur but also that other new interactions, when they occur, are determined quickly and resolved before patients are injured.

Questions

1. What is the safest mechanism for decreasing the mucosal irritation produced by drugs such as aspirin?
2. What types of nutrients decrease the absorption of antibiotics such as tetracyclines?

3. Why should natural licorice be avoided in patients with cardiovascular diseases?
4. What is the relationship between oral contraceptives and the development of anemia?
5. What nutrient deficiencies are associated with chronic alcohol ingestion?
6. What possible nutritional complications may arise in patients being treated for peptic ulcers with antacids?
7. What is the consequence of a decrease in the synthesis of vitamin K?

REFERENCES

1. Lehmann, P. Food and drug interactions. *FDA Consumer,* HEW Publication No. (FDA) 78-3070, U.S. Government Printing Office. Mar. 1978.
2. Pierpaoli, P. G. Drug therapy and diet. *Drug Intelligence and Clinical Pharmacy* **6:** 89–99, 1972.
3. Cooper, J. W. Food-drug interactions. *U.S. Pharmacist* **1:** 17–28, 1976.
4. Hartshorn. E. A. Food and drug interactions. *Journal of the American Dietetic Association* **70:** 15–19, 1977.
5. Conney, A. H. Pharmacological implications of microsomal enzyme induction. *Pharmacol. Rev.* **19:** 317–366, 1967.
6. Rubin, E., H. Gang, P. S. Misra, and C. S. Lieber. Inhibition of drug metabolism by acute ethanol intoxication: A hepatic microsomal mechanism. *Am. J. Med.* **49:** 801, 1970.
7. Kater, R. M. H., G. Roggin, F. Tobon, P. Zieve, and F. L. Iber. Increased rate of clearance of drugs from the circulation of alcoholics. *Am. J. Med. Sci.* **258:** 35, 1969.
8. Seixas, F. A. Alcohol and its drug interactions. *Annals of Int. Med.* **83:** 86, 1975.
9. Meyler, L. Side effects of drugs. *Exerpta Medica Foundation,* vol. 5, New York, 1966.
10. Weinsier, R. L. Fasting—A review with emphasis on the electrolytes. *Am. J. Med.* **50:** 233–240, 1971.
11. Leafy vegetables in diet alter prothrombin time in patients taking anticoagulant drugs. (Medical News) *J. Am. Med. Assoc.* **187:** 27, 1964.
12. Longstreth, G. F. and A. D. Neucomer. Drug-induced malabsorption. *Mayo Clinic Proc.* **50:** 284–293, 1975.
13. Christakis, G. and A. Miridjanian, Diets, drugs and their relationships. *J. Am. Dietetic Assoc.* **52:** 22, 1958.
14. Waxman, S. et al. Drugs, toxins and dietary amino acids affecting vitamin B_{12} or folic acid absorption. *Am. J. Med.* **48:** 600, 1970.
15. Roe, D. A. Drug-induced nutritional deficiencies. Westport, CN: AVI Publishing Co., 1976.
16. Dobbins, W. O. Drug-induced steatorrhea. *Gastroenterology* **54:** 1193–1195, 1968.
17. Levine, R. A. Steatorrhea induced by para-aminosalicylic acid. *Ann. Int. Med.* **68:** 1265–1270, 1968.

18. Palva, I. P. and O. Heinivaara. Drug induced malabsorption of vitamin B_{12}. Experimental studies with PAS-fed mice. *Acta Med. Int. Fenn.* **54:** 37–38, 1965.

19. Sinclair, L. Rickets from liquid paraffin. *Lancet* **1:** 792, 1967.

20. Hashim, S. A., S. S. Bergen, Jr., and T. B. Van Tallie. Experimental steatorrhea induced in man by bile acid sequestrant. *Proc. Soc. Exp. Biol. Med.* **106:** 173–175, 1961.

21. Heaton, K. W., J. V. Lever, and D. Barnard. Osteomalacia associated with cholestyramine therapy for postileectomy diarrhea. *Gastroenterology* **62:** 642–646, 1972.

22. Visintine, R. E. et al. Xanthomatous biliary cirrhosis treated with cholestyramine, a bile-acid-absorbing resin. *Lancet* **2:** 341–343, 1961.

23. Toghill, P. J. and P. G. Smith. Folate deficiency and the pill. *Br. Med. J.* **1:** 608, 1971.

24. Wood, J. K., A. H. Goldstone, and N. C. Allan. Folic acid and the pill. *Scand. J. Haematol.* **9:** 539–544, 1972.

25. Maxwell, J. D. et al. Folate deficiency after anticonvulsant drugs: An effect on hepatic enzyme induction? *Br. Med. J.* **1:** 297–299, 1972.

26. Bloom, W. L. and D. Finchum. Osteomalacia with pseudofractures caused by the ingestion of aluminum hydroxide. *J. Am. Med. Assoc.* **174:** 1327–1330, 1960.

27. Fagan, L. Griseofulvin and dysgeusia: Implications? (letters) *Ann. Intern. Med.* **74:** 795–796, 1971.

RECOMMENDED READINGS

Roe, D. A. *Drug-induced Nutritional Deficiencies.* Westport, CN: The AVI Publishing Co., 1976.

Hathcock, J. N. and J. Coon. *Nutrition and Drug Interrelations.* New York: Academic Press, 1978.

CHAPTER 12

Nutritional Care of Patients

HOSPITAL MALNUTRITION

The discovery in the mid-1970s that up to one-half of all hospitalized patients surveyed gave evidence of a significant degree of malnutrition was a startling and distressing revelation to health professionals in the United States (1–4). Such a discovery was an indictment of all health professionals but particularly of physicians and dietitians—of physicians because they carry the overall responsibility for the patient's welfare and of dietitians because they are charged with the nutritional care of the patient. How is it possible that individuals could become malnourished in modern hospitals which theoretically have all the personnel and equipment to provide excellent care of patients?

Probably the factor that has contributed most to the neglect of the patient's nutritional status is lack of communication and collaboration among the various health professionals. Although communication and collaboration are recognized as essential for optimal patient care, unfortunately health professionals usually have not been educated to approach disease states with a focus on the patient as a whole. Instead, members of the various health disciplines have inadvertently been taught that their role in health care is to address only those specific problems of the disease state for which their specialized education has prepared them. Nor does the administrative structure of the hospital promote communication and collaboration among health professionals. Although all services in the hospital are designed to meet needs of patients and should be interdependent, these services all too often operate almost like separate entities. Rapport between nurses and dietitians is often poor; nurses and dietitians stand in awe of the physicians and frequently fail to report important observations about patients or to question orders that appear inappropriate. Health professionals in general know so little about the contributions each discipline can make to patient care that they fail to utilize adequately the services of each other.

Most other health professionals, such as physicians (especially surgeons) and nurses have viewed dietitians not so much as fellow health professionals but as those hospital personnel employed to feed patients and staff. This attitude is easy to understand because traditionally the dietary department has been primarily a food service department, a support service, the responsibility of which is making sure that all patients are fed during their hospital stay and that hospital personnel are provided good meals. Because some patients require modified diets, the role of the therapeutic dietitian has been to see that these particular patients are fed adequately during their hospitalization and educated about their special diet as they are prepared for discharge.

An outgrowth of this attitude toward dietitians has been for most other health professionals to equate "nutrition" with serving the patient a tray and to consider it of little importance in treatment of patients, particularly those not requiring modified diets. The lack of importance afforded adequate nutrition by health professionals in the overall care of patients has been evidenced by their failure to emphasize the value of recording height and weight for every patient and of monitoring a patient's food intake in response to an unusual weight change. The thinking of most health professionals as well as much of the lay public has been so oriented toward the fast-acting "miracle drugs" and dramatic surgical procedures that anything as basic as good nutrition has failed to be recognized as essential to quality patient care (4).

Therapeutic or clinical dietitians, although convinced of the importance of good nutrition in patient care, have failed to be assertive in seeing that patients are provided appropriate nutritional care. Their lack of assertiveness has many causes, a few of which include: the attitude of medical and surgical personnel toward nutrition and dietitians (as described above); the dietitians' uncertainty about their own knowledge; the traditional role of dietitians in the hospital coupled with their relatively few number and possible poor communication with administrative dietitians (or food service managers) and food service workers; lack of flexibility in working hours which often prevents optimal contacts with patients and their families; failure to recognize the essentiality of establishing excellent rapport with the nursing staff whose interest can assure implementation of patients' nutritional care plans.

Instead of taking the lead in providing nutritional care of patients, most dietitians have allowed their functions to be dictated by hospital policies and procedures and by direct orders from physicians.

IMPETUS FOR IMPROVED NUTRITIONAL CARE OF PATIENTS

In recent years a pronounced change in attitude toward the importance of nutrition in the treatment of patients has occurred among physicians and other health professionals for several reasons:

1. Dudrick and Rhoads (5) demonstrated the dramatic improvement that could be obtained in severely debilitated patients by providing the needed nutrients parenterally. The literature is now full of reports from numerous clinicians who have shown that aggressive nutritional support can improve the patient's ability to withstand stress of disease and/or surgery.
2. Clinicians interested in nutrition (1–3) made known the high incidence of malnutrition among medical and surgical patients because of lack of attention to basic nutrient needs of patients although their primary disease states were being treated vigorously.
3. Better products and improved techniques have become available for the enteral and parenteral feeding of patients who could not take adequate amounts of food orally.
4. Concern over the high cost of hospitalization encouraged investigations of every possible means of decreasing the need for hospital admission and/or shortening of hospital stay. Well-nourished persons as a group have fewer and shorter hospital stays; persons nourished properly during hospitalization demonstrate lower mortality rates and an increased speed of recovery (4). Complications of malnutrition contribute to both increased mortality rate and extended hospital stays among affected patients because malnourishment causes delayed wound healing, depressed cell-mediated immunity, and increased susceptibility to infection (6).
5. The role of the dietitian in the hospital is changing due to modifications made in his/her educational preparation and to the emergence of the health team concept which emphasizes need for integrated planning among health professionals to promote the welfare of the patient. Dietitians are being recognized as valuable members of the health care team and are welcome (in most instances!) to operate as such.
6. Hospital accreditation policies are mandating that dietitians be involved in patient assessment and care and that this involvement be evidenced by dietitians' notes on medical records.

The present opportunities for the dietitian to become an integral part of the health care team are golden, and dietitians must make sure that these opportunities are seized. *Should another health professional be required to fill the void left by the unavailability of a dietitian on the team, there is always the strong possibility that the need for a dietitian will be forgotten.* Administrators of dietary departments may need to rework their priorities (and time schedules) in order to make sure that qualified dietitians are functioning as active members of health care teams, involved not only in nutritional assessment and care of patients (including the monitoring of food intake) but also in nutrition education activities for patients and health team members alike. Working hours need to be made more flexible with one dietitian always on call. Other health team members need to know that a dietitian is as near as the closest phone.

ASSESSMENT OF NUTRITIONAL STATUS AND PREPARATION OF NUTRITIONAL CARE PLAN

All health professionals concerned with patient management should be involved in the assessment of the nutrition status of the patient and identification of his/her needs. One of the major purposes of the nutritional assessment is to determine the status of the somatic protein compartment (i.e., lean body mass) the visceral protein compartment (i.e., plasma, albumin, and immuno proteins), and the fat stores. In the semi-starved state associated with illness or stress, glycogen stores are quickly depleted and energy is supplied through catabolism of stored fat along with some catabolism of somatic and visceral proteins.

Although free fatty acids mobilized from fat stores can provide energy, they cannot provide the glucose needed to keep blood sugar at a normal level; only the glycerol portion of the fat molecule is a glucose precursor. Consequently, somatic protein must be catabolized to produce the amino acids needed for gluconeogenesis and for the synthesis of visceral proteins, which have a very rapid turnover rate. Patients in good nutritional status, with adequate protein reserves, are able to catabolize somatic protein for a period of time without ill effects. The depleted patient or the patient confronted with a long-term or multiple trauma, however, is not so fortunate. Although the same demands are made on his/her body for energy and as a source of amino acids, the patient may have insufficient protein reserves to respond optimally to stress. There is a likelihood of impairment in visceral protein synthesis, which is essential for proper wound healing and antibody formation; therefore, recovery from trauma is impeded. Another important consequence of a depleted somatic protein compartment is the effect on respiratory and pulmonary function. A patient's ability to cough and perform respiratory toilet is significant in preventing pneumonia.

The possible consequences of a poor nutritional status emphasize how important it is that nutritional assessments be made on all patients. Some assessments may be brief and others quite detailed, but all patients should receive some sort of screening for nutritional status.

Assessments are made by the physician through the use of three tools: the history, physical examination, and laboratory data. These same three tools can be used effectively by other health professionals as well. Impressions gained by the various members of the health care team throughout the patient's hospital stay should be communicated orally through *team conferences* and *medical work rounds* as well as being recorded in the medical record. Optimal patient care requires an operative, interested health care team including at least a physician, nurse, dietitian, and pharmacist. Whenever possible a social worker and physical therapist also should participate in team conferences and medical work rounds.

The first step in the development of a nutritional care plan for the newly admitted patient is a compilation of measurements, both anthropometric and biochemical, which are indices of the patient's overall nutritional status. Depending on the detail required, indices can include *accurate* height/weight measurements, triceps skin fold, midarm muscle circumference, serum albumin, total lymphocyte count, serum transferrin and total iron binding capacity, a 24-hour creatinine, and some antigen skin testing. Anthropometric measurements can be made and pertinent lab data compiled by a trained health professional, preferably the dietitian. How accurately the assessment reflects the true status of the patient depends to a great degree upon the astuteness of the data gatherer. Therefore, the dietitian to be efficient as a data gatherer must be aware of the many factors that may influence the various measurements. For example, anthropometric measurements can be affected by the presence of edema, paralysis, or a recent muscle-building program; serum albumin can be altered by stress, edema, ascites, overhydration, transfusions, and liver disease. Dietitians also should be cognizant of the possibility of false positive or false negative antigen skin tests. A wide variety of drugs including aspirin and alcohol depress cellular immunity. Furthermore, dietitians should be familiar enough with the significance of various lab values to be able to suggest appropriate tests for an individual whose nutritional status is in question.

All parameters listed above for determination of nutritional status may be unnecessary in the majority of patients; the only measurements that *must* be recorded for every patient are height and weight. The decision about the other indices needed will be based on information gathered from the history and physical examination. If a patient's weight for height is within normal range ($\pm 10\%$)*, there is no history of recent unusual weight loss or gain, no indication of bizarre or drastically altered eating habits, or no history of prolonged therapy with drugs known to compromise nutritional status, an extensive nutrition profile is probably unnecessary. Nevertheless, even a patient who is apparently well nourished upon admission should be evaluated within 10 days (and periodically thereafter) should his/her hospitalization exceed this limit.

---

* A quick method for calculating Ideal Body Weight (IBW) for the patient of average or medium frame:
Males: 106 lbs for 5 ft; 6 lbs for each additional inch in height.
Females: 100 lbs for 5 ft; 5 lbs for each additional inch.

Ideally for all patients a nutritional care plan should be developed. Perhaps the plan will require a great deal of study or be quite simple; nevertheless, this should be a service afforded every patient. Education in normal nutrition, that is, principles and scientific bases for improved selection, care, and preparation of foods; dangers associated with fad diets; importance of diet and exercise in fitness; the amount of sodium, fat, cholesterol, and fiber contained in various foods may prove quite valuable for the apparently well-nourished patient. Nutrition education can be instrumental in the maintenance of health and in decreasing the number of hospitalizations.

In order to institute as soon as possible an individualized nutritional care plan for the new patient, the dietitian should visit him/her within 24 hours of admission. Before making that visit, however, the dietitian should learn all that he/she can about the patient so that the visit may be kept brief and still be quite productive. During the visit the dietitian should use all his/her interviewing skills* in order to make the visit a pleasant interlude for the patient. Gathering information on his/her eating habits and observing casually any overt physical signs that may have relevance for nutritional status should be accomplished without causing any apprehension on the part of the patient. Some of the dietary information to be sought and physical signs to be observed in order to develop a general impression of nutritional status are listed in Table 12.1.

Information gained from this visit should be reviewed by the dietitian in light of the physician's medical history, various clinical findings, and pertinent lab values obtained on the patient. The medical history should include a specific checklist for helping identify patients at risk nutritionally, such as those who use alcohol excessively or who have a chronic disease of the gastrointestinal tract. Butterworth (4) prepared a comprehensive list of possible conditions that should be checked shortly after the patient is admitted. Dietitians should familiarize themselves with this list and if a similar one has not been included in the medical history, they should take the responsibility for obtaining this information from the patient.

If the patient is identified as one who is at high risk nutritionally, a much more in-depth study by the dietitian may be necessary before appropriate nutritional therapy can be proposed. On the other hand, should the patient appear to have relatively mild or no nutrition-related health problems, the dietitian can formulate and begin immediately implementation of the nutritional care plan.

Formulation of an effective nutritional care plan for optimal patient management requires skills in problem solving as illustrated in Figure

---

* An excellent reference for the dietitian on interviewing is the American Dietetic Association Cassette entitled *Dietary Interviewing* by Joan Weise, Ph.D., 1976.

Table 12.1 Information Sought During Dietitian's Initial Visit to Patient

Questions
1. Where and with whom does patient have most of his/her meals?
2. Has food intake been unusual in any way during the last few weeks?
3. Has there been any noticeable weight loss or weight gain during last few weeks?
4. Has constipation or diarrhea been a problem lately?
5. Is there any difficulty in chewing, e.g., sore gums, ill-fitting dentures?
6. Does food taste or smell any different lately?
7. Has there been any nausea and/or vomiting lately?
8. What nonprescription drugs are ingested routinely, e.g., aspirin, antacids, laxatives, etc?
9. What beverages are favorites? (Try to determine use of alcoholic beverages without using terms "liquor, beer, whiskey".)
10. When was last meal? What did it consist of? (Brief description of food eaten.)

General impressions
1. Any evidence of bilateral angular stomatitis and/or blepharitis?
2. Any evidence of cheilosis?
3. Any evidence of glossitis?
4. Any evidence of enlarged thyroid gland?
5. Any evidence of petechiae?
6. Any evidence of pellagrous dermatosis?
7. General impressions of appearance that may have nutritional implications:
   a. Hair and nails (dull, dry hair; spoon-shaped nails)
   b. Skin appears tight and drawn; possibly dry, flaky, or discolored
   c. Muscle turgor (wasted muscles, flabby skin)
   d. Body composition

12.1. The plan is dynamic, changing as the patient's condition changes. All data used in the formulation of a nutritional care plan should be organized in such a fashion that statement of nutrition-related problems is readily accomplished. Each identified problem should be given the SOAP* treatment in order that the dietitian's involvment in the care of the patient can be recorded appropriately. One extremely important aspect of the dietitian's involvement with the patient is the plan for educating the patient about any nutrition-related problem and about the responsibility that the patient himself/herself has in management of the problem. A suggested form for dietitians to use in formulation of an uncomplicated nutritional care plan is presented in Table 12.2.

For patients whose history and physical examination suggest that an in-depth profile on their nutritional and metabolic status be developed, formulation of the nutritional care plan (or nutritional therapy) is more complicated and requires use of an additional form such as the one presented in Table 12.3.

---

* SOAP is an acronym for *S*ubjective Information, *O*bjective Information, *A*ssessment and *P*lans of Action.

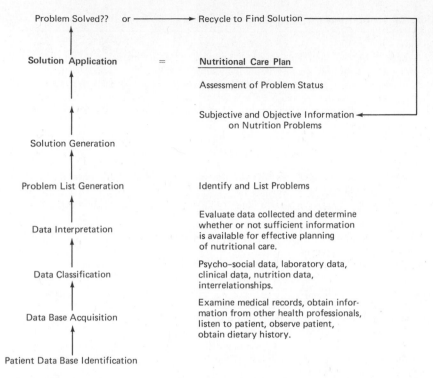

Figure 12.1 diagram content:

Problem Solved??   or ————→ Recycle to Find Solution —————

Solution Application   =   <u>Nutritional Care Plan</u>

Assessment of Problem Status

Subjective and Objective Information ◄—
            on Nutrition Problems

Solution Generation

Problem List Generation   Identify and List Problems

Data Interpretation   Evaluate data collected and determine whether or not sufficient information is available for effective planning of nutritional care.

Data Classification   Psycho–social data, laboratory data, clinical data, nutrition data, interrelationships.

Data Base Acquisition   Examine medical records, obtain information from other health professionals, listen to patient, observe patient, obtain dietary history.

Patient Data Base Identification

Figure 12.1 Steps in formation of patient nutritional care plan (problem solving technique).

High risk patients who most often require the in-depth profile include (7):

1. Patients who are obese or extremely underweight (i.e., ±20% ideal body weight). According to Blackburn (6) probably the most common type of malnutrition encountered in the hospital is that of the fat person who is depleted of visceral proteins but because of his/her size fails to attract attention to his/her nutrient needs. The extremely underweight patient is more visible in his/her needs and is particularly vulnerable because of limited reserves of both somatic and visceral proteins.
2. Patients who for a variety of reasons have failed to ingest adequate amounts of food or who have suffered from severe to moderate maldigestion and/or malabsorption.
3. Patients with increased metabolic requirements due to natural causes, such as pregnancy and rapid growth, or due to disease or trauma, such as fever, sepsis, burns.
4. Patients with continued external losses of body constituents, such as draining fistulas, exudative enteropathies, chronic blood loss, chronic renal dialysis.

5. Patients taking for long periods of time any medication that alters nutrient requirements and/or metabolism.
6. Patients who are likely to be unable to consume food orally for as long as 10 days because of head and/or neck trauma, gastrointestinal surgery. Patients undergoing elective gastrointestinal surgery may need substantial nutrition support before surgery as well as after because of their frequent inability to consume adequate diets prior to hospital admittance.

Although vitamin and mineral deficiencies may exist among hospitalized patients and all health professionals should be on the alert for evidence of such deficiencies, once identified, these problems can be alleviated much more rapidly than can the more commonly occurring protein–calorie malnutrition. Blackburn (8) has identified the types of protein–calorie malnutrition as (1) visceral attrition state (adult kwashiorkor), (2) adult marasmus or cachexia, and (3) intermediate state (kwashiorkor–marasmus mix). Classification depends on the adequacy or inadequacy of the visceral proteins, somatic proteins, and/or fat stores.

Adequacy of somatic proteins can be determined through height/weight measurements, midarm circumference, midarm muscle circumference and creatinine/height index, while fat stores are estimated by tricep skinfold measurements.

Visceral proteins are measured by means of serum albumin, serum transferrin (or total iron Binding capacity), and total lymphocyte count. Whenever the lymphocyte count is below normal, an impaired cellular immunity is possible. For this reason certain skin test antigens (9) are injected intradermally and read after 24 hours and 48 hours. An induration area of <5 mm indicates the patient's inability to recognize foreign protein. This test correlates well with morbidity or mortality and therefore is an excellent marker of nutritional status and/or progress in nutritional rehabilitation.

Estimation of the patient's nitrogen balance gives an indication of the degree of catabolism occurring, thereby providing information needed for calculating his/her protein and caloric needs. Calculation of a patient's needs is also possible through determination of his/her basal energy expenditure (BEE)* (9). Basal energy expenditure is derived from Harris-Benedict standards based on surface area plus age and sex. When metabolism is normal, maintenance nutrition can be accomplished by 30 to 35 kilocalories per kilogram body weight per day with a nitrogen:calorie ratio of 1:300. In the hypercatabolic state, patients will require approximately 40 to 50 kilocalories per kilogram body weight per day and a nitrogen:cal-

---

* BEE is figured as follows:
Male = 66 + [6.3 × body weight (lbs)] + [12.7 × height (in)] − (6.8 × years)
Female = 655 + [4.3 × weight (lbs)] + [4.7 × height (in)] − (4.7 × years)

Table 12.2 Nutritional Care Plan

Height _____

Weight _____

Ideal body wt. _____

Patient: _____ Sex: M F Age _____ Marital Status: S M D W Sep Admission Date: _____

Occupation: _____ Physician: _____ Diagnosis: _____

Sociological history (to include economic, cultural, family and personal data, etc.):

_____

Pertinent medical history:

_____

Pertinent laboratory values and their relationship to dietary care:

_____

Pertinent medications and their relationship to dietary care:

_____

List problems: Active	Inactive
Subjective	
Objective	
Assessment	
Plan of action	

Table 12.3 Nutrition Assessment Summary

Date of assessment ______

Patient ______ Room ______ Date of admission ______

Height ______ Ideal Body Weight (IBW)* ______ Weight on admission ______

Diagnosis ______ Physician ______

	Parameters	Patient values	Normal values	Degree of Depletion: None	Degree of Depletion: (>5–15%) Mild	Degree of Depletion: (>15–30%) Moderate	Degree of Depletion: (>30%) Severe
Somatic proteins and fat stores	Weight		*IBW				
	Triceps Skinfold (TSF)		Male: 12.5 mm Female: 16.5 mm				
	Midarm circumference (MAC)		Male: 25.3 cm Female: 23.2 cm				
	Midarm muscle circumference (MAMC) = MAC(cm) − [.314 × TSF(mm)]		Male: 21.4 Female: 18.0				
	Urinary creatinine		Refer to standards				
	Creatinine height index (CHI) $\text{CHI} = \frac{\text{Actual urinary creatinine}}{\text{Ideal urinary creatinine}} \times 100$		Refer to standards				

Visceral proteins	Lymphocytes, total count	1,500–3,000/mm
	Albumin, serum	4.0–5.5 g/dl
	Total iron binding capacity (TIBC)	240–410 /dl
	Serum transferrin	170–250 mg/dl
	Cell meditated immunity	>15 mm

Nutritional status: ☐ Normal   ☐ Marasmus (M)   ☐ Kwaskiorkor (K)
                                     Deficit in somatic proteins   Visceral proteins depressed
                                     Adequate in visceral proteins Somatic proteins and fat adequate

                                     ☐ Combination M–K
                                     Deficit in visceral and somatic proteins

Comments:

* Method for calculating IBW is found on page 417.

Table 12.3a Total Urinary Creatinine and Creatinine for Height

For Women

Height	Total mg creatinine/ 24 hours	Mg creatinine/ cm body height/ 24 hours
4'10" 147.3 cm	830	5.63
4'11" 149.9	851	5.68
5' 0" 152.4	875	5.74
5' 1" 154.9	900	5.81
5' 2" 157.5	925	5.87
5' 3" 160	949	5.93
5' 4" 162.6	977	6.01
5' 5" 165.1	1006	6.09
5' 6" 167.6	1044	6.23
5' 7" 170.2	1076	6.32
5' 8" 172.7	1109	6.42
5' 9" 175.3	1141	6.51
5'10" 177.8	1174	6.60
5'11" 180.3	1206	6.69
6' 0" 182.9	1240	6.78

For Men

Height	Total mg creatinine/ 24 hours	Mg creatinine/ cm body height/ 24 hours
5' 2" 157.5 cm	1288	8.17
5' 3" 160	1325	8.28
5' 4" 162.6	1359	8.36
5' 5" 165.1	1386	8.40
5' 6" 167.6	1426	8.51
5' 7" 170.2	1467	8.62
5' 8" 172.7	1513	8.76
5' 9" 175.3	1555	8.86
5'10" 177.8	1596	8.98
5'11" 180.3	1642	9.11
6' 0" 182.9	1691	9.24
6' 1" 185.4	1739	9.38
6' 2" 188	1785	9.49
6' 3" 190.5	1831	9.61
6' 4" 193	1891	9.80

orie ratio of 1:150 (6,8,10). Nitrogen provided in amounts greater than this appears to afford no additional benefits.

Guidelines have been established for estimating needs of the patient who requires only maintenance therapy as well as those of patients requiring anabolic therapy.

	Kilocalories/24 hours	*N/24 hours*
Maintenance	BEE × 1.22	(kcal÷300)g
Anabolic	(Oral) BEE × 1.54 ⎱	
	(IV) BEE × 1.76–2.0 ⎰	(kcal÷150)g

A word of caution needs to be inserted here concerning the danger of *overfeeding* the patient. No benefit is accrued from excessive weight gain during nutrition rehabilitation and can present quite a problem to the patient upon recovery. The dietitian should follow weight changes of the patient very carefully and whenever needed make appropriate recommendations to the physician.

In order to provide the optimal nutritional care of the patient, it is of particular importance that the nurse and dietitian work together so that the nursing care plan and nutritional care plan are integrated into a whole. Diagnostic procedures should be scheduled so as to interfere as little as possible with meal times (or nourishment plans), and when interference is unavoidable, arrangements should be made for replacement of nourishment missed. The magnitude of the problem of displaced meals was discovered in a study conducted by Butterworth and Prevost in 1973 (4) which revealed that, on the average for each hospitalization, meals for 3.1 complete days were missed because of diagnostic procedures and/or x-rays. When all practices reducing patient caloric intake were lumped together and averaged out according to hospital patient count, caloric deficit was estimated at 2600 kilocalories per patient per week. As mentioned earlier, one function of the dietitian should be to see that all missed meals are recorded so that replacements can be made.

MONITORING OF NUTRIENT INTAKE AND PROVIDING NUTRITION EDUCATION

Once the nutritional care plan has been formulated, it is the responsibility of the dietitian on the health care team to see that the patient is nourished appropriately. Nourishment may be provided orally, enterally, parenterally, or in combination. Only when the patient is fed totally by the parenteral route may the dietitian relinquish some of his/her responsibility. With the parenterally fed patient the responsibility should be shared by the physician, dietitian, and clinical pharmacist.

Because food has been their stock in trade, dietitians probably are still more comfortable in dealing with the patient who is fed orally than with one receiving enteral or parenteral feedings. Nevertheless, because of the new horizons in nutrition, the dietitian, in order to remain an integral member of the health care team, must become just as familiar with the composition and delivery systems of enteral and parenteral feedings as he/she is with the composition and delivery systems of ordinary foods. For the patient at high risk nutritionally it is essential that *daily nutrient intake* and weight be recorded. Making sure that these records are maintained should be a responsibility of both the dietitian and the nurse.

As was noted earlier, ideally every patient should have a nutritional care plan developed for him/her regardless of nutritional status. For the well-nourished patient this plan could be primarily education in normal nutrition. Visiting informally with the patient and listening carefully to his/her conversation and comments can allow the astute dietitian to identify the nutrition-related concerns of the patient and to institute valuable education.

For the patient who is at risk nutritionally but can take nourishment by the oral route, the dietitian should carefully monitor food intake and do everything possible to make sure that the patient is adequately nourished. In order to determine the amount of food the patient is consuming from his/her tray, it will be necessary for the dietitian to obtain assistance from nursing service. If an estimate of food intake will suffice, the nursing service can take responsibility for recording the approximate amount of various food items consumed by the patient. If, however, a reasonably accurate calorie and/or nutrient intake is needed, a method for securing this information that is appropriate for the specific institution will have to be formulated. Formulation of a workable method will take a good deal of study and imagination on the part of the dietitian and will necessitate obtaining as many suggestions as possible from the nursing service. Implementation of any method, no matter how good it appears on paper, will require cooperation from the nursing service. It is to be hoped that, through the efforts of the dietitian and nurse, notations can be made on the medical record that will apprise the physician in charge of the caloric and nutrient intake of patients at risk.

Many patients who need high caloric, high protein intakes find it very difficult to consume a sufficient amount of food at meal times. For these patients (weight loss > 10 percent of ideal body weight; serum albumin < 3.4 g), the dietitian has the responsibility of finding an acceptable supplementary liquid formula that is also sufficiently high in calories and all needed nutrients. Whenever possible, the dietitian should enlist the patient's help in carrying out this responsibility.

Several commercially available dietary supplements and defined formula diets are listed in Table 12.4. Also included in the table are the composition and possible uses of each product. The dietitian must be knowledgeable about the content and proposed usage of all available supplements and be familiar with their taste. When the taste of a nutritionally desirable formula is found unacceptable to the patient, the dietitian should experiment with several different formulas of similar composition to find one that is acceptable, or more nearly acceptable. Formulas can be made more nearly acceptable through the use of various flavorings; particularly valuable agents are chocolate syrup, decaffeinated instant coffee and electrolyte-free chocolate, vanilla and fruit flavorings (6).

The dietitian and nurse must take responsibility in making sure that the patient consumes the approximate number of calories and/or nutrients as prescribed in the nutritional care plan but reinforcement of their efforts should be provided by other members of the health team as well. Additionally, patients must be visited regularly and educated concerning the importance of their nutrition therapy; accomplishment of this goal cannot depend upon the dietitian alone but requires involvement of all members of the health care team. Nevertheless, how well the patient is educated depends to a large degree upon the rapport established between dietitian and patient. Ingenuity on the part of the dietitian is also necessary in order to find methods by which patients can be encouraged to consume more calories. One dietitian (6) has found that the best way to get patients to take snacks between meals is to use foods that are sufficiently nonperishable that they can be kept by the bedside and nibbled on as desired throughout the day. This same dietitian has also discovered that patients who are dependent on liquid supplements for much of their caloric and nutrient intake can be encouraged to consume more of this supplement if it is kept at bedside in an ice bath. Such an arrangement eliminates the danger of the supplement not reaching the patient and prevents the patients from being faced with drinking 6 to 8 ounces of formula at one time. Instead, he/she can take frequent small drinks throughout the day. Here again it must be emphasized that any feeding technique of this sort depends on the nursing service to see that it is coordinated into the treatment plan.

Weight changes in the patient at risk nutritionally should be observed carefully by the dietitian. Should the prescribed nutritional care plan appear inappropriate (inadequate or overadequate) for maintaining or promoting nutritional rehabilitation, the dietitian has the responsibility of alerting the physician to this fact. The dietitian should at all times act as a patient advocate (4).

TUBE FEEDINGS AND DEFINED FORMULA DIETS

Whenever the patient appears to the dietitian to be unable to ingest orally his/her needed nutrients and calories, the dietitian should suggest the use

Table 12.4 Some Commercially Available Nutrition Supplements, Tube
Feedings, and Defined Formula Diets

Supplements	Cal/ml	mOsm/L	% Cal (Pro)	% Cal (CHO)	% Cal (Fat)	N:Cal
Citrotein	.53		24.1	73.2	2.3	1:93
Lanolac	.66		21.0	30.0	49.0	1:81
Meritene (liquid) vanilla, chocolate, eggnog	1.00	550	24.0	46.0	30.0	1:79
Sustacal (liquid) vanilla chocolate	1.00	638 616	24.0	55.0	21.0	1:79
Meritene powder + skim milk	1.00		35.9	62.4	1.7	1:43
Meritene powder + whole milk	1.00		26.4	44.8	28.8	1:48
Sustagen powder vanilla, chocolate (normal dilution)	1.80	721	24.0	68.0	8.0	1:79
Meal replacements (or tube feedings)						
Complete B	1.00	405	16.0	48.0	36.0	1:131
Ensure vanilla, black walnut	1.06	460	14.0	54.5	31.5	1:155
Isocal	1.05	350	13.0	50.0	37.0	1:169
Nutri-1000	1.06	400	13.0	40.0	47.0	1:167
Portagen	1.00	354	16.0	44.0	40.0	1:160
Precision-isotonic vanilla	1.00	300	12.0	60.0	28.0	1:183
Defined Formula Diets (Low residue, clear liquid)						
Flexical Orange Vanilla Banana Fruit Punch	1.00	805	9.0	61.0	30.0	1:264
Precision L-R Cherry Lemon Lime Orange	1.08	525	8.8	90.8	.65	1:258
Vivonex Vanilla Beef broth Orange Grape Tomato Chocolate	1.00	550	8.1	90.3	1.3	1:286

Table 12.4 Continued

Protein source	CHO source	Fat source	mEq Na/L	Specific characteristics and/or suggested use
Egg white solids	Sucrose Dextrin-maltose	Mono- and diglycerides	23.0	Protein, vitamin and mineral supplement
Casein	Lactose	Coconut oil	1.1	Protein supplement for sodium restricted diets
Skim milk Casein	Sucrose Lactose Corn syrup solids	Vegetable oil	40.5	Protein supplement
Skim milk	Sucrose Lactose Corn syrup solids	Partially hydrogenated soy oil	47.1	Protein supplement with low lactose content
Skim milk	Lactose Corn syrup solids	Cream (cow's milk)	39.1	Protein supplement with low fat content
Milk	Lactose Corn syrup solids	Cream (cow's milk)	39.1	Protein supplement
Powdered whole milk Nonfat dry milk	Glucose Lactose Corn syrup solids	Cream (cow's milk)	54.3	Protein supplement
Beef	Lactose Sucrose	Corn oil Beef fat	59.0	Tube feeding for anabolism
Casein Soy protein isolate	Sucrose Corn syrup solids	Corn oil	32.0	Tube or oral feeding (lactose-free) for anabolism
Casein Soy protein isolate	Glucose Corn syrup solids	MCT Soy oil	22.6	Isotonic tube feeding for anabolism
Skim milk	Glucose Sucrose Lactose Dextrin-maltose	Corn oil	23.0	Tube or oral feeding for anabolism
Casein	Sucrose Corn syrup solids	MCT Safflower oil	27.0	Oral feeding for anabolism (used in malabsorption of natural fats)
Egg albumin	Glucose Oligosaccharides Sucrose	Vegetable oil	34.0	Isotonic tube or oral feeding (lactose-free)
Hydrolyzed protein plus the amino acids: methionine tyrosine tryptophan	Sucrose Dextro-oligo-saccharides	MCT Partially hydrogenated soy oil	15.2	Protein source requires some digestion; 2.16% calories from linoleic acid; used for maintenance
Egg albumin	Maltose Dextrins	Safflower oil	27.4	Protein source requires some digestion; low osmolality; 0.48% calories from linoleic acid; used for maintenance
Crystalline amino acids	Maltose Dextrins	Safflower oil	37.3	Easily absorbed protein source of high biological value; 1.04% calories from linoleic acid; osmolality increased with flavoring; used for maintenance

Table 12.4 Continued

	Cal/ml	mOsm/L	% Cal (Pro)	% Cal (CHO)	% Cal (Fat)	N:Cal
Precision-HN Citrus fruit Vanilla	1.00	557	16.6	82.9	.42	1:125
Vivonex-HN Beef broth Orange Grape Strawberry	1.00	800	16.6	84.1	.78	1:127
Special DFD Aminade	2.02	1050	4.0	68.0	28.0	1:418

Source: Adapted from Blackburn, G. L. and B. R. Bistrian, Curative nutrition: protein–calorie management. In *Nutritional Support of Medical Practice,* Schneider et al., eds., Harper & Row, 1977.

of tube feedings perhaps only as an adjunctive measure or in some instances to replace oral feedings totally. The dietitian's responsibility for patients on tube feedings and/or defined formula diets is the same as it is for patients who can eat normally, that is, making sure that each patient is receiving the caloric and nutrient intake prescribed. It is necessary for the dietitian to be familiar with the various commercially available defined formula diets and tube feedings, being aware of their composition, calories per ml, osmolality, and indications for use. In order to have this information at his/her fingertips, the dietitian needs to have a very close working relationship with the clinical pharmacist. Critical considerations in the selection of an enteral solution include:

1. Suitability for method of administration, for example, acceptablility for oral use, desirable viscosity for feeding tube
2. Substrate source, that is, protein base, carbohydrate base, fat source
3. Calorie: volume ratio
4. Electrolyte content
5. Nitrogen: calorie ratio
6. Vitamin–mineral composition
7. Presence or absence of lactose
8. Residue content
9. Osmolality

A drawback of commercially prepared tube feeding formulas is their inflexibility of composition and their consequent inability to meet unique nutrient requirements. Because of this inflexibility in composition of commercial formulas, the dietitian may be called upon to use his/her imagination and expertise in devising a formula tailored to the needs of an individual patient. Several options are available, including modification of

Protein source	CHO source	Fat source	mEq Na/L	Specific characteristics and/or suggested use
Egg albumin	Maltose Dextrins	Safflower oil	40.5	Protein requires some digestion; low osmolality; 0.33% calories from linoleic acid; used for anabolism
Crystalline amino acids	Glucose Maltose	Safflower oil	27.4	Easily absorbed protein source; 0.62% calories from linoleic acid; used for anabolism
Essential amino acids	Sucrose Dextrins	Soybean oil	2.0	Low protein of high biological value and easily absorbed; used in renal failure; 11% calories from linoleic acid; contains no vitamins

commercially available formulas; preparation of blenderized formulas made from table foods; use of commercially available protein (or individual amino acids), carbohydrate, fat, vitamin, mineral, and trace element sources which can be mixed in appropriate proportions; combinations of any of the above.

In many situations modifying commercially available formulas or blenderized table foods can be accomplished with little difficulty. A variety of oils including corn, safflower, or medium-chain triglycerides can be added to a formula to boost calories. Corn syrup or commercially available caloric supplements, consisting mainly of carbohydrates, can also be used for boosting calories when carbohydrate is more desirable than fat. With the help of a qualified pharmacist, salts of the various electrolytes, individual amino acids, and vitamin, mineral, and trace element supplements can be added to a commercial formula or blenderized table food formula to bring it to the specific composition.

Formulas also can be prepared completely by the mixing of commercially available individual sources of protein, carbohydrate, fat, vitamins, and trace minerals. When using formulations of this kind, the dietitian must check the consistency of the formula to be sure that it will flow through the feeding tube; occasionally the use of emulsifiers may be necessary. It also may be important to verify the composition of the formula through laboratory testing. In addition, the patient must be carefully monitored to determine the appropriateness of the formula for his/her nutrient requirements (11).

Adjusting and creating appropriate tube feeding formulas is a challenge for the clinical dietitian, but with the increased use of enteral hyperalimentation, specifically tailored feedings will almost certainly be on the rise. Fortunately, the dietitian almost always has a qualified pharmacist available to whom he/she can turn for help. When specific feedings are formulated, extreme care must be exercised in order to prevent contamination of the solution. It is essential, therefore, for the dietitian to be cognizant of the possible limitations that may exist in the institution when he/she is making the decision about which forms of tube feedings can be safely and appropriately utilized.

When the appropriate feeding has been selected or formulated, the dietitian should make certain that the feeding is administered properly and the patient is receiving the correct volume. This responsibility requires that the dietitian be familiar with the various feeding tubes, such as the traditional Levin tube or the smaller, much more flexible mercury-weighted tube (Fig. 12.2) and with commonly employed feeding techniques, such as nasogastric feeding via gravity drip system or constant infusion pump (Fig. 12.3). The constant infusion pump standardizes the rate by which the formula is delivered but this constancy is impossible with the gravity drip method. In the gravity drip method the rate of formula flow depends upon gravity, the size of the tube, and the flow resistance as controlled by the attending nurse.

The dietitian also needs to be aware of the possible complications associated with enteral feeding, the probable cause or causes of each complication and how these complications can be corrected. Possible compli-

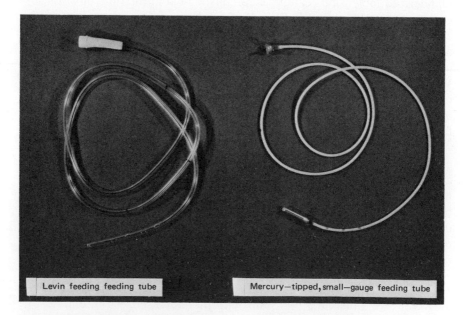

Levin feeding feeding tube   Mercury—tipped, small—gauge feeding tube

Figure 12.2 Comparison of traditional Levin feeding tube with the more recent, more easily inserted, mercury-tipped small gauge feeding tube.

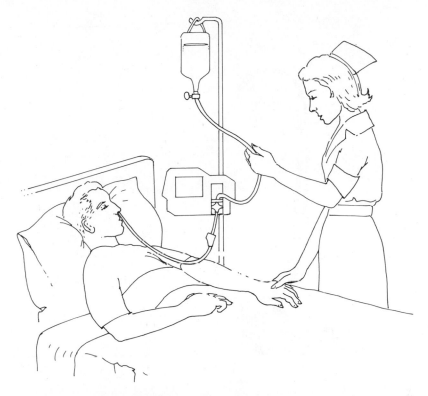

Figure 12.3 Nasogastric feeding via constant infusion pump.

cations of enteral feeding include aspiration of feeding, dehydration, diarrhea, cramps and/or distension. The danger of aspiration can be largely prevented through the use of a mercury-weighted tube that will insure the passage of the tube into the intestine (Fig. 12.4). A 30 degree elevation of the patient's bed is also very helpful in preventing the problem.

Dehydration is a particular danger in the comatose patient who is unable to express his/her feeling of thirst (see Chapter 4). Dehydration may be accompanied by a diarrhea due to the hyperosmolality of the tube feeding. Excessive amounts of protein in the feeding usually accounts for its hyperosmolality. Diarrhea has a number of possible causes other than the hyperosmolality of the feeding. Additional causes for diarrhea often accompanied by cramps and/or distension include improper insertion of feeding tube, administration of cold feedings, too rapid administration of formula, bacterial contamination of formula, and/or possible lactose intolerance on the part of the patient.

Before a definite determination can be made about the appropriate corrective action for the diarrheal condition, the possibilities of bacterial

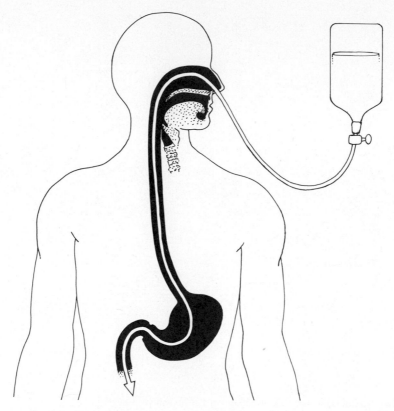

Figure 12.4 Enteral feeding through use of mercury weighted tube. The tube has been passed into jejunum.

contamination, lactose intolerance, and improper insertion of the feeding tube must be ruled out. Once these possibilities have been eliminated, the probable approach would be to (1) allow the formula to reach room tempature before administration; (2) administer a smaller volume of the formula at a lower concentration; (3) possibly add a bulk-forming agent to the feeding.

Most tube feedings are hyperosmolar; therefore, in order to prevent excessive fluid shifts, it is often necessary to begin administration with a formula diluted to about one-half strength and to give only 50 to 100 ml per hour until the patient can tolerate a higher osmolar load. Usually within three days the diet can have gradually increased to the desired volume and strength (6,12). An alternative approach to diluting the formula and taking 24 or more hours to reach a desirable caloric intake is the choice of an isotonic feeding which can be used full strength almost immediately (see Table 12.4).

Table 12.5 Conditions for Which Formula Defined (elemental)
Diets and/or Tube Feedings May Be Used

Defined-formula diets	Tube feedings
Preoperative bowel preparation	Head and neck cancer
Short gut syndrome	Trauma
Pancreatitis	Burns
Malabsorption syndrome	Central nervous system abnormalities
Inflammatory bowel disease	Preoperative anorexia
Postoperative jejunostomy	

Monitoring the progress of patients being fed by tube is also an important part of the dietitian's responsibility. Lab values of particular relevance are blood urea nitrogen (BUN), blood glucose, serum albumin, serum sodium, and urine specific gravity.

The dietitian's concern for hospital food safety extends to the care and delivery of all ingested foods including tube feedings. Therefore, he/she must be familiar with the techniques necessary for maintaining delivery systems free of bacterial contamination and make certain that these techniques are utilized at all times (4). Although patients are often encouraged to take defined formula diets orally, this method of delivery is rarely successful. The unpleasant odor and taste of the hydrolyzed protein cannot be totally disguised by any amount of flavoring; consequently, already anorectic patients usually find drinking these formulas an impossible task. Table 12.5 lists conditions in which tube feedings and defined formulas are most commonly used.

Quite often patients who are being maintained primarily on tube feedings are also being encouraged to take additional food by mouth. Getting the patient to the point that he/she can be maintained totally by oral feedings is the goal; therefore, the dietitian needs to tempt the patient's appetite as much as possible in order to speed up the transition period.

TOTAL PARENTERAL NUTRITION AND NUTRITION SUPPORT SERVICE

The type of nutritional therapy that has received the greatest amount of attention during the last few years is total parenteral nutrition (TPN), a technique introduced by Rhoads and Dudrick in the mid-1960s. Figure 12.5 illustrates the direct administration of feeding into central blood flow. Clinicians emphasize, however, that when the gastrointestinal tract works, it should be used rather than relying on TPN. TPN should be re-

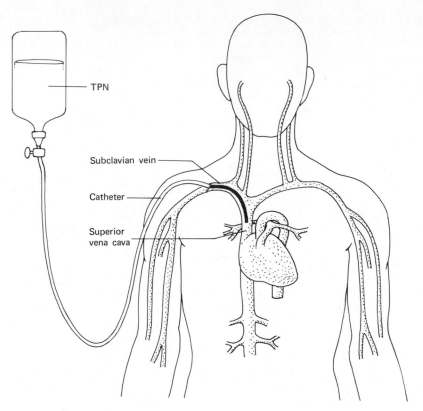

Figure 12.5 Administration of TPN through central venous catheter inserted into subclavian vein.

served for those patients who cannot get adequate nutrition by any other mode of administration. Table 12.6 lists some parenteral preparations available commercially and Table 12.7 gives conditions in which TPN may be the appropriate route of nourishment. Because these preparations contain only amino acids and selected electrolytes, they must be mixed with appropriate solutions of dextrose and have vitamins along with certain other electrolytes added to the solution. A typical "basic" formula used for an adult receiving TPN is given in Table 12.8. Over a three-day period the infusion rate of formula can be increased to 3000 ml daily; therefore, since each ml supplies approximately 1 kilocalorie, patients in need of rehabilitation can receive 3000 kilocalories per 24 hours.

The dramatic results obtained through TPN in the treatment of severely debilitated patients have mandated the formation of Nutrition Support Services (or Metabolic Support Services) in medical centers throughout the United States. The Nutrition (or Metabolic) Support Service is defined by Kaminski as "a group of multidisciplinary nutritional experts working as a team to provide specialized nutritional support for hospitalized patients" (13). Objectives of such a service include identification of patients in need of specialized nutritional support such as TPN, intravenous fat emulsions*, defined formula (or elemental) diets and tube feedings: monitoring nutritional therapy for malnourished patients; providing consultative services to hospital staff regarding specialized nutritional support; monitoring records of benefits and morbidity of patients receiving specialized nutritional support; providing cost analysis and quality control of various forms of nutritional support; instituting in-service education on identification and treatment of nutritional deficits (11).

The composition of the Nutrition (or Metabolic) Support Service may vary from hospital to hospital, but Kaminski recommends that the team include (as it does at St. Mary of Nazareth Hospital Center, Chicago) a physician, pharmacist, dietitian, nurse, physical therapist, hospital administrator, and secretary. Each team member has specific functions to perform so that all objectives as stated above can be met. The dietitian serves as the nutrition resource person and has the responsibility of performing nutritional assessments of patients, formulating special diets and assisting in the administration of tube feedings and defined formula diets, recommending TPN when patients are unable to be nourished adequately by the enteral route, and determining whether the nutrient needs of the patient are being met through TPN.

The dietitian who functions as a member of the Nutrition (Metabolic) Support Service must have developed skills in assessing nutritional status of patients, must possess a good working knowledge of nutrient metabolism, be familiar with the various laboratory tests that have significance for nutritional therapy, have the ability to function as a consultant and teacher and be very knowledgeable about the composition, value, and limitations of the various dietary supplements, defined formula diets, and tube feedings.

All hospitals will not be able to afford a Nutrition (Metabolic) Support Service of the composition recommended by Kaminski. Blackburn and Bistrian (10), nevertheless, stress the importance of an identifiable nutrition consultation service in *every* hospital because they estimate

---

* In the United States, intravenous fat emulsions (Intralipid, and more recently Liposyn) have been approved by the Food and Drug Administration only in recent years. Availability of 10% Intralipid (soybean oil) and Liposyn (safflower oil) solutions which provide 1.1 kcal/ml allows *peripheral* parenteral feedings which can supply approximately 1720 kilocalories in 3200 ml solution. Before introduction of these fat emulsions, calories could be provided only through dextrose and amino acids; therefore, no more than about 800 to possibly 1200 kilocalories could be safely provided in the same volume of fluid which usually is considered the maximum allowance of daily infusion. Figure 12.6 illustrates peripheral parenteral feeding by constant infusion pump.

Table 12.6 Commercially Available Parenteral Preparations (Amino Acid Infusions)

	Aminosyn 5% (Abbott)	Aminosyn 7% (Abbott)	Aminosyn 10% (Abbott)	Freamine II (McGaw)	Travesol 5.5% with electrolytes (Travenol)	Travesol 8.5% with electrolytes (Travenol)	Nephramine[1] (McGaw)	Aminosyn M[2] 3.5% (Abbott)	Travesol M[2] 3.5% with electrolytes (Travenol)
Protein concentration	*5%*	*7%*	*10%*	*8.5%*	*5.5%*	*8.5%*	*5.1%*	*3.5%*	*3.5%*
Nitrogen (gm/dl)	0.786	1.1	1.57	1.25	0.924	1.42	0.58	0.55	0.59
Amino acids —essential (mg/dl)									
Isoleucine	360	510	720	590	263	406	560	252	168
Leucine	470	660	940	770	340	526	880	329	217
Lysine	360	510	720	620	318	492	640	252	203
Methionine	200	280	400	450	318	492	880	140	203
Phenylalanine	220	310	440	480	340	526	880	154	217
Threonine	260	370	520	340	230	356	400	182	147
Tryptophan	80	120	160	130	99	152	200	56	63
Valine	400	560	800	560	252	390	650	280	161
Amino acids — nonessential (mg/dl)									
Alanine	640	900	1280	600	1140	1760		448	728
Arginine	490	690	980	310	570	880		343	364
Histidine[3]	150	210	300	240	241	372		105	154

Proline	430	610	860	950	230	356	300	147
Serine	210	300	420	500				147
Tyrosine	44	44	44		22	34	31	14
Amino acetic acid (glycine)	640	900	1280	1700	1140	1760	448	728
Glutamic acid								
Aspartic acid								
Cysteine				<20				
Electrolytes (mEq/L)								
Sodium			10	70	70	6	40	25
Potassium	5.4	5.4		60	60	60	18.4	15
Magnesium				10	10		3	5
Chloride				70	70	70	40	25
Acetate	*	*	*	100	135		27	54
Calcium								
Phosphate (mM/L)	*			10	30	30		7.5
Osmolality (mOsm/kg)	700	1000	850	850	1160	420	460	450

[1] Lysine acetate added in amount of 900 mg/dl. Each 250 ml. provide Rose's recommended intake of essential amino acids.
[2] Used primarily for peripheral parenteral infusions.
[3] Histidine is now considered essential for humans.
* Quantity not stated by manufacturer.

Table 12.7 Indications for Possible Use of Total Parenteral Nutrition (TPN)

1. *Surgical Indications*
    Enteric fistulas
    Trauma
    Burns
    Preoperative or postoperative cachexia
    Prolonged ileus
    Peritonitis
    Short bowel syndrome
2. *Gastrointestinal Diseases*
    Inflammatory bowel disease
    Pancreatitis
    Severe gastroenteritis
    Protein-losing enteropathy
    Colonic diverticulitis
    Malabsorption syndrome
	3. *Pediatric Indications*
	    Congenital anomalies
	    Extreme prematurity
	    Intractable diarrhea
	4. *Moderate to severe protein–calorie
	    malnutrition*
	5. *Miscellaneous Indications*
	    Cancer patients receiving adjuvant therapy
	    Renal failure
	    Reversible hepatic failure
	    Reversible coma
	    Anorexia nervosa
	    Hyperemesis gravidarum
	    Chronic respirator dependence
	    Cardiac cachexia

Table 12.8 Typical "Basic" Adult Formula for Central
Parenteral Nutrition

Total Volume	1000 ml
Protein (equivalent)	35 g (500 ml 7% Aminosyn)
Dextrose	250 g (500 ml 50% Dextrose)
Total kilocalories	990
Sodium	35 mEq
Potassium	36 mEq
Chloride	35 mEq
Acetate	74 mEq
Calcium	4.5 mEq
Magnesium	5 mEq
Phosphorus	9 mM
Multiple vitamin injection concentrate*	(1.6 ml)
Folic acid	200 mcg
Vitamin K_1	300 mcg
Vitamin B_{12}	10 mcg
Trace element package (0.3 ml):	
Zn	1 mg
Cu	133 mcg
Mn	140 mcg
Cr	1.13 mcg

* Multivitamin concentrate includes Vitamins A, D, C, E, thiamine, riboflavin, niacinamide, dexpanthenol, and pyridoxine. Only one multiple vitamin infusion is used regardless of the volume of parenteral formula required.

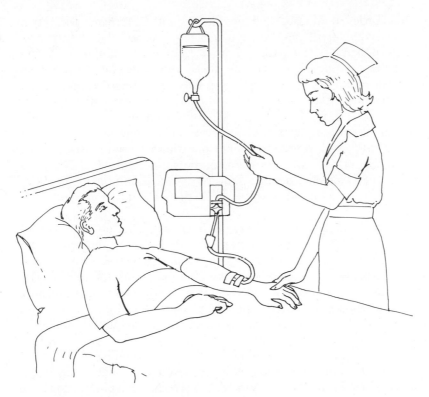

Figure 12.6 Peripheral parental feeding delivered by constant infusion pump.

that at least five percent of the patients in any acute care institution will require intensive nutritional support. The consultation service can be composed of a physician particularly interested in nutrition, a therapeutic dietitian, and a nurse-epidemiologist. The qualifications of the therapeutic dietitian functioning as a member of this consultation service would be the same as those required of the dietitian on a more sophisticated Support Service. TPN might be impossible in smaller hospitals, but the nutrition consultation service could make recommendations about disposition of those patients believed to need parenteral nutrition.

DISCHARGE AND FOLLOW-UP

The nutritional care of the patient cannot be confined solely to his/her hospitalization period. One of the most important duties of the dietitian is to prepare patients with nutrition-related health problems for discharge. Education of the patient should be occurring throughout his/her hospital stay and in order to educate (and most importantly, *motivate*) the patient appropriately, the dietitian should know as much as possible about the patient himself/herself, the patient's family situation, work and leisure habits, living conditions to which he/she is returning, and have a good picture of the patient's customary eating habits. Getting this information means frequent visits with the patient during which the patient is given opportunity to talk freely and ask questions; conversation with family members and frequently with the social worker; routine review of the patient's medical record. A food frequency questionnaire administered early during the patient's hospital stay can serve as a helpful educational tool and may assist in the identification of a nutrition-related problem. Throughout this teaching–learning process, the patient should be an active participant (14).

For each patient who is leaving the hospital with a nutrition-related problem requiring further management, the dietitian should write a discharge summary on the medical record in which is given the patient's condition at discharge and recommendations for follow-up. A copy of this discharge summary should go to the person or agency responsible for provision of follow-up care, such as private physician, visiting nurse, clinic dietitian or public health nutritionist. In order to be a facilitator in the follow-up care of individual patients, the dietitian not only needs a working knowledge of resources in the community but also should have a means of maintaining open communication with key resource people or agencies. Continuity of nutrition care is a deterrent to repeated hospitalizations and prevents many problems for the patient and health professionals alike should hospitalization reoccur.

CASE STUDY: PANCREATITIS

A 33 year-old white female was admitted to the hospital with severe abdominal pain, anorexia, nausea, and fever (102° F). The patient stated that she had experienced a 30-pound weight loss in the last two months and had noted the onset of foamy, light-colored, diarrheal stools. The patient had a history of depression, alcohol abuse, and cigarette abuse. Based on the history, the physician requested a nutritional assessment. Results of the nutritional assessment and laboratory tests were as follows:

Height 5′ 4″

Weight 87 pounds

Mid Upper Arm Circumference 21.8 cm

Triceps Skinfold Thickness 4 mm

Mid Upper Arm Muscle Circumference 20.5 cm

Hemoglobin 10.1 gm/dl

Hematocrit 30%

Total lymphocyte count 1127

Total protein 5.2 gm/dl

Albumin 2.8 gm/dl

Amylase (serum) 1175 units/dl

A diagnosis of pancreatitis and malnutrition was determined. The patient was placed on anticholinergics, nasogastric suction, and strict NPO (Nothing By Mouth). Ultrasound studies the following day showed the presence of a pseudocyst on the tail of the pancreas. Surgery was postponed until the patient could be repleted nutritionally on TPN. Enteral alimentation would be attempted as soon as possible after surgery.

Questions

1. What signs and symptoms suggested a diagnosis of pancreatitis?
2. What benefits are derived from keeping the patient with pancreatitis on anticholinergics, nasogastric suction, and strict NPO?
3. What factors in the patient's history suggested possible nutritional deficiencies?
4. Which biochemical parameters were indicative of malnutrition? Which anthropometric findings?
5. What advantages could be gained from postponing surgery?
6. What clinical signs will the physician use to determine when enteral feedings are possible?
7. What is an appropriate enteral feeding approach once oral feeding can be initiated?

Discussion

Severe abdominal pain, nausea, vomiting, and fever are characteristic symptoms of pancreatitis. Steatorrhea can occur when pancreatic lipase secretion is insufficient. Pseudocysts may develop due to pancreatic tissue necrosis and liquification. Alcoholism is common in the etiology of this disease.

Treatment is aimed at reducing stimulation of pancreatic secretions through the use of anticholinergics, continuous nasogastric suction, and adherence to strict NPO. All these measures decrease the amount of HCl which can enter the duodenum and stimulate secretion of HCO_3^- from the pancreas.

Alcohol abuse, anorexia, steatorrhea, and a 30-pound weight loss in two months are all factors suggestive of possible nutrient deficiencies. The suspicion of malnutrition is further substantiated by the anthropometric findings (all except height are below standard) and biochemical findings which are below normal (total protein, serum albumin, and total lymphocyte count). By postponing surgery, the chances of postoperative infection, mortality, and morbidity will be reduced and repletion of nutrient stores will help speed wound healing.

Following surgery enteral alimentation can be instituted with the return of active bowel sounds and a fall in serum amylase to normal or near normal levels (60–160 U/dl). Generally, the diet progresses from a clear liquid to a low fat, moderate protein diet. Additional fat can be added gradually as tolerated. Should anorexia persist, a nasogastric tube feeding will need to be initiated. As the patient's enteral intake improves, TPN should be gradually tapered off and finally discontinued. By the time the patient is discharged she should be on an oral maintenance diet.

REFERENCES

1. Butterworth, C. E. The skeleton in the hospital closet. *Nutrition Today* **9:** 4, Mar./Apr. 1974.
2. Bistrian, B. R., G. L. Blackburn, J. Vitale, D. Cochran, and J. Naylor. Prevalence of malnutrition in general medical patients. *J. Am. Med. Assoc.* **235:** 1567, Apr. 12, 1976.
3. Bistrian, B. R., G. L. Blackburn, E. Hallowell, and R. Heddle. Protein status of general surgical patients. *J. Am. Med. Assoc.* **230:** 858, Nov. 11, 1974.
4. Butterworth, C. E. Hospital malnutrition. Cassette-A-Month, Am. Diet. Assoc., 1976.
5. Dudrick, S. J. and J. E. Rhoads. New horizons for intravenous feeding. *J. Am. Med. Assoc.* **215:** 939, Feb. 1971.
6. Blackburn, G. L., R. Chernoff, L. Howard, and M. E. Shils. Malnutrition in the hospital. *Dialogues in Nutrition.* Health Learning Systems, Inc., June 1977.
7. Butterworth, C. E. and G. L. Blackburn. Hospital malnutrition and how to assess the nutritional status of a patient. *Nutrition Today* **10:** 8, Mar./Apr. 1975.
8. Blackburn, G. L. and B. R. Bistrian. Curative nutrition: Protein-calorie management. In *Nutritional Support of Medical Practice*, Schneider, Anderson, and Coursin, eds. New York: Harper and Row, 1977.
9. Kaminski, M. V. and A. L. Winborn. *Nutritional Assessment Guide.* Midwest Nutrition, Education and Research Foundation, Inc., 1978.
10. Blackburn, G. L. and B. R. Bistrian. Nutritional support resources in hospital practice. In *Nutritional Support of Medical Practice*, Schneider, Anderson, and Coursin, eds. New York: Harper and Row, 1977.
11. Chernoff, R. and A. Bloch. Liquid feedings: Considerations and alternatives. *J. Am. Med. Assoc.* **70:** 389, Apr. 1977.
12. Mitty, W. F., T. F. Nealon, and C. Grossi. Use of elemental diets in surgical cases. *Am. J. Gastroenterology* **65:** 297, Apr. 1976.

13. *Fundamental Principles and Applications of Nutritional Support; A Team Concept. Syllabus for Regional Seminar Program.* American Society Parenteral and Enteral Nutrition, 1978.
14. Mahoney, M. J. and A. W. Caggiula. Applying behavioral methods to nutritional counseling. *J. Am. Diet. Assoc.* **72:** 372, Apr. 1978.

RECOMMENDED READINGS

Grant, A. *Nutritional Assessment: Guidelines for Dietitians.* Seattle: Northwest Kidney Center, 1102 Columbia Street, 1977. (Price $6.50).

This is a "how-to" manual designed specifically for dietitians.

Shils, M. E., A. S. Block, and R. Chernoff. Liquid formulas for oral and tube feedings. *Clinical Bulletin* **6:** 151, 1976.

Clinical Bulletin is a publication of Memorial Sloan-Kettering Cancer Center. This particular issue provides comprehensive information on most of the commercially available liquid formulas.

CHAPTER 13

Current Nutrition-related Topics

NUTRITIONAL ANEMIAS

One hotly debated health topic is the significance of anemia, specifically iron deficiency anemia, to the overall health of the individual (1–4). Furthermore, public health measures for combating this type of anemia have caused battle lines to be drawn between noted nutritionists and equally noted hematologists (5,6).

The common occurrence of iron deficiency anemia among infants, young children, and females of childbearing age, however, should not preclude the fact that not only does more than one type of anemia exist but also there are many causes for its existence. One of these causes is nutritional in nature; a deficiency of various specific nutrients can interfere with the maturation of erythroid cells. The location of the defect in this maturation process determines which of the nutrients may be implicated in development of anemia. Some nutrients implicated directly in development of anemia include iron (as noted above), pyridoxine (vitamin B_6), pantothenic acid, folic acid, vitamin B_{12}, vitamin E, and protein. Other nutrients influencing the occurrence of anemia are copper, calcium, and ascorbic acid.

The proper maturation of erythroid cells is dependent upon both *normal hemoglobin synthesis and DNA replication* (7). A look at hemoglobin synthesis (Fig. 13.1)* allows identification of those steps in which a deficiency of certain nutrients could interfere with its production. Critical nutrients include pantothenic acid, pyridoxine, iron, protein, and possibly vitamin E:

1 Pantothenic acid is part of CoASH.
2 Pyridoxal phosphate is required cofactor of ALA synthetase.
3 Decreased activity of ALA dehydrase is associated with Vitamin E deficiency.
4 Fe^{2+} must be present for conversion of protoporphyrin into heme.
5 Globin peptide chains (protein) must be available for formation of hemoglobin.

* For structural formulas of various intermediary products in heme synthesis, see Chapter 3.

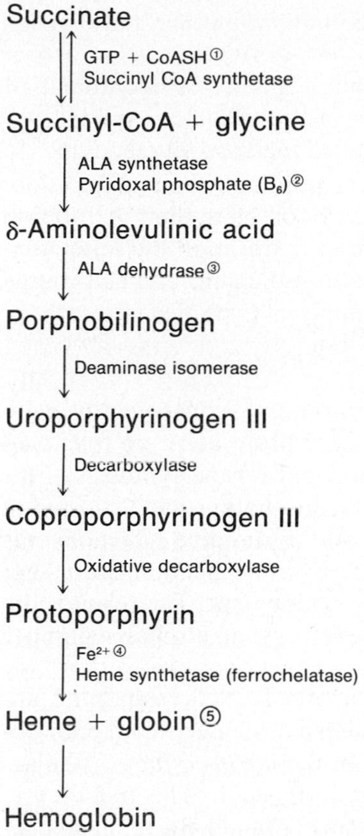

Succinate

$\quad$ GTP + CoASH ①
$\quad$ Succinyl CoA synthetase

Succinyl-CoA + glycine

$\quad$ ALA synthetase
$\quad$ Pyridoxal phosphate (B₆) ②

δ-Aminolevulinic acid

$\quad$ ALA dehydrase ③

Porphobilinogen

$\quad$ Deaminase isomerase

Uroporphyrinogen III

$\quad$ Decarboxylase

Coproporphyrinogen III

$\quad$ Oxidative decarboxylase

Protoporphyrin

$\quad$ Fe²⁺ ④
$\quad$ Heme synthetase (ferrochelatase)

Heme + globin ⑤

Hemoglobin

Figure 13.1 Hemoglobin synthesis, including identification of steps in which nutrient deficiency may inhibit production.

A deficiency of any nutrient required in hemoglobin synthesis could result in a microcytic, hypochromic anemia. Even with appropriate hemoglobin synthesis, erythroid cell maturation is dependent on normal cell division, that is, DNA replication. The series of events leading up to the emergence of the mature reticulocyte into systemic circulation emphasizes the importance of normal DNA replication (8):

1. Stem cells in bone marrow are converted into *pronormoblasts* by action of hormone, erythropoietin (see Chapter 10 for discussion of formation of this hormone). Division of the pronormoblasts into *basophilic normoblasts* represents the first of the four stages required for the maturation of erythroid cells. During this first stage of maturation the synthesis of hemoglobin begins.
2. In Stage II, two more cell divisions produce *polychromatophetic normoblasts I* and *II* which are characterized by increased hemoglobin

content but decreased RNA. This cycle ends in another cell division which leads into Stage III.

3. The cells resulting from this final division are called "orthochromatic" normoblasts. During Stage III the nuclei of the cells are expelled.

4. The cells now are in Stage IV and are called marrow reticulocytes. In the ensuing 48 hours, these reticulocytes continue their maturation, and are released into circulation where they complete their maturation into erythrocytes. During this final stage of maturation the mitochondria break up and their contents diffuse out of the cell. The cell is now essentially a bag of hemoglobin with a supply of enzymes to last it approximately 120 days.

Nutrients associated with DNA replication and, consequently, with appropriate cell division and maturation of erythroid cells are folic acid and vitamin B_{12}. These two vitamins are necessary for the synthesis of the pyrimidine *thymine* (a component of DNA) from the pyrimidine *uracil* (a component of RNA). Discussion of purine and pyrimidine metabolism is included in Chapter 3. Failure of appropriate DNA replication causes nuclear maturation to lag behind cytoplasmic development. The result is the production of large red blood cells which are fewer than normal in number (macrocytic or megaloblastic anemia).

In the past, an inadequate intake of vitamin B_{12} has been quite unusual. In most instances any deficiency has been associated with poor absorption of the vitamin due to the absence of the *intrinsic factor*, the secretion of which parallels that of hydrochloric acid. The macrocytic anemia caused by the body's inability to absorb vitamin B_{12} is called *pernicious anemia*, a condition that is accompanied by neurologic damage.

Presently, however, some concern exists over the possibility of an actual deficiency in vitamin B_{12} intake among strict vegans. The primary concern is for children born to strict vegans who may be breastfed or given vegetable-based formulas not supplemented with vitamin B_{12}.

Macrocytic anemia due to folate deficiency is relatively common and is often found among pregnant women, particularly during the third trimester of pregnancy. Folic acid intake among the general population is usually marginal and little can be stored in the body because it is a water-soluble vitamin. A deficiency of this vitamin can arise rather suddenly due to increased metabolic demands, decreased absorption, or decreased intake.

The synergism that exists between vitamin B_{12} and folic acid has long been recognized but its exact mechanism is poorly understood. However, one theory (9) is that methylcobalamin, an active form of vitamin B_{12}, is an essential cofactor in conversion of homocysteine to methionine. In this reaction the methyl group is lost and must be regenerated from N^5-methyl tetrahydrofolic acid (N^5-methyl-Fh_4), the principle form of folic acid in serum. The regeneration of methylcobalamin also allows N^5-methyl-Fh_4 to be converted to tetrahydrofolic acid (Fh_4) which is needed for the formation of N^5, N^{10}-methylene-Fh_4. N^5, N^{10}-methylene-Fh_4, in turn, is the cofactor essential for the conversion of uracil to thymine. Therefore, a deficiency of vitamin B_{12} might reduce the activity of folic acid by decreasing the amount of N^5, N^{10}-methylene-Fh_4 which could be produced.

Macrocytic anemia, whether due to a deficiency of folic acid or vitamin B_{12}, can be corrected by massive doses of folic acid; however, the neurologic symptoms of pernicious anemia can be reversed only through injections of vitamin B_{12}.

Among the additional nutrients that influence the development of anemia are calcium, copper, and ascorbic acid. *Calcium* is necessary for the binding of the intrinsic factor (IF)–vitamin B_{12} complex to the mucosal wall of the distal ileum for absorption; *copper* is needed for the proper absorption and utilization of iron; *ascorbic acid* reduces ferric iron to its ferrous state, thereby facilitating absorption. Ascorbic acid may also be important in keeping folic acid in its active reduced form.

Vitamin E deficiency in addition to being implicated in anemias resulting from defective heme formation is associated with hemolytic anemia sometimes encountered in the premature infant. A deficiency of vitamin E allows oxidation of the lipids in erythrocyte membranes, thereby causing destruction of red blood cells.

OSTEOPOROSIS

The term *osteoporosis* describes a disease state characterized by decreased bone mass per unit volume. Often the bone mass is so decreased that adequate mechanical support can no longer be provided and spontaneous fractures occur. Although bone formation appears to be normal in osteoporotics, their rate of bone resorption is accelerated, thereby reducing total bone mass.

Osteoporosis is actually an umbrella term referring to a whole group of diseases with diverse etiology, but the most common osteoporosis is that found in elderly adults, particularly women. Because the etiology of this particular disease state in uncertain, appropriate therapy is a debatable subject (10,11).

The life cycle of bone mass can be divided into three phases (11): (1) Phase I extends through the years of skeletal growth during which time both bone mass and bone density may increase; (2) Phase II follows cessation of growth and continues approximately 15 years, a period of stability for bone mass and bone density; (3) Phase III begins about age 35 years at which time bone resorption outstrips bone formation, thereby favoring a progressive and cumulative erosion of bone mass.

This propensity for adult bone loss appears to be universal but the female is usually more seriously affected than the male because she not only has a smaller total bone mass and density throughout the life cycle but also her postmenopausal decreased estrogen production accelerates bone loss. An additional factor that can increase bone loss in any individual of any age or sex is immobility.

As previously stated, the correct therapy for osteoporosis is a debatable subject. Therapy is designed either to correct hormonal imbalances, to improve nutritional status, or to combat mobility impediments.

Although increased parathyroid hormone activity associated with a decreased renal function (a normal aspect of aging) has been demonstrated in elderly osteoporotics (12), estrogen rather than calcitonin has been used more often in hormonal therapy. The rationale for its use is that menopause causes estrogen deficiency; therefore, estrogen replacement is necessary. Trials with estrogen therapy, however, have shown this treatment to be of dubious efficacy. Furthermore, the possible relationship between estrogen therapy and carcinogenesis makes this particular mode of treatment suspect.

Improvement of nutritional status as a mode of combating osteoporosis has revolved around increased intake of calcium and fluorine. Nevertheless, there is evidence to suggest that a decreased intake of phosphorus also may be instrumental in combating calcium loss from bones. Some osteoporotics have shown increased bone regeneration and high calcium retention when placed on generous intakes of calcium (13). When increased calcium intake is accompanied by fluoride, even more bone regeneration appears possible (14,15). The problem with fluoride dosage, however, is that the level that appears effective in bone regeneration lies within the range that may cause fluorosis.

Negative mineral balances have long been associated with immobility or failure to subject bones to pressure. Therefore, it can be hypothesized that increased physical activity decreases bone loss in all individuals, including the elderly. One such study with elderly subjects supporting this hypothesis has been reported in the literature (16).

Sandler (11) points out that, although the propensity for adult bone loss does exist, this bone loss is not inevitable as has been demonstrated by various investigators (17,18). The author proposes, therefore, that possible prevention of osteoporosis should receive as much scrutiny as its treatment which up to now has been ineffective. The belief is expressed that a good life-style that promotes overall good health through good nutrition, sufficient rest, and adequate physical activity may prevent an "obligatory" bone loss in the aged.

NUTRITION AND CANCER

Of very current interest is the possible interrelationship between food habits and the incidence of cancer which is the number two cause of death in the United States.

Food, an important aspect of any environment, is being scrutinized closely for its possible carcinogenic effect because epidemiologic studies have strongly suggested that specific neoplasms are related more to environmental factors than to genetic ones. Much of the American population believes that foods, particularly food additives, are a cause of cancer (19).

Some food additives have been found to be carcinogenic in experimental animals (e.g., saccharin) and through epidemiologic studies have been linked to human neoplasms (e.g., nitrates and nitrites in stomach cancer). Although certain food additives may be suspect, no potential carcinogen has been allowed as a new additive since the 1958 amendment to the Federal Food, Drug and Cosmetic Act. The so-called Delaney clause of this amendment is responsible for the ban of all possible carcinogens regardless of how remote the possibility of tumorigenesis may be in humans. Food additives under scrutiny at the present time, therefore, are those which were in general use before 1958 and were generally regarded as safe (GRAS list). A select committee on GRAS substances of the Federation of American Societies for Experimental Biology (FASEB) was appointed in 1972 to evaluate these substances and the 351 items reviewed to date have been grouped into the following categories (20):

1. *Nonhazardous when used at current level or at level that might reasonably be expected in future.* Seventy-one percent of GRAS substances have been placed in this category.
2. *Nonhazardous at present level of use but additional data needed to determine effects of a significant increase in consumption.* About 15 percent of GRAS items are categorized in this way, including such additives as natural gums, agar-agar, sulfur dioxide, licorice, sucrose, and corn syrup.
3. *No evidence of hazard when used at current levels but uncertainties exist and additional studies are needed promptly.* Six percent GRAS additives must be thus classified and include such items as butylated hydroxytoluene (BHT), carrageenan, and nutmeg.
4. *Adverse effects to public health when used at current levels and safer usage conditions need to be established.* This is, of course, the category about which there is most concern and four percent of GRAS additives fall under this classification. Examples of additives in this category include monosodium glutamate and hydrolyzed vegetable protein in baby foods; also the nitrates used for color and preservation.

5. *Insufficient data upon which to base an evaluation.* Four percent of GRAS additives fall in this category, examples of which are certain glycerides, japan wax for food packaging, and carnauba wax to polish fruits and vegetables.

Relationship Between Diet And Development Of Cancer

Food additives, however, comprise only *one* of the *many* groups of possible carcinogens that humans may ingest. A few of the other possible carcinogens in the diet include: (1) *polycyclic hydrocarbons* produced when meats are smoked or grilled; (2) *aflatoxin,* a naturally occurring potent carcinogen which is produced by strains of *Aspergillus flavus,* growing on nuts, grains, beans, corn, and milk products stored in warm, humid atmospheres; (3) *asbestos,* a powerful carcinogen for humans found in many water supplies; (4) *certain toxic and carcinogenic heavy metals,* such as arsenic, beryllium, cadmium, lead, and nickel, which are important industrially and, consequently, have the potential for entering both food and water supplies (21). Nor are the plants themselves without danger. Even plants grown under ideal conditions and subjected to no processing have been found to contain naturally occurring carcinogens.

Many researchers, however, believe that the main influence of ingested food upon carcinogenesis is not direct, but instead is one of modifying cellular reactions, thereby providing a more favorable environment for cancer development. A possible example of such a dietary modifying factor is excessive fat intake which experimental and epidemiologic studies have shown to be correlated with the development of colon, breast, endometrial, and prostate cancer (22,23). Additionally, epidemiologic studies provide evidence for a negative correlation between fiber intake and colon cancer (24,25). Independent of fat intake, overnutrition in itself apparently increases the risk of many types of cancer, perhaps through its effect on endocrine production (20,23).

Other identified relationships between dietary intake and development of cancer include the following (23):

1. Development of oral and esophageal cancer is correlated with excessive consumption of alcohol in combination with heavy tobacco usage.
2. Increased cancer of thyroid and upper gastrointestinal tract in populations with iodine and/or iron deficiency syndrome has been clinically recognized.
3. Increased evidence of cancer of the liver has been demonstrated in alcoholics who are also deficient in the B vitamins.

Neither the mechanisms of the effect of excesses or deficiencies of various nutrients on the development of cancer nor their predictability in car-

3308

BUSINESS REPLY MAIL

FIRST CLASS PERMIT NO. 22, CHICAGO, ILLINOIS

POSTAGE WILL BE PAID BY ADDRESSEE

**COLLEGE STORE SERVICE BUREAU
NATIONAL ASSOCIATION
OF COLLEGE STORES
528 E. LORAIN STREET
OBERLIN, OHIO 44074**

NO POSTAGE
NECESSARY
IF MAILED
IN THE
UNITED STATES

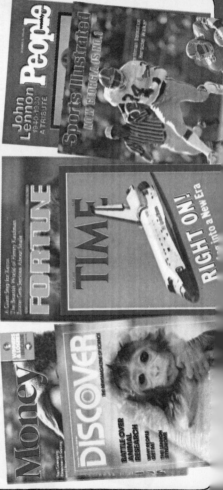

cinogenesis for individuals have been identified clearly. A great deal of research is needed in the area of nutrition and its relation to cancer development before any *definite* dietary changes can be recommended (23).

Certain nutrients may exert a protective effect against cancer, but a danger that always arises with experimental evidence for the possible therapeutic value of various nutrients is that the population *over reacts* and *over doses*. The fact that ascorbic acid can prevent the formation of nitrosamines from nitrites and therefore decreases the incidence of gastric cancer is exciting just as is the evidence that the correct level of vitamin A may protect against epithelial malignancies of lungs, bladder, and breasts (26). These discoveries, exciting as they are, presently do not warrant the ingestion of massive doses of these two vitamins as a cancer preventive.

In light of the present limited knowledge concerning nutrition and its relation to carcinogenesis, apparently the best preventive measure against the disease via the food intake route is consumption of a diet in which adequate levels of all nutrients are assured but overconsumption of calories is avoided. Although no *definite* dietary change can be recommended for cancer prevention, increasing complex carbohydrates as well as fruits and vegetables in the diet while decreasing comsumption of fats and refined carbohydrates possibly could prove beneficial (26).

Nutritional Status And Cancer

Although no definitive cause–effect relationship between nutrition and carcinogenesis has been determined, the effect of an extant cancer on the nutritional status of its host is easily identified. Here again, however, the picture is clouded because the mechanisms through which cancer makes its victims cachectic are poorly understood. Although most cancer patients are anorectic, their marked loss of both body fat and muscle mass is quite different from that found in simple starvation (27). The possibility exists that tumor-bearing organisms possess a substance not found in normal subjects that promotes breakdown of fat. Furthermore, certain cancer victims have been found to have a concentration and pattern of blood and tissue amino acids very different from those possessed by controls. Other frequently identified metabolic abnormalities in tumor-bearing animals and patients include: loss of liver glycogen, lowered level of insulin, diabetic glucose tolerance curve, increased activity in the Cori cycle, and increased insulin resistance (27).

Anorexia is common in cancer patients and can be caused not only by physical problems but also by psychological and emotional disturbances (28,29). Factors associated with decreased food intake and related to the physical condition of the tumor-bearing organism may include certain circulating chemicals, hormones, metabolites, concentration and pattern of amino acids not found in normal subjects. If the theoretical integrated system for food intake actually does exist, the above listed factors could provide negative inputs to food intake of the cancer patient. Although the exact cause of the anorexia is unclear, certain characteristics of cancer patients have been identified (28):

1. They experience an early satiation; therefore, only small amounts are eaten at any one time.
2. They frequently find they are able to eat much better earlier in the day than they can as the day progresses.
3. They are likely to develop abnormalities of taste; e.g., a slightly higher threshold for salt, a higher threshold for sweet, a lower threshold for bitter. Some patients have an aversion for meat and most of these patients have been found to have a lowered threshold for urea.

The anorexia of cancer patients can be worsened in many cases by the therapy employed to destroy tumor cells or arrest their growth. Radiotherapy directed at any part of the gastrointestinal tract, particularly in the area of the mouth, is likely to intensify anorexia and all chemotherapy agents cause a decreased desire for food (30).

Although all cancer patients are likely to exhibit some cachexia and anorexia, the severity of their deteriorating nutritional status is likely to be related to the organ system or systems affected by tumors. Whenever the gastrointestinal tract is invaded by cancer, the potential for severe nutrition problems exists even after the surgical excision of the tumor (31). Shils(32) outlines the many possible consequences of cancer treatment emphasizing the problems associated with surgical treatment of gastrointestinal cancer.

The most promising relationship between nutrition and cancer is the positive effect that improved nutritional status of the cancer victim can have not only on the course of tumor therapy but also on his/her overall quality of life.

Nutritional assessment (see Chapter 12) of the newly admitted cancer patient is a necessity in order to separate patients at no particular risk from those who have lost 10 percent or more of body weight and/or have such underlying problems as bowel obstruction or fistula. Such patients are at high risk of significant malnutrition and need to have aggressive nutrition therapy begun immediately (33). Additionally, all patients under treatment, regardless of their nutritional status on admission to the hospital, should have periodic nutritional assessments in order to delineate any possible deleterious consequences resulting from the therapeutic program. Depending upon the patient, the route of nutrition therapy may be oral, parenteral, or by tube. The methods selected will be determined primarily by the condition of the patient's gastrointestinal tract. There seems to be no question about the fact that the nutritionally repleted patient is better able to undergo surgery and to respond more favorably to chemotherapy or radiation therapy than is the patient who receives no nutritional therapy.

Oral feedings, whenever possible, are always preferable and prerequisites to any aggressive nutrition support via the oral route are subjective reports by the patient concerning his/her appetite and customary food intake. A dietary history should be obtained from the patient including recall of previous 24-hour food intake, general food frequency intake, and identification of those foods that are particularly liked or disliked. With this information at hand, the dietitian then makes every effort to see that the food served the patient is as appealing as possible to his/her appetite.

Research with patients undergoing radiation and chemotherapy has revealed the many taste changes that may occur in these patients (see page 456), and has allowed identification of those foods that are best accepted by a majority of these patients (33,34). It must be reemphasized, however, that each patient is an individual with his/her particular responses to food. Nevertheless, the foods most frequently requested by patients undergoing radiation and/or chemotherapy include cold clear liquids, carbonated liquids, flavored ices, jello, watermelon, grapes, and peeled cucumbers (34).

The acceptability of various nutrition supplements has been studied and identification of those best tolerated along with their preferred mode of preparation include (34):

Glucose polymers (Polycose, Controlyte) mixed with cold, clear liquids

Fruit-flavored albumin-based supplements, e.g., Precision LR, Citrotein, mixed with fruit-flavored beverages

Lactose-free soy bean formulas (Isocal, Ensure) served in their chocolate-flavored form.

Listed below are a few suggestions for increasing the food intake of cancer patients (34,35):

1. Provide patient with a good breakfast at least two hours before radiation or chemotherapy. Try to minimize nausea by encouraging the patient to rest after treatment and by providing antinausea drugs before any vomiting begins, thereby increasing possibility that the patient can eat something at the next meal.
2. Carefully select the types of foods that are offered the patient. Individual likes and dislikes are always kept in mind but some general suggestions for food preparation include:
   a. Use of cold protein items; such as, salad plates of fruit and cheese, and meat salads.
   b. Use of cold snacks high in protein; such as ice cream and salted nuts.
   c. Adjustment of seasoning to improve flavor of foods for patient; for example, additional amounts of salt and/or sugar, use of lemon juice and variety of spices.

3. Provide the patient optimum and extended exposure to food service during the evening in order to maintain a relaxed atmosphere in which he/she will be encouraged to eat.
4. Make available a 'family' kitchen in which familiar or ethnic foods may be prepared for the patient by members of his/her family.

Some excellent publications are available for the nutritional management of cancer patients. Two such publications are *A Guide to Good Nutrition: During and After Chemotherapy and Radiation* and *Health Through Nutrition: A Comprehensive Guide for the Cancer Patient* (36,37).

Nowhere is the care of the "whole" patient more important than in the support of the cancer victim. This support in order to be effective must by given by a team of interdisciplinary health professionals, one of whom is the dietitian/nutritionist. The aim of this team of professionals is to improve the quality of life for the patient by offering means by which he/she may be rehabilitated and/or encouraged to maximize his/her potential (38,39). Team members participate in regularly scheduled planning conferences and walking rounds, both of which promote communication among the various health professionals to the definite benefit of the patient. Family members of the patient are also involved in overall care and this involvement is important for the patient both psychologically and physically.

The dietitian/nutritionist approaches each patient on an individual basis, making every effort to encourage an adequate consumption of food and engaging in much education of the patient concerning his/her therapy and why eating is so important to therapy success.

Because the nutritional status of the cancer patient may decline rapidly once he/she goes home and is no longer seen on a daily basis, an essential part of every cancer patient's discharge plan is a comprehensive nutritional support and follow-up procedure (23). Before any patient is discharged, he/she should be consuming orally approximately 1500 to 2000 calories per day. This means that for those patients who have been receiving nutrition support through tube feedings and/or the parenteral route, much effort must be exerted to encourage the patient to eat. The dietitian may make a contract with the patient: The dietitian must supply the food that the patient wants while the patient must eat those foods supplied (39). Additionally, the family may be encouraged to bring in any food that the patient will eat, or if a "family kitchen" is available in the hospital, to prepare ethnic foods that would have special appeal for the patient.

Once the patient has reached an oral intake of 1500 to 2000 kilocalories per day and can be discharged, follow-up visits for the purpose of nutritional assessment must be planned on a regular basis. Recommended intakes of calories and protein per kilogram body weight for patients who need to be maintained at current nutritional status approximate 30 to 35 kilocalories and 1 to 1.5 grams, respectively. For those patients who need continued repletion, the recommended intakes are higher: 40 to 45 kilocalories and 1.5 to 2 grams protein per kilogram ideal body weight (23).

NUTRITION AND THE BRAIN

Probably the most recent area of intensive nutrition-related research is examination of the possible connection between nutrition and neurotransmitter metabolism in the brain. Since the discovery by Fernstrom and Wurtman (40) that the amount of carbohydrate and fat in a meal can influence the production by the brain of the neurotransmitter, serotonin, from tryptophan, much research has been directed toward identifying any behavior changes in the organism that can be related to its nutrition via various neurotransmitters. The most obvious way by which nutrition can affect brain transmitter synthesis is by altering the availability of the transmitter precursors to the brain. These transmitter precursors in most instances are the amino acids, for example, tryptophan from which serotonin is produced and tyrosine which gives rise to the catecholamines, dopamine and norepinephrine. A non-amino acid precursor is choline which gives rise to the neurotransmitter, acetylcholine. A diet high in lecithin of which choline is a component can eventually cause a rise in the amount of acetylcholine in the brain.

Other nutrients whose supply to the brain has been suggested possibly to influence brain function via neurotransmitters are iron and the vitamins, pyridoxine and niacin (41,42). The neurotransmitters not only may be influenced by the nutritional status of the organism but also may be instrumental themselves in regulating the food intake of the organism (43). Of particular interest is the possible relationship between neurotransmitter metabolism and anorexia nervosa (44).

VITAMIN C—NUTRIENT OR DRUG?

Megadosage of vitamin C as recommended by such giants of science as Linus Pauling has been responsible for the very close scrutiny to which ascorbic acid has been subjected for the last decade or so. Advances have been made in the understanding of this organic compound but many uncertainties still remain.

Virtues of the Vitamin

Although it cannot be said that the precise biochemical role of ascorbic acid is fully understood, many of the physiologic effects of its deficiency have been well documented. For instance, a vitamin lack impairs the normal formation of intercellular substance throughout the body, including collagen, bone matrix, and tooth dentin. A striking pathological change resulting from this defect is a weakening of the endothelial wall of the capillaries due to a reduction in the amount of intercellular substance. Therefore, the clinical manifestations of scurvy—hemorrhaging from mucous membranes of the mouth and gastrointestinal tract, anemia, pains in the joints, and defects in skeletal calcification—can all be related to the association of vitamin C and normal connective tissue metabolism. This function of ascorbic acid also accounts for its requirement for normal wound healing. In a study reviewed by Schwartz (45), incisional wounds were inflicted on volunteers who had been frankly deprived of vitamin C for three months. At that time, the plasma ascorbate level had been zero for 44 days and the buffy coat (leucocyte) concentration (a better indicator of tissue stores) was four mg/dl. There was no impairment of wound healing. However, three months later, with the plasma level at zero for 141 days and the buffy coat concentration zero for 61 days, normal healing was not observed. At this point, the volunteers had exhibited symptoms of scurvy. Therefore, it is apparent that while the vitamin is essential for normal wound healing, only at deficiency (scorbutic) levels is impairment evident.

Another beneficial function of vitamin C, seemingly apart from its antiscurvy property, is that it facilitates the transformation of cholesterol into bile acids in the liver. In a study using guinea pigs (46), cholesterol accumulated in the serum of the animals if they were deprived of an adequate vitamin C intake. In the reference cited, the author refers to a correlative study on humans that demonstrates a relationship between serum cholesterol and vitamin C intake. Vitamin C is known to be required for certain hydroxylation reactions, particularly the hydroxylation of proline to hydroxyproline and of lysine to hydroxylysine. The hydroxylated forms of these amino acids are found in collagen, thus accounting for the role of the vitamin in maintaining normal connective tissue. Because hydroxylation of the steroid nucleus is involved in the transformation of cholesterol to bile acids, this may explain the role of ascorbate in this transformation, although further investigation will be necessary to establish the precise function. The inference from these studies is that inadequate vitamin C intake, by elevating serum cholesterol, may predispose to atherosclerosis and cardiovascular disease.

An additional hydroxylation reaction in which ascorbate is known to participate is in the pathway of tyrosine metabolism. The specific reaction is the hydroxylation of the phenolic ring of p-hydroxyphenylpyruvic acid to form 2,5-dihydroxyphenylactic acid (homogentisic acid). p-Hydroxyphenylpyruvic acid has been found to accumulate in ascorbate-deficient guinea pigs and infants administered tyrosine.

Ascorbic acid is a strong reducing agent, or antioxidant, a property that can be disadvantageous (to be discussed later) if large amounts are consumed. However, its reducing property is also beneficial in certain physiological processes, such as in the absorption of dietary iron. Iron is absorbed in the ferrous (Fe^{+2}) state rather than the ferric (Fe^{+3}) form, and the reducing capability of ascorbate accounts for the enhanced absorption of the metal in the presence of the vitamin. One study (47) showed that there was a two-fold increase in iron absorption if 280 mg of supplemental vitamin C were taken at breakfast only, but that there was a three-fold increase if the same daily amount of vitamin C was taken in divided doses at each meal. The beneficial effect of the vitamin is therefore evident in certain cases of iron deficiency, but the author was quick to point out the risks associated with this enhancement if the individual suffered from such diseases as idiopathic hemochromatosis, thalassemia major, and sideroblastic anemia, in which the absorption of iron is already excessive.

There has also been interest in ascorbate's ability, as an antioxidant, to prevent or at least minimize the formation of carcinogenic substances from dietary material. Nitroso-compounds, for example, which are known to be carcinogenic in aminal studies, can be formed from the reaction of nitrites with certain amino compounds *in vivo*. The nitrites are formed from the oxidation of nitrates which are commonly incorporated into foodstuffs used in human nutrition. The proposed beneficial effect of ascorbate in this sequence of events is that it can prevent the oxidation of nitrate to nitrite (48). In another investigation (49), ascorbic acid was found to prevent the oxidation of the tryptophan metabolite, 3-hydroxy-anthranilic acid, to a product that has carcinogenic activity. The author proposed the administration of one gram vitamin daily to high risk individuals who are regularly exposed to such carcinogens as a prophylaxis against bladder cancer. Further research will be necessary to determine the extent to which vitamin C participates in the reduction-oxidation reactions of normal metabolism.

Possible Complications of Megadosing

A megadose refers to the ingestion of a substance in a quantity greatly exceeding that which is considered adequate for maintaining normal metabolism. In case of vitamin C, only about 10 mg per day are necessary to prevent the symptoms of scurvy, and presumably to sustain the biochemical reactions, discussed above, in which the vitamin participates. It has been estimated that a dietary intake of 100 to 150 mg/day is a "saturating" level, meaning that the concentration of vitamin C in the tissues is maximized at this daily dose, and that there will be no additional uptake of the vitamin if the dosage is increased.

In recent years there has emerged the popularized belief that mega-doses of ascorbic acid, taken on a continuous basis, may reduce the likeli-hood of contracting a head cold or other upper respiratory disorders, or alleviate the symptoms of the affliction, or both. The impetus for this belief came primarily from Dr. Linus Pauling's book, *Vitamin C and the Common Cold* (50), which was published in 1970, and in which the author proposed that megadoses of vitamin C were effective as a prophylaxis against the common cold. This allegation will be explored later in this dis-cussion. Needless to say, the appeal of self-prescribing a readily avail-able, inexpensive drug that might ward off the common cold was far reaching, and the publication wooed millions into a "megadose mania." The practice of consuming large quantities of ascorbate on a regular basis may, at least for a certain segment of the population, carry with it serious risks. It is important, however, to recognize that some of the complica-tions to be described are exceedingly rare, and that a given report of a complication may have been based on one or perhaps just a few cases.

Formation of Stones. Ascorbic acid is normally converted to a small extent into oxalate. Studies have shown that the level of urine oxalate rises slightly but significantly with large doses of vitamin C. In one such study (51), the interesting observation was made that one subject had a 10-fold increase in urinary oxalate after consuming four g vitamin C/day for just seven days. The authors proposed an enzyme-induction mechanism to ex-plain the excessive formation of oxalate. In the same study it was found that three out of 67 subjects tested displayed this enzymatic irregularity. Because oxalate salts represent the major portion of urinary calculi, sub-jects with this metabolic peculiarity would likely be predisposed to renal stone formation if they were taking megadoses of vitamin C.

There has been at least one case of enteric stone formation in a pa-tient taking large doses of vitamin C (52). An exploratory laparotomy per-formed on the patient, following complaints of persistent abdominal pain, revealed many stones in the ileocecal region of the bowel, some the size of large marbles. Chemical analysis revealed the composition of the stones to be largely ascorbate. The patient claimed to have been taking 300 mg per day over a long period of time, but increased the intake to five grams per day whenever cold symptoms were sensed. The reason for this unusual complication is not clear.

Vitamin B$_{12}$ Destruction. Following the observation that hospital patients taking one gram of ascorbate daily by prescription had low serum vitamin B$_{12}$ levels, a study (53) was carried out to determine the effect on dietary vitamin B$_{12}$ of the coingestion of "pharmacologic" doses of vitamin C. Vitamin C was added in varying amounts to food preparations homogen-ized to mimic the digestive process, and following incubation the vitamin

B_{12} content was determined. It was found that the amount of B_{12} destroyed correlated directly with the amount of vitamin C added to the food, and that as little as 500 mg of vitamin C destroyed 95 percent of the vitamin B_{12} in a "meal" regarded as having a moderate B_{12} content. Because this destruction occurs only when both vitamins are present together suggests that the effect could be circumvented by taking the vitamin C two or more hours after eating. However, the author pointed out that this would still destroy a substantial amount of the vitamin B_{12} normally excreted into the intestine via the bile, and which would normally be reabsorbed.

Interferences with Clinical Tests. A common problem in clinical testing is the presence of interfering substances in the specimen which affect the chemical reaction by which the assay is carried out. The result of such interference is either a falsely low or falsely high assay result depending on the nature of the interference. Interfering compounds must therefore be removed from the specimen prior to the determination, or the effect of the interference must somehow be corrected for in the quantitative calculation. Ascorbic acid and its metabolites display diverse chemical reactivity due to various functional groups within the molecules, and therefore the presence of ascorbate and its metabolites in serum or urine can affect tests conducted on these specimens. It is true also that the higher the concentration of ascorbate, the more pronounced its interference effect. Needless to say, unless an attending physician is aware of a patient's elevated ascorbate, and therefore able to make an appropriate correction, misinformation would be obtained from the test, and a correct diagnosis delayed.

Some of the routine tests that are affected by the presence of vitamin C are listed below. The list is referenced for the benefit of those readers who are interested in the mechanism of the interference and if uncorrected test results would be falsely high or low.

Bilirubin (54,55)

Transaminases (55,56)

Lactate dehydrogenase (55)

Glucose (57)

Uric acid (58)

17-Hydroxycorticosteroids (59)

Urobilinogen (60)

Occult stool blood (61)

Deficiency Symptoms Following Cessation of Megadose Intake. In an interesting study on the long-term ingestion of megadoses of vitamin C (62), an ascorbate-deficiency syndrome could be induced in volunteers who returned to a normal diet following the daily intake of gram quantities of the vitamin. It was observed in this study that plasma and erythrocyte levels of vitamin C decreased during a short-term vitamin C loading test, and that urinary excretion correspondingly increased. Upon cessation of the megadose, the high rate of renal clearance apparently continued with a resultant depletion of tissue vitamin C stores and the appearance of deficiency symptoms. In a self-experiment, one of the investigators consumed between 10 and 15 g of vitamin C daily for two weeks, then abruptly returned to a normal diet with no supplementary vitamin C. A few weeks later he experienced swelling and bleeding of gums, loosening of teeth, muscle pain, and other scurvylike symptoms. The symptoms could be reversed by a return to small amounts of supplementary vitamin C.

Risk/Benefit Ratio of Megadosing

It is evident from the results of the experimental investigations described above that supplemental megadoses of vitamin C are linked with a certain calculated risk. Megadosing of the vitamin has, of course, become popular because of the alleged benefit of the vitamin in reducing the incidence of the common cold and/or alleviating its symptoms. If the allegation is true, the advantages of megadosing may outweigh the risk of complications. But if the allegation is untrue, the public has been deluded into investing millions of dollars in an expensive, worthless morning ritual that could result in serious medical adversity. Where does the truth lie?

Research designed to answer the question is problematical because of the difficulty in quantitating the results of a study. For instance, the incidence of upper respiratory tract infections within a medicated group compared with a control or placebo group is not difficult to measure, but to quantitate the *severity* of the condition, investigators must rely solely on how the patient says he or she "feels." In spite of this subjectivity of data interpretation, studies with a sound scientific approach have emerged.

One of the early studies on the prophylactic effect of large daily doses of vitamin C was conducted on students at a ski school in the Swiss Alps (63). It was one of very few studies in which there appeared to be a positive prophylactic effect of the vitamin, yet it was probably instrumental in prompting the writing of the Pauling book that has already been referred to. It is felt by some, though not definitely established, that a greater intake of ascorbate may be required to maintain "saturation levels" of the vitamin in conditions of acute illness or severe environmental stress such as extreme cold or physical exertion. It will be recalled (p. 461) that as little as 100 to 150 mg per day is normally sufficient to maintain tissue saturation. The subjects in the study cited would, of course, have been exposed to environmental stress from the standpoint of both temperature and exertion. At any rate, nearly all subsequent investigations on a "less-stressed" population have failed to provide clear-cut evidence for prophylactic or therapeutic benefits from ascorbate excess.

A now well-known Canadian study (64–66) compared prophylactic doses of 250, 1000, and 2000 mg per day in one group of subjects over an extended period with a nonmedicated control group. Evaluated were the number of episodes of illness, the days spent indoors because of illness, and the days during which nasal symptoms were apparent. No statistical difference was observed between the two groups. The same investigators compared the effect of a combination of both prophylactic and therapeutic vitamin C regimen with nonmedicated controls. The medicated group received as much as four grams at the onset of illness in addition to the regular one gram per day prophylactic dose. There did seem to be a reduction in severity as measured by the days confined to the house, but there was no alleviation of nasal symptoms when compared with the unmedicated group.

In 1975, Dykes (67) reviewed nine relevant studies from 1940 to 1975, and concluded, "A review of the controlled studies of the efficacy of ascorbic acid in the prophylaxis and therapy of the common cold that meet some reasonable criteria of design reveal little convincing evidence to support claims of clinically-important efficacy". The authors stress the distortion of meaningful data due to the subjectivity of "patient" response and the judgment on the part of the investigators.

A double-blind study (68) designed to determine the therapeutic value only of large doses of vitamin C was recently reported. When symptoms suggestive of a cold appeared, husband and wife pairs were instructed to consume three grams of the vitamin daily for three days. Husbands and wives of the control group were given placebo to be taken in the event of symptoms. Illnesses were divided according to symptoms into simple head colds and chest colds, and the volunteers were asked to record the number of days that the symptoms persisted. In the simple cold evaluation, the men in the medicated group did report fewer number of days of illness than the men in the placebo group. Strangely, however, the women reported the opposite effect, with placebo volunteers enduring the simple cold symptoms for a fewer number of days than those receiving the vitamin megadose. In the chest cold category of illness, both men and women in the vitamin C medicated group actually reported a longer mean duration of illness than the placebo subjects.

In another comprehensive program (69) to assess the therapeutic efficacy of vitamin C in allaying common cold discomforts, 1524 volunteers agreed to consume 10 grams of the vitamin during a two and one-half day period when cold symptoms were first noticed. Of this number, 482 developed colds. Among those developing colds, active (medicated) and placebo groups were established, and the subjects were requested to quantitate their symptoms on the basis of duration in days. Symptoms quantitated included runny nose, muscular aches, days in bed, and days off work. The authors found that there was no difference in the medicated and placebo groups based on these criteria. They concluded that "Ascorbic acid is of no value in the treatment of the common cold; its preventive effect, in any, is not such as to justify its general use as a prophylactic measure."

In summary, various publications appearing in the 1960s and early 1970s alluding to the positive effect of megadoses of ascorbic acid in reducing the incidence and severity of upper respiratory distress have lead to a large scale, indiscriminate consumption of the vitamin. The results of scientifically sound research efforts designed to assess this allegation have appeared in the literature during the past several years. The data indicate that:

1. Vitamin C megadoses taken when symptoms of a cold are first noticed have virtually no therapeutic benefit in alleviating the symptoms of the illness.
2. There may be a statistical reduction in the incidence of the common cold among those who take vitamin C prophylactically, although the effect is minimal if it indeed exists at all. Furthermore, daily doses of two grams per day do not appear to be any more effective than 250 mg per day (one-fourth the dosage) in prophylactic benefit.

Additionally, although vitamin C is a natural nutrient with a high degree of water solubility which facilitates its excretion and prevents tissue accumulation, the consumption of large doses on a regular basis is not without serious risk. It is questionable therefore if this risk, although small, is worth taking in view of the inappreciable benefits of the megadose.

Questions

1. How can a deficiency of iron or pyridoxal phosphate cause a microcytic anemia while a deficiency of folate or vitamin B_{12} can result in macrocytic anemia?
2. Explain the possible mechanism by which vitamin B_{12} exerts its synergistic effect in the maturation of erythrocytes.
3. Identify the possible relationship which may exist between osteoporosis and (a) hormonal status, (b) nutritional status, and/or (c) mobility level.
4. How does the present status of GRAS substances differ from their status when the Food Additive Amendment was passed in 1958? To what factors may this difference be attributed?

5. Describe some of the characteristics of the anorexia associated with cancer and list means by which an increased food intake may be encouraged in the cancer patient.
6. Evaluate the risk/benefit ratio of megadosage of vitamin C.

REFERENCES

1. Elwood, P. C. Evaluation of the clinical importance of anemia. *Am. J. Clin. Nut.* **26:** 958, Sept. 1973.
2. Read, M. S. Malnutrition, hunger and behavior. *J. Am. Diet. Assoc.* **63:** 382, Oct. 1973.
3. Leibel, R. L. Behavioral and biochemical correlates of iron deficiency. *J. Am. Diet. Assoc.* **71:** 398, Oct. 1977.
4. Strauss, R. G. Iron deficiency, infections, and immune function: A reassessment. *Am. J. Clin. Nut.* **31:** 660, Apr. 1978.
5. Wintrobe, M. M. The proposed increase in the iron fortification of wheat products. *Nutrition Today* **8:** 18, Nov./Dec. 1973.
6. Anatomy of a decision. *Nutrition Today* **13:** 6, Jan./Feb. 1978.
7. Wintrobe, M. M., G. R. Lee, and H. F. Bunn. Pallor and anemia. In *Harrison's Principles of Internal Medicine.* Thorn et al., eds. 8th ed. New York: McGraw-Hill, 1977; pp. 288–294.
8. Williams, W. J., E. Beutler, A. J. Ersler, and R. W. Rundles. *Hematology* 2nd ed. New York: McGraw-Hill, 1977; pp. 104, 203–204.
9. Bunn, N. F., G. R. Lee, M. M. Wintrobe. Pernicious anemia and other megaloblastic anemias. In *Harrison's Principles of Internal Medicine,* Thorn et al. eds. 8th ed. New York: McGraw-Hill, 1977; pp. 1656–1664.
10. Krane, S. M. Metabolic bone disease. In *Harrison's Principles of Internal Medicine,* Thorn et al., eds. 8th ed. New York: McGraw-Hill, 1977; pp. 2028–2033.
11. Sandler, R. B. Etiology of primary osteoporosis: An hypothesis. *J. Am. Geriatrics Soc.* **XXVI:** 209, May 1978.
12. Berlyne, G. M., J. Ben-Ari, D. Galinsky, M. Hirsch, A. Kushelevsky, and R. Shainkin. The etiology of osteoporosis—the role of parathyroid hormone. *J. Am. Med. Assoc.* **229:** 1904, Sept. 30, 1974.
13. Albanese, A. A. Nutritional aspects of bone loss. *Food and Nutrition News* **47:** 1, Oct./Nov. 1975.
14. Hegsted, D. M. Mineral intake and bone loss. *Fed. Proc.* **26:** 1747, 1967.
15. Riggs, B. L. and J. Jowsey. Treatment of osteoporosis with fluoride. *Seminars Drug Treatment* **2:** 27, 1972.
16. Smith, E. L. and W. Reddan. Physical activity—a modality for bone accretion in the aged. *Am. J. Roentgenol.* **126:** 1297, 1976.
17. Garn, S. M., C. G. Rohmann, and P. Nolan. The developmental nature of bone changes during aging. In *Relations of Development and Aging,* J. E. Birren, ed. Springfield, IL: Charles C. Thomas, 1964.
18. Adams, P., G. T. Davies, and P. Sweatman. Osteoporosis and the effect of aging on bone mass in elderly men and women. *Quart. J. Med.* **39:** 601, 1970.

19. Public opinion divided on cancer causes. *Chemical and Engineering News,* Nov. 6, 1978, p. 6.
20. Irving, G. W. Safety evaluation of the food ingredients called GRAS. *Nutrition Reviews* **36:** 351, Dec. 1978.
21. Berg, J. W. Nutrition and cancer. *Seminars in Oncology* **3:** 17, Mar. 1976.
22. Carrol, K. K. Dietary factors in hormone-dependent cancers. In *Nutrition and Cancer,* M. Winick, ed. New York: John Wiley and Sons, 1977.
23. Feeding the cancer patient at home. *Dialogues in Nutrition, 2* (No.4), Health Learning Systems, Inc., N.J.: Bloomfield, June 1978.
24. Oace, S. M. Diet and cancer. *J. Nut. Ed.* **10:** 106, July/Sept. 1978.
25. Wynder, E. L. Dietary habits in cancer. (National Conference on Nutrition in Cancer), *Nut. Today* **13:** 8, Sept./Oct. 1978.
26. Young, V. R. Nutrients, vitamins and minerals in prevention of cancer. (National Conference on Nutrition in Cancer), *Nut. Today* **13:** 27, Sept./Oct. 1978.
27. Theologides, A. General effects of cancer—cachexia. (National Conference on Nutrition in Cancer), *Nut. Today* **13:** 10, Sept./Oct. 1978.
28. Theologides, A. Cancer cachexia. In *Nutrition and Cancer,* M. Winick, ed. New York: John Wiley and Sons, 1977.
29. DeWys, W. D. General effects of cancer—anorexia. (National Conference on Nutrition in Cancer), *Nut. Today* **13:** 10, Sept./Oct. 1978.
30. Donaldson, S. S. Chemotherapy and radiation. (National Conference on Nutrition in Cancer), *Nut. Today* **13:** 12, Sept./Oct. 1978.
31. Goodhart, R. S. and M. E. Shils. *Modern Nutrition in Health and Disease.* 5th ed. Philadelphia: Lea and Febiger, 1973; pp. 981–996.
32. Lawrence, W. Impaired organ system effects. (National Conference on Nutrition in Cancer), *Nut. Today* **13:** 11, Sept./Oct. 1978.
33. Shils, M. E. Principles of nutrition support. (National Conference on Nutrition in Cancer), *Nut. Today* **13:** 25, Sept./Oct. 1978.
34. Aker, S. N. Oral feeding in cancer. (National Conference on Nutrition in Cancer), *Nut. Today* **13:** 25, Sept./Oct. 1978.
35. Carson, J. S. and A. Gormican. Taste acuity and food attitudes of selected patients with cancer. *J. Am. Diet. Assoc.* **70:** 361, Apr. 1977.
36. Aker, S., G. Tilmont, and V. Harrison. *A Guide to Good Nutrition: During and After Chemotherapy and Radiation.* Medical Oncology Unit, Fred Hutchinson Cancer Research Center, 1124 Columbia Street, Seattle, Washington 98104, 1976.
37. Rosenbaum, E. H., C. A. Stitt, H. Drasin, and I. R. Rosenbaum. *Health Through Nutrition: A Comprehensive Guide for the Cancer Patient.* Alchemy Books, 681 Market, Room 755, San Francisco, CA 94105, 1979.
38. Pelham, M. C. and J. J. Wollard. Nutritional support of cancer patients. *Dietetic Currents—Ross Timesaver,* May/June 1978.
39. Carson, J. S. Nutrition in a team approach to rehabilitation of the patient with cancer. *J. Am. Diet. Assoc.* **72:** 407, Apr. 1978.
40. Fernstrom, J. D. and R. J. Wurtman. Nutrition and the brain. *Scient. Am.* **230:** 84, 1974.
41. Dickerson, J. W. T. and J. Wiryanti. Pellagra and mental disturbances. *Proc. Nut. Soc.* **37:** 167, 1978.

42. Youdin, M. B. H. and A. R. Green. Iron deficiency and neurotransmitter synthesis and function. *Proc. Nut. Soc.* **37:** 173, 1978.
43. Booth, D. A. Neurochemistry of appetite mechanisms. *Proc. Nut. Soc.* **37:** 181, 1978.
44. Crisp, A. H. Disturbances of neurotransmitter metabolism in anorexia nervosa. *Proc. Nut. Soc.* **37:** 201, 1978.
45. Schwartz, P. L. Ascorbic acid in wound healing—a review. *J. Am. Diet. Assoc.* **56:** 479–503, 1970.
46. Ginter, E. Cholesterol: Vitamin C controls its transformation to bile acids. *Science* **179:** 702–704, 1973.
47. Cook, J. D. and E. R. Monsen. Vitamin C, the common cold and iron absorption. *Am. J. Clin. Nutr.* **30:** 235–238, 1977.
48. Raineri, R. and J. H. Weisburger. Reduction of gastric carcinogens with ascorbic acid. *Ann. N.Y. Acad. Sci.* **258:** 181–189, 1975.
49. Schlegel, J. U. Proposed uses of ascorbic acid in prevention of bladder carcinoma. *Ann. N.Y. Acad. Sci.* **258:** 432–437, 1975.
50. Pauling, L. *Vitamin C and the Common Cold.* San Francisco: W. H. Freeman, 1970.
51. Briggs, M. Vitamin C-induced hyperoxaluria. *Lancet* **i:** 154, 1976.
52. Vickery, R. E. Unusual complication of excessive ingestion of vitamin C tablets. *Internat. Surg.* **58:** 422–423, 1973.
53. Herbert, V. and E. Jacob. Destruction of vitamin B_{12} by ascorbic acid. *JAMA* **230:** 241–242, 1974.
54. Briggs, M. H., P. Garcia-Webb, and J. Johnson. Dangers of excess vitamin C. *Med. J. Aust.* **ii:** 48–49, 1973.
55. Spiegel, H. E. and E. Pinili. Effects of vitamin C on SGOT, SGPT, LDH and bilirubin. *Med. J. Aust.* **ii:** 117, 1974.
56. Singh, H. P., M. A. Herbert, and M. H. Gault. Effect of some drugs on clinical laboratory values as determined by the Technicon SMA-12/60. *Clin. Chem.* **18:** 137–144, 1972.
57. Rodriquez, J. A., C. A. Robinson, M. S. Smith, and J. H. Frye. Evaluation of an automated glucose oxidase procedure. *Clin. Chem.* **21:** 1513–1514, 1975.
58. Carroll, J. A simplified alkaline phosphotungstate assay for uric acid in serum. *Clin. Chem.* **17:** 158, 1971.
59. Hansten, P. D. *Drug Interactions.* 2nd ed. Philadelphia: Lea and Febiger, 1972.
60. Milne, M. D. Influence of acid–base balance on efficacy and toxicity of drugs. *Proc. R. Soc. Med.* **58:** 961–963, 1965.
61. Jaffe, R. M., B. Kasten, D. S. Young, and J. D. MacLowry, Fake negative stool occult blood tests caused by ingestion of ascorbic acid (vitamin C). *Ann. Intern. Med.* **83:** 824, 1975.
62. Schrauzer, G. N. and W. J. Rhead. Ascorbic acid abuse: Effects of long-term ingestion of excessive amounts on blood levels and urinary excretion. *Internat. J. Vit. Nutr. Res.* **43:** 201, 1973.
63. Ritzel, G. *Helv. Med. Acta* **28:** 63, 1961.
64. Anderson, T. W., G. Suranyi, and G. H. Beaton. *Can. Med. Assoc. J.* **111:** 31, 1974.

65. Anderson, T. W., D. B. W. Reid, and G. H. Beaton. Vitamin C and the common cold: A double blind study. *Can. Med. Assoc. J.* **107:** 503, 1972.
66. Anderson, T. W., G. H. Beaton, P. N. Corey, and L. Spero. Winter illness and vitamin C: The effect of relatively low doses. *Can. Med. Assoc. J.* **112:** 823–826, 1975.
67. Dykes, M. H. M. and P. Meier. Ascorbic acid and the common cold. *JAMA* **231:** 1073–1079, 1975.
68. Elwood, P. C., S. J. Hughes, and A. S. St. Leger. A randomized controlled trial of the therapeutic effect of vitamin C in the common cold. *Practitioner* **218:** 133–137, 1977.
69. Tyrrell, D. A. J., J. W. Craig, T. W. Meade, and T. White. A trial of ascorbic acid in the treatment of the common cold. *Br. J. Prev. Soc. Med.* **31:** 189–191, 1977.

CHAPTER 14

The Chemical Basis
of Selected
Laboratory Tests

INTRODUCTION

The hospital laboratory is customarily sectioned according to the nature of the tests conducted on patients' specimens. Typically, the sections consist of:

1. Chemistry. This section utilizes specific chemical reactions to determine the concentration of certain substances in biological fluids.
2. Hematology. The tests conducted by this section encompass the examination of blood cells and the clotting mechanism.
3. Immunohematology. Also referred to as blood banking, this section determines the immunologic compatibility of cellular components in transfusions.
4. Microbiology. The isolation, identification, and antimicrobial sensitivity testing of pathogenic microorganisms is the major responsibility of this section.
5. Serology. The serology section detects or quantitates antibodies or antigens in a patient's serum by using immunological techniques.
6. Urinalysis. This section performs chemical tests and microscopic examinations primarily on urine specimens.

The medical technologists who carry out the tests are responsible not only for the physical performance of the tests but also for the proper handling of the patient's specimen and for applying sound quality control to assure the validity of the tests. The test results are interpreted by the attending physician.

Organic diseases, such as those described in the chapters dealing with the pancreas, cardiovascular system, liver, and kidney, cause disturbances in the concentration of substances in body fluids. Such disturbances are most commonly determined by the application of chemical tests performed by the chemistry section of the laboratory. It is the purpose of this chapter to acquaint the reader with the basis of the chemical tests that are of importance in diagnosing those diseases. Disease processes may cause an increase, or sometimes decrease, in the concentration of certain substances in serum or other fluids, and the diagnostic value of the laboratory tests is that they are designed to measure the concentration of the substances. A normal range of values has been established for all of the substances determined in the laboratory. Listings of normal values can be found in any text dealing with clinical chemical testing, and, therefore, will not be included here. Normal ranges of values should be established by each laboratory facility for its own reference, because values for a particular assay vary with age, sex, ethnic background, and even geographic location. Normal value ranges are generally established by determinations conducted on members of the hospital staff and on patients whose conditions would have no effect on the level of the substance in question.

To avoid dietary effects, specimens are routinely collected early in the morning after a 12-hour fast. The chemical basis of those tests referred to will be described briefly, but it must be understood that they are only representative of a larger number of tests by which a particular substance can be determined.

The great majority of chemical tests is based on the principle of colorimetry, which establishes a direct relationship between the concentration of a compound in solution and the amount of radiant energy (light) of a particular *wavelength* that it absorbs. Light is known to travel in a wavelike pattern. The distance from the peak of one wave to the peak of the next is called the wavelength and is expressed in units of length called nanometers (nm). In practice, the substance being measured is chemically converted into another substance capable of absorbing light of a particular wavelength when in solution. These absorbing compounds are referred to as *chromofores*, and each chromofore has a certain wavelength of light which it absorbs maximally. The range of wavelengths used almost exclusively in clinical assays lies between 300 and 700 nm. The essence of a colorimetric test, therefore, is to isolate from a source of light that range of wavelengths which is absorbable by the particular substance being measured and direct it through a solution of the substance. The greater the concentration of substance in the solution, say a diluted serum sample, the *less* light will exit from the solution because more of it is being absorbed. The light energy emerging from the solution is converted into electrical energy which can be monitored on various displays such as meters or digital readouts. Instruments called spectrophotometers furnish the light source, isolate the desired wavelengths of light, contain compartments for the test solutions, and convert the emergent light into recorded electrical energy, which is expressed as *absorbance*. The actual calculation of the concentrations can be made by comparing the absorbance of the unknown or test solution with that of a standard solution having a known concentration of the same substance. The validity of the calculation depends on the assumption that there is a direct and linear relationship between the concentration of a substance and the amount of light it absorbs. A substance that demonstrates this relationship is said to conform to *Beer's Law,* and when it does, an unknown concentration (C_u) is simply calculated by multiplying the ratio of the absorbance of the unknown (A_u) to the absorbance of the standard (A_{std}) by the concentration of the standard (C_{std}). Expressed as a formula:

$$C_u = \frac{A_u}{A_{std}} \times C_{std}$$

In modern, automated methods for determinations based on this principle, the mathematics are performed automatically by the instruments themselves which boldly display the numerical "answer."

DISEASES OF THE PANCREAS

The glucose tolerance test (GTT), diagnostic of diabetes, requires that a serum glucose determination be conducted periodically, during the course of several hours, after the patient has ingested a certain amount of glucose. The number of methods by which glucose can be measured is quite large, but so-called *enzymatic* methods, based on the production of chromofores by the action of enzymes on glucose, are most popular.

In the *glucose oxidase method,* the enzyme glucose oxidase converts the glucose in the sample to gluconic acid and hydrogen peroxide. The hydrogen peroxide, in the presence of a second enzyme, peroxidase, can oxidize certain organic dyes to a colored form. The depth of the color formed, quantitated colorimetrically as described above, therefore reflects indirectly the amount of glucose.

$$\text{Glucose} + O_2 \xrightarrow{\text{glucose oxidase}} \text{Gluconic acid} + H_2O_2$$

$$\underset{\text{(reduced form)}}{H_2O_2 + \text{Organic dye}} \xrightarrow{\text{peroxidase}} \underset{\substack{\text{(oxidized form)} \\ \text{(colored!)}}}{\text{Organic dye}}$$

Some instruments measure glucose by utilizing only the first reaction. Through the use of electrodes sensitive to oxygen in a solution, the rate of oxygen consumption (as the glucose is oxidized) can be monitored. The rate is proportional to the glucose concentration.

Another enzymatic method for glucose, the *hexokinase method,* introduces an intriguing and extremely popular approach to clinical chemical determinations over a broad base. It will be recalled from Chapter 3 that many dehydrogenases utilize nicotinamide adenine dinucleotide (NAD) as a coenzyme. The NAD becomes reduced to NADH as hydrogens are transferred to it from the substrate, or, in the reverse direction, a substrate may be reduced by a dehydrogenase as hydrogens are transferred to it from NADH.

$$\text{Reduced substrate} + \text{NAD} \xrightleftharpoons{\text{a dehydrogenase}} \text{Oxidized substrate} + \text{NADH}$$

The electronic shift that occurs when NAD accepts a hydrogen to become NADH (see structures on pps. 50–51) alters its spectral properties. NADH strongly absorbs light of 340 nm wavelength whereas NAD does not show this property. Therefore, by measuring the *increase* in absorbance at 340 nm (A_{340}) of a sample, the amount of NADH formed from NAD is indicated, and conversely, the *decrease* in A_{340} would reflect the amount of NADH converted to NAD. Most importantly, these coenzyme concentrations correspond directly with the substrate concentration because a one-to-one molar ratio exists. In the reaction shown above, for example, the A_{340} at the end of the reaction indicates the concentration of NADH, but it also measures the concentration of the *reduced substrate* because it is clear that NADH can only be formed from the reduction of NAD by the enzymatic transfer of hydrogens to the NAD from the reduced substrate. The same reasoning applies in the right-to-left reaction. The decrease in A_{340} measures the concentration of the oxidized form of the substrate as well as the simultaneous decrease in NADH. The hexokinase method for glucose is founded on this principle, and although the enzyme uses NADP rather than NAD, the same reasoning applies.

$$\text{Glucose} + \text{ATP} \xrightarrow{\text{hexokinase}} \text{Glucose 6-P} + \text{ADP}$$

$$\text{Glucose 6-P} + \text{NADP} \xrightarrow{\substack{\text{glucose 6-P} \\ \text{dehydrogenase}}} \text{6-Phosphogluconic acid} + \text{NADPH}$$

The reagents for the test, therefore, include ATP and NADP in addition to the two enzymes, and the concentration of glucose in the specimen corresponds to the concentration of NADPH formed, which in turn is measured by the solution's absorption of light at 340 nm.

A test known as the *glycosylated hemoglobin* (G-Hb) *test* has emerged as a significant and reliable test for diabetes, and most likely will become a routine procedure in most clinical labs. Serum glucose becomes nonenzymatically attached to hemoglobin A throughout the lifespan of the mature erythrocyte, and the resulting glycohemoglobin is referred to as the hemoglobin A_1 (HbA$_1$) fraction. Because the attachment occurs slowly and depends on the circulating level of blood glucose, the glycosylated hemoglobin level is thought to represent the time-averaged blood glucose level. For this reason, the test offers the clinician a true view of the glucose control of the patient over an extended period of time, and the test results would not be affected by recent changes in diet.

The basis of the test is to quantitate the HbA$_1$ (glycohemoglobin) fraction in a red cell hemolyzate prepared from the patient's blood. The fraction is separated from other hemoglobins by ion exchange chromatography and quantitated colorimetrically. The concentration of the HbA$_1$ fraction is expressed as a percent of the total hemoglobin, and in normal (nondiabetic) subjects should be below a certain value.

Exocrine disease of the pancreas such as pancreatitis can cause the release of pancreatic enzymes into the general circulation. Serum enzymes can be conveniently determined by incubating a serum sample with an excess of substrate (the substrate concentration must be high enough so as not to be rate limiting) and measuring the amount of product formed over a certain period of time. If the substrate is maintained in excess, then the rate of the reaction (product formed per unit time) is determined by the level of active enzyme in the serum specimen. Enzyme activity is usually expressed in terms of international units per liter of serum, or the equivalent, milliinternational units per ml (mU/ml). These units can be defined as the number of micromoles of substrate converted to product by the enzyme present in 1.0 liter of serum during a period of one minute. Even though only small volumes of serum are used for the tests (as little as 0.1 ml) the calculations are based on a liter because of the more convenient (larger) value for the number of units calculated. *Lipase* and *amylase* are the enzymes commonly assayed for the diagnosis of pancreatitis.

The substrate for lipase is triglyceride, and the specific substrate most commonly used is a fine emulsion of olive oil. The enzyme in the sample breaks down the oil droplets by hydrolyzing the triglycerides to free fatty acids, glycerol, and some monoglycerides. Two ways by which the rate of this reaction can be determined is to (1) quantitate the free fatty acids formed by titrating them with base in the presence of a suitable indicator or (2) measure the decrease in absorbance (actually light scattering) of the substrate emulsion as it is "cleared" by the enzyme. This latter method is an example of a *turbidometric* method.

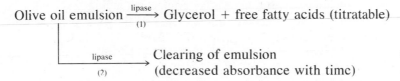

Amylase hydrolyzes starch to glucose and maltose units. As with lipase, the substrate for amylase (starch) is not water soluble and it forms large insoluble micelles in an aqueous medium. As enzymatic hydrolysis occurs, however, the fragmentation does produce soluble products. A very popular method for amylase assay is based on this fact. Starch to which a colored dye has been chemically bonded can be used as substrate. The dye is, therefore, insoluble prior to exposure to the enzyme, but as the enzyme hydrolyzes the starch, the resulting small starch fragments containing dye are water soluble and produce a clear blue solution, the concentration of which indicates the amount of amylase activity.

$$\text{Starch-dye complex} \xrightarrow{\text{amylase}} \text{Small Saccharide-dye fragments}$$
$$\text{(insoluble)} \qquad\qquad\qquad \text{(soluble)}$$

Other methods incorporate *maltase* as a reagent. This enzyme hydrolyzes the maltose formed in the reaction to glucose (see p. 72) so that glucose becomes the major product of the amylase hydrolysis of the starch. The glucose can then be measured by the hexokinase method (see p. 474).

DISEASES OF THE CARDIOVASCULAR SYSTEM

On page 232, reference was made to the fact that approximately 10 percent of all hypertension cases are attributable to known physiological causes. Among these causes, hyperfunction of the adrenal gland, producing abnormally high levels of mineralocorticoids such as aldosterone or the catecholamine hormones, epinephrine and norepinephrine, has been implicated in the disease.

The chemical assay of aldosterone is successfully carried out by the method of radioimmunoassay (RIA) or enzyme-linked immunoassay (EIA). These methods have become immensely important in clinical testing, and although they will be discussed here in connection with aldosterone determination, it is important to understand that the number of substances assayable by these methods is extremely large. This is particularly true for RIA; however, during recent years, EIA methods have undergone a precipitous rise in popularity. An in-depth description of the methods will not be attempted. Instead, only the salient features will be presented so as to at least acquaint the reader with general principles. An RIA procedure basically requires the following:

1. A radiolabeled preparation of the compound being assayed. These preparations are available commercially, and they are prepared by attaching to the compound radioactive isotopes of certain elements (usually iodine). The isotopes I-125 or I-131 emit gamma radiation which can be measured by counting devices called gamma counters. The intensity of the radiation is recorded by the counter as the units, *counts per minute (cpm)*. This radioactive compound is referred to as the *labeled antigen* for a reason that will be explained.
2. Antibodies formed against the compound being assayed. If the compound is injected in a suitable form into a foreign animal species such as a rabbit, the animal will produce *antibodies* against the compound in much the same manner as antibody production against invading viruses or bacteria. Because it elicited the production of antibodies in the animal, the compound is called an *antigen*. Antibodies are proteins (gamma globulins) that are capable of binding firmly, *but reversibly*, the compound (antigen) against which they were formed. These antibodies can be isolated from the rabbit's serum and used as a reagent in the test.

3. The patient's specimen, containing an unknown amount of the compound being determined. This form of compound is, of course, not radioactive, and is referred to as the *unlabeled antigen*.
4. Standards, containing known amounts of the compound (unlabeled antigen).
5. A means for separating the labeled antigen that is bound to antibody from the labeled antigen not bound to antibody.

In carrying out the test, a limited amount of antibody is incubated with a certain amount of labeled antigen. The proportions are such that roughly half of the labeled antigen is bound to antibody, the other half being free. In other words, only enough antibody is present to bind half of the labeled antigen. At this point, if the bound and free forms of the labeled antigen were separated and their radioactivity (cpm) separately determined, it would logically be found that about 50 percent of the total radioactivity would be bound label and 50 percent would be as free label. This represents the percent bound, of labeled, *in the absence* of any unlabeled antigen. In practice, a small amount of the patient's serum is incubated along with the antibody and the labeled antigen. There is now a certain amount of unlabeled antigen in the system competing with the labeled antigen for the limited number of antibody combining sites, and because the antibody does not distinguish between the two forms of the antigen, the unlabeled antigen can occupy antibody-combining sites that would have been occupied by labeled antigen had there been no unlabeled antigen present. This competition therefore results in a displacement of a certain amount of labeled antigen from the bound form to the free form, *and the more unlabeled antigen (substance being determined) present in the system, the more labeled antigen will be in the free form*. It remains to separate the bound and free forms of labeled antigen and determine the radioactivity in each. Whereas approximately 50 percent of labeled antigen was bound in the absence of unlabeled antigen, it follows that a *lower* percent bound will result when unlabeled antigen is present. *The percent of labeled antigen bound decreases as the unlabeled antigen concentration increases.* The substance can be quantitated by comparing the percent bound labeled antigen in the presence of known concentrations of the substance with the percent bound in the presence of the test specimen.

Closely allied in principle with RIA procedures are the enzyme immunoassays (EIA) which share with RIA the great versatility and sensitivity of the method. There are several variations of the EIA procedure itself, but the common feature is that the activity of a reagent enzyme is a function of the concentration of the compound that is being assayed. In one variation of the method, for instance, antibodies specific for the compound are fixed to the surface of an insoluble carrier, for example the walls of the tube in which the reaction is to take place. Into the tube is placed a reagent consisting of a conjugate of the compound being determined and an enzyme. The conjugate therefore is an enzyme-labeled antigen and functions in the test similarly to the labeled antigen of the RIA test, except that in RIA the "label" is a radioactive element rather than an enzyme. Although the compound is attached to the enzyme, it is still free to react with its specific antibody on the tube wall. If free compound (from the specimen or standards) is added to the reaction mixture, a competition between the free compound and the enzyme-labeled compound results, and *the higher the concentration of free compound, the less enzyme will be attached to the antibodies on the tube wall.* Following the incubation of specimen or standards with the enzyme-labeled compound in the tube, the contents are decanted from the tube and replaced with a solution of the substrate for the enzyme. An enzyme-substrate system is selected so that the product of the reaction is conveniently measured colorimetrically. In summation, the greater the amount of compound being determined, the less enzyme is attached to the tube wall through the compound-specific antibodies; and the less enzyme on the tube, the less conversion of substrate to product takes place. As with RIA, quantitative calculations are based on a comparison of residual enzymatic activity between sample and standards.

If hypertension is caused by a pheochromocytoma, a tumor of the adrenal medulla, there will be an overproduction of the gland's hormones, epinephrine and norepinephrine. The determination in urine of these hormones and their chief metabolite, vanilmandelic acid (VMA), is diagnostic of this condition. The hormones themselves are assayed *fluorometrically* following their chemical conversion to fluorescent substances. Fluorescence refers to the emission of light, usually in the visible range of the spectrum, as a result of the irradiation of a substance with ultraviolet light. The intensity of the emitted light is proportional to the concentration of the fluorescent compound.

$$\left.\begin{array}{l}\text{Epinephrine}\\\text{Norepinephrine}\end{array}\right\}\xrightarrow[\substack{\text{oxidation at}\\\text{alkaline pH}}]{}\left\{\begin{array}{l}\text{Adrenolutin}\\\text{Noradrenolutin}\end{array}\right.$$

Adrenolutin and noradrenolutin fluoresce when exposed to ultraviolet light, providing an indirect method for quantitating the hormones. The determination of VMA requires that the urine specimen be treated with sodium periodate ($NaIO_4$) which converts the VMA in the specimen to *vanillin*. The vanillin can then be extracted from the urine and quantitated spectrophotometrically as discussed in the introduction to this chapter.

$$\text{Vanilmandelic acid}\xrightarrow[NaIO_4]{}\text{Vanillin}$$

The fact that inflammation, ischemia, or necrosis can cause the release of enzymes from the cells of the affected tissue has already been cited in the text. The phenomenon is exemplified by the release of the cardiac enzymes, creatine kinase (CK), lactate dehydrogenase (LDH), and aspartate amino transferase (AST) as a result of a myocardial infarction. The determination of "total" serum CK or LDH is suitable only as a screening test because the enzymes are functioning in various tissues and organs. Tissue specificity is improved by separating the isoenzyme fractions of these enzymes and determining the relative concentrations of each. Therefore, for each of these two enzymes, a method for the "total" enzyme will be presented as well as the means by which the isoenzymes are separated and estimated.

Creatine kinase catalyzes the reversible reaction shown.

$$
\begin{array}{ccc}
\underset{\text{Creatine}}{\underset{\displaystyle \mathrm{H_3C-N-CH_2-COO^-}}{\overset{\displaystyle \mathrm{C-NH_2}}{\overset{\displaystyle \overset{+}{N}H_2}{\parallel}}}}
& + \text{ ATP } \overset{\text{CK}}{\longleftrightarrow}
& \underset{\text{Creatine Phosphate}}{\underset{\displaystyle \mathrm{H_3C-N-CH_2-COO^-}}{\overset{\displaystyle \mathrm{C-N\!\sim\!P}}{\overset{\displaystyle \overset{+}{N}H_2 \;\;\; H}{\parallel}}}}
& + \text{ ADP}
\end{array}
$$

The assay of total serum CK is preferably based on the reverse (right to left) reaction. The serum specimen is incubated with an excess of creatine phosphate and ADP, the rate of the reaction being determined only by the amount of CK in the sample. The ATP formed is used to phosphorylate glucose in the presence of the enzyme hexokinase, added as a reagent. The glucose 6-phosphate formed in this second reaction is then oxidized by a third enzyme, glucose 6-phosphate dehydrogenase, to 6-phosphogluconate. The dehydrogenase utilizes NADP as a coenzyme which becomes reduced to NADPH in the reaction, so that the primary (CK) reaction can be monitored by the increase in absorbance at 340 nm. (see p. 474). The coupled reactions are as follows:

$$\text{Creatine phosphate} + \text{ADP} \xrightarrow{\text{creatine kinase}} \text{Creatine} + \text{ATP}$$

$$\text{ATP} + \text{Glucose} \xrightarrow{\text{hexokinase}} \text{Glucose 6-P} + \text{ADP}$$

$$\text{Glucose 6-P} + \text{NADP} \xrightarrow{\text{glucose 6-P dehydrogenase}} \text{6-P Gluconic acid} + \text{NADPH}$$

Necessary reagents, therefore, include creatine phosphate, ADP, glucose, hexokinase, NADP, and glucose 6-P dehydrogenase. With all these in excess, the overall rate (measured by NADPH formation) is controlled only by the enzyme being determined, creatine kinase.

Serum CK may derive from skeletal muscle and brain as well as cardiac tissue. Therefore the isoenzyme specific for the heart must be separately quantitated for a positive diagnosis of myocardial infarction. Isoenzymes have subtle structural differences that permit their separation. The preferred method of separation is by *electrophoresis*, which effects separation in an electric field by taking advantage of the differences in net charge among the isoenzymes. The difference arises from the variable amino acid composition among the isoenzymes, in particular the amino acids that carry electrical charges on their side chains (see discussion on protein structure, Chapter 2). If the isoenzymes are placed in an electric field, the one with the greatest net negative charge will migrate most rapidly toward the positive electrode and the one with the lowest net negative charge moves slowest in that direction. In practice, the serum is applied to a solid supporting medium which contacts buffer reservoirs in which the electrodes are immersed. The support itself is wetted with the buffer to complete the electrical circuit. Current is applied for a certain period of time at the end of which the supporting strip is stained with a solution chemically compounded to reveal the regions of specific enzymatic activity. For example, the stain used to visualize the CK isoenzymes includes all the reagents used in the total CK method described above plus a dye which can be reduced to a deeply colored product by NADPH. Therefore, wherever there is enzymatic activity on the strip, the NADPH produced will create a region of color. The intensity of the color tells how much enzyme was functioning in that region. Creatine kinase is a dimer of two protein chains designated as M chains and B chains. The isoenzymes have different combinations of these chains. For example, the isoenzyme from skeletal muscle has two M chains and is referred to as the "MM band" after electrophoresis, heart CK consists of one M and one B chain and is called the MB band. Brain CK gives rise to the BB band. Electrophoretically, the MM band migrates most rapidly, the BB band moves slowest, and the MB band migrates to a point intermediate between the two. In the diagnosis of myocardial infarction (MI) it is the MB band, of course, which is of primary interest, and its concentration relative to the other bands can be estimated by scanning the bands with an instrument called a densitometer. The greater the color formed within a band, the greater the peak height of the densitometer scan. A comparison of a normal and typical MI scan is shown in Figure 14.1.

Lactate dehydrogenase (LDH) serum level also increases following an MI. Compared with CK, the LDH rises later, after the episode, but remains elevated for a longer period of time. The enzyme catalyzes the reversible reaction.

$$\underset{\text{Lactate}}{CH_3-\overset{\overset{\displaystyle OH}{|}}{CH}-COO^-} + NAD \xrightarrow{\;LDH\;} \underset{\text{Pyruvate}}{CH_3-\overset{\overset{\displaystyle O}{||}}{C}-COO^-} + NADH$$

The conversion of lactate to pyruvate is called the forward reaction and is measured by the increase in A_{340} (NADH) when an excess of lactate and NAD is incubated with the serum. The reverse reaction (pyruvate to lac-

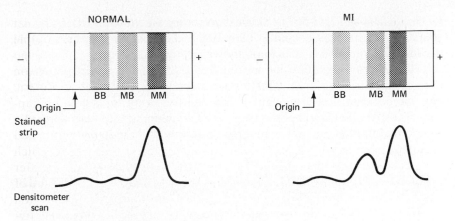

Figure 14.1 Typical creatine kinase isoenzyme patterns of a normal serum and a postmyocardial infarction serum.

tate) can also be used to determine LDH by reacting the serum sample with an excess of pyruvate and NADH. In this case the rate of the reaction is followed by a decrease in A_{340}.

Lactate dehydrogenase is active in many tissues and it therefore becomes necessary to carry out an isoenzyme test. Five LDH isoenzymes are separable by electrophoresis, and the bands are visualized and quantitated in the same manner as described for the CK isoenzymes. The fastest migrating isoenzyme (greatest net negative charge) is called LDH-1 and it is this fraction that is associated with heart muscle. The remaining four fractions migrate with the following decreasing order of mobility: LDH-2,

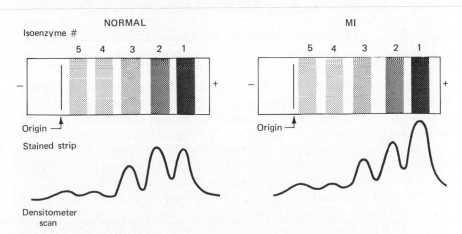

Figure 14.2 Typical lactate dehydrogenase isoenzyme patterns of a normal serum and a postmyocardial infarction serum.

LDH-3, LDH-4, LDH-5. The slowest migrating isoenzyme (LDH-5) is associated with liver tissue and its elevation is diagnostic of diseases of that organ. Normal and MI scans are shown in Fig. 14.2.

The enzyme aspartate amino transferase (AST), also called glutamate oxaloacetate transaminase (GOT) is also considered a "cardiac profile" enzyme because it is significantly elevated following myocardial infarction. The enzyme catalyzes the transfer of an amino group from aspartate to α-ketoglutarate, and in the reverse direction, from glutamate to oxaloacetate as shown.

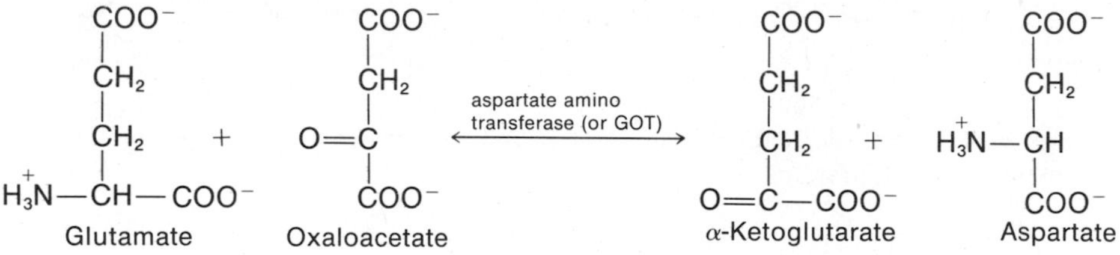

$$
\underset{\text{Glutamate}}{
\begin{array}{c}
COO^- \\
| \\
CH_2 \\
| \\
CH_2 \\
| \\
\overset{+}{H_3N}-CH-COO^-
\end{array}
}
\; + \;
\underset{\text{Oxaloacetate}}{
\begin{array}{c}
COO^- \\
| \\
CH_2 \\
| \\
O{=}C \\
| \\
COO^-
\end{array}
}
\; \underset{\text{transferase (or GOT)}}{\overset{\text{aspartate amino}}{\longleftrightarrow}} \;
\underset{\text{α-Ketoglutarate}}{
\begin{array}{c}
COO^- \\
| \\
CH_2 \\
| \\
CH_2 \\
| \\
O{=}C-COO^-
\end{array}
}
\; + \;
\underset{\text{Aspartate}}{
\begin{array}{c}
COO^- \\
| \\
CH_2 \\
| \\
\overset{+}{H_3N}-CH \\
| \\
COO^-
\end{array}
}
$$

The right-to-left reaction as shown is applied in determining enzyme activity. The serum is reacted with α-ketoglutarate and aspartate, and a coupled reaction catalyzed by malate dehydrogenase converts the oxaloacetate formed to malate. In the coupled reaction shown below, NADH is oxidized to NAD, and the primary (AST) reaction can therefore be indirectly measured by the rate of decrease in absorbance at 340 nm.

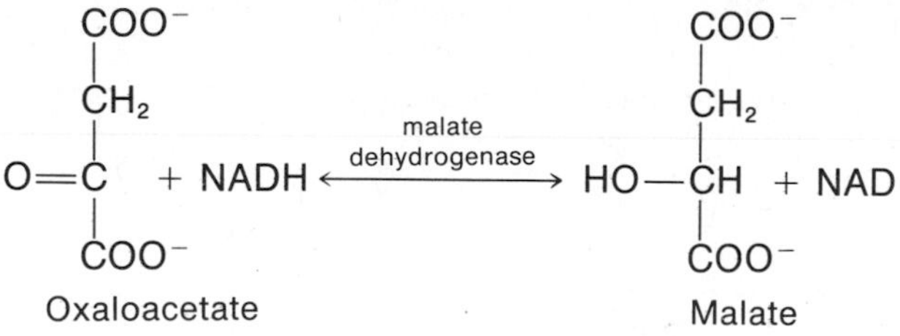

$$
\underset{\text{Oxaloacetate}}{
\begin{array}{c}
COO^- \\
| \\
CH_2 \\
| \\
O{=}C \\
| \\
COO^-
\end{array}
}
\; + \; NADH \;
\underset{\text{dehydrogenase}}{\overset{\text{malate}}{\longleftrightarrow}} \;
\underset{\text{Malate}}{
\begin{array}{c}
COO^- \\
| \\
CH_2 \\
| \\
HO{-}CH \\
| \\
COO^-
\end{array}
}
\; + \; NAD
$$

Atherosclerosis, discussed in Chapter 7, has an unknown etiology, but the disease is characterized by the deposition of lipid material within arterial walls, frequently accompanied by calcification of the tissue in later stages. High levels of serum lipids are regarded as an indicator of the individual's predisposition to future atherosclerotic disease. Certain lipid fractions such as cholesterol (total), high density lipoprotein cholesterol (HDLC), and tryglycerides are routinely assayed to assess this risk.

The newer methods for triglyceride determinations utilize specific enzymes as reagents purchased by the clinical laboratory in the form of kits. Although there are several enzymatic methods in use, the one described here typifies enzymatic methods and illustrates the principle. Regardless of the method employed, a common first step is to hydrolyze the triglycerides to glycerol and fatty acids, with subsequent determination of the glycerol formed.

(1) Triglycerides $\xrightarrow{\text{lipase}}$ Glycerol + Fatty Acids
(in sample)

(2) 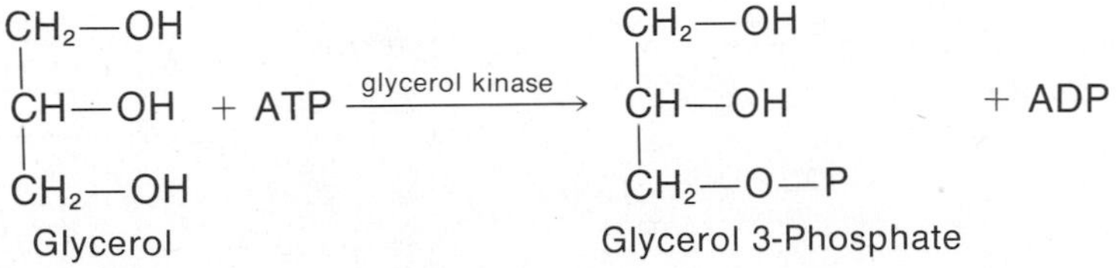
$$\begin{array}{l} CH_2{-}OH \\ | \\ CH{-}OH \quad + \text{ ATP} \\ | \\ CH_2{-}OH \\ \text{Glycerol} \end{array} \xrightarrow{\text{glycerol kinase}} \begin{array}{l} CH_2{-}OH \\ | \\ CH{-}OH \\ | \\ CH_2{-}O{-}P \\ \text{Glycerol 3-Phosphate} \end{array} \quad + \text{ ADP}$$

(3)
$$\begin{array}{l} CH_2{-}OH \\ | \\ CH{-}OH \\ | \\ CH_2{-}O{-}P \\ \text{Glycerol 3-Phosphate} \end{array} + \text{ NAD} \xrightarrow[\text{dehydrogenase}]{\text{glycerol phosphate}} \begin{array}{l} CH_2{-}OH \\ | \\ C{=}O \\ | \\ CH_2{-}O{-}P \\ \text{Dihydroxyacetone} \\ \text{phosphate} \end{array} + \text{ NADH}$$

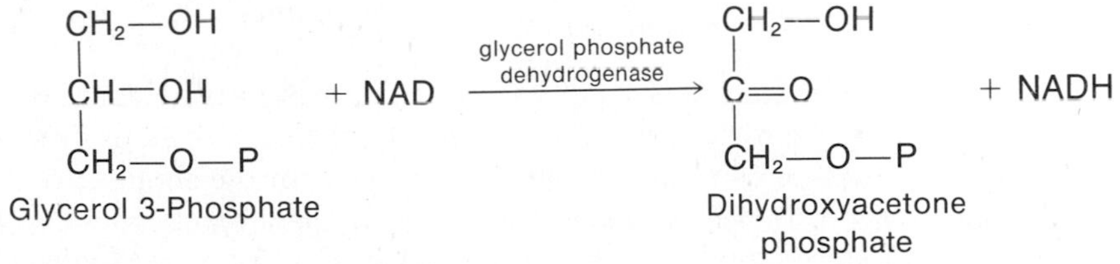

This represents still another example of how enzymatic reactions can be coupled in such a way that an absorbance at 340 nm (NADH) correlates with the concentration of the substance being measured.

Another method for triglycerides that will be illustrated because of its common usage is a colorimetric method that does not use enzymes as reagents.

(1) Triglycerides $\xrightarrow[\text{(saponification)}]{\text{alcoholic KOH}}$ Glycerol + Fatty acids
(in sample)

(2) Glycerol + Sodium periodate $\rightarrow$ 2 Formaldehyde + Formic acid

(3) Formaldehyde + NH_4^+ + Acetyl acetone $\rightarrow$ A diacetyl lutidine
(yellow color)

In this method, the concentration of the triglycerides is proportional to the intensity of the yellow color produced. A disadvantage of the method is that the hydrolysis (step 1) would also liberate glycerol from glycerophosphatides (see structures, pps. 30–33) causing erroneously high results for triglycerides. It is therefore necessary to remove the glycerophosphatides from the specimen prior to the hydrolysis.

The oldest and still most widely used method for determining total serum cholesterol is based on the formation of a green chromofore, quantitated colorimetrically, when the cholesterol in the sample is reacted with concentrated sulfuric acid in an anhydrous environment. The reaction is called the Liebermann-Burchard reaction. The structure of the chromofore itself is not precisely understood.

More recently an enzymatic method for cholesterol had been used successfully, and avoiding the use of the corrosive reagents of the Liebermann-Burchard reaction is a great advantage in itself. The basis of the method is shown below.

(1) Cholesterol and $\xrightarrow{\text{cholesterol esterase}}$ Free cholesterol
      cholesterol esters

(2) Cholesterol + O_2 $\xrightarrow{\text{cholesterol oxidase}}$ Cholest-4-ene-3-one + H_2O_2

(3) H_2O_2 + 4-Aminoantipyrene + phenol $\xrightarrow{\text{Peroxidase}}$
$$\text{Quinoneimine dye} + H_2O$$
$$\text{(colored)}$$

Two-thirds of the serum cholesterol exists as esters of fatty acids. In reaction (1), utilizing the hydrolase, cholesterol esterase, all cholesterol esters are converted to free cholesterol. This is necessary for the cholesterol oxidase reaction (reaction 2). The principle of the coupled reactions is analogous to the glucose oxidase method for glucose (p. 473) in that hydrogen peroxide (H_2O_2) formed in the reaction oxidizes a dye to a colored form.

A test that has recently come to be regarded as a much better indicator of the risk of cardiovascular disease is the determination of that portion of serum cholesterol associated with the high density lipoproteins relative to that associated with the low density lipoprotein fraction. The test involves the selective precipitation of the low density lipoproteins from diluted serum leaving the high density fraction in the supernatant. Precipitating agents such as phosphotungstate-Mg, heparin-Mg, and dextran sulfate have been used with varying degrees of success in precipitating the low density lipoproteins. Following centrifugation of the mixture, the supernatant is carefully separated from the precipitate, and the cholesterol concentration in the supernatant determined by one of the methods described. This gives the high density lipoprotein cholesterol value (HDLC). The cholesterol in the precipitated low density lipoproteins is generally not determined directly but is estimated from a mathematical relationship that exists among the total cholesterol, HDLC, and LDLC. The risk factor for cardiovascular disease *decreases* as the HDLC/LDLC ratio *increases*.

DISEASES OF THE LIVER

A large number of tests for assessing liver function is available to the clinician. Moreover, the tests are designed to measure various aspects of hepatic function, thereby enhancing the diagnostic value of their results.

The serum bilirubin test indicates the liver's ability to conjugate and excrete bilrubin formed from the catabolism of heme, as discussed on page 105. Bilirubin, both the conjugated and unconjugated forms, is nearly always determined by converting it into a chromoforic diazo derivative using the reagent diazotized sulfanilic acid. The reaction of this reagent with conjugated bilirubin is shown in Figure 14.3. The symbol G represents glucuronic acid residues, P = propionic acid, M = methyl, and V = vinyl side chains. The reaction between conjugated Bilirubin and diazotized sulfanilic acid occurs quickly, usually within one minute from the time the serum and reagents are mixed. Furthermore, because of the water solubility of the bilirubin conjugate, the reaction occurs directly in the aqueous medium. For this reason, the conjugate is referred to as *direct bilirubin*. Unconjugated bilirubin reacts with diazotized sulfanilic acid in the same manner as the conjugated form. However, because it is not as water soluble, and because it is more tightly associated with the serum protein albumin, reagents must be included that both dissociate the molecule from albumin and solubilize it. Methanol or the combination of caffeine and sodium benzoate is able to accomplish this. If the serum is treated with caffeine and sodium benzoate prior to the reaction with diazotized sulfanilic acid, the *total* bilirubin will, of course, be determined, i.e., both unconjugated and conjugated forms. The unconjugated bilirubin value is obtained by subtracting the conjugated (direct) value from the "total" value. Because the unconjugated bilirubin therefore is not determined directly, it is termed *indirect bilirubin*.

Certain enzymes show elevated serum levels as a result of hepatic disease. Generally they can be broken down into two categories according to the clinical significance of their assay results:

1. Those that are indicative of cholestasis. As bile is produced by the liver cells it enters small capillaries called canaliculi, which join to form larger ducts, which in turn combine to make the large common bile duct. The conditions in which the flow of bile is obstructed anywhere within the biliary network is called cholestasis.
2. Those that reflect primarily parenchymal cell damage, as in the case of acute hepatitis.

The list of enzymes related to liver function is very long, and methods for the assay of only several of the enzymes, representative of both categories, will be described here.

Among the cholestasis-indicating enzymes are alkaline phosphatase, 5'-nucleotidase, and γ-glutamyl transferase. Alkaline phosphatase is a nonspecific esterase, capable of hydrolyzing phosphate ester bonds. The substrate generally selected for its assay is p-nitrophenyl phosphate. This is because, while the substrate itself is colorless, the product (p-nitro-

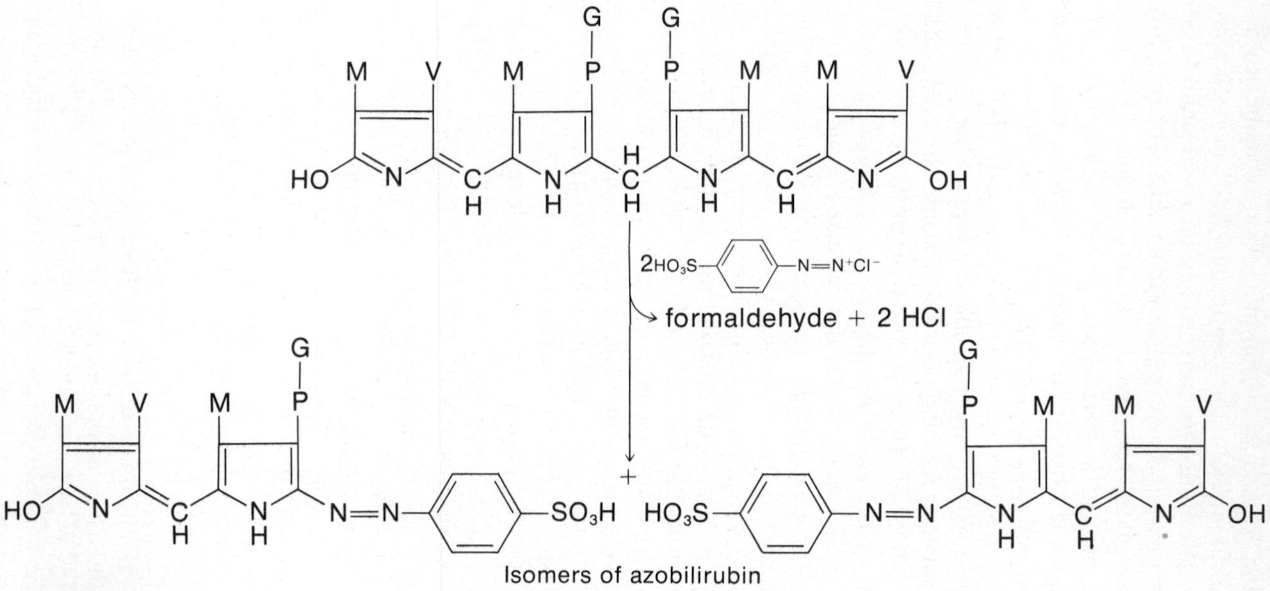

Figure 14.3 The formation of the chromofore azobilirubin by the reaction of conjugated bilirubin with diazotized sulfanilic acid.

phenol) has a deep yellow color, thereby providing a convenient means for measuring the rate of the reaction.

| p-nitrophenyl phosphate | alkaline phosphatase → | p-nitrophenol (yellow) | Inorganic phosphate |

Alkaline phosphatase is found in high concentration in bone, intestine, and placenta as well as liver, and liver specificity, therefore, can only be accomplished through an isoenzyme study of the enzyme. Serum is electrophoresed as described for the CK isoenzyme separation (pps. 479–480) and stained with chromogenic substrate specific for alkaline phosphatase. The distribution of the three major isoenzymes would be as shown in Figure 14.4. The concentration of the liver fraction is estimated from the depth of the color in that band.

Another cholestasis-indicating enzyme is 5′-nucleotidase. Like alkaline phosphatase, this enzyme is also a phosphatase but it is much more specific in its activity, because it acts only on nucleoside 5′-phosphates, releasing inorganic phosphate. The substrate generally used for its assay is adenosine monophosphate (AMP). In the presence of an excess of AMP, the enzymatic activity is accordingly monitored by the absorbance of the blue color produced through the reactions indicated (see p. 488).

There is a uniqueness about the enzyme γ-glutamyl transferase that warrants its mention here. In addition to its being a cholestasis-indicating enzyme, it is also useful for detecting early alcoholic cirrhosis. In fact, its serum levels are frequently elevated in those who drink heavily, even without the clinical manifestation of cirrhosis. The function of the en-

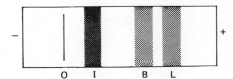

Figure 14.4 The distribution of the major isoenzymes of alkaline phosphatase following electrophoretic separation.
I = intestine
B = bone
L = liver fractions
O(Origin) represents the point of sample application

(1)

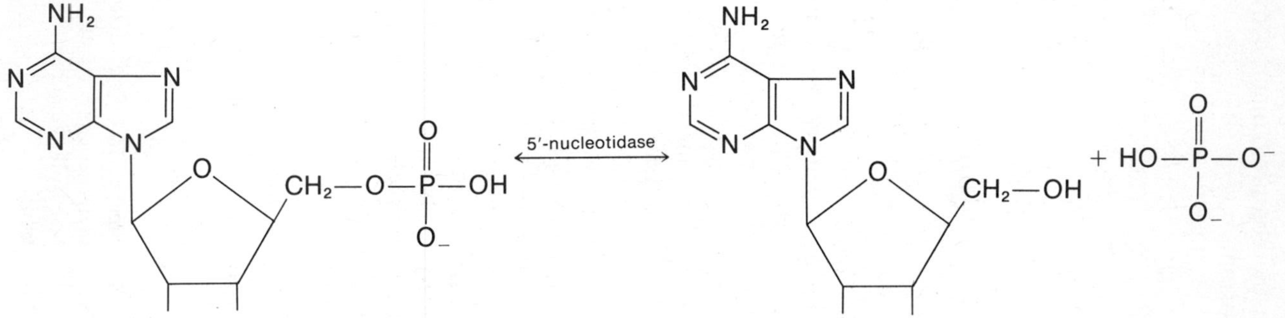

NH₂

Adenosine Monophosphate

$5'$-nucleotidase

NH₂

Adenosine

$+ \; HO$

(2)

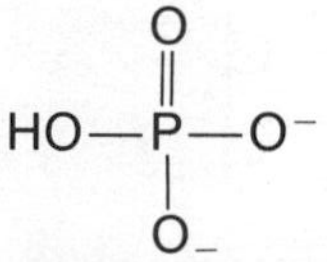

$HO-P-O^-$ + ammonium molybdate $\longrightarrow$ ammonium phosphomolybdate

(3) ammonium phosphomolybdate $\xrightarrow{\text{reducing agent}}$ blue molybdenum chromofore

zyme is to transfer the γ-glutamyl group from a peptide to a suitable amino group acceptor. The following reaction is used to establish its activity in serum. The portions of substrate and product enclosed by the dotted line is the unit transferred by the enzyme. Glycylglycine serves as the acceptor of the unit.

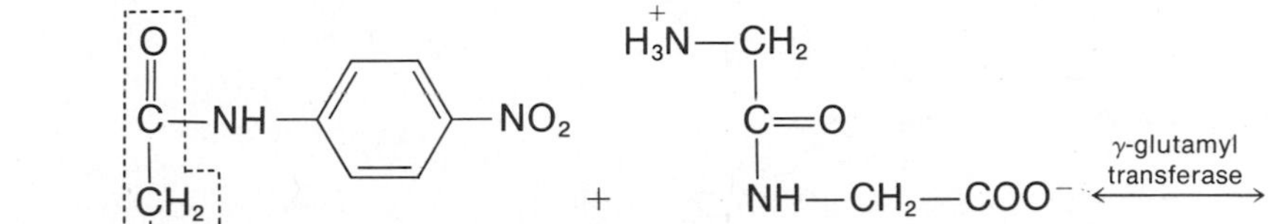

$$
\begin{array}{c}
\text{O} \\
\parallel \\
\text{C}-\text{NH}-\bigcirc-\text{NO}_2 \\
\mid \\
\text{CH}_2 \\
\mid \\
\text{CH}_2 \\
\mid \\
\overset{+}{\text{H}_3\text{N}}-\text{CH}-\text{COO}^-
\end{array}
\quad + \quad
\begin{array}{c}
\overset{+}{\text{H}_3\text{N}}-\text{CH}_2 \\
\mid \\
\text{C}=\text{O} \\
\mid \\
\text{NH}-\text{CH}_2-\text{COO}^-
\end{array}
\quad \underset{\longleftrightarrow}{\overset{\gamma\text{-glutamyl transferase}}{}}
$$

γ-Glutamyl-
p-nitroanilide   Glycylglycine

$$
\begin{array}{c}
\text{O} \\
\parallel \\
\text{C}-\text{NH}-\text{CH}_2 \\
\mid \qquad\qquad \mid \\
\text{CH}_2 \qquad \text{C}=\text{O} \\
\mid \qquad\qquad \mid \\
\text{CH}_2 \qquad \text{NH}-\text{CH}_2-\text{COO}^- \\
\mid \\
\overset{+}{\text{H}_3\text{N}}-\text{CH}-\text{COO}^-
\end{array}
\quad + \quad
\begin{array}{c}
\text{NH}_2 \\
\bigcirc \\
\text{NO}_2
\end{array}
$$

γ-Glutamyl-
glycylglycine   p-Nitroaniline
                     (yellow)

The increase in absorbance due to the formation of the yellow p-nitroaniline is measured spectrophotometrically.

Lactate dehydrogenase and alanine amino transferase (ALT), also named glutamate pyruvate transaminase (GPT), remain normal or are only marginally elevated in cases of biliary obstruction. However, in cases of acute hepatitis and certain other necrotic diseases of the liver in which there is associated cellular damage, these enzymes may show a marked increase in the serum.

The lactate dehydrogenase assay becomes liver-specific only by separating the isoenzymes and ascertaining the concentration of the LDH-5 isoenzyme. The separation and quantitation of the LDH isoenzymes has already been discussed under the diagnosis of myocardial infarction, pages 480–481.

The reaction catalyzed by alanine amino transferase is quite similar to the aspartate amino transferase transamination (p. 482) except for the substitution of alanine for aspartate as substrate. The enzyme catalyzes the transfer of the amino group of alanine to the keto group of α-ketoglutarate.

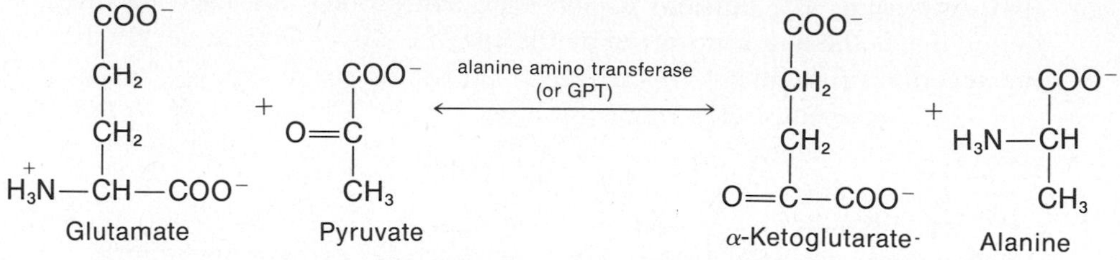

$$
\begin{array}{c}
\text{COO}^- \\
|\\
\text{CH}_2 \\
|\\
\text{CH}_2 \\
|\\
\overset{+}{\text{H}_3}\text{N}-\text{CH}-\text{COO}^- \\
\text{Glutamate}
\end{array}
+
\begin{array}{c}
\text{COO}^- \\
|\\
\text{O}=\text{C} \\
|\\
\text{CH}_3 \\
\text{Pyruvate}
\end{array}
\underset{\xrightarrow{\hspace{2cm}}}{\overset{\text{alanine amino transferase}}{\underset{\text{(or GPT)}}{\xleftarrow{\hspace{2cm}}}}}
\begin{array}{c}
\text{COO}^- \\
|\\
\text{CH}_2 \\
|\\
\text{CH}_2 \\
|\\
\text{O}=\text{C}-\text{COO}^- \\
\alpha\text{-Ketoglutarate-}
\end{array}
+
\begin{array}{c}
\text{COO}^- \\
|\\
\text{H}_3\text{N}-\text{CH} \\
|\\
\text{CH}_3 \\
\text{Alanine}
\end{array}
$$

The reaction applied for the assay of the enzyme is the right to left reaction as shown. As in the AST (GOT) reaction, a dehydrogenase reaction is coupled with the primary reaction so that the reaction can be followed by a change in A_{340}. Specifically, the pyruvate formed is converted to lactate by incorporating lactate dehydrogenase as a reagent. In this case, absorbance decreases as NADH is oxidized to NAD.

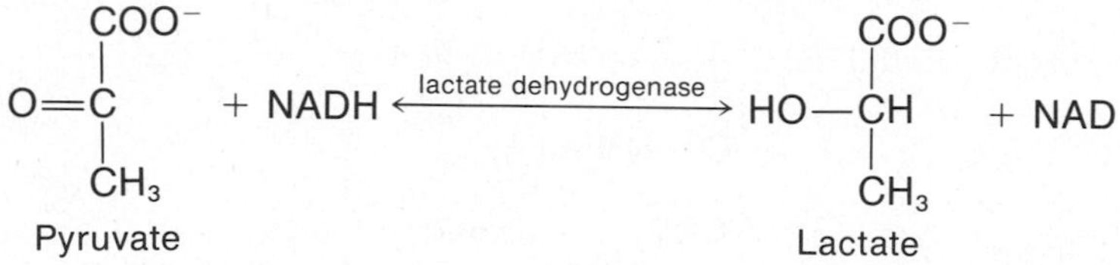

$$
\begin{array}{c}
\text{COO}^- \\
|\\
\text{O}=\text{C} \\
|\\
\text{CH}_3 \\
\text{Pyruvate}
\end{array}
+ \text{NADH}
\underset{\xrightarrow{\hspace{2cm}}}{\overset{\text{lactate dehydrogenase}}{\xleftarrow{\hspace{2cm}}}}
\begin{array}{c}
\text{COO}^- \\
|\\
\text{HO}-\text{CH} \\
|\\
\text{CH}_3 \\
\text{Lactate}
\end{array}
+ \text{NAD}
$$

It will be remembered from the discussion on amino acid metabolism in Chapter 3 that the liver is responsible for the excretion of ammonia. It does this by incorporating it into urea through carbamyl phosphate, and into glutamate, forming glutamine. In the event of severe impairment of liver function, the hepatic cells may lose their ability to carry out these reactions. The result is an accumulation of ammonium ion, the toxicity of which is attributed to its interference with Krebs cycle reactions, the brain being particularly susceptible. The condition is known as *hepatic coma,* and is diagnosed by the determination of serum ammonia, which can be carried out according to the following reaction.

$$\alpha\text{-ketoglutarate} + \text{NH}_3 + \text{NADH} \underset{\xrightarrow{\hspace{1.5cm}}}{\overset{\text{glutamate dehydrogenase}}{\xleftarrow{\hspace{1.5cm}}}} \text{Glutamate} + \text{NAD}$$

With α-ketoglutarate and NADH in excess, the rate of the reaction is established by the concentration of ammonia, and is measured by the decrease in A_{340}.

DISEASES OF THE KIDNEY

Kidney function tests are of three general types, (1) those that assess glomerular filtration, (2) those measuring tubular secretion, and (3) those that measure the concentrating ability of the tubules. The glomerular filtrate becomes more concentrated as it passes through the tubules of the nephron due to the tubular reabsorption of water. Reabsorption of water is primarily under the influence of the pituitary hormone, vasopressin, also referred to as antidiuretic hormone (ADH).

A normal concentration of urine can be determined by measuring its osmolality, a property dependent on the concentration of solutes in the urine. An instrument called an osmometer is used to measure osmolality. It is based on the depression of the freezing point of the urine as the solute concentration increases.

Most tests designed to measure tubular secretion involve injecting intravenously substances that are excreted primarily by the mechanism of tubular secretion. Examples of such substances are p-aminohippurate and phenolsulfonphthalein. Following injection, the urinary excretion of the compound is determined over a period of a few hours. A certain percentage of the total amount injected should have been excreted during this time if tubular secretion were normal.

The basis of glomerular filtration tests is to determine the serum concentration of compounds that are normally cleared from the circulation by glomerular filtration. Diseases such as glomerulonephritis and chronic nephritis, which interfere with the filtration process, cause retention of such substances in the serum and consequently elevated concentrations. Urea and creatinine are routinely assayed for this purpose. Urea is the chief breakdown product of proteins and is normally excreted in large amounts (30 g/d) in the urine. Two methods for its determination in serum will be discussed.

$$(1) \quad H_2N-\underset{\substack{\| \\ O}}{C}-NH_2 + 2H_2O + H^+ \xrightarrow{\text{urease}} 2NH_4^+ + HCO_3^-$$

Urea

$$(2) \quad NH_4^+ + OH^- \longrightarrow NH_3 + H_2O$$

(3) NH_3 + NaOCl + 2 (phenol) $\longrightarrow$ Indophenol (blue)

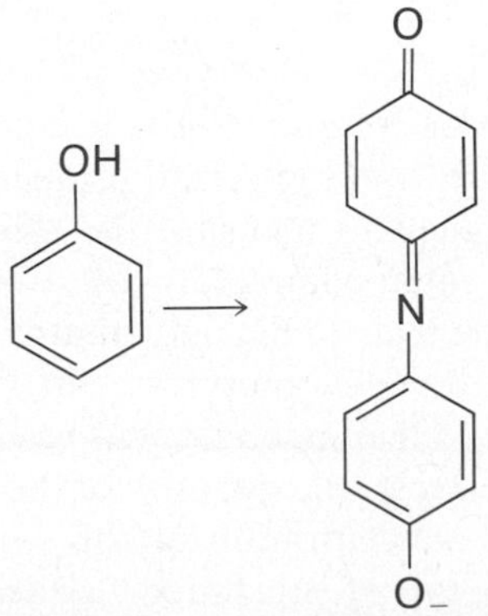

| Sodium Hypochlorite | Phenol | Indophenol (blue) |

In this series of reactions, urea is first hydrolyzed to ammonium ions and bicarbonate by the specific enzyme, urease. The ammonium formed reacts with phenol in the presence of alkaline hypochlorite to yield blue indophenol which is measured spectrophotometrically. In a more widely used method, urea is reacted directly with diacetyl to form a diazine chromofore.

$$CH_3-\overset{\overset{\text{O}}{\|}}{C}-\overset{\overset{\text{N--OH}}{\|}}{C}-CH_3 + H_2O \longrightarrow CH_3-\overset{\overset{\text{O}}{\|}}{C}-\overset{\overset{\text{O}}{\|}}{C}-CH_3 + \quad H\overset{.}{O}NH_2$$

Diacetyl Monoxime $\qquad\qquad\qquad$ Diacetyl $\qquad\qquad$ Hydroxylamine

$$CH_3-\overset{\overset{\text{O}}{\|}}{C}-\overset{\overset{\text{O}}{\|}}{C}-CH_3 + H_2N-\overset{\overset{\text{O}}{\|}}{C}-NH_2 \longrightarrow CH_3-\overset{N}{\underset{\overset{\|}{}}{C}}\overset{\overset{\overset{\text{O}}{\|}}{C}}{}\overset{N}{\underset{\overset{\|}{}}{C}}-CH_3 \quad + \; 2H_2O$$

Diacetyl $\qquad\qquad$ Urea $\qquad\qquad\qquad\qquad$ A Diazine
$\qquad\qquad\qquad\qquad\qquad\qquad\qquad\qquad\qquad\qquad\qquad$ (yellow)

Creatinine is the excretory form of creatine which is found in high concentrations in muscle as its phosphorylated derivative, creatine phosphate. The creatinine is removed from the circulation by glomerular filtration. The only time-tested method for serum creatinine assay has been the reaction of the compound with an alkaline picrate reagent, producing a yellow chromofore, the structure of which has not been ascertained.

$$\overset{\overset{\text{NH}_2{}^+}{\|}}{\underset{\underset{H_3C-N-CH_2}{|}}{C-NH}}\overset{}{\underset{C=O}{\diagdown}}\;+\;\;\; \begin{matrix}OH\\ O_2N\diagup\diagdown NO_2\\ ||\\ \diagdown\diagup\\ NO_2 \end{matrix} \quad \xrightarrow{\text{(NaOH)}} \text{Yellow Chromofore}$$

$\qquad$ Creatinine $\qquad\qquad\qquad$ Picric Acid

Tests known as *clearance tests* are much more sensitive in detecting early renal disease than the serum urea and creatinine tests. If the clearance test is designed to measure the effectiveness of filtration, a compound that is excreted completely, or at least predominately, by this process is used for the test. Inulin and creatinine are among those compounds that are suitable for clearance tests for measuring glomerular filtration. The principle of a clearance test will be described.

In a clearance test, the quantity of the substance excreted in the urine is related to the concentration of the same substance in the serum (or plasma). The amount of substance "cleared" by the kidney is expressed as that volume of plasma which contains the quantity of the substance excreted in the urine in a period of one minute. Mathematically, the relationship may be expressed as:

$$\text{Clearance (ml/min)} = \frac{U}{P} \times V \times \frac{1.73}{A}$$

where U = the concentration of the substance in urine
P = the concentration of the substance in plasma
V = the urine volume per minute, expressed in ml
A = the body surface area, expressed in sq meters

Clearance rate is proportional to the size of the kidney and the body surface area, hence the need for including the factor 1.73/A in the calculation. The value for A is conveniently determined from nomograms which relate the body surface area to the weight and height of the patient. If plasma concentration of the substance relative to that of urine concentration is abnormally high, the clearance will therefore be low, indicated improvement of glomerular filtration.

The reader is again reminded that only tests that relate to the diseases discussed in previous chapters have been described here. A compendium of the many tests that can be performed in a clinical laboratory can be found in the text, Clinical Diagnosis, and Management, Todd, Sanford, and Davidsohn, edited by J. B. Henry, 16th ed., 1979, W. B. Saunders Co.

Questions

1. Why would the results of a serum urea assay be questionable as a renal test if the patient had been on a low carbohydrate, high protein diet?
2. In performing a test for serum amylase, it is important that the technologist avoid pipetting the specimen or any of the reagents by mouth. Why is this precaution necessary?
3. Most of the enzymes that are assayed in the diagnosis of possible tissue damage are cytoplasmic enzymes. Why are mitochondrial enzymes not as clinically significant in such diagnosis?
4. A jogger who had just run 10 miles was admitted to a hospital emergency room complaining of chest pains. Why would the results of a total creatine kinase (CK) test only be misleading in the diagnosis of myocardial infarction? What would have been a more meaningful test?
5. The following results were obtained on two patients:

	Mr. Jones	Mr. Smith
Total cholesterol (mg/dl)	200	280
HDLC (mg/dl)	20	40
LDLC (mg/dl)	160	180

Which patient is the more likely candidate for cardiovascular disease? Why?

INDEX